PREVENTION
in Clinical Oral
Health Care

PREVENTION
in Clinical Oral
Health Care

DAVID P. CAPPELLI, DMD, MPH, PhD
Associate Professor, Department of Community Dentistry
Director, Dental Public Health Residency Program
The University of Texas Health Science Center at San Antonio, Dental School
San Antonio, Texas

CONNIE C. MOBLEY, PhD, RD
Acting Associate Dean of Research
Professor, Department of Professional Studies
School of Dental Medicine
University of Nevada Las Vegas
Las Vegas, Nevada

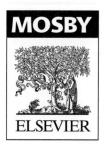

MOSBY

ELSEVIER

MOSBY
ELSEVIER

11830 Westline Industrial Drive
St. Louis, Missouri 63146

PREVENTION IN CLINICAL ORAL HEALTH CARE   ISBN: 978-0-323-03695-5
Copyright © 2008 by Mosby, Inc., an affiliate of Elsevier Inc.

Notice

ISBN: 978-0-323-03695-5

Vice President and Publisher: Linda Duncan
Senior Editor: John Dolan
Managing Editor: Jaime Pendill
Publishing Services Manager: Julie Eddy
Project Manager: Andrea Campbell
Cover Designer: Paula Catalano
Interior Designer: Paula Catalano

Printed in the United States of America

Last digit is the print number: 9 8 7 6 5 4 3 2 1

Contributors

Avni Adhvaryu Bhatt, BS, RDH
Research Assistant
Department of Orthodontics
The University of Texas Health Science Center at
    San Antonio, Dental School
San Antonio, Texas

Linda D. Boyd, RDH, RD, EdD
Assistant Professor and Chair
Department of Dental Hygiene
Georgia Perimeter College
Dunwoody, Georgia

John P. Brown, BDSc, MS, PhD
Professor and Chair 1984-2006
Department of Community Dentistry
The University of Texas Health Science Center at
    San Antonio, Dental School
San Antonio, Texas

Magda A. de la Torre, RDH, MPH
Assistant Professor
Department of Dental Hygiene
The University of Texas Health Science Center at
    San Antonio, School of Allied Health
San Antonio, Texas

Becky DeSpain Eden, BSDH, Med
Associate Professor
Department of Public Health Sciences
Baylor College of Dentistry
Texas A&M University System Health Science Center
Dallas, Texas

Michael W. J. Dodds, BDS, PhD
Sr. Principal Technology Scientist
Global Technology
Wm Wrigley Jr. Company
Chicago, Illinois

Georgia Dounis, DDS, MS
Associate Professor
Department of Clinical Sciences
School of Dental Medicine
University of Nevada Las Vegas
Las Vegas, Nevada

Cara Brigham Gonzales, DDS, PhD
Clinical Instructor
Department of Dental Diagnostic Science
The University of Texas Health Science Center at
    San Antonio, Dental School
San Antonio, Texas

John P. Hatch, PhD
Professor
Department of Psychiatry and Orthodontics
The University of Texas Health Science Center at
    San Antonio, Dental School
San Antonio, Texas

Arthur H. Jeske, DMD, PhD
Professor and Chair
Department of Restorative Dentistry and Biomaterials
University of Texas Dental Branch – Houston
Houston, Texas

Daniel L. Jones, DDS, PhD
Professor and Chair
Department of Public Health Sciences
Baylor College of Dentistry
Texas A&M University System Health Science Center
Dallas, Texas

John Wesley Karotkin, DDS
Resident
Department of Orthodontics
Temple University
Philadelphia, PA

Mildred A. McClain, PhD
Assistant Professor and Community Outreach
    Coordinator
Department of Professional Studies
School of Dental Medicine
University of Nevada Las Vegas
Las Vegas, Nevada

Elaheh Mohebzad, DDS
Resident
Department of Orthodontics
The University of Texas Health Science Center at
    San Antonio, Dental School
San Antonio, Texas

Karen F. Novak, DDS, MS, PhD
Associate Professor and Director of Graduate Studies
Division of Periodontology
Center for Oral Health Research
University of Kentucky
Lexington, Kentucky

Diane Rigassio Radler, PhD, RD
Assistant Professor
Graduate Programs in Clinical Nutrition
School of Health Related Professions
University of Medicine and Dentistry of New Jersey
Newark, NJ

John Rugh, PhD
Professor and Chair
Department of Orthodontics
The University of Texas Health Science Center at
    San Antonio, Dental School
San Antonio, Texas

Victor A. Sandoval, DDS, MPH
Professor and Chair
Department of Professional Studies
School of Dental Medicine
The University of Nevada Las Vegas
Las Vegas, Nevada

Jay D. Shulman, DMD, MSPH
Associate Professor and Director, Dental Public Health
    Residency Program
Department of Public Health Sciences
Baylor College of Dentistry
Texas A&M University System Health Science Center
Dallas, Texas

Cynthia Stegeman, RDH, MEd, RD, CDE
Associate Professor
Dental Hygiene Program
University of Cincinnati–Raymond Walters College
Cincinnati, Ohio

Jane E. M. Steffensen, MPH, CHES
Associate Professor
Department of Community Dentistry
The University of Texas Health Science Center at
    San Antonio, Dental School
San Antonio, Texas

Riva Touger-Decker, PhD, RD, FADA
Professor and Director
Graduate Programs in Clinical Nutrition
School of Health Related Professions Division of
    Nutrition
New Jersey Dental School
Newark, New Jersey

K. Vendrell Rankin, DDS
Professor and Associate Chair
Director, Tobacco Cessation Clinic
Department of Public Health Sciences
Baylor College of Dentistry
Texas A&M University System Health Science Center
Dallas, Texas

Foreword

How fitting! The authors of this important new text selected the quotation from G. V. Black, written in 1896, to begin the introduction to *Prevention in Clinical Oral Health Care* (see page xiii): "The day is surely coming... when we will be engaged in practicing preventive, rather than reparative dentistry."[1] The concepts of prevention and preservation of tooth structure using conservative restorative therapies are not new. However, advances in science continually improve our understanding of the epidemiology of and risk factors for oral conditions, and their importance to the overall health and well being of patients and populations. This book edited by Professors David Cappelli and Connie Mobley provides an important bridge from the earlier work of G. V. Black to our most current understanding of the epidemiology of oral diseases, risk-based assessment and prevention strategies. Through this text, readers are provided contemporary information about oral health and prevention, and are then challenged to effectively incorporate these concepts into practice. The advice provided is sound, and follows the guidelines and recommendations based on the synthesis of available literature and from numerous national reports including *Oral Health in America: A Report of the Surgeon General,*[2] the *Healthy People 2010*[3] objectives and the Future of Dentistry Report.[4] Cappelli, Mobley and the contributing authors challenge all members of the dental team to incorporate prevention into evidence based clinical practice and to work together in a cost-effective manner to improve the overall health and well-being of both people and populations.

This book is well organized into four parts. The first section focuses on a comprehensive review of the epidemiology and biology of the most common oral conditions—dental caries, periodontal diseases and oral cancer. Most notably, the authors update the readers of our progress towards meeting national health objectives for these conditions, helping use understand the challenges and opportunities for improving oral health status with emphasis on these three clinical conditions. Likewise, the readers are provided a foundation for understanding the interrelationships between these oral conditions and systemic health.

The second part of the book provides an important foundation for assessing risk factors for caries, periodontal diseases and oral cancer, and includes an important chapter on the synergism between pharmacology and oral health. Together, the four chapters of this section provide a comprehensive understanding of assessment strategies for these common oral conditions. Risk assessment and disease detection, coupled with a comprehensive understanding of the etiology, biology and epidemiology of oral conditions can greatly assist in clinical approaches to prevention and therapeutic interventions intended to optimize oral health. The chapter highlighting the adverse affects of drugs on the oral cavity is especially important given the aging of our population and the growing number of available drug therapies being prescribed, particularly for the treatment of chronic health conditions.

The third section of the book provides a critical link between the various assessment strategies and the development of a customized patient care plan to achieve and sustain oral health. As the authors point out, "information gathering and the application of information to create an individual plan of prevention is not readily embraced as a component of dental practice." As the reader completes this section, he or she should ask, "Why isn't this strategy commonly applied in dentistry," and more importantly, "How can I apply these approaches to improve the oral health of my patients?" As with all health promotion and disease prevention activities, and broad understanding of the behavioral sciences, patient motivational strategies, assessment and selection of appropriate tests and interventions based on the best available science constitutes ideal clinical practice with the emphasis on the maintenance of health. The chapters addressing the special needs of fearful patients and those of various ethnic and cultural backgrounds are particularly useful to practice in our increasingly diverse society.

The book's final section addresses the practical aspects of prevention and practice, ranging from the more global perspectives of health promotion and disease prevention, to chapters that specifically address prevention strategies for caries, periodontal diseases and oral cancer. Given the emerging evidence supporting the critical link between oral and systemic health, the authors wisely include a chapter on "Prevention Strategies for the Oral Components of Systemic Conditions." Likewise, some of the most underserved patients in society are those with special needs including developmental disabilities and dementia, and those patients residing in nursing and other specialized facilities. The final chapter focusing on the prevention needs for special populations is an important contribution to our understanding of strategies to improve the oral health of these individuals.

Throughout this textbook, Professors Cappelli and Mobley provide a framework to integrate clinical prevention and population health into clinical practice, and focus the text on clinical preventive services and health promotion based on the best available science. They bring together recommendations from many sources in a well organized format, opening the door and inviting the readers to not only understand the concepts presented, but to incorporate them into clinical practice with the goal of improving the oral health of patients and populations. I sincerely hope that all who read this book—students, patients, and practitioners—find a way to respond to the author's call for action and fulfill G. V. Black's vision that "we will be

engaged in practicing preventive, rather than reparative dentistry."

Teresa A. Dolan, DDS, MPH
Professor and Dean
University of Florida College of Dentistry
Health Science Center
Gainesville, Florida

REFERENCES

1. Black GV (1896). Taken from: Elderton RJ. IADR Year of oral health lecture, J Dent Res 73:179406, 1994.
2. U.S. Department of Health and Human Services. Oral Health in America: A Report of the Surgeon General. Rockville MD, U.S. Department of Health and Human Services, National Institutes of Dental and Craniofacial Research, National Institutes of Health, 2000.
3. U.S. Department of Health and Human Services. Healthy People 2010. McLean, VA, International Medical Publishing, 2000.
4. American Dental Association. Future of dentistry: today's vision tomorrow's reality. Chicago, IL, 2001, ADA.

Preface

Prevention in Clinical Oral Health Care was written to address a growing body of science and evidence between oral health status and microbiology, physiology, psychology, human behavior, sociology, and genetics. Advancing knowledge in the art and practice of preventive dentistry demands change in the traditional model of prevention practice. The dental professional is being challenged to join the ranks of health care providers who base clinical practice on models of health promotion and disease prevention as well as treatment. We tried to provide the reader with a guidepost to integrate this new paradigm of prevention into the clinical oral health practice arena.

The genesis of this textbook evolved from a long history of scientific discourse about concepts in caries prevention in the Department of Community Dentistry at the University of Texas Health Science Center at San Antonio. As parallel evidence has developed in support of oral-systemic linkages, it became clear that the past and future roles of the dental professional would need to meld into one oral medicine practice encompassing not only restorative dental treatment but prevention of oral and systemic diseases and general health promotion. We integrated the concept of risk for disease and the relative environmental and behavioral choices into prevention as an approach to compress and possibly prevent the advent of oral diseases. We addressed the universal approach to prevention, where, for example, all patients visit the dentist every six months for a dental cleaning and fluoride treatment whether they had or had not experienced active oral disease in the past 5 years. This model is used routinely in practice, yet lacks a sound evidence-based rationale. Therefore, a primary goal of this book is to explain the concept of risk-based prevention and to provide practical strategies for risk reduction that enable patients to be active participants in guiding the course of their health outcomes.

The purpose of the textbook is to provide a systematic approach to applications of risk-based prevention in clinical practice. *Prevention in Clinical Oral Health Care* is divided into sections that allow the reader and the student to examine and adopt a methodology for prescribing prevention for the individual patient based on their needs and health history. This book specifically addresses the three major oral diseases: dental caries, periodontal disease, and oral cancer. It is organized to present a scientific understanding of each disease mechanism, possible causes

and, the synergy between the disease and populations. This material is provided in Chapters 1-3. This is followed by Chapters 4-6 that provide the basis and strategies for conducting individual assessments for the development of longitudinal patient care plans. Thus once multiple factors, including environmental, behavioral and motivational elements, are identified they may be linked with a patient's disease profile. Chapter 7 describes the role of pharmacotherapies in disease risk and disease prevention. The third major section (Chapter 8-13) of this book examines the role of the provider in understanding the person's disease, obtaining additional information to assess risk, counseling the individual, moving the person toward change, and enhancing adherence to prevention protocols. The book looks at issues that provide barriers to change, including cultural perceptions and dental anxiety. Lastly, the final section focuses on health promotion and prevention of oral diseases that can be used to keep individuals healthy and to reduce their burden of oral disease. Chapters 14-19 examine prevention strategies for each of the three diseases and prevention for special population groups.

This textbook provides a roadmap for teaching oral disease prevention and for integrating it into dental/dental hygiene school curricula. In light of the current evolving science relating oral health to systemic health, the practice of prevention of oral diseases has become the equal of immunization and the promotion of lifestyles that include weight management and physical activity. Risk-based prevention should become an integrated component in the treatment plan of every dental patient and positions the dental professional among health care providers who adhere to a comprehensive patient care model.

While this textbook is similar in some aspects to other prevention textbooks, it has some unique and expanded key and radical differences. For example, the concept of risk-based prevention is submitted as an evidence based concept. Furthermore the book provides working models for incorporating risk assessment and prevention planning into practice. A second unique feature is the integration of patient counseling and behavioral modification into the prevention schema. Since these oral diseases have a causal link to certain behaviors, counseling and motivating a person to adopt healthier behaviors is important in oral disease risk reduction. Lastly, this textbook explores issues that affect adherence to preventive programs: cultural differences and dental anxiety. The book is meant to be a practical application of the preventive science.

We believe in the multidisciplinary team approach to oral health care. Dental professionals find themselves working with a multitude of professionals in maintaining the health of individuals. Dietitians, occupational therapists, nurses, and physician assistants are our partners in patient care. Collaboration between the dentist, dental hygienist and dental assistant is critical to a successful preventive outcome in the clinical setting. Therefore, we chose to use the term 'dental professional' to include dentists, dental hygienists and dental assistants and reflect the collaboration of professionals in patient care. However, we feel strongly that this textbook is meant for a broader audience than persons trained in the delivery of oral health services. We wrote this book for all professionals who address the unmet need for treatment of oral disease.

We want to recognize the contribution of John P. Brown, BDSc, MS, PhD, to the science of risk-based assessment. Dr. Brown developed a caries risk model in 1988 and integrated this model into the clinical teaching program at The University of Texas Health Science Center at San Antonio. We came to understand the science of risk-based prevention through our work with John. He is a visionary and scholar who is responsible for the genesis of this book. We want to thank John for his insight and guidance over the years and underscore his contribution to this work.

We want to thank those people who provided their assistance and support during the development and production of this book. We wish to thank the following individuals/friends who assisted with this project (alphabetically): Diana Balderas, Kenneth Anthony Bolin, Darla Doerffler, Scott Eddy, James Lalumandier, Nora Olivo, and Janie Silvaggio. We want to extend a personal thank you to our families, who were supportive as we worked on this project, especially our spouses, Patricia Cappelli and Roy Mobley.

Reflecting the technology of the 21st century, we have a webpage on the Evolve website: http://evolve. elsevier.com/cappelli/prevention. Through the webpage, students can reference relevant websites and periodic content updates. Evolve resources for instructors include an electronic test bank (Exam View) and all images from the textbook. We are interested in your thoughts and comments and invite you to communicate these to us on the Evolve site. We promise to consider your comments in the following edition(s).

It is our hope that this textbook provides you with a renewed sense of purpose in addressing prevention in your clinical practice and in meeting the individual needs of your patient family.

David P. Cappelli

Connie C. Mobley

Contents

Introduction
Integrating Preventive Strategies into Clinical Practice

DAVID P. CAPPELLI AND CONNIE C. MOBLEY

"The day is surely coming…when we will be engaged
in practicing preventive, rather than reparative dentistry."

This quotation originated from a lecture by G. V. Black in 1896[1] as he considered the future of dentistry. More than 100 years later, we continue to emphasize reparative over preventive dentistry in clinical practice. While dental professionals practice prevention, the prevention is rarely based upon the needs of the individual or addresses risk for future disease. Prevention in the clinical setting is largely dependent upon procedures that the professional provides to the patient. Oral health professionals are often unequipped to address changes in negative oral health behaviors, unwilling to work with the individual as a partner in maintaining their own oral health, or extending care to include the patient's general health. Yet, studies demonstrate that changes in deleterious health behaviors are effective in reducing the disease burden[2].

National attempts have been made to emphasize the role of prevention in health practice, including oral health practice. *Healthy People* objectives were created to provide benchmarks to reduce the disease burden in the United States, including oral disease, and to emphasize preventive practices, such as sealants, oral cancer screening and community water fluoridation.[3] The objectives focus on increasing health care infrastructure, delivering oral health preventive services, and reducing disease in the population. *Healthy People* objectives were devised to drive both public policy and clinical practice to reach the preventive goals. Logic dictates that individual care plans must be effective if the collective positive population outcomes can be self evident. The numbers do not reflect achievement yet. Each practitioner, in each respective discipline is challenged to meet the goals on a daily basis in delivery of health care. Prevention can not be ignored if the nation expects to meet these goals.

A spotlight on oral health as a national problem came with the publication of *Oral Health in America: A Report of the Surgeon General*, which was unveiled in 2000.[4] The report identified disparities in the burden of oral disease and lack of access to adequate oral health care services. The Surgeon General's Report cited eight major findings: (1) oral disease and disorders affect health and well-being throughout life; (2) safe and effective measures exist to prevent the most common dental diseases; (3) lifestyle behaviors that affect general health, such as tobacco use, alcohol use, and dietary choices affect oral and craniofacial health; (4) there are profound and consequential oral health disparities within the U.S. population; (5) more information is needed to improve oral health and eliminate health disparities; (6) the mouth reflects general health and well-being; (7) oral diseases and conditions are associated with other health problems; and (8) scientific research is the key to the reduction in the burden of diseases that affect the face, mouth and teeth.[4] Three overarching themes arise from these findings: (1) oral diseases are largely preventable; (2) oral disease impacts overall health and quality of life; and (3) there are disparities within the U.S. population to achieving optimal oral health.

The Future of Dentistry Report (2001) identified the need for comprehensive training of dental students in preventive services.[5] This observation supports the Report of the Surgeon General and identifies that oral diseases are largely preventable. This report noted that "improved health and quality of life" was achievable for all "through optimal oral health." The report focused on addressing oral health needs and strengthening preventive measures, calling for the development of national and global health policies to promote preventive strategies.[5]

The Clinical Preventive Dentistry Leadership Conference (2002) focused on the role of oral disease prevention and oral health promotion in dental education.[6] Taking the mantel from the Surgeon General's

Report and the Future of Dentistry Report, the conference sought to incorporate systematic teaching of longitudinal assessment and prevention. This conference worked from the premise that oral health can be achieved and is possible for all persons living in the US. This conference focused on the integration of disease prevention in the practice of oral health care.

The Clinical Prevention and Population Health Framework was unveiled in 2004.[7] This document originated from of the Healthy People Curriculum Task Force, which was composed of professionals in prevention from a cross-section of health disciplines, including dentistry. This report outlines a framework to integrate prevention into the overall health care curricula. The framework takes the goals/objectives cited in the reports above and provides a curriculum framework to integrate prevention into overall oral health care for the patient.

The Framework seeks to integrate clinical prevention and population health into clinical practice and consists of four domains: (1) evidence based practice, (2) clinical preventive services-health promotion, (3) health systems and health policy, and (4) community aspects of practice. This book focuses on the first two domains of the framework.

The reports cited above provide a future perspective on the role of prevention in clinical practice and suggest that at the present time, prevention is not well-integrated into clinical practice. This textbook brings together the recommendations from these national reports and provides an educational basis to teach a preventive strategy for the individual based upon risk. As the foundational knowledge is developing in this area, the interpretation of oral health into general health becomes more important.

Systemic relationships with oral disease are increasingly substantiated in the literature. Periodontal disease has been linked with diabetes,[8] cardiovascular disease,[9] preterm birth/low birth weight infants,[10] and other negative health events. Oral diseases are increasingly shown to be related to negative lifestyle behaviors. Caries is linked with obesity and poor dietary choices,[11] while the evidence for the link between oral cancer and tobacco and alcohol use[12] is well substantiated. As the science in these oral-systemic linkages develops, the role of the dental professional in oral disease prevention and overall health promotion must reflect the change in the science. The relationship of oral disease and systemic disease will require that the dental professional be a partner with the physician and patient in maintaining health and reducing systemic consequences from oral infections. Recognizing that oral diseases are biobehavioral in nature, the dental professional will need to be able to address those factors that are integral in the disease process, to counsel the patient about those behaviors, to motivate the patient to change negative behaviors and to apply prevention based upon the risk for future disease.

Third-party payers are becoming acutely aware that the promotion of prevention leads to a decrease in overall health care costs and an improvement in the quality of life. People are becoming increasingly knowledgeable about their role in maintaining their health, including their oral health. The increasing awareness from providers, third party payers, and consumers about the value of prevention will lead to a change in the practice of the healing arts. Dental professionals need to be at the forefront of this movement and to identify their role in maintaining the overall health of the patient.

The primary drawback to the practice of prevention is reimbursement. Prevention is generally reimbursed by third-party payers at a lesser rate than is treatment. This factor can drive treatment over prevention in clinical practice and has resulted in our current model for the provision of oral health care. While this is true, dentistry is a monopoly and with that comes a greater social responsibility. It is important for the current model to change in favor of prevention and for prevention to be integrated into the overall practice schema. Dental professionals are bound to provide the best service options for those persons under their care. Therefore, the current paradigm (making money through treatment) should be secondary to preventing disease (lose money in prescribing prevention and reduce the burden of disease). If the patient becomes more important than the number of procedures, the rewards can be measured in the long standing relationship a practitioner develops with his patients.

The role of the professional school in the milieu of patient, provider and third-party is to train the oral health provider to integrate prevention into the overall care plan and to evaluate preventive strategies in health. At each visit, the student should evaluate adherence to preventive strategies, modify the plan of prevention as needed and conduct periodic risk reassessment. Continued motivational techniques should be utilized to move the patient toward adoption of positive oral health behaviors. This activity should be incorporated into the routine patient visit. This protocol should become a part of the routine teaching expectation for each patient and reinforced by clinical faculty. The textbook provides a framework from which to teach these principles.

"The secrets of the means for the prevention of dental and oral abnormalities may remain hidden indefinitely unless dental schools actively institute a search for them."[13]

This quotation by William J. Gies (1926) defines the hope of dental education in the process of prevention. Clearly, Dr.Gies identified the role of oral health education to hold up the banner of preventive dentistry and to promote disease prevention over disease treatment. Since we reference this quotation today, it is apparent that many education programs fall short in accomplishing this goal. Following the framework outlined in the Clinical Prevention and Population Health,[7] this book attempts to advance the science in clinical prevention and to use evidence-based methods to provide a basis for prevention education.

Clearly, schools have a primary responsibility to lead in changing the paradigm of prevention in oral health care. The change in practice should be incorporated into both didactic and clinical teaching and through all the years of education. Also, prevention should be included in all phases of practice, including specialty practice and should be applied for each patient. As the prevalence of oral diseases diminishes in the population, we will focus on prevention rather than treatment. This shift toward prevention will change practice from a predominantly surgical model to more of a medical model of care, with an emphasis on the behavioral domain.

We disagree with Dr. Gies in that the means of prevention are largely known, but rarely employed to sufficiently change the outcome of disease over time. *Prevention in Clinical Oral Health Care* attempts to address this discrepancy and to provide a template that can be used to apply prevention into practice. The horizon may reveal new and exciting technologies, practices, and scientific frameworks for the role of prevention in health care. The economics of health care may be the ultimate force that puts prevention in the forefront. This book opens the door for what may be on the future cusp of dental clinical practice.

References

1. Black, GV, 1896. Taken from: Elderton RJ. IADR year of oral health lecture, *J Dent Res* 73:1794-1796, 1994.
2. Thomas DE, Elliott EJ, Naughton GA. Exercise for type 2 diabetes mellitus. *Cochrane Database of Systematic Reviews.* Issue 3; Art No. CD002968. DOI: 10.1002/14651858.CD002968.pub 2, 2006.
3. U.S. Department of Health and Human Services. *Healthy People 2010.* McLean, VA, International Medical Publishing, 2000.
4. U.S. Department of Health and Human Services. Oral Health in America: A Report of the Surgeon General. Rockville, MD, U.S. Department of Health and Human Services, National Institutes of Dental and Craniofacial Research, National Institutes of Health, 2000.
5. American Dental Association. *Future of Dentistry: Today's Vision Tomorrow's Reality,* Chicago, IL, 2001.
6. Brown JP, Hudepohl N, Spolsky V et al. Proceedings of the Clinical Preventive Dentistry Conference, December 11-13, 2002. *J Dent Ed,* (in press).
7. Allen J, Barwick TA, Cashman S et al. Clinical prevention and population health: Curriculum framework for health professions, *Am J Prev Med* 27:471-476, 2004.
8. Mealey BL. Diabetes and periodontal disease: A two way street, *JADA* 137 (Suppl):26S-31S, 2006.
9. Geismar K, Stoltze K, Sigurd B et al. Periodontal disease and coronary heart disease, *J Periodontol* 77:1547-1554, 2006.
10. Offenbacher S, Boggess KA, Murtha AP et al. Progressive periodontal disease and risk of very preterm delivery, *Obstet Gynecol.* 107:29-36, 2006.
11. Mobley CC. Lifestyle interventions for 'diabesity': the state of the science, *Compend Continu Educ Dent* 25:207-208, 211-212, 214-218, 2004.
12. Morse DE, Kerr AR. Disparities in oral and pharyngeal cancer incidence, mortality and survival among black and white Americans, *JADA* 37:203-212, 2006.
13. Gies WJ. Dental education in the United States and Canada. Bulletin 19. The Carnegie Foundation for the Advancement of Teaching, New York, New York.

Part *I*

Epidemiology and Prevention Theory

Chapter 1

Epidemiology of Dental Caries

JAY D. SHULMAN AND DAVID P. CAPPELLI

LEARNING OBJECTIVES

Upon completion of this chapter, the learner will be able to:
- Explain the biological process of caries development
- Describe etiological factors associated with caries
- Examine population-based measures of dental caries
- Discuss trends in caries prevalence
- Outline the *Healthy People 2010* caries objectives

KEY TERMS

Caries balance
Confidence limits
Decayed, Missing, Filled (DMF)
Demineralization
Dental caries
Enamel caries
Early childhood caries
National Health and Nutrition Examination Survey (NHANES)
Remineralization

Dental caries remains the most prevalent chronic childhood disease and is five times more prevalent than asthma.[1] This chapter provides foundational knowledge about the prevalence and trends of dental caries in the population, and explores population-based measurement systems. Dental caries is described as a disease process and the causal profile of the disease is outlined. Surveillance methods and disease trends in the U.S. population for both children and adults are described by using data from several national surveys. The **National Health and Nutrition Examination Survey** (NHANES) series comprises NHANES I (1971 to 1974),[2] NHANES III (1988 to 1994),[3] and NHANES (1999 to present).[4]

CARIES EPIDEMIOLOGY

Dental caries is a diet-dependent, transmissible, microbiologically mediated disease.[6] Similar to periodontal disease, it follows both an infectious and chronic disease model. The microorganisms that cause dental caries are transmitted vertically from mother to child soon after tooth eruption.[7] Studies indicate that the greater the delay in transmission, the lesser the caries burden through life.[7] Once caries is established, prevention focuses on the mitigation of risk factors that contribute to disease. Dental caries is caused by the interrelationship of multiple factors over time (Figure 1-1). These factors were described by Keyes in the 1960s using a Venn diagram (see Figure 4-1) of intersecting causal circles.[8] Modifications of this model appear in the literature, but all have their basis in the original Venn diagram. The cause of dental caries is related to a number of factors that are categorized into

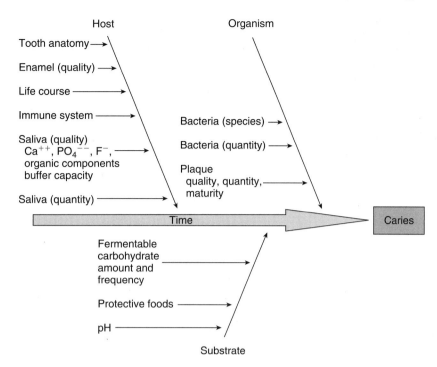

Figure 1-1   Diagrammatic presentation of factors involved in caries development, including substrate, host, and organism over time.

host susceptibility, microorganism, and substrate. All of these factors must intersect during a defined period of time, along a continuum, for caries to occur.

Dental caries is a dynamic process of **demineralization** and **remineralization** of tooth structure[9] in which oral biofilms mature and remain on the tooth for a prolonged period of time.[10] Early detection methods (described in Chapter 4) allow incipient lesions to be identified before the caries spreads into the dentin. Evidence-based prevention strategies allow intervention at this early stage to reduce tooth morbidity or mortality. These strategies, described in Chapter 15, include the use of fluoride and dental sealants to inhibit the progress of caries. This phenomenon has been described in the literature as caries balance.[11]

Caries balance (Figure 1-2) suggests that the process of demineralization and remineralization occurs as a dynamic between pathological and protective factors.[12] In a state of equilibrium, these factors are in balance. The demineralization process predominates when the pathological factors outweigh the preventive factors. If this process continues unchecked, a carious lesion can form. The key is to intervene and reduce the effect of these factors through a process of risk assessment and prevention planning. Similarly, the remineralization factors predominate when the preventive factors supersede the pathological factors. The list of pathological factors is adapted from the original Keyes concept and includes exposure to fermentable carbohydrates, decrease in salivary flow, and an increase in oral pathogens. Caries induction and progression are related to exposure to sugars and other fermentable carbohydrates. The role of diet in caries formation

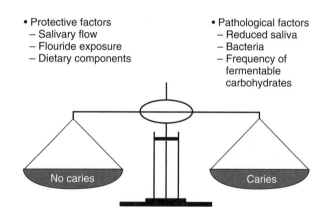

• Protective factors
  – Salivary flow
  – Flouride exposure
  – Dietary components

• Pathological factors
  – Reduced saliva
  – Bacteria
  – Frequency of fermentable carbohydrates

Figure 1-2   The caries balance concept. Relationship between pathological and protective factors in caries development. (Adapted from Featherstone JDB: Caries prevention and reversal based on the caries balance, *Pediatr Dent* 28:128-132, 2006.)

is presented in Chapter 8. Sufficient salivary flow is important to maintain mechanical cleansing of the oral cavity, to buffer against the acids produced by the organisms in the plaque, and to facilitate the host response to the pathogenic microorganisms in the plaque. Acidogenic bacteria have been implicated as an indicator in the formation of dental caries. Therefore, the proliferation of these organisms can be linked to the formation of a carious lesion.[12]

This balance between pathological and preventive factors is an ongoing process of demineralization and remineralization. Dental caries is a process or continuum of events over time (Figure 1-3). This cycle of demineralization

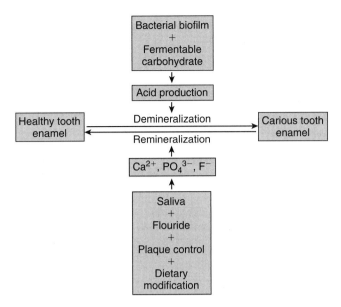

Figure 1-3 Diagram of the continuum of demineralization and remineralization in caries. (Adapted from Kidd EAM, Joyston Bechal S: *Essentials of dental caries, the disease and its management,* ed 2, New York, 1997, Oxford University Press.)

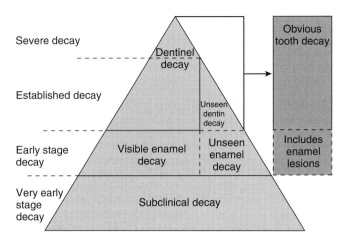

Figure 1-4 Diagram of the iceberg metaphor for dental caries identifying the stages of caries scored at different diagnostic thresholds. (Adapted from Pitts NB: Are we ready to move from operative to non-operative/preventive treatment of caries in clinical practice? *Caries Res* 38:294-304, 2004.)

and remineralization is affected by the presence of inciting factors, cariogenic bacteria and fermentable carbohydrates, and the balance with protective factors, including saliva, fluoride exposure, plaque control, and healthy diet. Over time, this demineralization-remineralization phenomenon can lead to cavitation, reversal of the lesion, or a static state with neither mineral loss nor gain.[10]

The current trend in caries reduction is away from the surgical model (replacement of the diseased tooth structure with a restorative material) to a primarily medical model—a preventive approach. The classic restorative approach to treat the disease removes diseased tissue, but in and of itself, does not provide a cure. Studies demonstrate that once a restoration is placed, the tooth is more vulnerable to future replacement of the restoration with loss of additional tooth structure.[13] The preventive approach seeks to identify factors associated with a patient's disease and to prevent the disease from occurring over the patient's life span.[14] Protective factors include adequate exposure to fluoride, maintenance of salivary flow, and use of antimicrobials.[12] The role of fluorides and antimicrobials in caries prevention is described in Chapter 15. Although not exclusive, these protective factors should be considered in the development of a risk-based plan of prevention.

The role of prevention and maintenance of tooth structure is demonstrated in the "iceberg of dental caries," proposed by Pitts.[15] An adaptation of this model appears in Figure 1-4. This model outlines a care philosophy that focuses on primary and secondary prevention (remineralization) rather than tertiary prevention (restoration). This adapted design notes that subclinical carious lesions may need no intervention, depending on the patient's caries risk status. For patients with a moderate or high caries risk, however, identification of these lesions may be a marker for disease activity for which preventive therapies can be applied. A discussion of the association between risk and prevention for dental caries is provided in Chapters 4 and 15. Preventive approaches to the carious lesion can be applied until the lesion is detectable in dentin. Early identification of the carious lesion and prompt prevention can reduce the need for restorative care.

THE SCIENCE OF CARIES

The interplay of diet, bacteria, and caries has a sound scientific basis. A study by Kite et al. showed that rats fed a cariogenic diet by stomach tube did not develop caries, and animals fed the same diet by mouth did develop caries.[16] The study concluded that cariogenic foods that can be fermented by bacteria to acids in the mouth are essential to caries development. This finding led to the acidogenic theory of caries.[17] Rather than the result of systemic or developmental effects, caries was shown to be a diet-dependent, infectious disease.[18]

Gnotobiotic (germ-free, monoculture) animal studies by Keyes and Fitzgerald[8] showed that caries did not develop in the absence of bacteria. This study suggested that a group of organisms could be responsible for caries formation, rather than a single organism. Caries is now thought to be linked to the acquisition of a consortium of bacteria, indicator organisms, as a mostly vertically transmitted infection from mothers to infants, but not as a horizontally infectious, chronic disease.[7]

TYPES OF CARIES

Enamel caries, the earliest sign of demineralization, is seen as a white-spot lesion. These lesions are small areas of surface demineralization under the dental plaque. Plaque covering the lesion allows the lesion to develop if the plaque remains undisturbed for an extended period. Similarly, the cavitated lesion harbors the organisms within the biofilm and supports the continuation of the caries process. The carious site provides an ecological niche in which the plaque organisms adapt to the lower pH.[10]

Dental caries is traditionally identified by the tooth surface on which the demineralization or cavitation is observed. For epidemiological purposes, it is often classified by surface type. Four surface types are traditionally used to define caries: (1) pits and fissure or occlusal caries, (2) smooth surface lesions, (3) approximal lesions, and (4) root caries. One type of caries, early childhood caries (ECC), is defined by the patient's age and the disease presentation.

Pits and fissures are located on the occlusal surfaces of premolars and molars, lingual surfaces of maxillary incisors, buccal surfaces of mandibular molars, and lingual surfaces of mandibular molars. Carious lesions can form in the grooves or pits and fissures that cover the occlusal surface. Early caries in children's permanent teeth is usually seen in the pits and fissures. This observation may be related to the tooth morphology and difficulty in maintaining hygiene because of the tooth's posterior position. Smooth surfaces include the facial and lingual surfaces and exclude pits and fissures. Approximal lesions occur between the contacts of two adjacent teeth. Although these are on a smooth surface, they are traditionally discussed independently of smooth surface lesions. Root surfaces are the most susceptible surfaces to caries. In the healthy mouth, they are protected from the oral environment by the gingival attachment. When the gingiva moves apically, usually as the result of periodontal disease, the cementum, a softer tissue than enamel, is highly susceptible to caries.

Early childhood caries, formerly called "baby bottle tooth decay" or "nursing caries," occurs in the primary teeth in infants. Although no universal definition exists, early childhood caries (ECC) is usually defined as a lesion that occurs in the six anterior teeth of the maxilla or mandible. Some definitions include primary molars as well. The pathological presentation is similar to caries in permanent teeth with observance of the white-spot lesion, usually on the maxillary incisors. The carious lesion will spread along the maxilla, first infecting the incisors. ECC is a rapidly progressing form of dental caries that can result in complete destruction of the crown of the tooth if left unchecked. In the most severe forms of this disease, destruction of the maxillary teeth is followed by the destruction of the lower molars.[20] This form of caries has been associated with behaviors, especially *ad libitum* bottle or "sippy cup" feeding and prolonged exposure to sweetened drinks in the bottle or cup.

POPULATION-BASED MEASURES OF CARIES

An important distinction should be made between caries diagnosis in clinical practice and caries assessment in a population-based or community survey. In clinical practice the unit of analysis is the patient, and in public health practice the unit of analysis is the community, that is, a geographically defined area[21] such as a school, city, county, state, or nation. The goal of caries diagnosis is to develop a treatment plan for a patient, and the goal of assessment or survey is to characterize caries experience in a community. Therefore, the tools described in the text that follows are not meant to be sufficiently sensitive to diagnose dental caries, but are intended to describe the extent of disease in a given population at a defined point in time.

Because the epidemiologic assessment must be performed quickly, a visual-tactile method is generally used to identify dental caries. For example, the ongoing (1999 to present) NHANES,[4] NHANES I,[2] and NHANES III,[3] used only a mirror, No. 23 dental explorer, and a light source.[22] Caries was recorded when the "explorer catches after insertion with moderate, firm pressure," accompanied by either a softness at the base and/or an opacity adjacent to the area, providing evidence of undermined or demineralized enamel.[23] Contemporary thought in caries science favors minimal use of explorers for caries diagnosis. Studies show that little sensitivity is gained from using an explorer for caries detection. Furthermore, deep pits and fissures can lead to false positive diagnoses when an explorer is used. Routine use of an explorer can disrupt remineralizing enamel, leading to the transfer of pathogenic bacteria from one site to another, and can damage intact enamel structure. Therefore, studies use visual identification of caries for both the individual patient and for population-based surveys.

Other approaches to caries measurement distinguish between noncavitated (D1) and cavitated (D2) lesions,[24] and the approach used by the World Health Organization[25] adds a third category, caries into dentin (D3). The distinction between noncavitated (D1) and cavitated (D2/D3) lesions makes it possible to study surface-specific progression and reversals of lesions over time.[26]

Coronal Caries

The **Decayed, Missing, and Filled Teeth (DMFT)** index has been used since the 1930s[27] and today is the predominant population-based measure of caries experience worldwide. This index gives the sum of an individual's decayed, missing, and filled permanent teeth or surfaces (DMFS). For example, an individual with two decayed, three filled, and one missing tooth has a DMFT of 6. It is important to note that the DMF score is a count that does not indicate the number of teeth that are at risk or the number of sound teeth. Moreover, the DMF does not distinguish between the mix of decayed, missing, and filled teeth or surfaces and whether teeth are lost for reasons other than caries; therefore, the validity of the DMF is reduced. All teeth with the exception of third molars are included, so for an adult, DMFT ranges from zero to 28, and DMFS ranges from zero to 128 with molars and premolars having 5 surfaces and incisors and canines having 4 surfaces. This index accounts for teeth that are restored and missing, and those teeth that are decayed. The DMF is irreversible so that an individual's DMF score cannot decrease. For population-based measures, the sum of all DMFT/S scores is divided by the number of individuals in the total sample. It is important to note that DMF counts are highly skewed with a mode of zero, and linear models are generally not appropriate when a DMF count is a dependent variable.[28]

Although the DMF provides an indicator of both current and past caries experience, individual variables (decayed/missing/filled) can be separated in the data collection process. One limitation is that DMF gives an equal weight to decayed teeth and well-restored teeth. The DMF index has rules that apply to scoring an individual tooth or surface. Each tooth (DMFT) or surface (DMFS) may be counted only once, and decayed, even secondary caries, takes precedence over filled teeth/surfaces.

A similar approach is used for the primary dentition, which consists of a maximum of 20 teeth. The "d" and "f" of the def represent decayed and filled primary (deciduous) teeth, whereas the "e" represents teeth that should be/were extracted. The dmf is often used before teeth begin to exfoliate and the df is often used after exfoliation begins.[29] Although all of these indices appear in the literature in studies of the primary dentition, the index used must be cited when data are compared. Because it is assumed that all missing teeth and all restorations are the result of caries, the DMF score will be overstated to the extent that (1) teeth are missing because of trauma, orthodontic extractions, or periodontal disease; (2) restorations were placed for esthetic reasons or preventive resin restorations; and (3) early lesions that could have remineralized were restored.

In addition to the aggregate measurements, other useful measures can be derived from the DMF. The proportion of a population that is caries free (DMF=0) is commonly used to describe the extent to which the caries burden is concentrated in a subpopulation. Dental professionals may be able to tell which component of the DMF is decayed compared with filled teeth. Separation of the data provides a better indicator of the current caries burden and past history. Although the DMF does not provide a valid indication of treatment need, the proportion of the DMF that is decay (D/DMF) is a surrogate for unmet treatment need and the proportion of the DMF that is filled (F/DMF) can be viewed as a measure of access to care.

The Basic Screening Survey (BSS) was developed by the American Association of State and Territorial Dental Directors (ASTDD) in 1999.[30] The survey method was created in response to the diverse collection of data among different states and the lack of any standardized method to collect oral health information. The BSS provides a simple method to collect oral health information that can be compared among states. The BSS has three distinct advantages. First, the BSS was developed so that the same information is collected locally, regionally, statewide, and nationally. Second, the BSS can be used to collect information on preschool children, school children, and adults in a short time period. Third, trained nonoral health care professionals (e.g., school nurses) can be trained to use this method to collect data.

Protocols are available to describe the collection process for all three groups.[30] Demographic information is collected for all groups. In preschool children, the BSS measures untreated caries, caries experience, and early childhood caries. The BSS protocol for school children measures untreated caries and caries experience as well as the presence of sealants on first permanent molars. For adults, caries experience, untreated caries, and number of teeth are evaluated. In all cases, an assessment of treatment urgency is noted.

The BSS has limitations. The collection of data by trained nondental health professionals introduces a question about the validity of the information. Although the calibration of examiners is possible, any lack of calibration could make comparison among the different reference groups suspect. The BSS provides an estimate of disease burden that can be used in surveillance programs and program planning.

Early Childhood Caries

As discussed earlier in this chapter, early childhood caries (ECC) occurs in the primary teeth.[31] A report from a workshop sponsored by the National Institute of Dental and Craniofacial Research suggests that ECC be defined as one or more df surfaces in any child younger than 71 months of age. Severe early childhood caries (S-ECC) is defined as one or more smooth dmf surfaces in children younger than 36 months of age or one or more cavitated, filled, or missing (because of caries) smooth surfaces in the primary maxillary anterior teeth or a DMFS greater than or equal to 4, 5, and 6, for children 3, 4, and 5 years of age, respectively.[32] Figure 1-5 applies this taxonomy to data from NHANES III[33] and NHANES 1999-2002.[4] The proportion of children with ECC has declined from 1988 to 1999, and the proportion of ECC that is severe (S-ECC) declined only among Mexican Americans.

Root Caries

Root caries is caries of the cementum and dentin on the root surface. These mineralized tissues are softer than enamel. The lesion starts at or below the cemento-enamel junction (CEJ), a region that is irregular and prone to retain bacteria.[34] In the normal periodontium, the CEJ

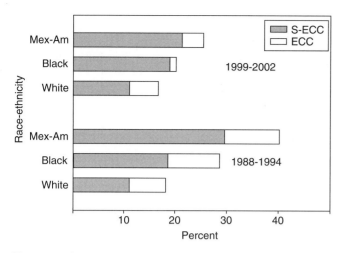

Figure 1-5 Prevalence of early childhood caries (ECC) and severe early childhood caries (S-ECC), U.S. children 2 to 6 years of age by race-ethnicity, 1988-1994 and 1999-2002. (From NHANES III 1988-1994 and NHANES 1999-2002 {unpublished data}.)

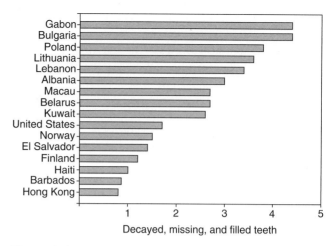

Figure 1-6 Decayed, missing, and filled teeth (DMFT), children 12 years of age, 2000-2001 in selected worldwide locations. (From World Health Organization: *Oral health surveys—basic methods,* ed 4, Geneva, 1997, WHO.)

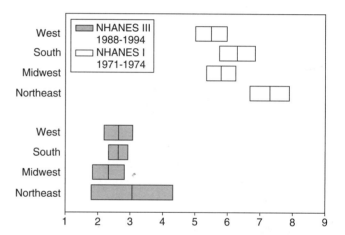

Figure 1-7 Mean decayed, missing, and filled permanent teeth and 95% confidence limits for U.S. regions in youths 12 to 17 years of age, 1971-1974 and 1988-1994. (From NHANES I 1971-1974 and NHANES III 1988-1994 {unpublished data}.)

region is protected from the oral environment by the gingival attachment; however, as the gingiva moves apically (recedes), the root surface becomes visible in the oral cavity.[35] Gingival recession commonly occurs with aging. Causes of gingival recession include deposition of plaque and calculus, occlusal trauma,[36] toothbrush trauma, and other oral hygiene practices.[37] Once the protection of the gingival tissue is lost, the tooth becomes vulnerable to colonization with plaque biofilm and is exposed to the inciting factors for caries.

Used to describe the prevalence of root caries in the population, the Root Caries Index (RCI) is based on the DMF index. The difference between the RCI and DMF is that the RCI uses the number of teeth at risk in the denominator. Therefore, the RCI provides a proportion for each individual and can be applied to the entire population. The index is calculated as the number of root surfaces that are decayed or filled, divided by the number of surfaces exposed because of gingival recession (surfaces with loss of attachment). This index, like other indices used to describe populations, has some limitations.

Definitions of Risk

No discussion of the biology of a disease is complete without a discussion of its correlates. These can be divided into risk factors and risk indicators.[38] A risk factor is an environmental, behavioral, or biological factor, confirmed by temporal sequence, usually in longitudinal studies, which if present directly increases the probability of a disease occurring, and if absent or removed, reduces the probability.[39] A risk indicator is a factor believed to be associated with a disease that has not been demonstrated by longitudinal studies (temporal sequence has not been established).[21] Risk factors and indicators can be categorized as (1) those beyond an individual's

ability to control: nonmodifiable or sociodemographic factors such as age, gender, and race/ethnicity[21]; (2) those within the individual's control, such as lifestyle; and (3) those that are part of the environment, such as fluoride concentration of community water. This chapter will discuss sociodemographic risk factors, and the others will be addressed in Chapter 4.

Geographic Variation

Caries prevalence varies substantially worldwide (Figure 1-6) with a greater than fourfold difference between the areas of highest and lowest prevalence.[40] Studies have shown regional variation within the United States. Figure 1-7 and subsequent figures uses horizontal bars with the mean and 95% **confidence limits**. If a mean is within the 95% confidence interval of another mean, the difference between the means is not statistically significant at two-sided α=0.05. For example, the mean DMFT for the West region in 1971-1974 is less than the lower bound of the 95% confidence interval for the South region (Figure 1-7). Consequently, the means for the two regions are statistically different at the two-sided α=0.05 level. Despite the substantial decline in caries prevalence between 1971 and 1974 and 1988 and 1994, the Northeast continues to have significantly more caries burden than other U.S. regions. The Western United States has a lower prevalence of caries. Although not proven, this trend may reflect the fact that the population in the Northeastern United States tends to be older and less affluent than that in the Western United States.

Secular Trends

Caries prevalence declined substantially in the second half of the 20th century in the United States,[41-44] Western Europe,[45] and most of the world.[40] A comparison of data from four U.S. nationwide oral examinations[4,33,46-48] from 1963 to 2002 shows a marked decrease in caries experience among children and youths (Figure 1-8). This decline can also be seen in the primary dentition (Figure 1-9) although the difference is statistically significant only for 4-year-olds. Table 1-1 shows a substantial increase in the proportion of caries-free individuals between 1988 and 1994 and between 1999 anxd 2002. Most of the reduction in caries prevalence has been in smooth surfaces so that pit and fissure lesions are now a greater proportion of all lesions.[29] This trend is attributed to exposure to fluorides, primarily through community water fluoridation, which has its greatest effect on smooth surfaces.

Sociodemographic Factors

Age. Caries experience is cumulative and DMF increases with age (Figure 1-10). The longer a tooth is exposed to the oral environment, the more time for the caries process to work. Disease progression decreases with

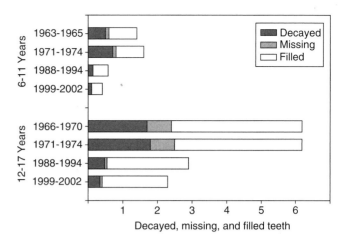

Figure 1-8 Decayed, missing, and filled permanent teeth, and components, U.S. children and youth, 1963-2002. (From Decayed, missing, and filled teeth among children: United States NHANES I 1971-1974, NHANES III 1988-1994, and NHANES 1999-2002 {unpublished data}.)

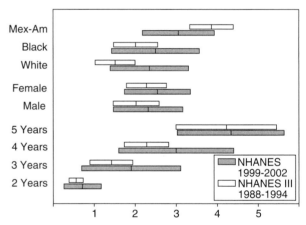

Figure 1-9 Mean decayed and filled primary surfaces and 95% confidence limits in children 2 to 5 years of age, 1988-1994 and 1999-2002. (From NHANES III 1988-1994 and NHANES 1999-2002.)

TABLE 1-1

CHANGES IN PROPORTION OF INDIVIDUALS WITHOUT CARIES EXPOSURE BETWEEN 1988-1994 AND 1999-2002

	NHANES III (1988-1994)		*NHANES (1999-2002)*	
AGE (Y)	CARIES-FREE (%)	95% CONFIDENCE LIMIT	CARIES-FREE (%)	95% CONFIDENCE LIMIT
6-11	76.6	73.30, 79.57	88.6	86.43, 90.52
12-17	33.7	29.63, 38.00	64.5	60.55, 68.26
18-24	17.2	14.33, 20.52	49.3	44.62, 54.00
25-34	6.3	4.95, 8.05	33.7	29.68, 38.08
35-44	4.8	3.26, 6.89	22.3	19.32, 25.60

(Modified from NHANES III 1988-1994 and NHANES 1999-2002 {unpublished data}.)

increasing age. The greater disease burden is seen in the younger population. Although DMF increases with age, the contribution of decay decreases and that of the filled and missing components increases. As individuals age, there is an increase in tooth loss caused by periodontal disease, making the DMF less sensitive as a measure of caries experience alone. Because the prevalence of gingival recession increases with age, root surface caries primarily affects middle-aged and older adults (Figure 1-11).

Dental caries is increasing among the elderly (Chapter 19). This phenomenon may be attributed to the fact that more adults are retaining their teeth through the life span. Studies show that the elderly are experiencing dental caries at a greater rate than children.[49] Certain risk factors are associated with aspects of aging, including xerostomia. As our medication history becomes increasingly complex, diminished salivary function may result from these drugs (Chapter 7), placing the patient at increased risk for caries. In addition, a decrease in motor skills can impact the effectiveness of oral hygiene practices. Changes in diet can affect caries risk status. Although aging alone does not increase the risk for future caries, certain factors associated with aging can have a profound effect on caries risk status.

Gender. Although gender, in itself, is not a risk factor for caries, tooth eruption begins and is completed earlier in girls, thus their teeth are exposed to the oral environment longer.[29] Figure 1-12 shows that females had more decayed and filled surfaces than males in two national surveys. The risk for dental caries is a function of the time a tooth is exposed to the oral environment. Therefore, the difference in dfs in the primary dentition may be caused by the longer exposure time. This relationship is demonstrated in the permanent dentition (Figure 1-13)

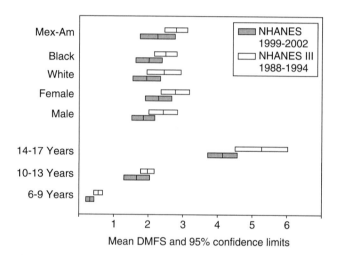

Figure 1-12 Mean decayed, missing, and filled permanent coronal surfaces and 95% confidence limits in U.S. children and youths, 1988-1994 and 1999-2002. (From NHANES III and NHANES 1999-2002 {unpublished data}.)

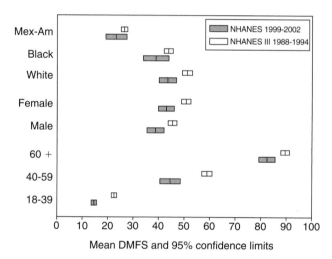

Figure 1-10 Decayed, missing, and filled permanent surfaces, United States, 1999-2002. (From NHANES 1999-2002 {unpublished data}.)

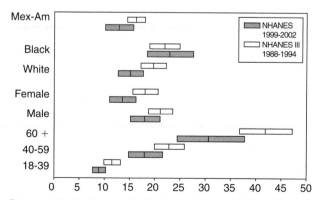

Figure 1-11 Prevalence of decayed or filled root surfaces by age, gender, and race-ethnicity, 1988-1994 and 1999-2002. (From NHANES III and NHANES 1999-2002 {unpublished data}.)

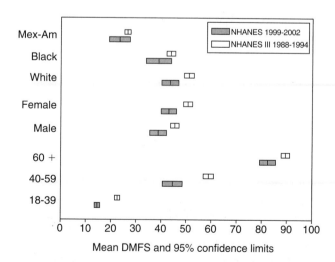

Figure 1-13 Mean decayed, missing, and filled permanent coronal surfaces and 95 percent confidence limits by age gender and race-ethnicity, U.S. adults, 1988-1994 and 1999-2002. (From NHANES III and NHANES 1999-2002 {unpublished data}.)

although not for root caries (see Figure 1-11), which affect more males than females in both surveys. This observation may be attributable to differences in the prevalence of periodontal attachment loss, which is greater in males.

Traditionally, this difference in caries prevalence by gender was explained by differences in treatment seeking behavior. In NHANES III, adolescent males and females (age 12 to 17 years) had similar rates of decayed teeth; however, females had more filled surfaces than males.[50] Whatever the reason for this difference in caries prevalence between males and females, no data exist to support differences in caries susceptibility by gender.

Race and ethnicity. Race and ethnicity (race-ethnicity or race/ethnicity) are related concepts[51] that are commonly used to explain health disparities. Although they are not synonymous with socioeconomic status (SES) or social class, epidemiologists commonly group them together as a surrogate for low SES,[52] because blacks and Hispanics in the United States are disproportionately poor. The burden of caries is higher for blacks compared with whites for caries of the deciduous (see Figures 1-5 and 1-9) dentition, coronal (see Figure 1-12), and root (see Figure 1-11) surfaces. Although a general decline in caries prevalence occurred from 1988-1994 and 1999-2002, black children experienced a slight (although not statistically significant) increase in the prevalence of caries.[53]

Although caries is declining among the U.S. population as a whole, certain groups, including racial and ethnic minorities, experience disparities in caries burden. Although poverty is certainly a covariate in this association, disparities exist in levels of untreated caries among nonpoor blacks and Hispanics when compared with whites.[1] This trend in caries prevalence spans all age groups.

Income. Although caries experience does not differ markedly by income level (see Figure 1-10), the proportion of DMF attributable to decayed and missing teeth decreases as income level increases. Individuals with incomes less than 130% of the federal poverty level had more untreated decay than those with higher incomes and when the decay is treated, the treatment was more likely to be an extraction (Figure 1-14). This disparity was addressed in the 2000 Surgeon General's Report on Oral Health.[1]

Concentration of caries. Although the overall prevalence of caries in the United States has decreased during the past 50 years (see Figure 1-8), the reduction in the caries burden has not been shared equally. Figure 1-15 is a Lorenz curve that shows the distribution of DMFT in U.S. children in three national surveys. The distribution of DMFT is measured by the Gini coefficient: the area between the Lorenz curve (which plots cumulative DMFT proportion of children, against the cumulative share of DMFT) and the 45-degree line (the equality line). The values range from 0 in the case of perfect

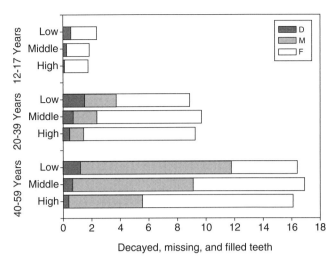

Low: Family income < 130% federal poverty threshold
Middle: Family income between 130% and 350% of federal poverty threshold
High: Family income > 350% federal poverty threshold

Figure 1-14 Decayed, missing, and filled permanent teeth, and components, U.S. adults, by age and income level. (From NHANES III, 1988-1994 {unpublished data}.)

equality (for example, 10% of the population has 10% of the DMFT, 20% has 20% of the DMFT, and so on) to 100 in the case of perfect inequality. Although the proportion of children with a DMFT of 0 has decreased from approximately 70% in the early 1970s to 30% in 1999-2002, the remaining DMFT has become increasingly concentrated. This relationship is depicted by the 45-degree line on Figure 1-15 (the equality line). In 1971-1974, the area under the equality line, represented by the Gini Index, has increased markedly to the point that in 1999-2002, all of the DMFT was concentrated in 30% of U.S. children, who are differentially nonwhite and poor.[54]

Life course. Adverse occurrences during gestation, such as maternal undernutrition, have been shown to be associated with chronic disease that develops in adults.[55] This life course concept may be responsible for increased caries susceptibility caused by either increased prevalence of hypoplastic enamel or decreased immune system function. Life course theory has been used to explain the associations among sugar consumption, tooth brushing, and dental attendance in adolescents born in low socioeconomic circumstances.[56] Some studies have found an association between low birth weight (<2500 g) and caries of the primary dentition,[57-60] and others have not.[61,62] Associations between low birthweight and short stature (surrogates for adverse fetal and post-fetal development) with caries in the permanent dentition have been reported.[63,64]

Healthy People 2010

Healthy People 2010[65] outlines national health objectives for the first decade of the twenty-first century. Table 1-2 lists the *Healthy People 2010* objectives as they relate to caries

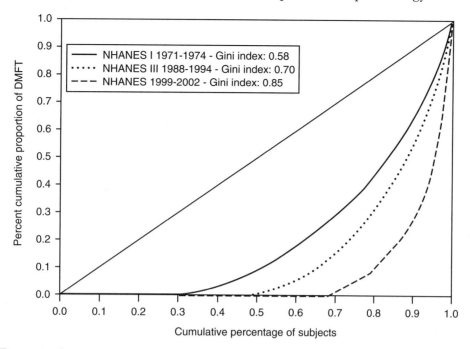

Figure 1-15   Lorenz curve showing the distribution of DMFT in U.S. children in three national surveys.

TABLE 1-2

PROGRESS TOWARD MEETING *HEALTHY PEOPLE 2010* CARIES OBJECTIVES

HEALTHY PEOPLE 2010 CARIES-RELATED OBJECTIVES	BASELINE 1988-1994 (%)	2010 TARGET (%)	STATUS 1999-2004 (0%)	DIFFERENCE (%)
21-1a: Reduce the proportion of children (2-4 years) with dental caries experience in their primary teeth.	18.5	11	23.7	5.2*
21-1b: Reduce the proportion of children (6-8 years) with dental caries experience in their primary and permanent teeth.	51.6	42	53.2	1.6
21-1c: Reduce the proportion of adolescents (15 years) with dental caries experience in their permanent teeth.	61.2	51	56.1	−5.1
21-2a: Reduce the proportion of young children (2-4 years) with untreated dental decay in their primary teeth.	15.9	9	18.9	3.0
21-2b: Reduce the proportion of children (6-8 years) with untreated dental decay in primary and permanent teeth.	28.5	21	29.2	0.7
21-2c: Reduce the proportion of adolescents (15 years) with untreated dental decay in their permanent teeth.	19.8	15	18.2	−1.6
21-2d: Reduce the proportion of adults (35-44 years) with untreated dental decay.	26.9	15	27.8	0.9
21-3: Increase the proportion of adults (35-44 years) who have never had a permanent tooth extracted because of dental caries or periodontal disease	30.1	42	38.4	8.3*

*$p < 0.05$.
Shaded cells indicate that the trend is moving away from the *Healthy People 2010* target.
(Modified from *Healthy People 2010* and NHANES 1999-2004.[4])

with baselines (generally derived from NHANES III[3]) and targets for 2010. Based on NHANES 1999-2004 data,[4] caries trends between 1988-1994 and 1999-2004 have not been uniform and some are trending away from the targets (shaded cells). Overall, the proportion of children 2-11 years of age with caries experience (dft > 0) has increased from 40.0% to 42.2%, with a more marked increase among children 2-5 years of age from 24% to 28%.[4] On the other hand, the prevalence of caries in permanent teeth of adolescents 12-19 years of age has decreased from approximately 68% in 1988-1994 to 59% in 1999-2004.[4] Finally, there were statistically significant declines in overall DMFT scores and root caries prevalence for adults between the two study periods.[4]

While some progress has been made from NHANES III to NHANES 1999-2004, it has been primarily in the permanent dentition. How much of this progress is the result of a general decline in caries prevalence during the decade between the studies, and how much is the result of preventive interventions such as community water fluoridation and the increased use of pit and fissure sealants is difficult to determine. A popular emphasis on health and wellness, including the maintenance of oral health during an individual's lifetime, certainly contributes to this effect. Therefore, one can assume that an increased emphasis on prevention has contributed to a decline in caries prevalence.

SUMMARY

Dental caries is a chronic, diet-dependent, bacterial disease that spans the course of life. The impact of dental caries is profound and can result in considerable pain and expensive treatment. Although the prevalence of dental caries is declining, the fact that people living in the United States are keeping their teeth throughout their life contributes to an increased risk for this disease. The trend toward improved overall health is reflected in better oral health, but the disease of dental caries is increasing in prevalence among older persons. Therefore, targeted prevention is the key to maintaining health in the population. This goal can best be achieved by a preventive program based on an understanding of risk and trends in the population.

REFERENCES

1. U.S. Department of Health and Human Services: *Oral health in America: a report of the Surgeon General*, Rockville, MD, 2000, U.S. Department of Health and Human Services, National Institutes of Dental and Craniofacial Research, National Institutes of Health.
2. National Center for Health Statistics: National health and nutrition examination survey, 1971-1974, U.S. Department of Health and Human Services (DHHS), Centers for Disease Control and Prevention (website): http://www.cdc.gov/nchs/about/major/nhanes/nhanesi.htm. Accessed May 7, 2007.
3. National Center for Health Statistics: National health and nutrition examination survey, 1988-1994, U.S. Department of Health and Human Services (DHHS), Centers for Disease Control and Prevention (website): http://www.cdc.gov/nchs/about/major/nhanes/nh3data.htm. Accessed May 7, 2007.
4. Dye BA, Tan S, Smith V et al.: Trends in oral health status: United States, 1988-1994 and 1999-2004. National Center for Health Statistics, *Vital Health Stat* 11(248), 2007.
5. Glantz SA: *Primer of biostatistics*, ed 5, New York, 2002, McGraw-Hill, p. 209-210.
6. Fejerskov O, Kidd EAM, editors: *Dental caries: the disease and its clinical management*, Copenhagen, 2003, Blackwell Monksgaard.
7. Caufield PW, Griffen AL: Dental caries: an infectious and transmissible disease, *Pediatr Clin North Am* 47:1001-1019, 2000.
8. Keyes PH: Present and future measure of dental caries control, *JADA* 79:1395-1404, 1969.
9. Featherstone JDB: The continuum of dental caries-evidence for a dynamic disease process, *J Dent Res* 83:C39-C42, 2004.
10. Selwitz RH, Ismail AI, Pitts NB: Dental caries, *Lancet* 369:51-59, 2007.
11. Featherstone JDB: Prevention and reversal of dental caries: role of low level fluoride, *Community Dent Oral Epidemiol* 27:31-40, 1999.
12. Featherstone JDB: Caries prevention and reversal based on the caries balance, *Pediatric Dent* 28:128-132, 2006.
13. Elderton RJ: Clinical studies concerning re-restoration of teeth, *Adv Dent Res* 4:4-9, 1990.
14. Pitts NB: Are we ready to move from operative to non-operative/preventive treatment of caries in clinical practice? *Caries Res* 38:294-304, 2004.
15. Pitts NB, Longbottom C: Preventive care advised (PCA)/Operative care advised (OCA) — Categorizing caries by the management option, *Commun Dent Oral Epidemiol* 23:55-59, 1995.
16. Kite OW, Shaw JH, Sognnaes RF: The prevention of experimental tooth decay by tube-feeding, *J Nutr* 42:89-105, 1950.
17. Miller WD: *The microorganisms of the human mouth*. (Original publication 1890, Philadelphia, PA.) Reprinted by Karger, Basel, Switzerland, 1973.
18. Steinman RR, Haley MI: Early administration of various carbohydrates and subsequent dental caries in the rat, *J Dent Res* 36:532-535, 1957.
19. Fitzgerald RJ, Keyes PH: Demonstration of the etiologic role of streptococci in experimental caries in the hamster, *JADA* 61:9-19, 1960.
20. De Grauwe A, Aps JK, Martens IC: Early childhood caries (ECC): what's in a name? *Eur J Paediatric Dent* 5:62-70, 2004.
21. Burt BA: Concepts of risk assessment in dental public health, *Commun Dent Oral Epidemiol*, 33:240-247, 2005.
22. Westat, Inc. National health and nutrition examination survey. Dental examiners procedure manual (Revised, January 2001). Rockville, MD: Westat, Inc.
23. Westat, Inc. National health and nutrition examination survey III: Oral examination component. Rockville, MD: Westat, Inc., 5-41, 1992.
24. Canadian Dental Association: *National epidemiology project*, Canada, 1990, National Health Research and Development Program.
25. World Health Organization: *Oral health surveys-basic methods*, ed 4, Geneva, 1997, WHO.

26. Maupomé G, Shulman JD, Clark DC et al.: Tooth-surface progression and reversal changes in fluoridated and no-longer fluoridated communities over a 3-year period, *Caries Res* 35:95-105, 2001.
27. Klein H, Palmer CR, Knutson JW: Studies on dental caries: I. Dental status and dental needs of elementary school children, *Public Health Rep* 53:751-765, 1938.
28. Lewsey JD, Gilthorpe MS, Bulman JS et al.: Is modeling dental caries a 'normal' thing to do? *Commun Dent Health* 17:212-217, 1999.
29. Burt BA, Eklund SA: *Dentistry, dental practice and the community*, ed 6, St Louis, 2005, Mosby.
30. American State and Territorial Dental Directors (ASTDD): ASTDD Basic Screening Survey. Revised 2003 (website): http://www.astdd.org/index.php?template=basic_screening.html. Accessed January 2007.
31. Kaste LM, Drury TF, Horowitz AM et al.: An evaluation of NHANES III estimates of early childhood caries, *J Public Health Dent* 59:198-200, 1999.
32. Drury TF, Horowitz AM, Ismail AI et al.: Diagnosing and reporting early childhood caries for research purposes, *J Public Health Dent* 59:192-197, 1999.
33. National Center for Health Statistics: Third National Health and Nutrition Examination Survey, 1988-1994, NHANES III Examination and Adult Data Files (CD-ROM), 1997. Hyattsville, MD, Dept. of Health and Human Services (DHHS), Centers for Disease Control and Prevention.
34. Fejerskov O, Nyvad B, Kidd EAM: Clinical and histologic manifestations of dental caries. In Fejerskov O, Kidd E, editors: *Dental caries: the disease and its clinical management*, Oxford, 2003, Blackwell Munksgaard.
35. Haffajee AD, Socransky SS, Goodson JM: Clinical parameters as predictors of destructive disease activity, *J Clin Periodontol* 10:257-265, 1983.
36. Novaes AB, Ruben M, Kon S et al.: The development of the periodontal cleft. A clinical and histopathological study, *J Periodontol* 46:701-709, 1975.
37. Gorman WJ: Prevalence and etiology of gingival recession, *J Periodontol* 38:316-322, 1967.
38. Burt BA: Definitions of risk, *J Dent Educ* 65:1007-1008, 2001.
39. Beck JD: Risk revisited, *Commun Dent Oral Epidemiol* 26:220-225, 1998.
40. World Health Organization: WHO oral health country/area profile programme. Caries for 12-year-olds by country/area (website): http://www.whocollab.od.mah.se/countriesalphab.html. Accessed January 31, 2007.
41. Brown LJ, Wall TP, Lazar V: Trends in untreated caries in permanent teeth of children 6 to 18 years old, *J Am Dent Assoc* 130:1637-1644, 1999.
42. Brown LJ, Wall TP, Lazar V: Trends in untreated caries in primary teeth of children 2 to 10 years old, *Am Dent Assoc* 131:93-100, 2000.
43. Brown LJ, Wall TP, Lazar V: Trends in total caries experience: permanent and primary teeth, *J Am Dent Assoc* 131:223-231, 2000.
44. Brown LJ, Wall TP, Lazar V: Trends in caries among adults 18 to 45 years old, *J Am Dent Assoc* 133:827-834, 2002.
45. Marthaler TM: Changes in dental caries 1953-2003, *Caries Res* 38:173-181, 2004.
46. Kelly JE, Scanlon JV: Decayed, missing, and filled teeth among children: United States, *Vital and Health Statistics*, Series 11 No. 106, DHEW Pub. No. (HSM) 72-1003, Washington, DC, 1971, U.S. Government Printing Office.
47. Kelly JE, Harvey CR: Decayed, missing, and filled teeth among youths 12-17 years: United States, Vital and Health Statistics, Series 11 No. 144, DHEW Pub. No. (HRA) 75-1626. Washington, DC, U.S. Government Printing Office, 1974.
48. Decayed, missing, and filled teeth among persons 1-74 years, United States, 1971-1974. *Vital and Health Statistics*. Series 11 No. 223. DHHS Pub. No. (DHHS Pub. No. PHS 81-1673). Washington, DC, U.S. Government Printing Office, 1981.
49. Griffin SO, Griffin PM, Swann J et al.: Estimating rates of new root caries in older adults, *J Dent Res* 83:634-638, 2004.
50. Kaste LM, Selwitz RH, Oldakowski RJ et al.: Coronal caries in the primary and permanent dentition of children and adolescents 1-17 years of age: United States, 1988-1991, *J Dent Res*, 75(spec issue):631-641, 1996.
51. Lin SS, Kelsey JL: Use of race and ethnicity in epidemiologic research: concepts, methodological issues, and suggestions for research, *Epidemiol Rev* 22:187-199, 2000.
52. Lillie-Blanton M, Parsons PE, Dievler A: Racial differences in health: not just black and white, but shades of gray, *Annu Rev Public Health* 17:411-448, 1996.
53. Vargas CM, Crall JJ, Schneider DA: Sociodemographic distribution of pediatric dental caries: NHANES III, 1988-1994, *JADA* 129:1229-1238, 1998.
54. Beltrán-Aguilar ED, Barker LK, Canto MT et al.: Surveillance for dental caries, dental sealants, tooth retention, edentulism, and enamel fluorosis—United States, 1988-1994 and 1999-2002, *MMWR* 54:31-44, 2005.
55. Kuh D, Ben-Shlomo Y: Introduction. In Kuh D, Ben-Shlomo Y, editors: *Life course approach to chronic disease epidemiology*, Oxford, 2004, Oxford University Press, pp 1-14.
56. Nicolau B, Marcenes W, Bartley M et al.: A life course approach to assessing causes of dental caries experience: The relationship between biological, behavioural, socio-economic and psychological conditions and caries in adolescents, *Caries Res* 37:319-326, 2003.
57. Lai PY, Seow WK, Tudehope DI et al.: Enamel hypoplasia and dental caries in very-low birth weight children: a case-controlled, longitudinal study, *Pediatr Dent* 19:42-49, 1997.
58. Li Y, Navia JM, Bian JY: Caries experience in deciduous dentition of rural Chinese children 3-5 years old in relation to the presence or absence of enamel hypoplasia, *Caries Res* 30:8-15, 1996.
59. Fearne JM, Bryan EM, Elliman AM et al.: Enamel defects in the primary dentition of children born weighing less than 2000 g, *Br Dent J* 168:433-437, 1990.
60. Needleman HL, Allred E, Bellinger D et al.: Antecedents and correlates of hypoplastic enamel defects of primary incisors, *Pediatr Dent* 14:158-166, 1992.
61. Burt BA, Pai S: Does low birth weight increase the risk of caries? A systematic review, *J Dent Educ* 10:1024-1027, 2001.
62. Shulman JD: Is there an association between low birth weight and caries in the primary dentition? *Caries Res* 39:161-167, 2005.
63. Nicolau B, Marcenes W, Bartley M et al.: A life course approach to assessing causes of dental caries experience: the relationship between biological, behavioural, socio-economic and psychological conditions and caries in adolescents, *Caries Res* 37:319-326, 2003.
64. Peres MA, Latorre MRDO, Sheiham A et al.: Social and biological early life influences on severity of dental caries in children aged 6 years, *Commun Dent Oral Epidemiol* 33:53-63, 2005.
65. U.S. Department of Health and Human Services: *Healthy People 2010, ed 2, with understanding and improving health and objectives for improving health*, 2 vols, Washington, DC, 2000, U.S. Government Printing Office.

Chapter 2

Epidemiology/Biology of Periodontal Diseases

DAVID P. CAPPELLI AND JAY D. SHULMAN

NORMAL PERIODONTAL STRUCTURE

GINGIVITIS

PERIODONTAL DISEASE

MEASUREMENT SYSTEMS TO DESCRIBE
PERIODONTAL DISEASE

TRENDS AND PREVALENCE OF GINGIVAL
INFLAMMATION AND DESTRUCTIVE
PERIODONTAL DISEASE IN THE
UNITED STATES

DEMOGRAPHICS

ETIOLOGY OF PERIODONTAL DISEASES

ORAL-SYSTEMIC LINKAGES

CONCLUSION

LEARNING OBJECTIVES

Upon completion of this chapter, the learner will be able to:
- Describe healthy periodontal structures and the pathogenesis of periodontal disease
- Identify measures of periodontal disease used to describe individuals and populations
- Explain the etiology of periodontal disease
- Examine trends in periodontal disease prevalence in populations

KEY TERMS

Alveolar process
Biofilm
Cementum
Endotoxin
Gingival crevicular fluid (GCF)
Gingivitis (gingival inflammation)
Gram-negative bacteria
Immunoglobulin
Inflammatory mediators
Lipopolysaccharide (LPS)
Periodontal disease (periodontitis)
Periodontium
Polymorphonuclear leukocytes (PMN)

Periodontal diseases include a group of chronic inflammatory diseases that affect the supporting tissues of the periodontium, including bone, gingival tissue, and the periodontal ligament.[1] By definition, **periodontal disease** is an inflammatory disease of the supporting tissues of the teeth caused by specific microorganisms or groups of microorganisms, resulting in a progressive destruction of the periodontal ligament and alveolar bone with pocket formation, recession, or both.[1] This definition describes both nondestructive periodontal diseases (gingivitis) and more destructive forms of the disease **(periodontitis)**. Similar to dental caries, periodontal diseases are associated with several microbiological species that have been implicated as potentially causal in this relationship. Oral inflammation, in response to bacterial proliferation in the biofilm, is identified as another component in this hypothesized causal model.

Periodontal diseases are routinely "subdivided" into two distinct categories on the basis of the destructive nature of the disease. **Gingivitis** or **gingival inflammation** is defined as an inflammation of the soft tissue without apical migration of the junctional epithelium. It is reversible, nondestructive in nature, and does not result in the loss of periodontal structures.[2] Similar to gingivitis, periodontitis is an inflammatory disease; however, a component of the inflammatory process in periodontitis results in the apical migration of the

TABLE 2-1

CLASSIFICATION OF PERIODONTAL DISEASES

CATEGORIES	CLINICAL MANIFESTATION
I. Gingival diseases	Dental plaque-induced gingival diseases Nonplaque-induced gingival lesions
II. Chronic periodontitis	Localized Generalized
III. Aggressive periodontitis	Localized Generalized
IV. Periodontitis as a manifestation of a systemic disease	Associated with a disorder Associated with a genetic disorder
V. Necrotizing periodontal diseases	Necrotizing ulcerative gingivitis Necrotizing ulcerative periodontitis
VI. Abscesses of the periodontium	Gingival abscess Periodontal abscess Pericoronal abscess
VII. Periodontitis associated with endodontic lesions	Combined periodontic-endodontic lesions
VIII. Developmental or acquired deformities and conditions	Localized tooth-related factors that modify or predispose to plaque induced gingival diseases/periodontitis Mucogingival deformities and conditions around teeth Mucogingival deformities and conditions on edentulous ridges Occlusal trauma

(From Armitage, GC: Development of a classification system for periodontal diseases and conditions, *Ann Periodontol* 4:1-6, 1999.)

junctional epithelium. This event manifests clinically with the destruction of the connective tissue attachment and loss of alveolar bone.[3]

Before 1999, the classification of periodontal diseases focused on destructive disease at the exclusion of gingival inflammatory disease and heavily weighted age of onset and rates of disease progression.[1] The new classification system (Table 2-1) emphasizes the multifactorial and complex nature of the disease processes and categorizes disease on the basis of clinical manifestation rather than age of onset.[1]

NORMAL PERIODONTAL STRUCTURE

The **periodontium** is composed of the gingiva, periodontal ligament, cementum, and alveolar bone with the accompanying vascular and nerve supply. This complex organ is unique in that it provides a portal to the systemic organism through the extensive vasculature of the gingival tissue, which covers the alveolar process. When healthy, the tissue has a scalloped border with a thin edge and is usually pink in color, although variations in color are evident among different races/ethnicities. The free gingiva

extends from the gingival margin to the free gingival groove, including the interdental papilla (Figure 2-1). In health, the interdental papillae fill the interproximal space and extend to the contact of the two adjacent teeth. At the contact, a slight "dip" occurs in the tissue beneath the contact, which is referred to as the col. The col is most prominent in the posterior teeth, both in the maxilla and mandible, where the contact is the widest. The mucogingival line demarcates the attached gingiva. The attached gingiva, in a healthy state, is firm against the periosteum with the presence of stippling. Because of the ease of visualization and relationship to the more destructive disease process, changes in the gingival tissues are used routinely to measure changes in gingival health.

Cementum is a thin cellular layer that covers the root surface and acts to protect the tooth against outside insult. The cementum acts as an attachment to the periodontal ligament. The periodontal ligament connects the tooth to the alveolar bone. Because the periodontal ligament is visible radiographically, an increase in the width of the ligament can indicate disease.

The **alveolar process** is composed of three distinct structures, the alveolar bone proper (lamina dura), trabecular bone, and compact bone. The bone maintains the tooth in place in the oral cavity. Bone configuration

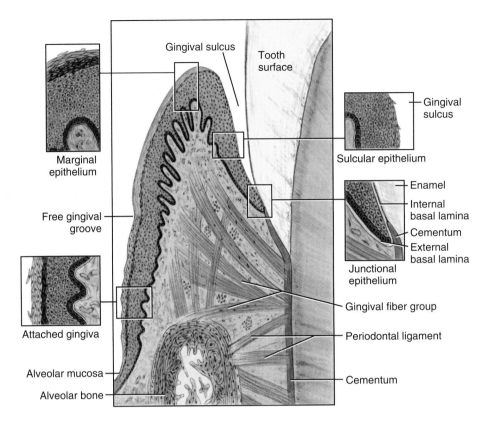

Figure 2-1 Periodontal structure. The periodontium consists of the cementum, periodontal ligament, lamina dura, and cancellous bone. The periodontal structures are covered by soft tissue: both free and attached gingiva. The attached gingival is keratinized and meets the free gingiva at the mucogingival junction. The gingival sulcus contains gingival crevicular fluid, which provides a reservoir for immune cells and inflammatory mediators. (From Bath-Balogh M, Fehrenbach MJ: *Illustrated dental embryology, histology, and anatomy,* ed 2, Philadelphia, 2006, Saunders.)

follows the shape of the tooth root. The lamina dura is radiographically distinct and is covered by compact bone. The lamina dura serves to anchor the periodontal ligament fibers. The compact bone and lamina dura overlay a complex pattern of trabecular bone. The configuration of bone corresponds to the course of the cementoenamel junction of the teeth.

Vascular supply is provided in the maxilla by the superior alveolar artery, and the inferior alveolar artery provides supply in the mandible. Branches of these arteries supply the highly vascular gingival tissue, bone, and supporting structures. The maxillary vasculature comprises the terminal branches of the dental artery, posterior alveolar artery, infraorbital artery, and greater palatine artery, which are terminal branches of the inferior alveolar artery and posterior alveolar arteries. The branches of the facial artery, mental artery, buccal artery, and sublingual artery comprise the mandibular vasculature. These vessels provide a complex, interdependent vascular network.

Lymphatic drainage through the submandibular lymph nodes is accomplished for most of the periodontal tissues. Submental lymph nodes and cervical lymph nodes play a lesser role in the lymphatic drainage of the oral cavity.

GINGIVITIS

Plaque-associated gingivitis is caused by an accumulation of dental biofilms (plaque) on the tooth surface.[4] Although plaque-associated gingivitis is the most prevalent form of the disease, gingival inflammation includes acute necrotizing ulcerative, hormonal, drug-induced, and desquamative gingivitis.[5] This discussion will focus on plaque-associated gingivitis. The response to this **biofilm** is an inflammation of the surrounding local gingival and periodontal tissues (Figure 2-2). The inflammatory response subsides after the removal of the bacterial plaque that colonizes the tooth surface.[4] Although the presence of the dental biofilm is necessary for gingivitis to occur, the duration and intensity of the inflammatory response varies between individuals and even among different teeth in the oral cavity.[6,7] Although gingivitis is a precursor to a more destructive disease process, not all patients who express gingival inflammation will progress to that state. This fact, along with the difference in the inflammation, suggests that a subset of patients express differences in levels of response to the biofilm. Epidemiological investigations indicate that approximately

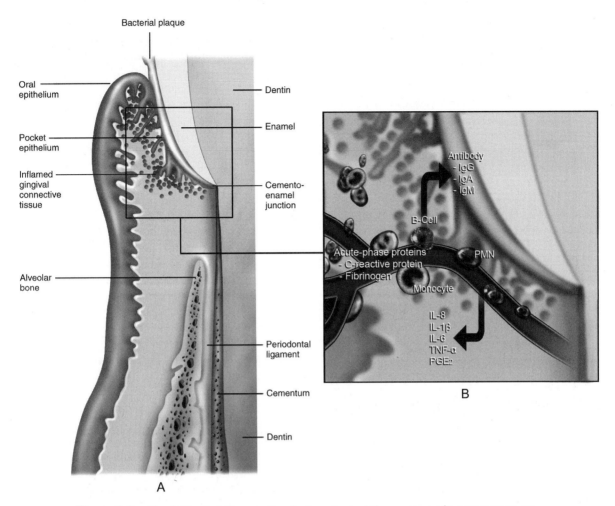

Figure 2-2 Gingivitis. A, Inflammation in the gingival tissue occurs in response to an increase in bacterial plaque. B, The immune system is upregulated with an increase in numbers of immune cells (PMNs, monocytes) and cytokines. An increase in acute phase proteins (CRP, fibrinogen) is seen in response to the biological challenge. The early inflammatory response is to contain the infection and to remove damaged tissue. As the inflammation becomes increasingly chronic, continued stimulation results in an altered immune response. (A, From Rose LF, Mealey BL, Genco RJ, et al. *Periodontics: Medicine, Surgery and Implants.* St. Louis, 2004, Elsevier-Mosby. B, Original art by Mr. Scott A. Eddy)

35% of persons in the United States are at risk for expression of a more destructive disease.[8]

Specific bacterial species are associated with gingival inflammation. Gingivitis occurs when the microbial ecology shifts from a predominance of gram-positive microorganisms, such as *Actinomyces, Lactobacillus,* and *Streptococcus,* to **gram-negative bacteria,** which include *Porphyromonas, Prevotella, Aggregatibacter,* and *Bacteroides.* As the disease progresses, maturation of the biofilm occurs. Initially, the biofilm is colonized with mostly streptococci species. As the inflammation progresses, *Actinomyces* species predominate in the biofilm, and have been shown to be associated with an increasing plaque mass.[9] An increase in the number of *Prevotella* and *Porphyromonas* species is associated with an increase in gingival inflammation.[10] In sites with gingivitis, increases have been observed in *Fusobacterium nucleatum, Treponema,* and *Eubacterium.*[11] An increase in gingival bleeding correlates with an increasing colonization with *Actinomyces* spp.[10]

The concomitant host response to the microbial challenge marks the progression from an acute gingivitis to a chronic inflammation. Initially, when gram-positive organisms colonize the biofilm, an infiltration of biologically active mediators occurs, including tumor necrosis factor (TNF) α, prostaglandin (PG) E_2, interleukin (IL)-1β, IL-8, and metalloproteinases (MMPs). One outcome of an upregulation of these proteins is an increase in chemotaxis of polymorphonuclear leukocytes (PMNs) and the initiation of the cellular immune response.[12]

Clinical signs/symptoms that indicate this disease include rubor (a change in color), tumor (swelling), calor (temperature), dolor (pain), and the presence of bleeding. Histopathology demonstrates a predominance of inflammatory infiltrates into the gingival tissues. Although the disease is reversible, treatment philosophy is based largely on the potential of gingival inflammation to progress into destructive periodontal disease.

PERIODONTAL DISEASE

Periodontal disease may manifest as several unique conditions, including chronic periodontitis, aggressive periodontitis, necrotizing forms of periodontal disease, or periodontal disease associated with or as a manifestation of systemic disease (see Table 2-1). Chronic periodontitis is the most prevalent form of this destructive disease. This disease is characterized by bursts of activity with periods of quiescence.[13] Similar to gingivitis, destructive periodontal diseases are inflammatory diseases that are accompanied by destruction of the periodontal tissue with apical migration of the connective tissue attachment and loss of the alveolar bone.[14] As with its precursor, gingivitis, periodontal disease is a consequence of maturation of the microorganisms that colonize the dental biofilm and the host response that results from this colonization.[15] Several bacterial species are commonly associated with this mixed infection. A predominant group of microorganisms identified as the "red complex"[16] have been implicated in the disease. Organisms in the "red complex" include *Tannerella forsythia, Porphyromonas gingivalis,* and *Treponema denticola.* In addition, other microorganisms are implicated in the destructive process, including *Aggregatibacter actinomycetemcomitans* (formerly *Actinobacillus actinomycetemcomitans*), *Fusobacterium nucleatum, Campylobacter rectus,* and *Prevotella intermedia.*[16,17] The capability of these species to produce **endotoxin** is implicated in the tissue destruction, resulting in bone resorption and the induction of the host immune response. In a subset of patients who initially express chronic gingival inflammation, the disease progresses to periodontitis with destruction of the alveolar bone and apical migration of the periodontal attachment. Although several hypotheses for this mechanism are proposed, the exact causal framework has yet to be elucidated.

Although multiple risk factors are associated with the disease, the primary etiology of all forms of periodontitis is a shift in the subgingival bacterial ecology to colonization of predominantly gram-negative microorganisms. Although pathogenic microorganisms are necessary, this shift to a more periodontopathogenic environment alone is not a sufficient cause for disease to occur. The susceptibility of the host is also important in this schema. The induction and progression of destructive periodontal disease can be influenced by multiple variables, including genetics, lifestyle behaviors, comorbidities, and socioeconomic factors. These factors are discussed in Chapter 5.

The pathway of progression from gingivitis to periodontitis begins when the supragingival plaque that is evident in gingivitis becomes established and matures (Figure 2-3). When the microorganisms overwhelm the local host response, periodontopathogenic bacteria migrate subgingivally and establish in the subgingival niche.[16] The initial lesion, defined by subclinical gingivitis appears 2 to 4 days after the colonization of the gingival sulcus.[19] Clinically, these changes manifest as vasculitis,

exudation of serous fluid from the gingival sulcus (gingival crevicular fluid, or GCF), increased migration of **polymorphonuclear leukocytes (PMNs)** into the sulcus, alteration of the junctional epithelium at the base of the pocket, and the dissolution of perivascular collagen.[19] Within 4 to 7 days after the formation of the initial lesion, the early lesion forms in response to accumulation of bacterial plaque. The early lesion is characterized by an accumulation of leukocytes at the site of acute inflammation, cytopathic alterations of the resident fibroblasts, increased collagen loss within the marginal gingival, and proliferation of basal cells of the junctional epithelium.[19]

If left undisturbed, the inflammatory reaction in response to the insult leads to the formation of the established lesion. The established lesion develops within 2 to 3 weeks after the onset of plaque accumulation. Plasma cells predominate in the established lesion, and the presence of **immunoglobulins** within the connective tissue and junctional epithelium can be observed.[19] Histologically, continued collagen destruction occurs, accompanied by proliferation, apical migration, and lateral extension of the junctional epithelium. Clinically, the presence of early pocketing may be noted. At this stage, the periodontal lesion may be confined to the marginal and coronal portions of the gingiva or it may progress to an advanced stage. The disease may remain confined indefinitely or may become advanced at any time that the nidus remains intact. The advanced lesion is similar to the established lesion; however, clinical manifestation at this stage is more pronounced with the loss of alveolar bone, periodontal ligament, and the formation of periodontal pockets. Unlike the previous stages, the advanced lesion, once formed, can progress and the associated bone destruction may result in eventual tooth loss.[19]

In classic epidemiological studies, Löe and colleagues demonstrated that, if left untreated, periodontal disease progresses with time.[20] They studied a Norwegian population receiving dental care and a Sri Lankan population with no access to routine dental care.[21] By age 40 years, the Sri Lankan population demonstrated a threefold to fourfold increase in attachment loss when compared with the Norwegian group. Another finding from this study demonstrated an inherent ability in the host to respond to the insult. Although most of the Sri Lankan study participants expressed severe inflammation with accompanying biofilm, not all had the same extent or severity of periodontal disease, as defined by clinical loss of attachment (LOA). Three different subgroups emerged from this study. Approximately 8% of the population expressed a rapidly progressive disease (mean LOA, 13 mm), 81% had a moderately progressive disease (mean LOA, 7 mm), and 11% were defined as stable or not progressing.[20] In conclusion, 89% of the Sri Lankan population had a severe periodontal disease that progressed at a more rapid rate than a Norwegian population that received routine oral health care.[20] These findings suggest that specific groups are at

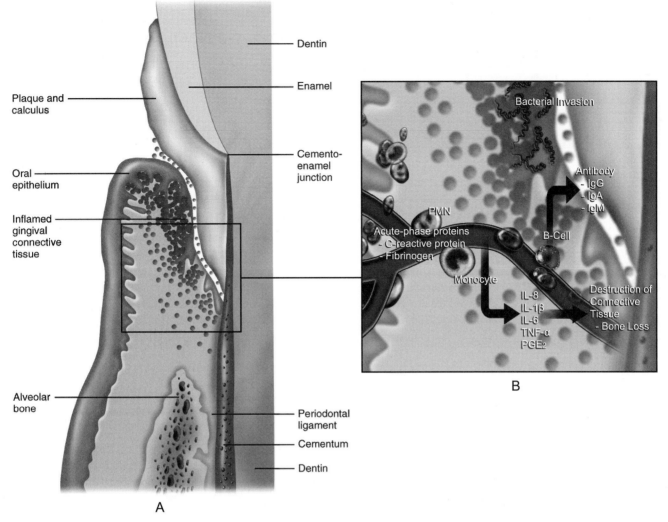

Figure 2-3 Periodontitis. A, The clinical presentation of periodontitis includes inflammation of the gingival tissue with loss of bone, destruction of connective tissue and apical migration of the epithelium. B, In response to an increasing pathogenic microflora, chronic inflammation and bacterial invasion of the gingival tissue stimulates a continued cellular and humoral immune response with the production of cytokines/chemokines and acute phase proteins. Activation of the inflammatory and innate immune response results in collateral damage of the local tissues, as the immune system attempts to manage the infection and achieve homeostasis. (A, Redrawn from Armitage GC: *Biologic Basis of Periodontal Maintenance Therapy,* Berkeley, 1980, Praxis Publishing. B, Original art by Mr. Scott A. Eddy)

greater risk for disease and validate the importance of routine prevention.

MEASUREMENT SYSTEMS TO DESCRIBE PERIODONTAL DISEASE

From an epidemiological perspective, the lack of a single measure of periodontal disease in population-based research impacts the ability to obtain consistent, reliable data. The prevalence of disease in a population depends on the threshold chosen. Studies have shown that the prevalence of disease ranges from 99%, with a loss of attachment greater than 1 mm,[22] to 7% of the population, with a loss of attachment greater than 7 mm.[23] At a threshold of 3 mm, the prevalence of attachment loss was 53.1%.[23]

Gingivitis is diagnosed by the presence of bleeding, redness, edema, ulceration, or an increase in thickening of the gingival tissue. The most accepted index for measuring the prevalence of gingivitis is the presence, extent, or severity of bleeding.[24] Several measures of bleeding have been used clinically and in research; however, no single measure for inflammation has been accepted as the standard. In epidemiological studies, several indices exist that can be used to define inflammation. The Gingival Index (GI) scores each site on a 0 to 3 scale, with 0 being normal and 3 being severe inflammation characterized by edema, redness, swelling, and spontaneous bleeding[4] (Table 2-2). This measurement is based on the presence or absence of bleeding on gentle probing. Four sites are

TABLE 2-2

INDICES USED TO MEASURE GINGIVITIS AND PERIODONTITIS IN POPULATIONS AND THE CRITERIA DEFINED FOR EACH SCALE OF MEASUREMENT

INDEX	SCALE
Plaque index (PlI)	0 = No plaque in the gingival area. 1 = A thin film of plaque adhering to the free gingival margin and adjacent to the area of the tooth. The plaque is not readily visible, but is recognized by running a periodontal probe across the tooth surface. 2 = Moderate accumulation of plaque on the gingival margin, within the gingival pocket, and/or adjacent to the tooth surface, which can be observed visually. 3 = Abundance of soft matter within the gingival pocket and/or adjacent to the tooth surface.
Gingival index (GI)	0 = Healthy gingiva. 1 = Mild inflammation: characterized by a slight change in color, edema. No bleeding observed on gentle probing. 2 = Moderate inflammation: characterized by redness, edema, and glazing. Bleeding on probing observed. 3 = Severe inflammation: characterized by marked redness and edema. Ulceration with a tendency toward spontaneous bleeding.
Modified gingival index (MGI)	0 = Absence of inflammation. 1 = Mild inflammation: characterized by a slight change in texture of any portion of, but not the entire marginal or papillary gingival unit. 2 = Mild inflammation: criteria as above, but involving the entire marginal or papillary gingival unit. 3 = Moderate inflammation: characterized by glazing, redness, edema, and/or hypertrophy of the marginal or papillary gingival unit. 4 = Severe inflammation: marked redness, edema, and/or hypertrophy of the marginal or papillary gingival unit, spontaneous bleeding, or ulceration.
Community periodontal index (CPI)	0 = Healthy gingiva. 1 = Bleeding observed after gentle probing or by visualization. 2 = Calculus felt during probing, but all of the black area of the probe remains visible (3.5-5.5 mm from ball tip). 3 = Pocket 4 or 5 mm (gingival margin situated on black area of probe, approximately 3.5-5.5 mm from the probe tip). 4 = Pocket > 6 mm (black area of probe is not visible).
Periodontal screening and recording (PSR)	0 = Healthy gingiva. Colored area of the probe remains visible, and no evidence of calculus or defective margins is detected. 1 = Colored area of the probe remains visible and no evidence of calculus or defective margins is detected, but bleeding on probing is noted. 2 = Colored area of the probe remains visible and calculus or defective margins is detected. 3 = Colored area of the probe remains partly visible (probe depth between 3.5-5.5 mm). 4 = Colored area of the probe completely disappears (probe depth > 5.5 mm).

scored for each tooth and can be averaged to produce a mean value for the individual tooth. The Eastman Interdental Bleeding (EIB) Index also uses bleeding as a measure of inflammation.[25] The EIB involves insertion of a wooden interdental cleaner in the interproximal space and depression of the tissues approximately 1 to 2 mm. The cleaner is inserted parallel to the occlusal plane to reduce potential trauma to the tissues. Bleeding is recorded if present after approximately 15 seconds. Both of these indices require careful drying of the teeth and gingiva before scoring.[25]

Indices that rely solely on bleeding as a measure of gingival inflammation have limited use in public health practice. Invasive measures, such as bleeding, are often inappropriate for field conditions. The Modified Gingival Index (MGI) uses a visual scale to assess gingival health.[26] The MGI relies on a visual assessment of gingival changes to measure the severity of inflammation. Five categories, using a 0-4 scale, score the marginal and papillary gingival tissue based on color, texture, edema, and spontaneous bleeding (see Table 2-2). Using this index, 108 sites are scored per person (52 papillary and 56 marginal sites).

Plaque indices have been used as a marker for the presence of gingivitis, because supragingival plaque is a known risk factor for inflammation. The most frequently referenced measure of supragingival plaque is the Plaque Index or PlI.[27] The PlI is similar to the Gingival Index and uses an ordinal scale of 0 to 3. Similar to the GI, the PlI is scored on four sites per tooth. The PlI considers only the thickness of the plaque along the gingival margin without regard to the extension of the plaque. The PlI initially relies on visual measures to assess the presence of plaque. If the plaque cannot be observed visually, a periodontal probe is wiped along the gingival margin to detect the presence of plaque. Similar to the gingival indices, drying of the teeth before examination is recommended before measurement of the PlI. The scale for scoring the PlI is presented in Table 2-2.

The status of the oral health of the U.S. population was obtained in the National Health and Nutrition Examination Survey (NHANES). Several NHANES were conducted, including NHANES I from 1971 to 1974, NHANES III from 1988 to 1994, and NHANES from 1999 to 2002. The periodontal measures used in NHANES I varied considerably from the subsequent NHANES surveys. Although NHANES I relied on a visual index of periodontal health (Periodontal Index, PI) on all teeth,[28] NHANES III data were obtained through direct clinical examination of the periodontal structures measuring probing depths and clinical attachment loss.

The PI uses an ordinal scale to weigh each of the following disease classifications: mild gingivitis, gingivitis, gingivitis with pocket formation, and advanced destruction with loss of masticatory function, drifting of teeth, and increased mobility. This index relies solely on a visual inspection rather than probing or clinical attachment loss measures.

One modification of the PI is the Periodontal Disease Index (PDI). The PDI is unique in that it provides an estimate of periodontal disease for the entire mouth by measuring selected index teeth.[29] Partial mouth recording using a periodontal probe is routinely used in epidemiological investigations to measure the prevalence of periodontal disease in a population. The PDI is the most widely recognized partial mouth recording protocol. The six selected teeth scored to assess the extent and severity of periodontal disease are the maxillary right first molar (#3), maxillary left central incisor (#9), the maxillary left first bicuspid (#12), the mandibular left first molar (#19), the mandibular right central incisor (#25), and the mandibular left first bicuspid (#28). These teeth have been shown to provide an accurate representation of the periodontal status of the individual.[29]

Periodontal Screening and Recording (PSR) is an adaptation of the original Community Periodontal Index (CPI, formerly CPITN). The CPITN was developed by the World Health Organization in an attempt to standardize the measurement of periodontal disease prevalence.[30] For both indices, a special periodontal probe is used. The probe has a 0.5-mm ball on its tip with color-coded banding that extends from 3.5 to 5.5 mm from the tip of the probe. Although each tooth is measured, each sextant of the mouth is given a code reflecting the greatest probe depth value. Codes, ranging from 0 to 4, are determined for each sextant (see Table 2-2). Code X is used for an edentulous sextant. This method is effective in screening for disease and for measuring the prevalence of disease in populations.

The measurement of periodontal disease is determined through a complete clinical examination and the measurement of the clinical attachment level around each tooth. The clinical attachment level (CAL) is calculated by measuring the probing pocket depth and the recession measurement from the cementoenamel junction (CEJ) as a fixed reference point. Destructive periodontal disease is, then, traditionally defined clinically by increased loss of attachment as measured from the CEJ to the base of the pocket. The measure of loss of attachment is used, because longitudinal comparison over time is more reliable than other methods. Increasing pocket probing depths continue to be used to define periodontal disease. Probing depth is measured from the crest of the free gingival margin to the base of the pocket. As a record of destructive disease, this measure is less reliable than other measures, because it records both true bone loss and tissue inflammation.

Clinical loss of attachment and probing depths are usually recorded at six sites per tooth (mesiobuccal, buccal/facial, distobuccal, mesiolingual, lingual, and distolingual). Measurements are made using one of several available graduated periodontal probes. Bleeding after probing is noted after recording the probing depth for each site.

Radiographic evidence of bone loss remains the most valid measure of destructive periodontal disease. The primary limitation to radiography is the difficulty in quantifying small changes in bone architecture longitudinally. Advances in technology in the area of both quantification of bone density change and standardization of radiographs have increased the reliability of this diagnostic tool; however, no universally accepted measure for bone density change has been adopted.

The ability to measure both the induction and progression of the disease process is critical to assessing risk and to applying prevention. Therefore, researchers have turned to laboratory assays in hopes of increasing both the validity and reliability of the measures that assess changes in periodontal health. One strategy is to examine changes in the local microbial ecology. Techniques are adopted to examine whether the site/tooth experiences colonization by more periodontopathogenic bacterial species, which can then be related to an increased future risk for disease. A second strategy involves changes in the local host response. **Gingival crevicular fluid (GCF)** is assayed to measure changes in mediators of inflammation that may be a marker for either the induction or progression of destructive disease process. Finally, genetic markers may be predictive of a greater risk for expression of periodontal disease. These methods are described in Chapter 9.

TRENDS AND PREVALENCE OF GINGIVAL INFLAMMATION AND DESTRUCTIVE PERIODONTAL DISEASE IN THE UNITED STATES

Although national studies of periodontal disease prevalence in the United States have been performed since 1959,[31] the results have been inconsistent, primarily because of the use of different assessment protocols.[32] Moreover, unlike most diseases in which a generally accepted operational or case definition exists, prevalence studies of periodontal disease vary widely in the threshold for disease. For example, Borrell et al. defined a periodontitis case as an adult with "at least 3 sites of LOA ≥ 4 mm and at least 2 sites with PD ≥ 3 mm"[32] and *Healthy People 2010* defined destructive periodontal disease as the presence of attachment loss greater than or equal to 4 mm in at least one site.[33] Strength of association between demographic and behavioral factors and periodontal disease is sensitive to the periodontal disease case definition.[34]

To illustrate sociodemographic and temporal factors associated with destructive periodontal disease, we use the case definition of *Healthy People 2010*: loss of attachment greater than or equal to 4 mm in at least one site (midfacial and mesial facial line angles) for a randomly selected maxillary and mandibular quadrant in adults 35 to 44 years of age.[35] These measures are available in NHANES III[36] and NHANES 1999 to 2004.[37]

Table 2-3 shows that increased periodontal disease prevalence is associated with being black or Mexican-American, male, having a low education level, and smoking more than 10 cigarettes per day. These findings are consistent in both the 1988-1994 and 1999-2004 studies (see Table 2-3, Column A, B). These trends generally hold for individuals who smoked 10 or fewer cigarettes per day (see Table 2-3, Column E, F). On the other hand, these differences were

TABLE 2-3

PREVALENCE OF ONE OR MORE SITES WITH AT LEAST 4 MM CLINICAL ATTACHMENT LOSS BY CIGARETTE SMOKING STATUS, 1988-1994 AND 1999-2002, U.S. ADULTS 35 TO 44 YEARS OF AGE. ADJUSTED FOR COMPLEX SAMPLE DESIGN (STATA 9.0, COLLEGE STATION, TX)

	1988-1994	1999-2002	1988-1994	1999-2002	1988-1994	1999-2002
	ALL SUBJECTS		SMOKES >10 CIGARETTES/DAY		SMOKES ≤10 CIGARETTES/DAY	
	A	B	C	D	E	F
Race/Ethnicity	19.8‡	16.83‡	38.3	12.9	14.7‡	24.8*
Black	30.3	26.42	47.3	20.0	26.5	38.9
White (non-Hispanic)	17.9	15.14	37.1	11.0	12.0	23.5
Mexican-American	24.0	17.71	42.9	15.3	22.4	9.4
Gender	20.2‡	21.4*	39.2	25.2	9.5‡	15.3
Male	27.2	14.1	42.6	26.3	22.1	19.6
Female	13.9	17.9	34.8	23.6	15.2	11.9
Education level	20.2‡	17.9‡	39.2	25.2	15.1‡	15.3‡
Less than high school	31.7	31.8	43.2	25.2	26.2	28.3
High school graduate	26.0	20.5	42.4	30.2	19.4	20.7
At least some college	13.5	12.8	32.4	20.2	10.5	10.5
% Federal poverty level	20.0‡	17.6‡	38.7	20.8	15.1‡	15.4†
<150	32.1	28.6	48.0	33.3	25.9	28.5
150 to <300	21.7	19.6	32.8	19.4	18.2	16.0
≥300	14.9	12.1	38.4	13.7	10.3	10.8
Smokes >10 cigarettes/day	20.2	17.4*				
Yes	15.2	25.2				
No	39.2	15.3				

*Chi square test: $p < 0.05$.
†Chi square test: $p < 0.01$.
‡Chi square test: $p < 0.001$.

not statistically significant in individuals who smoke more than 10 cigarettes per day (see Table 2-3, Column C, D).

Bleeding on gentle insertion of a periodontal probe (bleeding on probing or BOP) can be expressed as the presence or absence of BOP, the mean number of BOP sites per mouth, or the percent of measured sites with BOP. Table 2-4 shows that among all subjects, gingivitis prevalence was significantly different by race/ethnicity, gender, education, and income level. Smokers of more than 10 cigarettes per day had decreased prevalence of gingivitis than subjects who smoked 10 or fewer cigarettes per day. As with periodontal disease (see Table 2-3), these relationships held for subjects who smoked 10 or fewer cigarettes per day but were not statistically significant among subjects who smoked more than 10 cigarettes per day. This finding suggests that the effect of smoking is so strong that it overshadowed the effects of sociodemographic variables.

DEMOGRAPHICS

The prevalence of chronic periodontitis increases with age, and the disease usually becomes clinically significant only in adults. Increasing age is correlated with an increased prevalence of periodontal disease, as well as an increase in both the extent and severity of the disease.

Approximately 35.7% of adults aged 30 to 39 years experienced greater than 3 mm of attachment loss compared with 89.2% for those individuals aged 80 to 90 years.[23] In a study that evaluated the prevalence, severity, and extent of periodontal disease in an employed United States population, loss of attachment greater than 1 mm was found in 99% of the subjects.[22] Approximately 44% of people aged 18 to 64 years exhibited attachment loss at one or more sites, with an average of 3.4 affected sites per person.

Other studies suggest an aging pattern in which periodontal disease is expressed through adulthood to age 50 years. After that time, the disease appears to stabilize somewhat through the aging process. Pocket depth measures of 4 mm or greater increased in the population to age 50 years and then remained stable or experienced a slight decrease through the end of life.[8] A similar pattern is observed with moderate and advanced periodontal disease and may suggest a unique relationship between disease severity and aging.

As is observed in most oral diseases, chronic periodontal disease is more common in males than in females. When compared with females, males expressed more disease as measured by greater loss of attachment and deeper pocket depths. This association spanned all ages, except in ages 85 to 90 years, when males had better periodontal health than females, but also had greater tooth loss

TABLE 2-4

PREVALENCE (PERCENT) OF ONE OR MORE SITES WITH GINGIVAL BLEEDING ON PROBING BY CIGARETTE SMOKING STATUS, 1988-1994, U.S. ADULTS 35 TO 44 YEARS OF AGE. ADJUSTED FOR COMPLEX SAMPLE DESIGN (STATA 9.0)

	1988-1994 ALL SUBJECTS	1988-1994 SMOKES >10 CIGARETTES/DAY	1988-1994 SMOKES ≤10 CIGARETTES/DAY
Race/Ethnicity	47.0[†]	38.4	49.3*
Black	51.2	45.8	52.2
White (non-Hispanic)	45.3	37.0	47.8
Mexican-American	60.9	56.8	61.2
Gender	48.3*	39.0	50.7[†]
Male	52.2	37.8	56.5
Female	44.7	40.6	45.7
Education level	48.2[‡]	39.0	50.5[‡]
Less than high school	60.5	42.0	68.2
High school graduate	52.4	38.0	58.0
At least some college	42.3	38.4	43.0
% Federal poverty level	48.5[‡]	38.4	51.0[‡]
<150	59.9	47.1	64.8
150 to <300	53.5	45.8	55.5
≥300	41.7	27.8	44.5
Smokes >10 cigarettes/day	48.4[†]		
Yes	39.0		
No	50.7		

*Chi-square test: $p < 0.05$.
[†]Chi-square test: $p < 0.01$.
[‡]Chi-square test: $p < 0.001$.

than females. Men also expressed a more severe periodontal disease than women.[38]

Differences exist among the major racial/ethnic groups in the United States. African-Americans experience the highest prevalence of chronic periodontal disease and the greatest severity of disease. Compared with white Americans, Mexican-Americans have both a higher prevalence and more severe disease presentation.[23] A similar racial/ethnic breakdown appears in aggressive forms of the disease.[39]

Gingival inflammation, as measured by bleeding on probing, was observed in approximately 50% of the adult U.S. population.[8] Both the extent and severity of the inflammation increased with age and this increase in prevalence by age was more dramatic in those with more sites of inflammation. As noted in periodontal disease patterns, males expressed a higher prevalence of bleeding than females. Gingivitis was more prevalent in Mexican-Americans than either African-Americans or whites, respectively.[8]

Associations with socioeconomic variables and periodontal disease are not as clear as for other oral diseases. Because socioeconomic variables are linked with health behaviors, including oral hygiene behaviors and access to care, gingival inflammation is related to lower socioeconomic status, including income and education. Studies suggest an association between lower socioeconomic status and periodontal disease,[40] but this association is not clear.

ETIOLOGY OF PERIODONTAL DISEASES

Because periodontal disease follows an infectious disease paradigm, the role of the certain bacteria and the induction of an immune response to that insult are primary to the clinical manifestation of the disease process. As a chronic disease, the disease process is a bit more complex than the traditional infectious disease model with many factors contributing to the induction and progression of periodontal disease. Because periodontal disease is multifactorial, we must also consider the impact of lifestyle behaviors, systemic and genetic determinants, and social and cultural factors in this causal framework. These factors are discussed in Chapter 5.

Although several bacteria have been implicated in the onset and progression of chronic periodontal disease, to date, none of the organisms have been identified as causal. Only *Aggregatibacter actinomycetemcomitans* has been causally linked to aggressive periodontitis previously identified as local juvenile periodontitis (LJP).[41] The inability to identify a specific microbiological causal link to chronic periodontitis has led to speculation that, rather than one organism, a consortium of microbiota play a role in the formation of the disease.

The host response to the bacterial colonization of the subgingival niche is a complex reaction of local and systemic defenses. In response to the colonization of the subgingival pocket, an enhanced host response occurs, both humoral and cellular.[42] Host defenses are manifested by changes in cytokines locally in the gingival crevicular fluid and systemically in the serum. Soon after subgingival colonization occurs, an influx of PMNs occurs which is accompanied by an increase in crevicular fluid. Gingival crevicular fluid is a serous exudate or transudate that collects in the gingival sulcus. The interchange of fluid between the vasculature in the gingival tissue and the gingival sulcus allows immune cells to be delivered to the site. **Inflammatory mediators** can be produced in the crevicular fluid that is independent of the systemic concentration. This mechanism of action produces a localized response to the bacterial insult.

One theory suggests that the activated host response, including production of cytotoxic proteins, results in the loss of periodontal structures with the manifestation of clinical periodontal disease. When the dental plaque matures, a chronic inflammatory response replaces the initial acute response. An increase in cellular immunity occurs with the infiltration of T cells, PMNs, and monocytes into the gingival sulcus. An increase in collagenase activity results from the induction of cellular immunity and the proliferation of PMNs, macrophages, and fibroblasts (see Figure 2-3).

As the cellular immune response matures, several mediators are released in response to the insult by the microorganisms cultivating the subgingival environment. Primarily released into the gingival crevicular fluid, inflammatory mediators, including TNFα, PG(E$_2$), interleukin (IL)-1α and β, and IL-6, are found in increased levels in response to increased inflammation.[43]

An increase in immunoglobulin levels occurs in response to the antigenic insult. In the oral cavity, the production of secretory immunoglobulin A (sIgA) in saliva provides the initial defense. Either opsinization of the bacteria occurs or the bacteria survive and are able to adhere to the mucosa and colonize in the resident biofilm. Initially, the response is predominantly a secretory response, with IgA as the primary antibody. After the organism invades the tissue, the humoral antibody response shifts to a serous response with IgG as the primary responder antibody. On invasion of the tissue, IgE is released, stimulating mast cells to release vasoconstrictive and chemotactic factors that draw plasma cells and PMNs to the local site. This event activates both the cellular and humoral response at the site of invasion. In response to the insult, plasma cells and lymphocytes produce IgG specific to the invading organism.

As the disease progresses, the host systemic response to the oral microorganisms can be identified in the systemic circulation.[44] Chronic gingival inflammation stimulates an acute-phase response with production of C-reactive protein (CRP), complement and fibrinogen by local cells, which further exacerbate the inflammatory response.[45] This process may contribute to the oral-systemic linkages that were reported in the literature. Clinically, chronic periodontal disease is defined by an inflammatory response resulting in a loss of bone and collagen.

ORAL-SYSTEMIC LINKAGES

Considerable interest in the possible association between periodontal disease and multiple systemic diseases has arisen in the scientific literature. A detailed description of these relationships is presented in Chapters 5 and 18. The strongest evidence for an association with periodontal disease is between diabetes (both type 1 and type 2).[46] Diabetes and the relationship to periodontal disease are well documented in the literature. The association appears to be bidirectional, that is, the severity of the diabetes is related to the severity of periodontal disease and the severity of the periodontal condition affects the ability to maintain adequate glycemic control.[47,48] The mechanism for this association, although unclear, appears to be related to both the bacterial infection and the host response to the insult.[49]

Periodontal disease has been linked with other systemic diseases. In cross-sectional and retrospective case-control studies, linkages have been suggested among periodontal disease and cardiovascular disease, osteoporosis, and negative birthing outcomes (preterm birth/low birth weight), among others.[50,51,52] Evidence to suggest a clear association is premature, and although it is plausible, insufficient evidence exists to confirm the associations or to identify a causal mechanism of action.

Although the mechanism of these relationships is largely unknown, theories have emerged to describe the systemic response to this oral infection. Although periodontal disease was long thought to be a localized or focal infection, this chronic insult is now thought to have systemic ramifications that impact general health outcomes. Because of the vascular nature of the gingival tissue and the chronic nature of periodontitis, the potential for translocation of the oral pathogens and their end products (i.e., **lipopolysaccharide [LPS]**, endotoxin) into the systemic circulation exists, resulting in a chronic subclinical sepsis. It has been suggested that the ulcerated epithelial surfaces within periodontal pockets (for untreated, moderate-to-advanced periodontitis) could range from 50 to 200 cm^2, although more conservative figures place it at only 8 to 20 cm^2 (x1, x2). Although the larger estimate is equivalent to ulcerated skin covering a forearm, even the smaller estimate is a considerable chronic infection insult to the host.[53,54]

The release of endotoxin or LPS may promote the release of biochemical mediators, which are associated with inflammation.[55] The hypothesis of these oral-systemic linkages is that a low-level chronic bacteremia results from the periodontal infection and contributes to the release of macromolecules, including LPS and endotoxin, that leads to an upregulation of cellular mediators, which contributes to the exacerbation of the systemic condition. Although the exact mechanism of these oral-systemic associations is unknown, this area of ongoing investigation will lead to an explanation of the causal pathway for these associations.

CONCLUSION

Understanding the epidemiology of periodontal disease will greatly enhance our ability to assess risk and to apply prevention. Population-based measures for gingivitis and periodontitis are not uniform or standardized, which hinders comparison across population groups. To adopt a standard of measure of periodontal health at the population level is critical to have a greater understanding of changes in this disease nationally. The prevalence of destructive periodontal disease has remained fairly stable over time, but as the population in the United States shifts to a more mature population, an increase in the number of cases is certainly anticipated. Ramifications of this increase will challenge oral health care providers, and with the suggested associations between oral and systemic disease, may have greater implications in overall health. Continued research into periodontal disease pathogenesis is instrumental in solidifying the oral-systemic connection. A greater knowledge in this area will assist with the creation of community-based prevention strategies that can reduce the prevalence and impact of these diseases.

REFERENCES

1. Armitage GC: Development of a classification system for periodontal diseases and conditions, *Ann Periodontol* 4:1-6, 1999.
2. Ciancio SG: Current status of indices of gingivitis, *J Clin Periodontol* 13:5375-5382, 1986.
3. Flemmig TF: Periodontitis, *Ann Periodontol* 4:412-438, 1999.
4. Silness J, Loe H: Periodontal diseases in pregnancy. II. Correlation between oral hygiene and periodontal condition, *Acta Odontol Scand* 22:121-135, 1964.
5. Steffensen B, Sottosanti JS: Prevention and treatment of plaque associated gingivitis. In Wilson TG, Kornman KS, editors: *Fundamentals of periodontics*, Chicago, 1996, Quintessence Publishing.
6. Page RC: Gingivitis, *J Clin Periodontol* 13:345-359, 1986.
7. Oliver RC, Brown LJ, Loe H: Periodontal diseases in the United States population, *J Periodontol* 69:269-276, 1998.
8. Albander JM: Periodontal diseases in North America, *Periodontol 2000* 29:31-69, 2002.
9. Loesche WJ, Syed SA: Bacteriology of human experimental gingivitis: effect of plaque gingivitis score, *Infect Immun* 21:3830-3839, 1978.
10. Syed SA, Loesche WJ: Bacteriology of human experimental gingivitis: effect of plaque age, *Infect Immun* 21:821-829, 1978.
11. Moore WEC, Moore LH, Ranney RR et al.: The microflora of periodontal sites showing active destructive progression, *J Clin Periodontol* 18:729-739, 1991.
12. Listgarten MA: Pathogenesis of periodontitis, *J Clin Periodontol* 13:418-425, 1986.
13. Socransky SS, Haffajee AD, Goodson JM et al.: New concepts of destructive periodontal disease, *J Clin Periodontol* 11:121-132, 1984.
14. Suzuki JB: Diagnosis and classification of periodontal diseases, *Dent Clin North Am* 32:2195-2216, 1988.

15. Kinane DF, Lappin DF: Clinical, pathological, and immunological aspects of periodontal disease, *Acta Odontol Scand* 59:3154-3160, 2001.

16. Holt SC, Ebersole JL: *Porphyromonas gingivalis, Treponema denticola, and Tannerella forsythia*: the 'red complex', a prototype polybacterial pathogenic consortium in periodontitis, *Periodontol 2000* 38:72-122, 2005.

17. Socransky SS, Haffajee AD: Microbial mechanisms in the pathogenesis of destructive periodontal diseases: a critical assessment, *J Periodontal Res* 26:195-202, 1991.

18. Ximenez-Fyvie LA, Haffajee AD, Socransky SS: Comparison of microbiota of supra- and subgingival plaque in health and periodontitis, *J Clin Periodontol* 27:648-657, 2000.

19. Page RC, Schroeder HE: Current status of the host response in chronic marginal periodontitis, *J Periodontol* 52:477-491, 1981.

20. Loe H, Anerud A, Boysen H et al.: Natural history of periodontal disease in man. The rate of periodontal destruction before age 40, *J Periodontol* 49:607-620, 1978.

21. Loe H, Anerud A, Boysen H et al.: Natural history of periodontal disease in man. Study design and baseline data, *J Periodontal Res* 13:550-562, 1978.

22. Brown LJ, Oliver RC, Loe H: Evaluating the status of US employed adults, *JAMA* 121:226-232, 1990.

23. Albander JM, Brunelle JA, Kingman A: Destructive periodontal disease in adults 30 years of age and older in the U.S. 1988-1994, *J Periodontol* 70:1-13, 1999.

24. Kingman A, Albandar JM: Methodological aspects of epidemiological studies of periodontal diseases, *Periodontol 2000* 29:11-30, 2002.

25. Caton J, Polson AM: The interdental bleeding index: a simplified procedure for monitoring gingival health, *Compend Contin Educ Dent* 6:88-92, 1985.

26. Lobene RR, Mankodi SS, Ciancio SG et al.: Correlation among gingival indices: a methodology study, *J Periodontol* 60:159-162, 1989.

27. Loe H: The gingival index, the plaque index, and the retention index systems, *J Periodontol* 38(suppl):610-616, 1967.

28. Russell AI: A system of classification and scoring for prevalence surveys of periodontal disease, *J Dent Res* 35:350-359, 1956.

29. Ramjford SP: Indices for prevalence and incidence of periodontal disease, *J Periodontol* 30:51-59, 1959.

30. Ainamo J, Ainamo A: Validity and relevance of the criteria of the CPITN, *Int Dent J* 1994:44(suppl):527-532.

31. U.S. Department of Health and Human Services (DHHS): National Center for Health Statistics. The First Health Examination Survey Datafile 1959-62. Public Use Data file Documentation. Hyattsville, MD, Centers for Disease Control and Prevention (website): http://www.cdc.gov/nchs/products/ elec_prods/subject/nhes1.htm.

32. Borrell LN, Burt BA, Taylor GW: Prevalence and trends in periodontis in the USA: from NHANES III to the NHANES, 1988-2000, *J Dent Res* 84:924-930, 2005.

33. Vargas C, Schober S, Gift H: Operational definitions for year 2000 objectives: priority area 13, oral health. Healthy people 2000 statistical notes, DHHS Publication No. (PHS) 97-1237 7-03987/97, 2005.

34. Dye BA, Selwitz RH: The relationship between selected measures of periodontal status and demographic and behavioral risk factors, *J Clin Periodontol* 32: 798-808, 2004.

35. U.S. Department of Health and Human Services: *Healthy People 2010, ed 2, with understanding and improving health and objectives for improving health,* 2 vols, Washington, DC, U.S. Government Printing Office, November, 2000.

36. National Center for Health Statistics: Third national health and nutrition examination survey, 1988-1994, Department of Health and Human Services (DHHS), Centers for Disease Control and Prevention (website): http://www.cdc.gov/nchs/about/major/nhanes/nh3data.htm. Accessed May 18, 2007.

37. National Center for Health Statistics: National health and nutrition examination survey, 1999-2004, Department of Health and Human Services (DHHS), Centers for Disease Control and Prevention (website):http://www.cdc.gov/nchs/about/major/nhanes/nhanes99-00. htm, http://www.cdc.gov/nchs/about/major/nhanes/nhanes01-02.htm, http://www.cdc.gov/nchs/about/major/nhanes/nhanes2003-3004/ nhanes03_04.htm. Accessed May 18, 2007.

38. Marcus SE, Drury TE, Brown LJ et al.: Tooth retention and tooth loss in the permanent dentition of adults: United States, 1988-1994, *J Dent Res* 75:684-695, 1996.

39. Albander JM, Brown LJ, Loe H: Clinical features of early onset periodontitis, *JADA* 128:1393-1399, 1997.

40. Anstrom AN, Rise J: Socioeconomic differences in patterns of health and oral health behavior in 25 year-old Norwegians, *Clin Oral Investig* 5:122-128, 2001.

41. Zambon JJ: Actinobacillus actinomycetemcomitans in human periodontal disease, *J Clin Periodontol* 12:1-20, 1985.

42. Page RC: The role of inflammatory mediators in the pathogenesis of periodontal disease, *J Periodontal Res* 26:230-242, 1991.

43. Ebersole JL, Cappelli D: Acute phase reactants in infectious and inflammatory diseases, *Periodontol 2000,* 23:19-49, 2000.

44. Ebersole JL, Cappelli D, Mathys EC et al.: Periodontitis in humans and nonhuman primates: Oral-systemic linkage inducing acute phase proteins, *Ann Periodontol* 7:102-111, 2002.

45. Ebersole JL, Machen RL, Steffen MJ et al.: Systemic acute phase reactants, C reactive protein and haptoglobin in adult periodontitis, *Clin Exp Immunol* 107:347-352, 1997.

46. Soskolne WA, Klinger A: The relationship between periodontal diseases and diabetes: an overview, *Ann Periodontol* 6:91-98, 2001.

47. Stewart JE, Wager KA, Friedlander AH et al.: The effect of periodontal treatment on glycemic control in patients with type 2 diabetes mellitus, *J Clin Periodontol* 28:306-310, 2001.

48. Grossi SG, Skrepcinski FB, DeCaro T et al.: Response to periodontal therapy in diabetics and smokers, *J Periodontol* 67: 1094-1102, 1996.

49. Lalla E, Lamster IB, Stern DM et al.: Receptor for advanced glycation end products, inflammation, and accelerated periodontal disease in diabetes: mechanisms and insights into therapeutic modalities, *Ann Periodontol* 6:113-118, 2001.

50. Offenbacher S, Katz V, Fertik G et al.: Periodontal disease as a possible risk factor for preterm low birth weight, *J Periodontol* 67:1103-1113, 1996.

51. Beck J, Garcia R, Heiss G et al.: Periodontal disease and cardiovascular disease, *J Periodontol* 67:1123-1137, 1996.

52. Offenbacher S: Periodontal diseases: pathogenesis, *Ann Periodontol* 1:821-878, 1996.

53. Hujoel PP, White BA, Garcia RI et al.: The dentogingival epithelial surface area revisited, *J Periodontal Res* 36:148-155, 2001.

54. Timothe P, Eke PI, Presson SM et al.: Reported patterns of dental utilization among pregnant women, *J Dent Res* 83(Spec Iss A), 2004.

55. Collins JG, Windley HW, Arnold RR et al.: Effects of *Porphyromonas gingivalis* infection on inflammatory mediator response and pregnancy outcome in hamsters, *Infect Immunity* 62:4356-4361, 1994.

Chapter 3

*E*pidemiology/Biology of Oral Cancer

JAY D. SHULMAN AND CARA BRIGHAM GONZALES

MALIGNANT TRANSFORMATION AND ORAL SQUAMOUS CELL CARCINOMA

Malignant Transformation
Types of Oral Cancers and Sites of Oral Squamous Cell Carcinoma in the Oral Cavity

DYSPLASIA, CLINICAL STAGING, AND PROGNOSIS

Oral Epithelial Dysplasia
Tumor, Node, Metastases Clinical Staging and Prognosis

CLINICAL PRESENTATION

Oral Leukoplakia
Erythroplakia
Oral Lichen Planus

CANCER SURVEILLANCE

Incidence and Mortality
Trends
Race
Strategies for Application in Practice

DETECTION

Clinical Examination
National Oral Health Objectives
Dental Care for OSCC Patients

LEARNING OBJECTIVES

Upon completion of this chapter, the learner will be able to:
- Describe the classification of cancers of the head and neck
- Discuss the pathogenesis of oral cancer
- Outline the concept of cancer staging
- Describe the clinical presentation of premalignant and malignant oral lesions
- Explain cancer surveillance in the United States
- Identify trends in oral cancer prevalence and mortality
- Identify *Healthy People 2010* oral cancer objectives

KEY TERMS

5-year relative survival rate
Age-adjusted mortality rate
Epithelial dysplasia
Erythroplakia
Oral cancer
Oral leukoplakia
Risk factors
Staging
Surveillance

Oral cancer includes cancer of the lips (excluding the skin of the lip), the floor of the mouth, the anterior two thirds of the tongue, the hard and soft palate, the gingiva, and the buccal mucosa. Oropharyngeal cancer adds the base of the tongue, the tonsil, and the posterior pharyngeal wall. The dental literature generally refers to cancers at sites in the top two tiers of Figure 3-1 as "oral," "oropharyngeal," or "oro/oropharyngeal." The focus of this

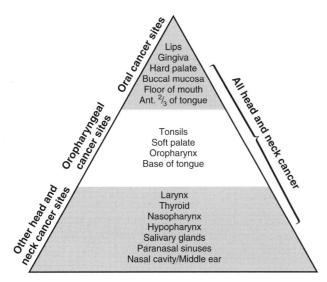

Figure 3-1 Head and neck cancer components. Head and neck cancer includes nonoral or oropharyngeal sites in the head and neck, oropharyngeal cancer sites, and oral cancer sites. Oropharyngeal cancers, which include both oral cancer sites and oropharyngeal cancer sites, account for 33.4% of all head and neck cancers. Oral cancer sites account for 16.4% of all cases of head and neck cancer. (From National Cancer Institute, DCCPS, Surveillance Research Program, Cancer Statistics Branch: Surveillance, Epidemiology, and End Results (SEER) Program SEER*Stat Database: Incidence - SEER 17 Regs Public-Use, Nov 2005 Sub (1973-2003 varying) - Linked To County Attributes - Total U.S., 1969-2003 Counties (website): (www.seer.cancer.gov) (Released April 2006, based on the November 2005 submission.) Accessed May 7, 2007.

chapter is cancers of the head and neck that dental professionals are trained to identify, specifically those shown in the top two tiers of Figure 3-1 with the exception of cancers of the hypopharynx, nasopharynx, and pyriform sinus. For simplicity, this chapter will refer to cancers at these sites as "oral cancers" unless site-specific designations are required.

Population-based research in the area of oral cancer refers to "cancers of the oral cavity and pharynx" frequently without identifying the component sites. In general, they comprise International Classification of Diseases Oncology (ICD-0-3) codes C00.0-C14.8, shown in Table 3-1.[1] Table 3-1 identifies the oral (n = 13,680) and pharyngeal (n = 17,310) sites that are commonly reported. Head and neck cancer (n = 41,419) adds the accessory sinuses, nasal cavity, and middle ear, larynx, and thyroid gland. Cancers of the oral cavity and pharynx comprise 42.8% of head and neck cancers. Although most oropharyngeal sites can be viewed or palpated during a standard oral examination, others, such as the nasopharynx, pyriform sinus, and hypopharynx cannot be easily visualized or palpated. Consequently, although cancers of the oral cavity and pharynx "are usually surface malignancies whose signs and symptoms can be recognized early"[2] identifying surface changes in these inaccessible sites, in which 13.9% of cancers in the oral cavity and pharynx occur, is difficult.

Oral cancers are the sixth most common sites for cancer in the world and have a high rate of morbidity and mortality, with more than 300,000 new cases and 200,000 deaths reported annually.[3] In the United States, the mouth and oropharynx is the tenth most common

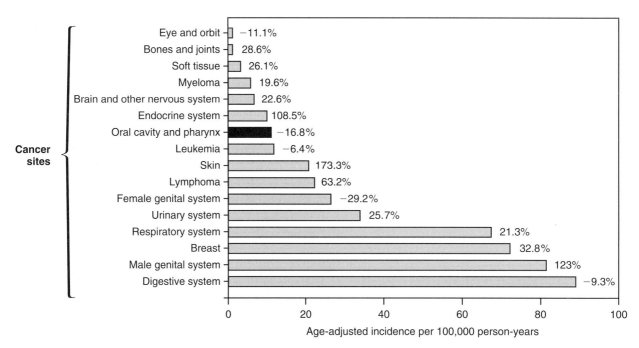

Figure 3-2 Age-adjusted, site-specific year 2002 cancer incidence rates and percent change from 1973. (From the Surveillance Epidemiology and End Results 9, National Cancer Institute, 2003.) (Released April 2006, based on the November 2005 submission.)

TABLE 3-1

ESTIMATED AGE-ADJUSTED HEAD AND NECK CANCER INCIDENCE RATES PER 100,000, BY ANATOMICAL SITE, 2006

ANATOMICAL SITE	ICD-0-3 CODE	Incidence per 100,000	
		COUNT	%
ORAL SITES		13,680	18.9
Hard palate	05.0	536	0.74
Gingiva	03.0-03.9	1139	1.57
Soft palate	05.1-05.9	1173	1.62
Buccal mucosa and other unspecified parts of mouth	06.0-06.9	1932	2.67
Floor of mouth	04.0-04.9	1999	2.76
Lip	00.0-00.9	2435	3.36
Tongue (other)	02.0-02.9	4466	6.17
PHARYNGEAL SITES		17,310	23.9
Hypopharynx	13.0-13.9	815	1.13
Pyriform sinus	12.9	1273	1.76
Oropharynx	10.0-10.9 14.0-14.8	1508	2.08
Nasopharynx	11.0-11.9	2100	2.90
Salivary glands	07.9-08.9	3451	4.77
Tongue (base)	01.9	3909	5.40
Tonsil	09.0-09.9	4254	5.87
OTHER HEAD AND NECK SITES		41,419	57.2
Nasal cavity / middle ear	30.0-30.1	784	1.08
Accessory sinuses	31.0-31.9	945	1.31
Larynx	32.0-32.9	9510	13.13
Thyroid	79.3	30,180	41.68

Estimated new head and neck cancer cases (2006). Head and neck cancer (n = 72,409) includes nonoral or oropharyngeal sites in the head and neck (n = 41,419), oropharyngeal cancer sites (n = 17,310), and oral cancer sites (n = 13,680). Projections for oral cavity and pharynx components made using SEER 2003 incidence rates.
(From National Cancer Institute, DCCPS, Surveillance Research Program, Cancer Statistics Branch: Surveillance, Epidemiology, and End Results (SEER) Program SEER*Stat Database: Incidence-SEER 17 Regs Public-Use, Nov 2005 Sub (1973-2003 varying) - linked to county attributes-Total U.S., 1969-2003 Counties (website): (www.seer.cancer.gov), released April 2006, based on the November 2005 submission.) Accessed May 7, 2007.

site (Figure 3-2), with an estimated 30,000 new cases and 7400 deaths.[3] Oral cancers, with the exception of cancers of the salivary glands, are primarily squamous cell carcinomas (OSCC), the primary cause of which is environmental exposure to carcinogens such as tobacco, alcohol, or chronic sunlight exposure.

Chapter 6 provides a comprehensive discussion of **risk factors** associated with oral cancer. Because of the associated morbidity and mortality, oral cancers are the most serious oral conditions that dentists are in the position to identify and many of these lesions are accessible to visual examination in the dental office. It should be noted that while malignant melanoma is not an 'oral' lesion, dental professionals should include the exposed skin of the head and neck area in any visual examination.

Advances in surgical techniques and chemoradiation therapy have greatly improved the outcome for early stage disease (stage I and II), however, the number of deaths caused by oral cancer has actually increased.

This increase is the result of both the prevalence of distant metastases and the recurrence of primary tumors. Approximately 66% of all new cases are at advanced stages III and IV at initial diagnosis.[3] When local control over the disease improves, a decrease in the number of cases with distant metastases and local recurrences is observed. To date, no medical advances have been effective in eradicating disseminated disease.

Early detection and treatment of stages I and II of the disease results in an improved prognosis for overall survival and increases the number of disease-free intervals. The 5-year overall survival—the proportion of individuals alive 5-years after diagnosis—for stages I and II disease is 82%.[1] If the disease spreads to regional lymph nodes, the 5-year survival rate is reduced to 51%.[3] Early detection and intervention, before advance stages (III and IV), are essential to improve prognosis and overall survival. Development of superior therapies for late stage disease is required to reduce mortality. Because a thorough oral examination is often a patient's first line of defense, it is crucial that dental practitioners understand the etiology, risk factors, modes of detection, and diagnosis of oral cancer, and incorporate this knowledge into their practice as a matter of routine standard of care.

MALIGNANT TRANSFORMATION AND ORAL SQUAMOUS CELL CARCINOMA

Malignant Transformation

Oral cancers, specifically oral squamous cell carcinoma (OSCC), are not linked to an inheritable genetic mutation.[6] Rather, environmental factors, such as chronic exposure to sunlight and repeated exposure to carcinogens (e.g., tobacco and ethanol) are the primary cause of OSCC. When exposed to carcinogens, cells in the oral cavity undergo genetic changes that lead to malignant transformation.

Malignant transformation is a multistep process. With time and repeated exposures, cells accumulate numerous genetic mutations that lead to increased cell proliferation and cellular immortalization (the ability to replicate indefinitely), which develop into invasive carcinomas that are capable of metastatic spread. Some of these genetic changes may be present in premalignant lesions that often appear as a small white patch lesion called oral leukoplakia. (These lesions are described later in the chapter.) When the cells accumulate multiple mutations and move from a premalignant state to a malignant state, changes can be observed, which are detected on biopsy and are diagnostic for cancer. Early lesions will display different grades of epithelial dysplasia, ranging from mild dysplasia to carcinoma *in situ*. A subpopulation of these abnormal cells may accumulate additional genetic mutations that enable them to break through the basement membrane. A lesion that has broken through the basement membrane is classified as carcinoma. Identifying premalignant lesions with the potential of malignant transformation is important to improve OSCC survival rates.

Types of Oral Cancers and Sites of Oral Squamous Cell Carcinoma in the Oral Cavity

Several tissue types exist in the oral cavity and oropharynx that may give rise to oral tumors. Rarer cancers found intraorally are malignant tumors of minor salivary glands, malignant melanoma, rhabdomyosarcoma, fibrosarcoma, leiomyosarcoma, Kaposi's sarcoma, and lymphoma.[8] OSCC makes up 90% of all oral cancers and is the focus of this discussion.

The three most common sites for OSCC, in order of prevalence, are the vermillion border of the lower lip, the floor of the mouth, and the lateral border of the tongue (Figures 3-3 to 3-6). Metastatic spread to regional nodes

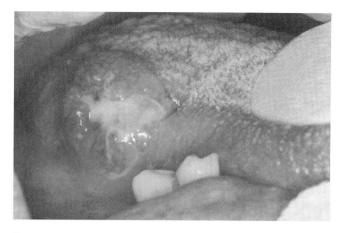

Figure 3-3 Squamous cell carcinoma. Ulcerated lesion of the ventral tongue/floor of mouth. (From Neville BW, Damm DD, Allen CM: *Oral and maxillofacial pathology,* ed 2, Philadelphia, 2002, Saunders.)

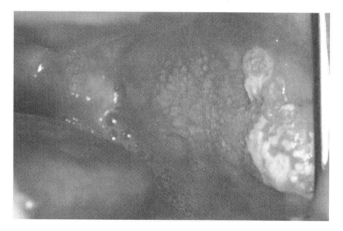

Figure 3-4 Squamous cell carcinoma. Exophytic, papillary mass of the buccal mucosa. (From Neville BW, Damm DD, Allen CM: *Oral and maxillofacial pathology,* ed 2, Philadelphia, 2002, Saunders.)

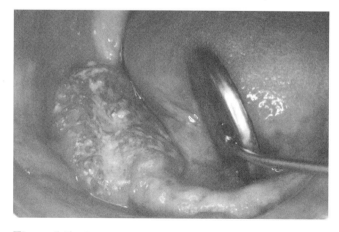

Figure 3-5 Squamous cell carcinoma. Deeply invasive and crater-like ulcer of the anterior floor of mouth and alveolar ridge. The lesion had eroded into the underlying mandible. (From Neville BW, Damm DD, Allen CM: *Oral and maxillofacial pathology,* ed 2, Philadelphia, 2002, Saunders.)

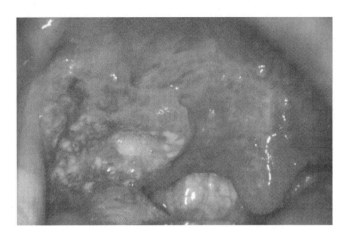

Figure 3-6 Squamous cell carcinoma. Red, granular lesion of the left lateral soft palate and tonsillar region. (From Neville BW, Damm DD, Allen CM: *Oral and maxillofacial pathology,* ed 2, Philadelphia, 2002, Saunders.)

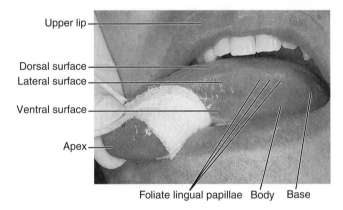

Upper lip

Dorsal surface
Lateral surface

Ventral surface

Apex

Foliate lingual papillae Body Base

Figure 3-7 Examination of the oral cavity. The tip of the tongue should be grasped with a piece of gauze and pulled out to each side. (From Fehrenbach MJ, Herring SW: *Illustrated anatomy of the head and neck,* ed 3, Philadelphia, 2007, Saunders.

is rarely detected in OSCC of the lip. In contrast, 50% of floor of the mouth tumors and 60% of tumors on the lateral border of the tongue will metastasize to regional lymph nodes. Therefore, examination of these sites should be performed routinely to identify and treat these lesions before invasive OSCC and metastatic spread (Figure 3-7).

DYSPLASIA, CLINICAL STAGING, AND PROGNOSIS
Oral Epithelial Dysplasia

Oral epithelial dysplasia is the earliest form of precancerous lesion. This term is applied to early cellular changes, also called atypia, that are associated with an increased risk of malignant potential.[12,13] The presence of epithelial dysplasia is the manifestation of the continuum

of clinical change that occurs as oral cancer develops and progresses with time.

Epithelial dysplasia is graded as mild, moderate, severe, and carcinoma *in situ*. Distinctions between mild, moderate, and severe are made on the basis of a histological examination. Knowledge of the degree of dysplasia assists with diagnostic decision-making and helps to predict whether the lesion will progress to cancer or will resolve on its own after removal of the irritant. Carcinoma *in situ* is the highest grade of dysplasia and consists of abnormal cells that have not invaded adjacent tissue. The risk of progressing to cancer is high but treatment at, or before, this stage is considerably more successful. A diagnosis of malignancy occurs when abnormal cells have invaded the underlying tissues and are identified on histological examination. Cells may vary in their appearance, but the less differentiated the cell, the higher the malignant potential.

Oral epithelial dysplasia does not follow a predictable sequential progression from mild to moderate to severe. It is not uncommon for a mild dysplasia to rapidly progress to an invasive carcinoma; however, not all epithelial dysplasias will develop into carcinoma. Carcinomas may arise from lesions in which epithelial dysplasia has not been diagnosed. Because of this unpredictable progression, biopsy of suspect lesions is essential to managing precancerous and cancerous lesions.

Tumor, Node, Metastases Clinical Staging and Prognosis

Establishing a prognosis for patients diagnosed with OSCC is based on clinical staging at the time of initial diagnosis. **Staging** provides a clinical estimate of how advanced the disease is and whether or not it has spread from the original site to regional lymph nodes, other parts of the body, or both. Tumor, node, metastases (TNM) is the traditional method of staging OSCC. TNM clinical staging is based on the **t**umor size, lymph **n**ode involvement, and distant **m**etastases, hence the name TNM staging.[14] Stages I and II are early stages in which the primary tumor is localized, small in size, and has not spread to regional lymph nodes or distant sites. Stages III and IV are advanced stages in which the tumor is either larger in size or has spread to distant sites of the body or lymph nodes. Patients diagnosed with a clinical TNM stage I disease have an 82% survival rate at 5 years, compared with stage III, which has a 51% survival rate at 5 years.[3]

The clinical TNM staging system is used to establish prognosis in oral cancer patients. The primary prognostic factor is metastases to regional lymph nodes. Both the presence and the number of lymph nodes with metastases predict the risk of distant metastases and the increased risk of local recurrences. Oral cancer patients with no lymph node metastases have a 75% 5-year survival rate compared with 49% for patients with at least one involved lymph node.[19] The prognosis for the patient worsens as the number of involved lymph nodes increases.[8,19]

CLINICAL PRESENTATION

Oral Leukoplakia

Oral leukoplakia is a clinical term used to describe a white patch lesion of unknown etiology that cannot be removed by rubbing. The diagnosis of oral leukoplakia is made when all other potential causes for a white patch lesion have been eliminated. The World Health Organization defines oral leukoplakia as "a predominantly white lesion of the oral mucosa that cannot be characterized as any other definable lesion."[12,13]

There is an association between tobacco use and the presence of leukoplakia. A large number of patients diagnosed with leukoplakia also have a history of using smoking or smokeless tobacco. Cessation of tobacco use results in the resolution of leukoplakias in many of these cases. Interestingly, tobacco-associated leukoplakias seem to have less malignant potential than leukoplakias found in patients that do not use tobacco. Silverman et al. (1984) analyzed malignant transformation in 257 patients with oral leukoplakia and determined that 12% of smokers (n = 183) developed carcinoma and 32% of nonsmokers (n = 74) developed carcinoma.[27]

Early identification of white patch lesions, characterizing the lesion as homogenous or non-homogenous, and having detailed knowledge of the patient's history of tobacco use is essential when treating oral leukoplakia. Homogenous lesions (Figure 3-8) are uniformly white. Nonhomogenous lesions have areas of redness interspersed within the white lesion, producing a lesion with a less uniform appearance (Figure 3-9). The presence of oral leukoplakia in a non-smoker should trigger clinicians to suspect that the lesion has a high malignant potential and to perform a biopsy for a definitive diagnosis. If the patient uses tobacco, these lesions can be followed over time. In the absence of tobacco use, the dental practitioner can determine if the lesion will resolve once the irritant is removed. It is impossible to visually determine which oral leukoplakia will transform into carcinoma. The only definitive way to differentiate a benign white patch lesion from a premalignant or malignant lesion is through biopsy.

Erythroplakia

Erythroplakia is a clinical term that describes a red lesion that cannot be defined clinically or pathologically as any other condition. Erythroplakias occur more frequently in older men and are found on the lateral border of the tongue, the floor of the mouth, the retromolar pad, and on the soft palate (Figure 3-10). Clinically, they appear as red macules or plaques with a soft, velvety texture that tend to bleed easily when rubbed.[14] These lesions are often painless, although some patients complain of soreness or burning sensations.

Erythroplakia is rare compared to oral leukoplakia. Histological examination of erythroplakia invariably

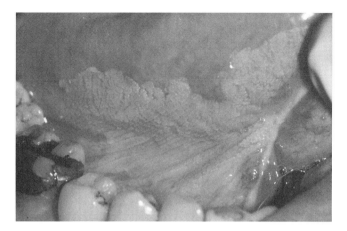

Figure 3-8   Leukoplakia. Area of leukoplakia on floor of the mouth and ventral aspect of the tongue. (From Neville BW, Damm DD, Allen CM: *Oral and maxillofacial pathology*, ed 2, Philadelphia, 2002, Saunders.)

Figure 3-9   Nonhomogenous leukoplakia. This mixed white and red lesion of the buccal mucosa showed moderate epithelial dysplasia. (From Neville BW, Damm DD, Allen CM: *Oral and maxillofacial pathology*, ed 2, Philadelphia, 2002, Saunders.)

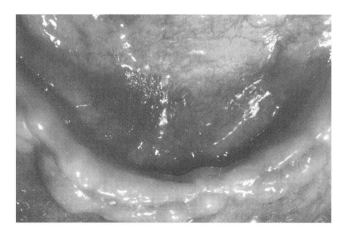

Figure 3-10   Erythoplakia. This small, subtle, red lesion on the right lateral border of the tongue shows carcinoma *in situ* on biopsy. (From Neville BW, Damm DD, Allen CM: *Oral and maxillofacial pathology*, ed 2, Philadelphia, 2002, Saunders.)

reveals epithelial dysplasia, carcinoma *in situ*, and even invasive OSCC, however.[8,13,14] These lesions should be biopsied at the earliest detection followed by definitive treatment. In nonhomogenous leukoplakias, the red component of the lesion is more likely to have dysplastic changes. Therefore, the red area of mixed lesions should always be included in the biopsy.

Oral Lichen Planus

Malignant transformation of lesions in patients with oral lichen planus (OLP), measured over a period of 6 months to more than 20 years, ranged from 0.4% to 3.3%, depending on the study.[28-30] The prevalence of oral cancer in these patients was greater than would be expected in the general population. Thus, an increased risk of associated malignancy appears to exist in patients with OLP. This risk appears to be greatest in the erosive form of OLP and in erythematous areas.

CANCER SURVEILLANCE

Surveillance is an essential public health activity[31] that includes identifying and monitoring short and long-term disease trends, and determining disease-related morbidity and mortality. Population-based cancer registries are the foundation for cancer surveillance, providing data about patterns and trends that enable individuals with cancer to be followed over time.[32] The preeminent source of cancer statistics in the United States is Surveillance,

Epidemiology, and End Results (SEER), a public domain database maintained by The National Cancer Institute. Since 1973, it has been the repository for data from population-based cancer registries. SEER 9 (1973 to present), SEER 13 (1992 to present), and SEER 17 (2000 to present), cover 9.5%, 13.8%, and 26.2% of the U.S. population, respectively.[33] Although the SEER cancer registries are not a random sample of the U.S. population,[34] they were chosen to be representative of the diversity of the U.S. population and are regarded as the gold standard for cancer surveillance. Among the data collected are patient demographics (place of birth, age at diagnosis, and gender), social characteristics (race, ethnicity, and geography), tumor characteristics (site, history, behavior, and staging), treatment, and follow-up.[32]

Incidence and Mortality

Oral cancer comprises 2.2% of all cancers reported in the United States,[3] and the incidence has decreased since 1973.[4] Compared with other cancers, the 5-year survival rate (59.4%) is low and has decreased only 7.8 percentage points since 1973 (Table 3-2). Worldwide, cancers of the oral cavity and pharynx were responsible for an estimated 2.1% of all cancer deaths; 3.0% of all new cancers in males, and 1.6% of deaths and 2.0% of cancers in 2002.[5]

An estimated 7430 individuals died in the United States in 2006 from cancers of the oral cavity and pharynx,[3] comprising 58.6% of all deaths from cancers of the head and neck (Table 3-3). Deaths attributed to cancer of

TABLE 3-2

COMPARISON OF TOTAL AND SITE-SPECIFIC SURVIVAL RATES FOR CANCERS OF THE ORAL CAVITY AND PHARYNX, DIAGNOSED IN 1973 AND 2003 (SOURCE, SEER 1973-2003)

	5-Year Relative Survival Rate								
	All			*White*			*Black*		
SITE	1973	2003	% CHANGE	1973	2003	% CHANGE	1973	2003	% CHANGE
All sites	51.6	59.4	13.1	52.7	62.5	18.6	36.1	36.2	0.3
Lip	96.6	92.4	−4.3	96.5	92.5	−4.1	100.0	100.0	0.0
Tongue	30.0	58.8	96.0	29.4	62.2	111.6	14.1	37.7	167.4
Salivary glands	71.3	72.7	2.0	70.7	70.0	−1.0	68.7	79.3	15.4
Floor of mouth	48.6	51.0	4.7	50.5	54.3	7.5	36.9	31.4	−14.9
Gingiva	50.7	56.1	10.7	49.5	58.8	18.8	38.5	29.7	−22.9
Tonsil	29.0	57.4	97.9	28.7	60.4	110.5	29.3	38.7	32.1
Oropharynx	18.0	36.6	103.3	19.8	42.6	115.2	*	*	*
Hypopharynx	15.7	36.1	129.9	16.4	37.7	129.9	16.1	25.1	55.9
Nasopharynx	37.8	40.5	6.7	40.3	43.5	7.4	36.0	35.6	0.0
Other oral cavity and pharynx	23.1	39.9	72.7	51.0	43.9	−13.9	*	18.3	*

*Insufficient data to compute.

TABLE 3-3

ESTIMATED AGE-ADJUSTED HEAD AND NECK CANCER MORTALITY RATES PER 100,000, BY ANATOMICAL SITE, 2006

ANATOMICAL SITE	ICD-0-3 CODE	Mortality	
		COUNT	%
ORAL SITES		**3124**	**24.66**
Lip	00.0-00.9	69	0.54
Floor of mouth	04.0-04.9	140	1.10
Gingiva and other mouth (includes soft and hard palate and buccal mucosa)	03.0-03.9 05.1-05.9	1124	
	06.0-06.9		8.87
Tongue	01.9-02.9	1791	14.14
PHARYNGEAL SITES		**4306**	**33.99**
Hypopharynx (includes pyriform sinus)	12.9 13.0-13.9	304	2.40
Nasopharynx	11.0-11.9	571	4.51
Tonsil	09.0-09.9	581	4.59
Oropharynx	10.0-10.9	598	4.72
Salivary glands	07.9-08.9	655	5.17
Other oral cavity and pharynx	14.0-14.8	1507	11.89
OTHER HEAD AND NECK SITES		**5240**	**41.36**
Nasal cavity/middle ear/sinuses	30.0-30.1 31.0-31.9	1082	8.54
Thyroid	79.3	1500	11.84
Larynx	32.0-32.9	3740	29.52

Estimated New Head and Neck Cancer Deaths (2006). Head and neck cancer (12,670 includes nonoral or oropharyngeal sites in the head and neck (n = 5240), oropharyngeal cancer sites (n = 4306), and oral cancer sites (n = 3124). Oropharyngeal cancers, which include both oral cancer sites and oropharyngeal cancer sites, account for 58.65% of all head and neck cancer deaths. Oral cancer sites account for 24.66% of all head and neck cancer deaths.

(From National Cancer Institute, DCCPS, Surveillance Research Program, Cancer Statistics Branch: Surveillance, Epidemiology, and End Results (SEER) Program SEER*Stat Database: Mortality-All COD, Public-Use With State, Total U.S. (1969-2003) (website): www.seer.cancer.gov, released April 2006. Underlying mortality data provided by National Center for Health Statistics (www.cdc.gov/nchs). Accessed May 7, 2007. Projections for oral cavity and pharynx components made using SEER 2003 incidence rates.

the nasopharynx, pyriform sinus, and hypopharynx comprised 11.8% of deaths associated with cancer of the oral cavity and pharynx. A comparison of site-specific incidence and mortality data show that although the cancers of the lip comprised 3.4% of head and neck cancers and 7.9% of cancers of the oral cavity and pharynx, they comprised 0.5% and 0.9%, of deaths, respectively. On the other hand, after cancer of the larynx, which accounted for 29.5% of head and neck cancer deaths, cancer of the other oral cavity and pharynx (11.9%) and cancer of the tongue (14.1%) had the highest **mortality rates**.[36]

In the United States, more than half the cancers of the oral cavity and pharynx occur at three sites: the tongue, tonsil, and salivary glands (see Table 3-1). Although the incidence of these cancers increased substantially between 1973 and 2003, the incidence of cancers of the lip, floor of the mouth, and gingiva has shown a marked decline (Table 3-4). Five-year relative survival varies among sites ranging from 36.1 percent for the hypopharynx to 92.4% for the lip (see Table 3-2).

The aggregate incidence of oral cancer varies substantially by gender and is 2.5 times higher in males than females[45] and this disparity is observed worldwide (Figure 3-11). Male-female site-specific incidence ratios vary and are particularly high for cancers of the base of the tongue (3.8:1), tonsil (3.4:1), lip (3.3:1), and floor of the mouth (2.3:1) (Figure 3-12). The hard palate is the only site where gender parity exists. The disparity between males and females has become less pronounced during the past 50 years because of the increase in the proportion of women who use tobacco products, drink alcohol, or both.[14]

TABLE 3-4

COMPARISON OF AGE-ADJUSTED TOTAL AND SITE-SPECIFIC ORAL CANCER INCIDENCE BY RACE BETWEEN 1973 AND 2003 (SOURCE, SEER 1973-2003)

| | Age-adjusted incidence per 100,000 person-years | | | | | | | | |
| | All | | | White | | | Black | | |
ANATOMICAL SITE	1973	2003	% CHANGE	1973	2003	% CHANGE	1973	2003	% CHANGE
All sites	13.5	11.2	−17.1*	13.4	11.1	−16.6*	12.7	12.1	−3.8*
Lip	2.9	0.8	−70.1*	3.1	1.0	−69.0*	0.4	0.1	−60.2
Base of tongue	0.8	1.4	62.4*	0.8	1.5	76.1	1.1	1.5	28.9
Tongue (other)	1.5	1.5	−2.3	1.5	1.5	3.5	1.0	1.0	−1.8*
Hard palate	0.2	0.2	12.4	0.2	0.2	1.1	0.1	0.3	224.1
Soft palate	0.8	0.6	−25.1*	0.8	0.6	−20.8*	1.4	0.9	−38.5*
Buccal mucosa and other unspecified parts of mouth	0.8	0.7	−18.8*	0.8	0.7	−20.8*	0.9	1.0	7.6
Floor of mouth	1.3	0.8	−49.4*	1.3	0.8	−46.9*	0.7	0.3	−42.3*
Gingiva	0.6	1.7	−0.5*	0.6	1.7	−0.2*	0.7	0.3	−60.7
Salivary glands	1.0	1.5	40.9*	1.0	1.5	50.8*	1.9	1.5	−23.8*
Tonsil	1.4	1.6	19.0*	1.3	1.7	27.0*	1.9	1.8	−4.9*
Oropharynx	0.5	0.5	−1.2	0.5	0.5	−6.3	0.4	1.0	139.8
Hypopharynx	0.3	0.3	−16.9*	0.3	0.3	−24.5*	0.3	0.6	129.6*
Nasopharynx	0.8	0.8	1.8	0.6	0.5	−24.7*	0.4	0.9	139.4
Pyriform sinus	0.6	0.4	−28.1*	0.6	0.4	−37.2*	0.4	0.8	115.0*

*Annual percent change significantly different from zero (*p* <0.05).

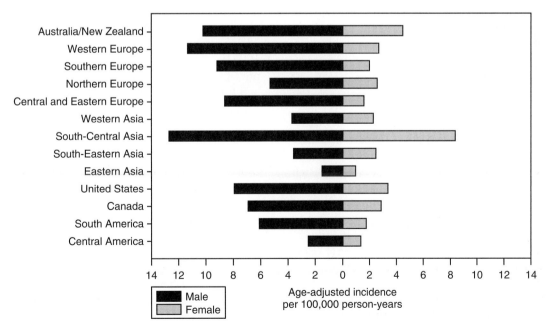

Figure 3-11 Age-adjusted oral cancer incidence by region and country, 1997 to 1999. Ferlay J, Bray F, Pisani P et al.: GLOBOCAN 2002: *Cancer incidence, mortality and prevalence worldwide IARC CancerBase, No. 5, version 2.0*, Lyon, France, 2004, IARC Press.

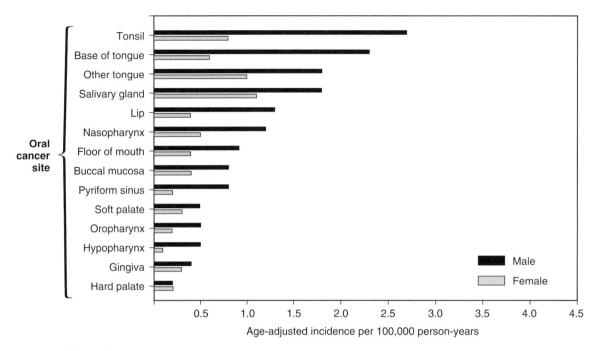

Figure 3-12   Age-adjusted, incidence site-specific, oral cancer incidence, 1998 to 2003, by gender. (From the Surveillance Epidemiology and End Results 9, National Cancer Institute, 2003. Released April 2006, based on the November 2005 submission.)

Five-year relative survival for oral cancer is low (59.4%) compared with other cancers, but survival rates have shown a modest (7.1%) improvement from 1973 to 2003 (Figure 3-13).[36] Aggregate survival rates mask substantial site-specific variations. Cancer of the lip has a 5-year survival rate greater than 90%, and cancers of the hypopharynx, oropharynx, and other oral cavity and pharynx have survival rates less than 40% (see Table 3-2).

Trends

Although apparent increases or decreases in cancer incidence with time may reflect changes in diagnostic methods or case reporting rather than true changes in cancer occurrence,[35] it is nonetheless useful to examine trends. Oral cancer incidence rates rose in the mid-1970s through the mid-1980s and declined from the mid-1980s to the present.[37] As with most forms of cancer, the incidence of oral cancer increases markedly with age (Figure 3-14). In 2003, 19.2% of oral cancers were diagnosed in individuals younger than 50 years of age, and 66.9% were diagnosed before age 70 years.[45] Males have more than three times the lifetime probability of developing oral cancer than females.[51] Cancer of the vermillion border of the lip is associated with chronic sunlight exposure and occurs primarily in white men who work in outdoor occupations, such as farmers.

Overall, oral cancer incidence has decreased from 1973 to 2003 (see Table 3-4), however, that belies the heterogeneity of the site-specific incidence trends. Although the incidence of cancers of the vermilion border of the lip,

floor of the mouth, and gingiva decreased substantially, cancers of the tongue, salivary glands, and tonsil increased. Consequently, reports of incidence or survival trends for oral cancer in the aggregate are misleading because they mask site-specific trends and combine the majority of sites that are predominantly OSCC with sites (i.e., salivary glands) that have different risk factors. Similarly, the 13.1% improvement between cases diagnosed in 1973 and 1998 is overshadowed by twofold increases in survival rates for cancers of the hypopharynx, oropharynx, tonsil, and tongue (see Table 3-2).

The proportion of individuals diagnosed at a late (distant) stage has declined from 15.0% in 1973 to 7.3% in 2003. Only 38.4% of oral cancers were diagnosed at an early (localized) stage in 2003 (Table 3-6), which corresponds to a 16% improvement since 1973. The 5-year survival rate for individuals diagnosed with oral cancers in 1998 was 79.7% if the cancer was localized, 46.1% if it was regional, and 21.6% if it was distant (see Table 3-6).

Race

The annual incidence of cancers of the oral cavity and pharynx is higher among blacks than whites (12.1 versus 11.1 per 100,000 population) (see Table 3-4). Blacks have a higher incidence of cancers of the hard palate, soft palate, buccal mucosa, salivary glands, tonsil, oropharynx, hypopharynx, nasopharynx, and pyriform sinus than whites. Although the incidence rate for black Americans is higher, the reduction in incidence from 1993 to 2003 was one fifth that of white Americans (see Table 3-5).

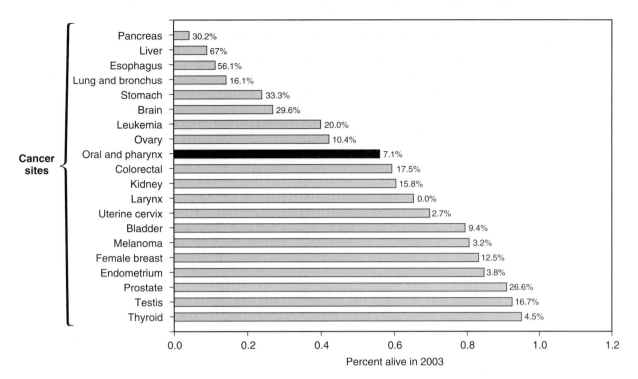

Figure 3-13   Age-adjusted, site-specific, 5-year survival for cancer diagnosed in 1997 and percent change from 1973. (From the Surveillance Epidemiology and End Results 9, National Cancer Institute, 2003. Released April 2006, based on the November 2005 submission.)

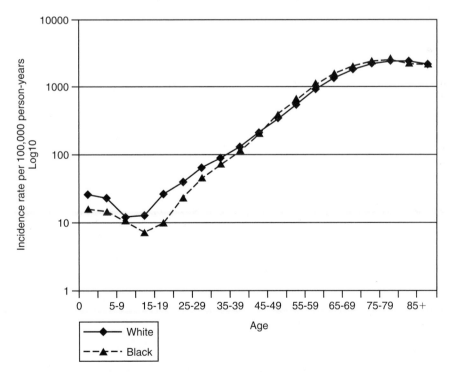

Figure 3-14   Age-adjusted oral cancer incidence per 100,000 person-years by race and age for year 2003 (From National Cancer Institute, DCCPS, Surveillance Research Program, Cancer Statistics Branch: Surveillance, Epidemiology, and End Results (SEER) Program DevCan database: SEER 17 Incidence and Mortality, 2000-2003 (website): (www.seer.cancer.gov), released June 2006, based on the November 2005 submission.) Underlying mortality data provided by NCHS (www.cdc.gov/nchs). Accessed May 7, 2007.

TABLE 3-5

SUMMARY OF GENDER AND RACE DISPARITIES RELATED TO CANCERS OF THE ORAL CAVITY AND PHARYNX (SOURCE, SEER 1973-2003 AND SEER 2000-2003)

MEASURE	Race / Ethnicity		Gender	
	WHITE	BLACK	MALE	FEMALE
Incidence trend, 1993-2003 (%)	−8.5	−1.7	−10.0	−4.5
5-year relative survival, 2003 (%)	58.0	37.5	53.9	60.4
5-year relative survival, 1993 (%)	55.5	30.7	51.3	58.2
Percent diagnosed at localized stage, 1993	41.0	25.7	36.6	42.3
Percent diagnosed at localized stage, 2003	36.9	20.3	31.1	43.2
Percent diagnosed at distant stage, 1993	8.4	15.0	18.5	8.4
Percent diagnosed at distant stage, 2003	10.3	16.2	11.7	8.9
Median age at diagnosis, 1993	65	55	61	67
Median age at diagnosis, 2003	63	57	60	65
Median age at death, 1993	68	56	62	68
Median age at death, 2003	67	60	61	72

Both oral cancer diagnosis and death from oral cancer occur at younger ages for blacks than for whites. Furthermore, black males have the highest probability of developing oral cancer until the eighth decade (Figure 3-15).

A substantial divergence existed in trends by race. Blacks have a substantially higher incidence rates for cancers of the oropharynx, tonsil and floor of the mouth (see Table 3-4). From 1973 to 2003, whites showed a substantial increase in cancers of the tongue, tonsil, and salivary glands and blacks showed a marked increase in cancers of the anterior tongue, oropharynx, nasopharynx, and pyriform sinus (see Table 3-4). During this time, whites showed modest decreases in incidence of cancers of the lip, floor of the mouth, and pyriform sinus, and blacks showed a modest decrease in cancers of the lip, gingiva, floor of the mouth, and soft palate.

In addition to having a higher incidence rate for many oral cancers, black Americans had significantly poorer 5-year survival rates than white Americans (Figure 3-16). This difference remains consistent over time. Blacks are diagnosed with oral cancer at later stages than whites (see Table 3-6). In 1973, 1998, and 2003, the proportion of

TABLE 3-6

COMPARISON OF 5-YEAR RELATIVE SURVIVAL RATES FOR CANCERS OF THE ORAL CAVITY AND PHARYNX DIAGNOSED IN 1973 AND 1998 BY RACE AND DISEASE STAGE (SOURCE, SEER 1973-2003, SEER 2000-2003)

RACE	Site					
	Localized		Regional		Distant	
	% IN STAGE	5-YEAR SURVIVAL	% IN STAGE	5-YEAR SURVIVAL	% IN STAGE	5-YEAR SURVIVAL
DIAGNOSED 1973	45.7	71.1	39.3	39.6	15.0	15.8
White	46.8	76.8	38.6	42.1	14.6	15.3
Black	36.8	57.4	41.5	31.3	21.7	14.8
DIAGNOSED 1998	36.4	79.7	53.8	46.1	9.8	21.6
White	38.9	80.6	51.4	46.5	9.7	21.3
Black	24.5	65.9	60.3	30.6	12.8	15.2
DIAGNOSED 2003	38.4		54.3		7.3	
White	36.9		53.3		10.3	
Black	20.3		63.5		16.2	

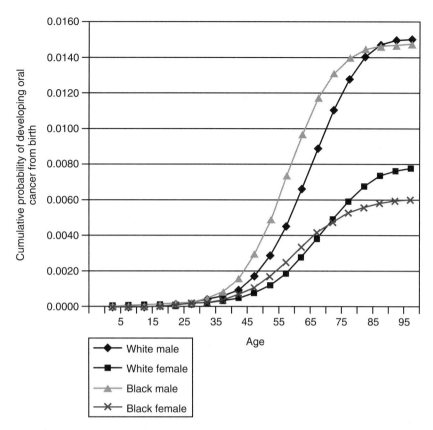

Figure 3-15 Cumulative probability of developing oral cancer by a given age based on 1999 to 2001 incidence data. (From the Surveillance Epidemiology and End Results 9, National Cancer Institute, 2003. Released April 2006, based on the November 2005 submission.)

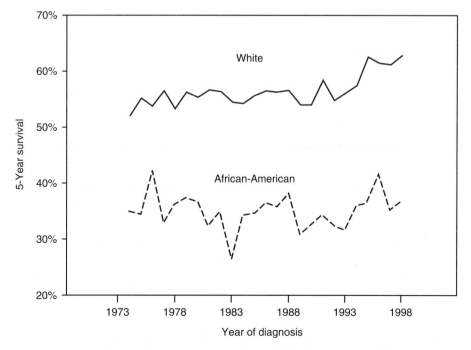

Figure 3-16 Cancers diagnosed in 1973-1998. Five-year oral cancer relative survival rate, by race. (From the Surveillance Epidemiology and End Results 9, National Cancer Institute, 2003. Released April 2006, based on the November 2005 submission.)

blacks diagnosed at an early stage was at least 10 percentage points lower than that of whites.

Marked differences exist for site-specific survival rates. Blacks have not experienced improvement in survival overall, but have seen marked improvements in survival rates for cancers of the hypopharynx, tongue, and tonsil (see Table 3-2). The reasons for these improvements in survival are complex; however, it is likely that increased awareness of oral cancer by dental professionals—especially for cancers of the tongue and tonsil—is a factor. Improvement in these site-specific survival rates is consistent with the increasing proportion of blacks diagnosed at earlier stages (see Table 3-6). Most recently 37.5% of blacks experienced a 5-year survival rate from oral cancer compared with 58.0% of whites (see Table 3-5). Although these findings are promising, the survival rate remains lower for blacks than for whites. During the past 20 years, survival rates for blacks have only improved by 7.8 percentage points (see Table 3-2). Blacks are younger at diagnosis and die from oral cancer at a substantially younger age than whites (see Table 3-5).

Table 3-2 shows trends in 5-year survival rates between 1973 and 2002. Although overall survival rates increased 13.1% from oral cancers diagnosed in 1973 to those diagnosed in 1998, the improvement can be attributed almost exclusively to increased survival rates among whites. Survival rates for black Americans decreased 0.3% compared with 18.6% for whites over the same time period. Black 5-year survival rates are consistently lower than those of whites for all sites except for cancer of the lip (Figure 3-17). Most troubling, incidence rates for cancers of the nasopharynx, hypopharynx, and oropharynx have more than doubled for black Americans from 1973 to 2003 (see Table 3-4). These cancers have the low survival rates (see Table 3-2), and because they are difficult to visualize, these lesions tend to be diagnosed at later stages.

Strategies for Application in Practice

Too often, oral cancer is not diagnosed until the patient is symptomatic. This delay may explain the fact that the majority of these cancers are identified at a late stage.[38] In fact, only 38.4% of oral cancers reported in 2003 were at the local stage; this represents a 16% improvement from 1973 (see Table 3-6). Because survival rates for many oral cancers that are diagnosed in the later stages are low, early diagnosis is important to improving survival rates. For example, the 5-year survival rate for oral cancer

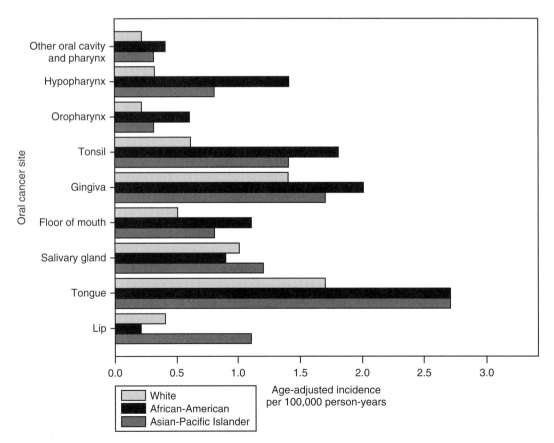

Figure 3-17   Age-adjusted, site-specific, 1998 to 2003 oral cancer incidence by race. (SEER 9 Regs Public-Use, Nov. 2005 Sub 1973-2003, linked to county attributes, total U.S., 1969-2003 Counties, www.seer.cancer.gov, released April 2006, based on the November 2005 submission.) Accessed May 9, 2007.

diagnosed at an early stage (local) in 1997 is 83.7 percent compared with 47.6% for regional and 25.6% for cancers at distant stages.[36] Less than 40% of oral cancers are diagnosed at the earliest stage, however (see Table 3-6).

Centers for Disease Control and Prevention surveys found that although 63.5% of adults reported having a dental examination within the past year (1996 survey),[39] only 16% (1998 survey) recalled receiving an examination "in which the doctor or dentist pulls on your tongue, sometimes with gauze wrapped around it, and feels under the tongue and inside the cheeks."[40] As mentioned previously in this chapter, this type of examination would not identify cancers of the nasopharynx, pyriform sinus, and hypopharynx.

DETECTION

Clinical Examination

Regular, thorough intraoral and extraoral examination by a dental professional is the most effective technique for early detection and prevention of most oral cancers. All patients should be examined annually, and those at higher risk should be given even closer, more frequent scrutiny. The profile of a high-risk patient includes increased age, usually older than 50 years, and any of the risk factors listed previously (for example, tobacco or alcohol use), either singly or in combination. Risk assessment for oral cancer is described in Chapter 6. Suspect lesions in females younger than the age of 50 years, with no history of alcohol or tobacco use, have a greater risk of malignant potential and often behave more aggressively. Lesions in this population of patients must be treated very quickly and aggressively.

It is important to comprehensively examine all areas of the oral cavity and vermilion border, especially the floor of the mouth and the lateral border of the tongue (see Figure 3-7). This examination should be done both visually and using palpation. All suspect lesions should be biopsied and sent for histological analysis. The role of the dentist in many cases is to diagnose oral cancer and coordinate care for surgical resection and adjunctive radiation, chemotherapy, or both.

National Oral Health Objectives

Healthy People is a set of national health objectives designed to identify the most significant preventable threats to health and to establish national goals to reduce these threats. These measurable objectives can be used to provide a framework for establishing prevention programs for the United States. Current *Healthy People* initiatives reflect efforts during the past two decades.[43]

In 1990, the Department of Health and Human Services published *Healthy People 2000*,[41] which describe national health promotion and disease prevention objectives for the year 2000. Two of the oral health objectives

were related to oral cancer. These two objectives are as follows:

1. *Reduce deaths resulting from cancer of the oral cavity and pharynx to no more than 10.5 per 100,000 men aged 45 to 74 years and to 4.1 per 100,000 women aged 45 to 74 years (baseline: 12.1 per 100,000 men and 4.1 per 100,000 women in 1987).*
   The final review of the objective found that male deaths per 100,000 were reduced from 13.6 in 1987 to 10.4 in 1998, and that for females declined from 4.8 to 3.4. The mortality rate for black males, however, (21.0 per 100,000) did not decline appreciably.[42]
2. *Increase to at least 40% the proportion of people aged 50 years and older visiting a primary care provider in the preceding year who have received oral, skin, and digital rectal examinations during one such visit.*

A small increase, from 9% (1992) to 13% (1998).[42]
Healthy People 2010 set out the national health promotion and disease prevention agenda for the first decade of the twenty-first century.[43] The following oral cancer goals were established:

1. *Reduce the annual **age-adjusted** oropharyngeal cancer death rate from 3.0 (1998) to 2.7 per 100,000 population (10% decrease).*
   The 2002 oral cancer death rate for 1998 to 2002 was 2.7% per 100,000 population.[44]
2. *Increase the proportion of oral and pharyngeal cancers (ICD codes, 140-149) detected at the earliest stage from a 35% baseline (SEER 9, 1990-1995).*
   The proportion of oral cancers diagnosed at the earliest stage, 1996 to 2002 was 40.2% (SEER 9).
3. *Increase the proportion of adults aged 40 years and older who report having had an examination to detect oral and pharyngeal cancer in the past 12 months from 13% (1998).*

This goal cannot be evaluated, because the 1998 study has not been repeated.

Dental Care for OSCC Patients

Many patients will be immunocompromised when they receive chemotherapy and will have an increased risk of developing caries and infection after radiation therapy. Dental providers are responsible for removing all sources of oral infection before the start of these treatments. Xerostomia (dry mouth), mucositis, and *Candida* infections are common sequelae of chemotherapy and radiation treatment. Dental professionals must work closely with these patients, and their physicians, in managing these common problems associated with OSCC treatment. Some patients will lose a portion of their mandible or maxilla. It is the dental practitioner that will assist with fabrication of prosthesis to assist in postsurgical eating and speaking. Last, the dental professional plays a crucial role in monitoring patients regularly for local recurrences and additional primary tumors.

REFERENCES

1. Fritz A, Percy C, Jack A et al.: *International classification of disease oncology, ed 3*, Geneva, 2000, World Health Organization.

2. Silverman S: Demographics and occurrences of oral and pharyngeal cancers. The outcomes, the trends, the challenges, *J Am Dent Assoc* 132:(suppl7S-11S), 2001.

3. Jemal A, Siegel R, Ward E et al.: Cancer statistics 2006, *CA Cancer J Clin* 56:106-130, 2006.

4. National Cancer Institute: Surveillance, Epidemiology, and End Results (SEER) Program SEER*Stat Database: Incidence SEER 9 Regs Public-Use, Nov. 2005 Sub 1973-2003, linked to county attributes, total U.S., 1969-2003 Counties, http//:www.seer.cancer.gov, released April 2006, based on the November 2005 submission. Accessed May 9, 2007.

5. Ferlay J, Bray F, Pisani P et al.: GLOBOCAN 2002: *Cancer incidence, mortality and prevalence worldwide IARC CancerBase, No. 5, version 2.0*, Lyon, France, 2004, IARC Press.

6. Lichtenstein P, Holm NV, Verkasalo PK et al.: Environmental and heritable factors in the causation of cancer: analysis of cohorts of twins from Sweden, Denmark, and Finland, *N Engl J Med* 343:78-85, 2000.

7. Sen S: Aneuploidy and cancer, *Curr Opin Oncol* 12:82-88, 2000.

8. Walker DM, Boey G, McDonald LA: The pathology of oral cancer, *Pathology* 35:5376-5383, 2003.

9. Gillison ML, Koch WM, Capone RB et al.: Evidence for a causal association between human papillomavirus and a subset of head and neck cancers, *J Natl Cancer Inst* 92:709-720, 2000.

10. Napier SS, Gormley JS, Newlands C et al.: Adenosquamous carcinoma. A rare neoplasm with an aggressive course, *Oral Surg Oral Med Oral Pathol* 79:607-611, 1995.

11. Ellis GL, Corio RL: Spindle cell carcinoma of the oral cavity: a clinicopathologic assessment of 59 cases, *Oral Surg Oral Med Oral Pathol* 50:523-534, 1980.

12. Reibel J: Prognosis of oral pre-malignant lesions: significance of clinical, histopathological, and molecular biological characteristic, *Crit Rev Oral Bio Med* 14:147-162, 2003.

13. Pindborg JJ, Reichart P, Smith CJ et al.: *World Health Organization: histological typing of cancer and precancer of the oral mucosa*, Berlin, 1997, Springer-Verlag.

14. Neville BW, Day TA: Oral cancer and precancerous lesions, *CA Canc J Clin* 52:195-215, 2002.

15. Bryne M, Koppang HS, Lilleng R et al.: New malignancy grading is a better prognostic indicator than Broders' grading in oral squamous cell carcinomas, *J Oral Pathol Med* 18:432-437, 1989.

16. Bryne M, Boysen M, Alfsen CG et al.: The invasive front of carcinomas. The most important area for tumor prognosis, *Anticancer Res* 18:4757-4764, 1998.

17. Anneroth G, Hansen LS: A methodologic study of histologic classification and grading of malignancy in oral squamous cell carcinoma, *Scand J Dent Res* 92:448-468, 1984.

18. Rapidis AD, Langdon JD, Patel MF et al.: STNMP. A new system for the clinico-pathological classification and identification of intra-oral carcinomata, *Cancer* 39:204-209, 1977.

19. Kalnins IK, Leonard AG, Sako K et al.: Correlation between prognosis and degree of lymph node involvement in carcinoma of the oral cavity, *Am J Surg* 134:450-454, 1977.

20. Suarez P, Batsakis JG, el-Naggar AK: Leukoplakia: still a gallimaufry or is progress being made?-a review, *Adv Anat Pathol* 137-155, 1998.

21. Pindborg JJ, Reichart PA, Smith CJ et al.: *Histological typing of cancer and precancer of the oral mucosa, ed 2*, London, 1997, Springer Verlag.

22. Lumerman H, Freedman P, Kerpel S: Oral epithelial dysplasia and the development of invasive squamous cell carcinoma, *Oral Surg Oral Med Oral Pathol Oral Radiol Endod* 79:321-329, 1995.

23. Sudbo J: Novel management of oral cancer: a paradigm of predictive oncology, *Clin Med Res* 2:233-242, 2004.

24. Pindborg JJ, Renstrup G, Poulsen HE et al.: Studies in oral leukoplakias. V. Clinical and histologic signs of malignancy, *Acta Odontol Scand* 21:407-414, 1963.

25. Axell T, Holmstrup P, Kramer IRH et al.: International seminar on oral leukoplakia and associated lesions related to tobacco habits, *Community Dent Oral Epidemiol* 12:145-154, 1984.

26. Holmstrup P, Vedtofte P, Reibel J et al.: Long-term treatment outcome of oral premalignant lesions, *Oral Oncol* 42:461-474, 2006.

27. Silverman S Jr, Gorsky M, Lozada F: Oral leukoplakia and malignant transformation, *Cancer* 53:563-68, 1984.

28. Silverman S Jr, Gorsky M, Lozada-Nur F et al.: A prospective study of findings and management in 214 patients with oral lichen planus, *Oral Surg Oral Med Oral Pathol* 72:665-670, 1991.

29. Chainani-Wu N, Silverman S Jr, Lozada-Nur F et al.: Oral lichen planus: patient profile, disease progression and treatment responses, *J Am Dent Assoc* 132:901-909, 2001.

30. Barnard NA, Scully C, Everson JAW: Oral cancer development in patients with oral lichen planus, *J Oral Pathol Med* 22:421-424, 1993.

31. Institute of Medicine: *The future of public health*, Washington, DC, 1988, National Academy Press.

32. Wingo PA, Howe HL, Thun MJ et al.: A national framework for cancer surveillance in the United States, *Cancer Causes Control* 6:2151-2170, 2005.

33. National Cancer Institute: Options for Accessing the Public-Use Data and SEER*Stat Software (website): http://seer.cancer.gov/publicdata/options.html. Accessed May 7, 2007.

34. Canto MT, Devesa SS: Oral cavity and pharynx cancer incidence rates in the United States, 1975-1988, *Oral Oncol* 38:610-617, 2002.

35. Lagiou P, Adami H: Burden of cancer. In Adami H, Hunter D, Trichopoulos D, editors: *Textbook of cancer epidemiology*, New York, 2002, Oxford University Press.

36. National Cancer Institute, DCCPS, Surveillance Research Program, Cancer Statistics Branch: Surveillance, Epidemiology, and End Results (SEER) Program SEER*Stat Database: Incidence - SEER 13 Regs Public-Use, Nov 2004 Sub (1973-2002 varying), (website): http//:www.seer.cancer.gov, released April 2005, based on the November 2004 submission. Accessed May 7, 2007.

37. Morse DE, Kerr R: Disparities in oral and pharyngeal cancer incidence, mortality, and survival among black and white Americans, *J Am Dent Assoc* 137:203-212, 2006.

38. Mashberg A, Samit A: Early diagnosis of asymptomatic oral and 3-oropharyngeal squamous cancers, *CA Cancer J Clin* 45:328-351, 1995.

39. Macek MD, Manski RJ, Vargas CM et al.: Comparing oral health care utilization estimates in the United States across three nationally representative surveys, *Health Serv Res* 37:2499-2521, 2002.

40. Neville BW, Day TA: Oral cancer and precancerous lesions, *CA Cancer J Clin* 52:195-215, 2002.

41. U. S. Department of Health and Human Services: *Healthy People 2000*, Washington DC, 1990, Government Printing Office, DHHS publication no (PHS) 91-50212.

42. National Center for Health Statistics: *Healthy People 2000 Final Review*, Hyattsville, MD, 2001, Public Health Service.

43. U.S. Department of Health and Human Services: *Healthy People 2010: Understanding and Improving Health*, ed 2, Washington, DC, 2000, U.S. Government Printing Office.

44. National Cancer Institute, DCCPS, Surveillance Research Program, Cancer Statistics Branch: Surveillance, Epidemiology, and End Results (SEER) Program SEER*Stat Database: Mortality-All COD, Public-Use With State, Total U.S., 1969-2002 (website): www.seer.cancer.gov, released April 2005. Underlying mortality data provided by NCHS (http://www.cdc.gov/nchs). Accessed May 7, 2007.

45. National Cancer Institute, DCCPS, Surveillance Research Program, Cancer Statistics Branch: Surveillance, Epidemiology, and End Results (SEER) Program DevCan database: SEER 17 Incidence and Mortality, 2000-2003, (website): (http://www.seer.cancer.gov), released June 2006, based on the November 2005 submission. Underlying mortality data provided by NCHS (http://www.cdc.gov/nchs). Accessed May 7, 2007.

46. Mao L, Lee JS, Fan YH et al.: Frequent microsatellite alterations at chromosomes 9p21 and 3p14 in oral premalignant lesions and their value in cancer risk assessment, *Nat Med* 2:682-685, 1996.

47. Reibel J: Prognosis of oral pre-malignant lesions: Significance of clinical, histopathological, and molecular biological characteristics, *Crit Rev Oral Biol Med* 14:47-62, 2003.

48. Wynder EL, Bross IJ: Aetiological factors in mouth cancer, *Br Med J* 1:1137-1143, 1957.

49. Mashberg A, Samit A: Early diagnosis of asymptomatic oral and oropharyngeal cancers, *CA Cancer J Clin* 45:328-351, 1995.

50. National Cancer Institute, DCCPS, Surveillance Research Program, Cancer Statistics Branch: Surveillance, Epidemiology, and End Results (SEER) Program SEER*Stat Database: Mortality - All COD, Public-Use With State, Total U.S.,1969-2002 (website): (http://www.seer.cancer.gov), released April 2005. Underlying mortality data provided by NCHS (http://www.cdc.gov/nchs). Accessed May 7, 2007.

51. National Cancer Institute, DCCPS, Surveillance Research Program, Cancer Statistics Branch: Surveillance, Epidemiology and End Results (SEER) Program DevCan database: SEER 17 Incidence and Mortality, 2000-2003, with Kaposi sarcoma and Mesothelioma (website): (http://www.seer.cancer.gov), released June, 2006, based on November 2005 submission. Underlying mortality data provided by NCIS (http://www.cdc.gov/nchs). Accessed May 7, 2007.

Risk-Based Prevention

Chapter 4

Dental Caries and Associated Risk Factors

JOHN P. BROWN AND MICHAEL W. J. DODDS

LEARNING OBJECTIVES

Upon completion of this chapter, the learner will be able to:
- Review the history of the science of dental caries etiology and risk assessment.
- Explain risk factors associated with dental caries.
- Describe different caries detection methods.
- Identify models that are available to assess caries risk.

KEY TERMS

Caries risk assessment
Fiber optic transillumination
Quantitative light fluorescence
Digital imaging fiber optic transillumination
Caries activity
Caries detection
Caries risk factors

Interest in caries risk prediction emerged because of the overall decline in caries during the latter part of the twentieth century.[1] The systematic understanding of dental caries evolved with the creation of the Venn diagram of major etiologic factors that described interrelationships among the causes of dental caries (Figure 4-1).[2] The application of this etiological framework to assess risk for future disease was not applied to clinical practice until the 1980s, however.[3] This diagram continues to be supported by scientific progress in the understanding of caries and in risk assessment.

Arguments have been raised against the risk-based approach to prevention. Veatch defended using the "whole population approach" to prevention. He based this argument on the ethical constructs of social justice and equity.[4] Batchelor and Sheiham[5] criticized the risk-based approach citing epidemiologic studies that show changes in the caries experience occur throughout populations and are not limited to subgroups. Based on these studies of populations, this argument is that individual risk assessment could ignore the needs of the majority of the population. These authors advocate from a health policy perspective rather than an individual risk-based approach. This position is not specific for dental caries, because the risk for any disease is difficult to assess.[6]

Risk-based prevention for oral disease is not dissimilar to approaches used in medicine. The discriminative ability of combinations of risk factors for heart disease, though modest, is better than that achieved using specific risk factors.[7] The argument that the sensitivity and specificity is not adequate to support risk-based prevention fails to recognize that the use of this approach in medicine has improved access to care and medical practice in recent decades.

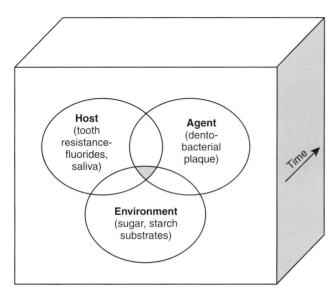

Figure 4-1   Traditional Venn diagram of caries causation.

Clinicians are drawn to risk-based prevention because they usually care for individual patients, rather than populations. Because of the multifactorial nature of caries and other oral diseases, a comprehensive preventive program at the patient level requires that the clinician examine all possible factors and assess etiology on an individual basis. As with other chronic disease prevention, the combination of population-based public health promotion and individual prevention holds the most promise. This chapter will identify risk factors and indicators that are associated with the induction, progression, and severity of dental caries in individuals. This chapter explains the mechanisms for these processes on the basis of the current science. The background, rationale, and description of the state of the science in oral health risk assessment are a major focus of this chapter. Several approaches to the assessment of caries risk are discussed.

HISTORY

Risk assessment has its foundation in a scientific understanding of caries etiology. The science of dental caries infers an association between risk factors or indicators and the disease. Keyes and Fitzgerald[8] showed that caries did not develop in the absence of bacteria. Their work demonstrated that a number of organisms were implicated, and that caries was not caused by a single pathogen. Dean and others helped to develop the notion of tooth susceptibility, especially as influenced by fluorides.[9] Kite, Shaw and Sognnaes showed that fermentable substrate in the mouth was necessary for caries to develop.[10] In recent years, a balanced approach to causation was emphasized, and the role of saliva, diet, and time, in relation to the microbiology and tooth resistance, were developed into a comprehensive explanatory framework.

Keyes' familiar Venn diagram that depicts the major etiologic factors in dental caries uses the well established notion of multilevel causal influences on health.[2] The area of each of the three circles within the Venn diagram represents the relative influence among each of three categories of etiologic factors (see Figure 4-1). The shaded area is designed to suggest the dynamic interaction of host, environment, and agent, and represents by its variable area the intensity of caries activity that can change with time when any or all of the factors change in response to altered environmental or genetic influences.

Until the 1970s, scientific interest focused on subgroups of the population who did not develop dental caries.[1] In 1977, a scientific conference that addressed methods of caries prediction[11] identified promising predictor variables reflected in the Venn diagram that included clinical, microbiological/biochemical, morphological, and nutritional factors. However, a coherent or systematic clinically applicable method was not proposed for clinical use at that time. In 1976, a highly systematized approach to clinical risk assessment was published. This assessment included gathering data from multiple sources to identify a detailed preventive history, elements of clinical observation, and longitudinal records so that one might implement a longitudinal evaluation.[12]

After landmark studies of associations between environmental and genetic variables with caries prediction in infants and children,[13-16] a short, practical, risk-based guide for caries prediction and prevention emerged.[3] Since that time, a risk-based approach to caries prevention for individuals has been advocated. The rationale for using a risk assessment approach is to tailor appropriate preventive strategies to the individual patient. Those patients who are at greater risk for disease require more aggressive intervention at more frequent intervals. In patients with on-going caries activity and progression, the desired intensity of prevention and frequency of reevaluation are recommended to be proportional to the degree of disease risk. Interventions should address the particular risk factors operating to promote the disease in the individual patient.

CARIES DETECTION METHODS

Absolutely essential to any risk-based system are valid and reliable methods of disease detection and recording.[17] Early and reliable means of detecting enamel and root caries incorporate both traditional **caries detection** approaches, such as visual and radiographic methods, and emerging new technologies. Although at present the new technologies may be used infrequently in clinical practice, these methods will become accepted as standards of care as new technologies and skills become more accessible, efficacious, and efficient.

Caries activity is a dynamic process of demineralization, stasis, and remineralization. To be able to accurately assess the dynamic state of a lesion, systematic, longitudinal clinical observation and documentation of an early carious lesion is necessary. A system of recording both the absence of caries lesions and caries at the early and later stages, and the ability to review and evaluate these records over time, is required. Electronic recordkeeping can facilitate this evaluation and can provide a visual representation that can serve as a means of communication with the patient about caries activity over time. Longitudinal assessment, which includes multiple measures over time of an existing caries lesion, is mandatory to determine caries activity, whether the lesion is demineralizing, static, or remineralizing, and to tailor prevention or treatment strategies. As the new caries detection systems become accepted and available, improved, valid, reliable, and efficient, caries detection standards will continue to emerge.[18,19]

Identification of individual risk factors can lead to specific preventive action when disease etiology is understood. **Risk factors** are causal, and risk markers or risk indicators reflect increased or decreased risk, but are not necessarily causal. An attribute or exposure that increases the probability of occurrence of a disease is a determinant. If the determinant (factor or marker) can be changed by an intervention it is said to be modifiable. If the determinant cannot be changed by an intervention, then the factor is nonmodifiable. Rationale for longitudinal assessment is supported by the reality that modifiable factors change continually during an individual's life course.

The basic test for determining the presence or absence of dental caries is a careful visual examination. A dental explorer (probe) should not be used routinely. Dental explorers can be used to remove dental plaque to enhance visualization, to detect, or confirm hidden approximal cavitation using a light touch, and to examine the dentin on the root surface to determine the texture and softness of root caries. Investigators have reported that the use of an explorer does not enhance the added validity or reliability in fissure caries detection when compared with visual examination alone.[17, 20] The lack of validity and reliability of the dental explorer when compared with visual examination has been established for 40 years.[21] Explorer use can result in false positive diagnoses of caries in which the fissure is deep and narrow. Vigorous use of an explorer to detect caries in fissures may result in fracture of the relatively intact surface zone of enamel into the body zone. The use of an explorer can produce cavitation, which may contribute to demineralization and inhibit remineralization.

Fiber optic transillumination (FOTI) can be used to enhance detection of approximal caries.[22] FOTI uses visible light to illuminate the approximal surface from which a lesion can be observed through the marginal ridge. Because decayed tooth structure has a lower index of light transmission than sound tooth structure, the FOTI image is observed as a darker zone surrounded by sound tooth structure. This examination is performed using the light from the hand piece coupler in the dental operatory with subdued room lighting and without the use of an operating light. The light source should be of the smallest possible diameter. Posterior approximal caries can be observed when the light probe is positioned above the gingival margin of the tooth. The light source should be directed perpendicular to the approximal area to prevent direct observation of the beam and allow diffraction between demineralized and sound tooth structure. This position allows the light to pass through the tooth structure. Approximal decay will produce a dark shadow on the occlusal marginal ridge. When dental caries is present, this tool is a highly accurate indicator of approximal caries. The observed image can be easily modified by reangulating the tip of the light probe to address any projection effects on perceived lesion depth.

Bitewing radiographic examination should be used when a reasonable expectation exists of aiding and contributing to detecting a carious lesion[18, 23] and within current radiation standards of practice.[24] A 12-month interval is usually considered appropriate when reassessing remineralization or stasis of a carious lesion and to examine the patient for further evidence of demineralization. Evidence of remineralization may not be evident either on visual or radiographic examination, but stasis or lack of lesion progression is a positive sign.

Digital radiographic images can be obtained by digitization of conventional film radiographs or by direct digital radiography. Digital radiography reduces the amount of radiation required to obtain an image. Digital intraoral radiographic systems appear to be as accurate as traditional radiographic methods for caries detection, even though the image quality may appear degraded upon visual examination.

A resurgence has occurred in electrical resistance tests for caries detection, especially for fissure caries.[23,25] These caries detection methods rely on detecting the increase in the conductivity of an electrical current that results from a decrease in the mineral content of carious enamel and dentin. Enamel demineralization results in increased porosity of the enamel structure. This increase in porosity is filled with fluid, which facilitates the conduction of an electrical current. The probe tip is placed in the fissure and the level of conductivity is recorded on a scale reflecting increased levels of demineralization.

Several light-based methods of caries detection are available. Current research on the validity and reliability of these tests identifies important issues that should be acknowledged to avoid poor treatment decisions. **Quantitative light fluorescence** (QLF) can be used for both the detection and monitoring of dental caries and serves as an indirect measure of enamel porosity and lesion severity. QLF relies on the natural fluorescence of the tooth to distinguish between carious and sound enamel. Fluorescence is a function of the light absorption and scattering properties that is inherent in the tooth mineral structure. This inherent fluorescence of the enamel is reduced by demineralization of the enamel structure. Therefore, QLF is a measure of the change in the demineralized enamel structure compared with the surrounding sound tooth structure. The demineralized tissue will appear darker when visualized with QLF because demineralized tissue reduces the penetration of light. A caries lesion is observed as a darker spot surrounded by highly luminescent sound enamel. Advantages of QLF are that this technology uses ordinary white light sources, and the contrast between carious and sound enamel makes earlier detection of lesions possible.

There are some limitations to QLF technology. QLF depends on a stable state of hydration of the tooth enamel. Reproducible hydration of tooth enamel is very difficult to maintain and achieve longitudinally, which can impact the measure of mineral status. QLF is not able to distinguish between active and arrested caries and between caries and stains on the tooth surface, increasing the rate of false positive diagnoses. QLF technology is presently limited to detection of caries on smooth surfaces. The presence of dental plaque and staining can limit its validity.

DIFOTI, digital imaging fiber optic transillumination, produces a high-contrast image of early caries, but is very susceptible to invalidation by both extrinsic and intrinsic staining.

The validity and reliability of early caries detection methods be understood. The mere detection of dental caries using these methods does not justify active treatment. The detection of caries can indicate the need to examine individual risk factors that contribute to the disease and suggest a change to current preventive strategies.

RISK FACTORS FOR DENTAL CARIES

When determining an individual patient's caries risk profile, etiological factors must be considered not as separate entities, but in combination. The approach depicted in Figure 4-2 emphasizes interactions, rather than a narrow focus on any one single factor. It likewise provides a graphic depiction of all factors involved in the caries process. A discussion of the individual components of caries etiology is merited to explain the independent and collective causal theories discussed in Chapter 1.

Dental caries is a multifactorial disease initiated by microbiological virulence and proliferation within the biofilm that is modified by salivary flow and composition, diet, and preventive strategies, including fluoride exposure.[26] It results from the interaction of four key risk factors: diet, tooth/host, and bacteria over time; therefore, intervention to change the balance of any of these four factors can theoretically lead to a reduction or increase in disease. This concept provides the basis for **caries risk assessment**.

As a biobehavioral disease process, the balance of these factors within the oral cavity relies on the presence or absence of preventive variables and modulators. Preventive variables that have a direct impact on caries risk include saliva flow, composition and buffer capacity, dietary

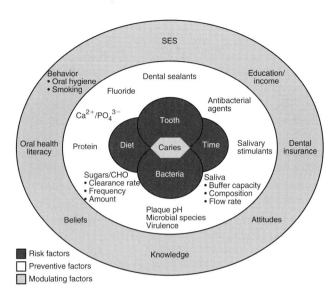

Figure 4-2 Factors involved in caries development. (Modified from Selwitz RH, Ismail AI, Pitts NB: Dental caries, *Lancet* 369:51-59, 2007.)

factors, exposure to fluoride, sealants, and antibacterial agents. These are discussed in detail in Chapters 9 and 15.

Modulators of dental caries identified in the model in Figure 4-2 include demographic factors that are specifically defined as income status, ownership of dental insurance, social status, and extent of education. Knowledge, attitudes and beliefs related to understanding of oral health concepts and the individual's role in their oral health have a direct impact on disease progression and reduction of caries risk. These behavioral modulators are discussed in Chapter 13, including an explanation of health literacy, the principles of which are often ignored. Behaviors, including oral hygiene practices, diet modification, and tobacco cessation, should be addressed by the dental professional. A review of these behavioral intervention strategies with scientific justification of efficacy is in Chapters 16 and 17.

Bacteria

The plaque biofilm is essential to caries; however, not all of the more than 300 species of bacteria found thus far in the plaque biofilm are cariogenic. With gene technology, additional oral bacterial species are being identified in plaque. Only a few species of microorganisms have been implicated in the caries process: mutans streptococci (*Streptococcus mutans, Streptococcus sobrinus*), *Lactobacillus* spp., and *Actinomyces*. Although their virulence varies, these organisms are indicator organisms. Bacteria live on the teeth in microcolonies that are encapsulated in an organic matrix of polysaccharides and proteins secreted by the cells, which provides protection from host defenses.[27] The cariogenic bacteria present in the biofilm mass ferment dietary sugars into weak acids that lower the plaque pH and cause demineralization. The demineralization process results in leaching of calcium and phosphate ions, which if continued, results in cavitation. Therefore, the trend has been to define caries not simply as a plaque-mediated disease, but rather as a disease associated with a specific pathogenic plaque—the so-called "specific plaque hypothesis."[28]

After early childhood, mutans streptococci are ubiquitous in the oral cavity and in the biofilm. Rather than an exogenous infection, dental caries results from an ecological imbalance of the virulence and proliferation of organisms in the oral cavity. This observation would suggest that risk assessment must address this homeostasis and the dental professional should work to restore balance rather than eradicate the bacteria.

Acquisition of these microorganisms occurs at a young age. Transmission of the bacteria is through a vertical pathway, typically from mother to child, and not horizontal, or person to person.[29] Therefore, dental caries is infectious and transmissible, but not communicable. Colonization typically occurs soon after the first tooth erupts in the oral cavity. Once introduced into the oral cavity, the bacteria colonize the erupting teeth that offer a perfect niche for colonization of the biofilm in large numbers. Kohler et al. and Caufield et al. demonstrated that the longer the delay in transmission to the child, the less caries prone the child is later in childhood.[16,29] Therefore, a direct association exists between the oral health of the mother and the caries risk for the child, because the mother's bacterial load and virulence is related to the time and intensity of the infant's acquisition of these organisms and the child's risk for caries. This important finding should be widely applied in programs to prevent early childhood caries (ECC).

Because of the nature of the bacteria in the oral cavity, the disease of dental caries occurs throughout the life span. Caries risk can be lowered through a systematic preventive approach that includes, when indicated, decreasing bacterial risk factors. This can be accomplished by diet modification, oral hygiene, and increasing the tooth resistance with fluorides and salivary stimulation.

Tooth/Host

The role of the tooth in biofilm formation, the susceptibility of the tooth in the caries process, and saliva as a source of maintaining integrity, are key factors in caries risk. Caries lesions are prone to develop where oral biofilms are allowed to mature and remain on the teeth for long periods of time. Teeth provide nonshedding surfaces for microbial colonization, and large numbers of bacteria accumulate in the biofilm of the tooth surface in both health and disease.[30] When discussing the role of the tooth in caries risk, consideration must be given to tooth morphology and caries history. Studies have shown that previous caries experience is an important consideration for caries risk and that the presence of caries, including early lesions, is most predictive of future caries

development.[31] Research suggests that determining caries activity, not just the presence of the lesions, may be important to predict caries[32]; however, the only way at present to determine lesion activity is by longitudinal assessment. These findings suggest that prevention and intervention in the disease process would contribute to a reduction in both disease burden and risk for future disease.

Dental caries predominates in specific teeth in both primary and permanent dentition.[33,34] In the primary dentition, early childhood caries is found most often on smooth surfaces.[35] Later in childhood, caries is most often found in pit and fissure surfaces.[33,36] Persons with deep and narrow pits and fissures are at increased risk for caries in those surfaces. These grooves are more retentive and difficult to clean using routine oral hygiene. Adults continue to be at risk for initial caries, in addition to secondary or recurrent caries that form around existing restorations. Because more elderly individuals are retaining their teeth, an increase in the prevalence of root caries has been observed.[26] Root caries develops after the root of the tooth is exposed following gingival recession. These observations underscore the role of the tooth morphology in caries development.

Fluoride bioavailability in plaque is important in tooth integrity. Fluoride provides resistance to demineralization, favoring remineralization of smaller, less acid soluble crystals. Saliva is an essential source of calcium and phosphate ions for remineralization. The role of saliva in supplying mineral stabilizing proteins, acid buffering, production of antibacterial enzymes, oral clearance, and lubrication are essential to oral health and the integrity of the oral cavity.

Diet

Caries is a diet- and biofilm-dependent oral disease. Sugar and other fermentable carbohydrate exposures are an essential etiological factor in caries development. Dietary fermentable carbohydrates act to change the biochemical and physiological composition in dental biofilm by bacterial fermentation and rapidly lowering plaque pH from a neutral state to 5.0 or below. Sucrose serves as a substrate for bacterial synthesis of insoluble glucans (extracellular polysaccharides) in dental plaque, thus promoting bacterial adherence to tooth surfaces.[37]

As a general rule, the cariogenic bacteria metabolize sugars to produce energy required for their growth and reproduction. The energy sources may be exogenous (from immediate food sources) or endogenous (from stored polysaccharides within biofilm). Cariogenic bacteria can metabolize any monosaccharides (glucose, fructose, and galactose) or disaccharides (sucrose and maltose) for energy. Cooked starches are an available source of glucose. The result of this sugar catabolism is the production of organic acids in the dental plaque fluid, which lower the plaque pH. When the pH decreases to approximately 5.2 to 5.5, the immediate tooth environment (interface between tooth and plaque) is no longer saturated with calcium and phosphate ions, and the tooth starts to demineralize. Once the decalcification reaches the dentin-enamel junction, acid decalcification of the dentin can progress, and the bacteria themselves later invade the protein of the dentin and destroy it through proteolysis.

Sucrose further reduces concentrations of calcium, inorganic phosphorus and fluoride ions that are important in maintaining mineral equilibrium between the tooth and the oral environment. Possible mechanisms for this process are hypothesized to be related to changes in and depletion of biofilm matrix structure, frequency of sucrose exposure, and changes in calcium-binding protein biofilm composition.[37]

A number of classic studies in specific human populations have shown a clear relationship between sucrose consumption and caries prevalence and incidence. These include the Vipeholm study from the 1940s,[38] the Hopewood House study from the 1960s,[39] and the Turku Sugar studies from the early 1970s.[40] The Vipeholm study remains the most influential study of diet and dental caries to date. This study showed that the quantity of sugar consumed and whether it was consumed with or between meals were important factors in caries development. Raw starches are considered less cariogenic than simple sugars such as sucrose, glucose, and fructose. Sucrose, in particular, promotes higher enamel mineral loss, and when combined with cooked starch enhances the cariogenic potential of starch.[41]

Eating patterns are as important as the quantity of fermentable carbohydrates consumed. Repeated cariogenic attacks produce the cumulative mineral loss that characterizes caries. Retentive foods such as dried fruit, highly processed grains, and some cooked starches, like potato chips, may be classified as "fermentable carbohydrates;" these include all sugars or cooked starches, which can be metabolized by oral bacteria to produce acids.[42] Snacking patterns, occupational and lifestyle changes, eating and drinking patterns, and oral hygiene practices may all potentially influence the role of diet in caries risk.

Other dietary considerations include the presence of protective factors in foods such as calcium, phosphate, fluoride, protein, and dietary fiber. Food form may also be important. Sugar in drinks appears to be somewhat less cariogenic than those in solid form such as candies. The increased frequency and duration of exposure to sugary drinks has been associated with sustained oral plaque pH below 5.0.[43] Also, the consumption of these drinks has dramatically risen and milk consumption has fallen. The sugar in beverages merits full consideration in assessing caries risk.

Attempts to develop a caries risk assessment model that adequately includes dietary assessment have been minimal. This textbook sets out to address this deficiency. Food choices and dietary patterns are essential determinants of dental caries. Conversely, the discomfort and possible tooth loss caused by caries can affect food choices and dietary patterns and may itself lead to dietary inadequacies and compromised nutritional status.

Any assessment of caries risk and etiology must include dietary factors that address the quantity and frequency of fermentable carbohydrate in the diet, the pattern of food and beverage consumption, and an identification of dietary food combinations. If screening and risk assessment indicate a need for more detailed dietary information, there are numerous approaches to dietary assessment listed in Table 8-4, which provides additional dietary information and complete dietary assessment.

Time

Dental caries is both multifactorial and modulated by time. Prevention requires longitudinal assessment and monitoring. The onset of this disease can progress from a preclinical phase of exposure to etiological bacteria and substrate with undetectable demineralization to gross cavitation of tooth structure and tooth loss. For caries to progress without remission, time to form a visible lesion and then a cavity is required. With the decline in caries prevalence, this time has increased. Therefore, time is on the side of the patient and dental professional, allowing for nonsurgical, preventive intervention. Development, equilibrium, progression, and remineralization may reoccur over a lifelong period; however, this can be controlled in several ways. Lifestyles and behaviors, including oral hygiene practices, use of preventive products, dietary choices, socioeconomic status, access to dental insurance, and dental attendance may vary throughout one's life course. Thus, caries risk assessment and reassessment must be an on-going and integral component of long-term dental patient care. As noted in Figure 4-2, time is a major factor in caries development.[26]

CARIES RISK ASSESSMENT MODELS

Caries risk assessment is a systematic process based on the patient's past and present caries experience and known risk factors or indicators for disease that attempt to categorize persons into risk groups with respect to the potential to develop new carious lesions over time. The use of risk assessment in the clinical management of caries is outlined in Box 4-1.

Risk-based systems of caries prevention have been widely proposed; however, no comprehensive and validated method to assess caries risk has been developed and adopted universally by dental professionals. The first practical clinical guide to modern caries risk assessment was developed by Krasse in 1985.[3] In the late 1980s and 1990s, dental schools began to adopt the risk-based approach in clinical teaching.[44,45] One of the first clinical caries risk assessment models described in the literature was developed at the University of Texas Health Science Center at San Antonio, Dental School.[44] The American Dental Association review of caries diagnosis and risk assessment was published in 1995.[46] In 1998, Brathall

BOX 4-1

PURPOSE OF CARIES RISK ASSESSMENT IN CLINICAL PRACTICE

- Evaluate the degree of the patient's risk of developing caries to determine the intensity of prevention and frequency of reevaluation/recall appointments.
- Identify the main etiological agents that contribute to past and present disease and which thus may contribute to future disease, to determine the specific type of appropriate interventions.
- Determine whether additional diagnostic or testing procedures are required.
- Aid in preventive or restorative treatment decisions, or both.
- Improve the reliability and the prognosis of the planned interventions.
- Provide a basis to explain and empower the patient on how to prevent dental caries and to communicate and facilitate needed change in health behaviors to prevent caries.
- Assess the efficacy of the interventions and preventive plan at reevaluation/recall appointments and adjust preventive strategies as needed.

(Modified from Fontana M, Zero DT: Assessing patients' caries risk, *JADA* 137:1231-1239, 2006.)

and others[47,48] published a web-based version of a caries risk-assessment program that was referred to as the Cariogram. This program was an online instrument used to determine the future probability estimates of developing dental caries by individuals.

Today, each of the U.S. military dental services uses a risk-based caries assessment model in their delivery of dental care. The U.S. Navy adopted past and present caries status in preventively oriented treatment planning,[49] and the U.S. Army[50] and Air Force[51] adopted a risk-based caries assessment protocol. The American Academy of Pediatric Dentistry developed a caries-risk assessment tool in 2002.[52] This Caries Risk Assessment Tool (CAT) takes a broad approach to risk assessment, considering the effect of both systemic disease and reported behavioral factors in the interpretation of caries risk. In 2003, the California Dental Association published a comprehensive caries risk assessment guide that targeted the adult patient.[53] This instrument was adopted by numerous dental schools located on the west coast of the United States. Caries Management by Risk Assessment (CAMBRA) attempts to address the management of caries in a systemic way.[53]

The risk assessment models that are currently used rely on a series of common elements; however, differences exist among the models because of differences in emphasis and interpretation of the science among the various designers. None of the existing caries risk assessment tools have fully demonstrated internal and external validity.

Caries risk assessment models use data gleaned from a patient's medical, dental, social, and preventive history; dietary screening; clinical determinants of caries status and history; salivary function assessment; and fluoride exposure. These variables are used to assess the patient's risk for future disease. One example of a caries risk assessment model used in San Antonio is presented in Figure 4-3.[44] The model was initially designed to categorize adult patients into four risk groups. Questions on dietry screening and salivary function have demonstrated internal validity.[54,57] However, attempts to further validate the entire model using a retrospective study of patient records proved unfeasible in a dental school population. This study sought to assess behavior change as an intermediate goal and disease prevention as an ultimate goal. The inability to validate this model was the result of a low recall rate and a loss to follow-up, which is typical in a dental school patient population. One possible solution to the inability to validate the model is the implementation of electronic record systems. Electronic records with an adequate level of detail and "smart systems" can "self-improve" the carries risk assessment method by progressively analyzing patient records over time.

Patient screening questions that contribute to the assessment of caries risk status should be incorporated in the initial diagnostic work-up. On the basis of the initial screening questions, additional testing may be indicated. Testing approaches specific to various outcomes are described in Chapter 9. Once any additional testing is completed, the information analyzed, and the patient's risk assessment status is determined, this status can be used to plan caries prevention. See Chapter 15 for a discussion of preventive strategies that may be included in a treatment plan.

Patient History

Identification of present and past individual preventive and health practices is essential to motivate patients to adopt healthy behaviors, reduce caries risk, and to improve their oral health. Consideration should be given to assess oral functional status and its impact on the patient's quality of life. Quality of life measures are important to the broader impact of oral function on daily living. Knowledge of individual patient health and disease history, attitudes toward health attainment and disease occurrence, and preventive and risky health behaviors need to be identified and evaluated. This evaluation requires that the health professional has a clear understanding of the patient's environmental and cultural context, so that cultural filters do not obscure knowledge, attitudes, or behaviors of the patient, or cause them to be misinterpreted. This topic is addressed in Chapter 13. Interpersonal communication skills can enhance the oral health professional's ability to successfully

Oral Health Evaluation

Caries Risk Assessment			
Dietary screening for caries risk		Date →	/ /
1	Do you eat food or drink sugar-sweetened beverages five or more times a day?	1 pt if yes	
2	Do you chew regular (non-sugar-free) gum?	1 pt if yes	
3	Do you drink any sugar-sweetened beverages between meals?	2 pts if yes	
4	Do you eat mints, candies, pastries, chips, crackers, etc., between meals?	2 pts if yes	
5	Do you drink milk or eat cheese every day?	1 pt if no	
Dietary screening total			
Caries indicators—consider clinical findings, radiographic interpretation, and other findings incorporated into caries charting approved by faculty. Use caries assessment and management decision trees.			
6	Are carious lesions present? (cavitated)	3 pts if yes	
7	Number of carious lesions (include coronal and root caries): (cavitated)	1 pt each	
8	Number of carious lesions limited to enamel (incipient, uncavitated) and incipient of root	1 pt each	
9	Five or more filled surfaces (amalgams, composites, crowns)?	2 pts if yes	
10	One or more teeth missing due to caries?	2 pts if yes	
Caries indicator total			
Fluoride exposure			
11	No fluoride from water, tablets, or drops?	1 pt	
12	No fluoride from regular personal use of toothpaste, rinse, or gel?	1 pt	
Caries Risk Assessment (Total of #1-12)			

Very high – CRA score >15 or >4 cavitated lesions	**Caries risk category at left**	
High – CRA score 10-15 or 3-4 cavitated lesions	**Caries risk category after indicated saliva tests (see below*)**	
Mod – CRA score 5-9		
Low – CRA score 4 or less		

Hyposalivation Screening (JADA 115: 581, 1987)		
13	Does your mouth feel dry when eating a meal?	Y/N
14	Do you have difficulty swallowing food?	Y/N
15	Do you have to sip liquids needed to aid in swallowing?	Y/N
16	Is the amount of saliva in your mouth "too little" most of the time?	Y/N

Indications for additional testing:

Diet

If Caries Risk Assessment is very high or high, or dietary screening total >3:

☐ Complete 24-hour recall diet diary

☐ Otherwise these additional dietary assessments are not indicated for caries.

The analysis of this dietary data and the dietary screening will lead to specific desirable dietary changes to be entered in the daily treatment record and acted on through patient counseling and reinforcement.

☐ A 3-day prospective diet diary may be required in consultation with faculty.

Saliva tests

If Caries Activity Total is >5, or Dietary Screening Total >3, or Hyposalivation Screening includes >1 'Yes':

☐ a) Determine unstimulated saliva flow rate AND

☐ b) Collect stimulated whole saliva for M. Strep count for lab OR

☐ Otherwise additional saliva tests are not indicated

a) _____ ml/min
b) _____ cfu/ml

* Revised Caries Risk Assessment

If (a) is <0.2 ml/min. or (b) >5.5 × 10^5 cfu/ml, raise caries risk category by one and enter new or unchanged category above, at "Caries risk category after indicated saliva tests."

Other Oral Health Risk Factors		
17	PSR or full periodontal evaluation indicates periodontal prevention will be required?	Y/N
18	Poor oral hygiene? (Plaque index >20%)	Y/N
19	Presence of any systemic disease which compromises oral health?	Y/N
20	Oral cancer risk factors? (alcohol, tobacco, sunlight, history of oral cancer)	Y/N
21	Risk of oral injury? (contact sport, no seatbelt use, physical abuse)	Y/N
22	Evidence of tooth erosion?	Y/N

Figure 4-3 Oral health evaluation. (Courtesy Department of Community Dentistry, University of Texas Health Science Center at San Antonio, San Antonio, TX.)

empower the patient to make appropriate health behavior choices. Motivational interviewing techniques are discussed in Chapter 11. As a component of communication, the dental professional needs to assess the patient's health literacy. The dental professional should acknowledge the patient's understanding and willingness to change when delivering the preventive message so that patient adherence will be enhanced. Considering the patient as a partner in the caries risk process can facilitate personalized health risk communication.

Many common diseases and drugs impact the health status of the oral cavity and caries risk. Endocrine and other disorders impact oral health status and are important in the determination of caries risk. Radiation therapy associated with management of head and neck cancer affects salivary gland function and necessitates special dietary regimens that may be caries preventive or inducing. Sugar-based medications given to chronically ill children can increase their risk for dental caries, and psychopharmaceutical drugs can reduce salivary flow. Details on the interactions between pharmacology and oral health status are discussed further in Chapter 7. The dental professional's awareness of a patient's medication and health status use and the implications for oral health is essential to caries risk assessment activities.

Dietary Screening

Evaluation of the dietary and nutritional issues associated with caries risk can be addressed in several ways. Dietary screening questions specifically designed to address caries risk are listed in Chapter 8 (see Figure 4-3 and Table 8-4). These five questions were validated[54] and meet minimum criteria for a predictive test (specificity 75%, sensitivity 77%). The individual questions were weighted for their impact. A total score greater than three identifies persons likely to be at increased caries risk due to diet. If so, a more detailed dietary evaluation is indicated. A 24-hour recall of dietary intake, including amounts, eating patterns, sugar, and fermentable carbohydrates consumed, will specifically identify a caries-promoting diet and indicate where individually tailored dietary intervention is most appropriate. It will also help to fit such changes into the diet as a whole, without confusing the patient. A more detailed assessment of diet is discussed in Chapter 8. Responses to the dietary screening questions may be subsequently modified in light of more detailed dietary assessment, and a full determination made of the total contribution to the overall caries risk assessment (CRA).

Caries Status and History

Present and past caries is considered a central indicator of overall and future caries risk. In considering the role of caries status and history in the caries risk assessment, the dental provider needs to determine from patient assessment: (1) number of past restorations, (2) current lesions, (3) stage of the lesions (enamel/dentin), and 4) history of extraction of teeth because of caries.

For the purposes of this text, the term caries activity reflects the remineralization, equilibrium, or demineralization process longitudinally over time. Assessment of activity depends on a carefully crafted clinical exam, testing, history taking, and comprehensive, systematic recording, including radiographs when appropriate. The importance of measuring caries activity makes longitudinal measurement of caries progression or stasis critical to the overall

plan of prevention. It is important to differntiate between the early lesion in enamel and the lesion clearly extending into dentin is important. Research shows that early caries lesions are more predictive than either filled surfaces or cavitated surfaces.[55] Appropriate visual, fiber optic transillumination (FOTI), radiographic, and other sufficiently valid and reliable tests of caries detection can be used to best assess caries, to identify early lesions, and to provide a baseline from which to assess future caries activity. Documentation should be detailed to allow comparison and longitudinal assessment when the patient is reevaluated in future encounters. Longitudinal assessment is the most indicative measure of caries progression, stasis, or remineralization, and is a true reflection of caries activity.

One assessment of past caries history is evident in the presence of existing restorations. Identifying the number of existing restorations and cavities alone, however, is insufficient information to determine overall caries risk status. Through an assessment of past and present caries and other disease indicators, a current estimation of risk can be made.

Fluoride Exposure

Assessment of fluoride exposure should be included in the assessment. All potential sources of fluoride, such as community water fluoridation and personal patterns of use of toothpaste with fluoride and from other sources should be included. These elements of the caries risk assessment protocol comply with the Centers for Disease Control and Prevention's Recommendations for Fluoride Use.[56] For children and adolescents who are not exposed to community water fluoridation, exposure to fluoride could include fluoride supplements. Over-the-counter rinses and gels should be considered in the overall assessment of past fluoride exposure, and frequency of professional fluoride application in the past should be included.

Salivary Assessment (Hyposalivation)

Four validated questions are included in a caries risk assessment (see Figure 4-3) as an indicator of low salivary function.[57] These are listed in Box 4-2. If the patient

---

BOX 4-2

Xerostomia Screening Questions

- Does your mouth feel dry when eating a meal?
- Do you have difficulty swallowing food?
- Do you have to sip liquids to aid in swallowing?
- Is the amount of saliva in your mouth "too little" most of the time?

(Modified from Fox PC, Busch KA, Baum BJ: Subjective reports of xerostomia and objective measures of salivary gland performance, *JADA* 115:581-584, 1987.)

experiences more than one of the symptoms or conditions, the patient may be considered to have salivary hypofunction and be at increased risk for dental caries. Additional testing to ascertain salivary flow rates may be initiated if the patient responds positively to any of the screening questions. The process for measuring unstimulated salivary flow rate is described in Chapter 9, as are several techniques to measure whole mouth levels of indicator cariogenic bacteria present in saliva.

Tooth Morphology

Tooth morphology relates to caries risk. Deep and retentive pits and fissures on occlusal tooth surfaces are at greater risk for caries. In adults, risk assessment activities should include an assessment of exposed root surfaces, caused by gingival recession, which may predispose a patient to root caries.

Indicator Bacterial Load

Estimates of mutans streptococci in whole stimulated saliva are indicative of caries risk, and the counts are typically stable over time. The negative predictive value is superior to the positive, so the validity and reliability of these counts help to identify individuals who are less likely to develop future caries. Another major use is to assess dietary adherence when major reductions in sweet food and drink intake have been recommended. With patient adherence to the recommended diet, high levels of mutans streptococci will fall. For these reasons and to identify those with high levels of these indicator bacteria, persons whose oral screening and history indicate a moderate or high caries risk should be tested for mutans streptococci bacterial load in saliva. Commercial kits are available to test indicator organisms. These methods are described in Chapter 9.

Caries Risk Assessment Method

At the conclusion of the information gathering steps in a caries risk assessment (CRA) protocol, an assessment of caries risk status should be made. This assessment should be used to place the patient into a caries risk category. On the basis of the number and severity of the risk factors, the patient is classified as low, moderate, or high risk for future caries development. Ultimately, a caries risk assessment is a systematic approach to identify all etiologic factors that promote caries for a person. This leads to the specific and individually tailored preventive interventions that are discussed in Chapter 15. For patients at low risk, this assessment will help confirm lack of etiological factors and basic caries preventive behaviors and measures can be reinforced.

SUMMARY

Dental caries, as a disease, affects persons across the lifespan and remains the most prevalent disease in the population. Although caries rates have declined in the US population, disparities in disease remain evident, and caries prevention and restoration remain one of the most common aspects of clinical dental practice. Although significant strides have been made in addressing this disease, risk-based approaches to address dental caries are necessary to identify those individuals at greatest risk and for efficient prevention. The dramatic reduction in disease among some segments of the population provides further opportunity to target and tailor successful prevention modalities. Caries risk assessment provides a springboard to engage the patient in defining and achieving mutual disease prevention goals. By understanding those factors that are related to each patient's disease, the dental practitioner can better monitor the outcomes of care, and improve the quality of dental care.

REFERENCES

1. Wolstemholme GEW, O'Connor J, eds: *Caries resistant teeth: 1964 CIBA foundation symposium,* London, 1965, Churchill.
2. Keyes PH: Present and future measures of dental caries control, *JADA* 79:1395-1404, 1969.
3. Krasse B: *Caries risk: a practical guide for assessment and control,* Chicago, 1985, Quintessence Publishing Company.
4. Veatch RM: Minority opinion: Dental sealants in the prevention of tooth decay. NIH Concensus Development Conference, *J Dent Ed* 48(Suppl 2):128, 1984.
5. Batchelor P, Sheiham A: The limitations of a "high risk" approach for the prevention of dental caries, *Commun Dent Oral Epidemiol* 30:302-312, 2002.
6. Hansen H: Caries prediction-state of the art (review), *Commun Dent Oral Epidemiol* 25:87-96, 1997.
7. Milne R, Gamble G, et al.: Disseminative ability of a risk-prediction tool derived from the Framingham Heart Study compared with single risk factors, *N Z Med J* 116:1185, 2003.
8. Fitzgerald RJ, Keyes PH: Demonstration of the etiological role of streptococci in experimental caries in the hamster, *JADA* 61:9-19, 1960.
9. Dean HT: Some reflections on the epidemiology of fluorine and dental health, *Am J Pub Health* 43:704-709, 1953.
10. Kite OW, Shaw JH, Sognnaes RF: The prevention of experimental tooth decay by tube-feeding, *J Nutr* 42(1):89-105,1950.
11. Bibby BG, Shern RJ, ed: *Methods of caries prediction, Oct. 3-5, 1977, Niagara Falls, N.Y.,* Washington, DC, 1978, Information Retrieval.
12. Mühlemann Hans R: *Introduction to oral preventive medicine: a program for the first clinical experience,* Chicago, 1976, Quintessence Publishing.
13. Kloch B, Krasse B: A comparison between different methods for prediction of caries activity, *Scand J Dent Res* 87:129-39, 1999.
14. Kohler B, Bratthall D, Krasse B: Preventive measures in mothers influence the establishment of a bacterium streptococcus mutans in their infants, *Arch Oral Biol* 28:225-31, 1983.
15. Kohler B, Andreen J, Jonsson B: The effect of caries-preventive measures in mothers on dental caries and the oral presence of the bacterial streptococcus mutans lactobacilli in their children, *Arch Oral Biol* 29:879-83, 1986.
16. Kohler B, Andreen I: Influence of caries prevention measures in mothers on cariogenic bacteria and caries experience in their children, *Arch Oral Biol* 39:907-11, 1994.
17. Brown JP: Dilemmas in caries diagnosis, *J Dent Educ* 57:407-443, 1993.

18. Tyvid B, Machiulakine V, Baelin V: Reliabilty of new caries diagnostic system differentiating between active and inactive caries lesion, *Caries Res* 33:252-260, 1999.

19. Pitts N: ICDAS—an international system for caries detection and assessment being developed to facilitiate caries, epidemiology, research and appropriate clinical management, *Community Dent Health* 21:193-198, 2004.

20. Lussi A: Validity of diagnostic and treatment decisions of future caries, *Caries Res* 25:296-303, 1991.

21. Slack GL: The technique of examination in clinical trials. In Jones PMC, ed: *Advances in fluoride research and dental caries prevention*, New York, 1966, Oxford Pergamon Press.

22. Davies GM, Worthington HV, Clarkson JE, et al: The use of fiber-optic transillumination in general dental practice, *Br Dent J* 19:145-147, 2001.

23. Dodds MWJ: Applications to current practice and need for research, *J Dent Educ* 57:433-438, 1997.

24. National Council on Radiation Protection and Measurements (NCRP): Radiation protection in dentistry: report 145, Bethesda, Md., 2003.

25. Wenzel A: New caries detection methods, *J Dent Educ* 57:428-432, 1993.

26. Selwitz RH, Ismail AI, Pitts NB: Dental caries, *Lancet* 369: 51-59, 2007.

27. Fejerskov O, Kidd EAM, eds: *Dental caries: the disease and its clinical management*, Copenhagen, 2003, Blackwell Munksgaard.

28. Loesche WJ: Clinical and microbiological aspects of chemotherapeutic agents used according to the specific plaque hypothesis, *J Dent Res* 58:2404-2412, 1979.

29. Caufield PW, Griffen AL: Dental caries: an infectious and transmissible disease, *Pediatr Clin North Am* 47:1001-1019, 2000.

30. Scheie A, Peterson F: The biofilm concept: consequences for future prophylaxis of oral diseases? *Crit Rev Oral Biol Med* 15:4-12, 2004.

31. National Institutes of Health: Diagnosis and management of dental caries throughout life. NIH Consensus Statement 26-28; 18(1):1-24, 2001.

32. Zero D, Fontana M, Lennon AM: Clinical applications and outcomes of using indicators of risk in caries management, *J Dent Educ* 65:1126-1132, 2001.

33. Anderson M: Risk assessment and epidemiology of dental caries: review of the literature, *Pediatr Dent* 24:377-385, 2002.

34. Brown LJ, Selwitz RH: The impact of recent changes in the epidemiology of dental caries on guidelines for the use of dental sealants, *J Public Health Dent* 55:274-291, 1995.

35. DeGrawe A, Aps JK, Martens IC: Early childhood caries (ECC): what's in a name? *Eur J Paediatr Dent* 5:62-70, 2004.

36. U.S. Department of Health and Human Services: Oral health in America: A report of the Surgeon General, Rockville, MD, 2000, National Institute of Dental and Craniofacial Research, National Institutes of Health.

37. Leme AFP, Koo H, Bellato CM et al.: The role of sucrose in cariogenic dental biofilm formation—new insight, *J Dent Res* 85:878-887, 2006.

38. Gustafsson BE, Quensel CE, Lanke SL: The Vipeholm dental caries study, *Acta Odontol Scand* 11:232-364, 1954.

39. Harris R, Nicoll AD, Adair PM et al.: Risk factors for dental caries in young children: a systematic review of the literature, *Community Dent Health* 21:71-85, 2004.

40. Scheinin A, Makinen KK: Turku sugar studies: an overview, *Acta Odont Scand* 34:405-408, 1976.

41. Ribeiro CC, Tabchoury CP, DelBelCury AA et al.: Effect of starch on cariogenic potential of sucrose, *Br J Nutr* 94:44-50, 2005.

42. Kandelman D: Sugar, alternative sweeteners and meal frequency in relation to caries prevention: new perspectives, *Br J Nutr* 77:S21-S28, 1997.

43. Fontana M, Zero DT: Assessing patients' caries risk, *JADA* 137:1231-1239, 2006.

44. Brown JP: Developing clinical teaching methods for caries risk assessments, *J Dent Educ* 59:928-985, 1995.

45. Benn DK: Practical evidence-based management of the early carious lesion, *J Dent Educ* 61:855-860, 1997.

46. Caries diagnosis and risk assessment: a review of preventive strategies and management, *JADA* 126(suppl):1S-24S, 1995.

47. Hansel-Petersson G, Carlsson P, Bratthall D: Caries risk assessment: a comparison between the computer program, Cariogram, dental students and dental instructors, *Euro J Dent Educ.* 2:184-190, 1988.

48. Bratthall D, Hansel-Petersson G: Cariogram—a multifactorial risk assessment model for a multifactorial disease, *Comm Dent Oral Epidemiol* 33:256-264, 2005.

49. Cook NB: Preventive oriented treatment planning, National Navy Medical Center, Learning Center (website): http://www.bethesda.med.navy.mil/patient/learning%Fcenter. Accessed November 2000.

50. Chaffin JG: Dental population health measures: supporting Army transformation, *Mil Med* 168:223-226, 2003.

51. King BB: Revised dental population health metrics guidelines (Updated for 1999), U.S. Air Force, January 2005.

52. American Academy of Pediatrics Dentistry: Policy statement on the use of a caries-risk assessment tool (website): http://www.aapd.org/media/policies_guidelines/P_cariesriskassess.pdf. 2002. Accessed June 27, 2007.

53. Featherstone JDB, Roth JR: Caries risk: moving from restoration toward prevention, *J Calif Dent Assoc* 31:123-161, 2003.

54. Mobley CC: Dietary analysis in restorative practice: the changing practice of restorative dentistry. In Duke ES, ed: Proceedings of the 5th annual Indiana conference, Indiana University School of Dentistry (Indianapolis, IN), pp. 139-156, 2002.

55. ter Pelkwijk A, van Palestein Helderman WH, van Dijk JWE: Caries experience in the deciduous dentition as predictor for caries in permanent dentition, *Caries Res* 24:65-71, 1990.

56. Recommendations for using fluoride to prevent and control dental caries in the United States. Centers for Disease Control and Prevention, *MMWR* 50(RR-14):1-42, August 17, 2001.

57. Fox PC, Busch KA, Baum BJ: Subjective reports for xerostomia and objective measures of salivary gland performance, *JADA* 115:581-584, 1987.

Chapter 5

Periodontal Disease and Associated Risk Factors

KAREN F. NOVAK

BACKGROUND

RISK FACTORS/INDICATORS FOR PERIODONTAL DISEASES

Local Factors
Environmental Factors
Systemic Factors
Economic Factors

RISK ASSESSMENT IN CLINICAL PRACTICE

CONCLUSION

LEARNING OBJECTIVES

Upon completion of this chapter, the learner will be able to:
- Outline the detection and diagnosis of periodontal diseases.
- Examine the local and environmental risk factors for periodontal diseases.
- Discuss the systemic risk factors for periodontal diseases.
- Describe the association between systemic diseases and periodontal diseases and importance in risk assessment.
- Apply risk assessment protocols to identify individuals at risk for periodontal diseases.

KEY TERMS

Modifiable risk factor
Nonmodifiable risk factor
Periodontal disease
Risk

Risk assessment
Risk indicator

Periodontitis affects approximately 35% of dentate United States adults aged 30 to 90 years, and approximately 13% have a moderate or severe form of the disease.[1] These statistics suggest that not everyone is equally susceptible to **periodontal diseases**. If susceptibility is not equal, then factors exist in tandem, which places certain individuals at an increased **risk** for disease. In this chapter, these factors are categorized as local, environmental, systemic, or economic (Figure 5-1). These factors also can be categorized as **nonmodifiable** and **modifiable**. By strict definition, however, a risk factor for disease must have been present before the onset of disease and must directly result in an increased likelihood of an individual being seen with the disease. In contrast, **risk indicators** can affect the course or progression of disease without truly being causal. These distinctions are less important than understanding that the presence of factors, indicators, or both, may increase the risk for the development of periodontal disease.

   Risk assessment includes identification of specific factors/indicators and an evaluation or judgment of their impact on the individual. The goal of risk assessment is to develop and implement strategies in those identified as being at risk for disease that will either prevent them from developing disease or improve the prognosis for those with existing disease.

BACKGROUND

Periodontal diseases are a heterogeneous group of disorders that can be divided into two broad groups: gingivitis and periodontitis. Both are inflammatory conditions usually initiated by a common primary etiologic agent: bacterial plaque. They differ, however, in the tissues involved

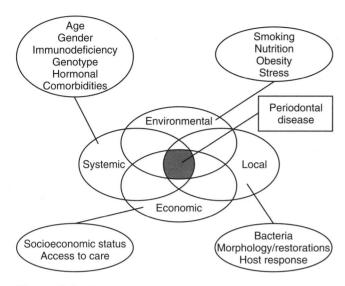

Figure 5-1 Risk model for periodontal disease.

and the extent of the inflammatory response. Gingivitis is confined to the gingival tissues and is reversible, and the inflammatory response in periodontitis damages not only the gingival tissues, but also the periodontal ligament, cementum, and alveolar bone. Periodontitis is therefore irreversible. The hallmarks of periodontitis are apical migration of the junctional epithelium and connective tissue attachment, with concomitant loss of alveolar bone.

Periodontitis can be further broken down into two major classifications: chronic periodontitis and aggressive periodontitis.[2] Both these forms of the disease can be further characterized by the extent of attachment loss (localized or generalized) and the severity of the disease (slight, moderate, or advanced). The majority of patients suffer from chronic periodontitis, a slowly progressive disease in which the presence of bacterial plaque and calculus clearly contributes to the risk for disease and disease progression. In contrast, aggressive periodontitis involves rapid attachment loss and bone destruction, often in the absence of significant amounts of microbial deposits. The localized form of aggressive periodontitis is a somewhat unique disease relative to other forms of periodontitis, because it usually occurs during adolescence; the subgingival microbiota demonstrates a high association with a single bacterium, *Actinobacillus actinomycetemcomitans* (currently named *Aggregatibacter actinomycetemcomitans*)[3]; bone resorption progresses at a rate 3 to 4 times faster than that observed for chronic periodontitis[4]; the disease may spontaneously arrest,[5] and it is localized to very specific teeth (first molars and incisors). Importantly, the disease tends to cluster in families suggesting the presence of a genetic predisposition.[6-12] A detailed description of the etiology of the disease is explored in Chapter 2.

In current practice, the primary means of detecting gingivitis and periodontitis include clinical assessment by using a periodontal probe to determine pocket depths and clinical attachment levels, and radiographic evaluation to determine alveolar bone levels. Evaluation of the results of the clinical and radiographic examinations, and information obtained from medical and dental histories, allows the clinician to establishment a diagnosis. Information obtained from the medical and dental histories, also allows the clinician to identify both modifiable and nonmodifiable risk factors/indicators that influence the patient's disease. This knowledge can be used to develop a plan of prevention tailored to the individual patient's needs.

RISK FACTORS/INDICATORS FOR PERIODONTAL DISEASES
Local Factors

Accumulation of a bacterial plaque biofilm at the gingival margin is the primary factor responsible for the initiation of gingivitis.[13] Studies conducted during the 1930s to 1970s emphasized the importance of the quantity of this microbial challenge to the disease process, leading to the development of the "nonspecific plaque hypothesis." In this model, individuals with significant amounts of plaque would be predicted to be at risk for developing significant disease, and those with limited accumulation would have little risk. This model was subsequently challenged, however, when investigators found that some patients exhibited severe loss of attachment in the absence of significant accumulations of bacterial plaque. This finding suggested that the quality of the plaque rather than the quantity was of prime importance in the disease process, a theory that became known as the "specific plaque hypothesis." This theory recognized that of the 500 to 700 different bacterial species present in the oral cavity,[14] only a limited number play a pivotal role in the initiation and progression of periodontal disease.[15-20] These organisms include three specific bacteria that have been identified as etiologic agents for periodontitis: *Porphyromonas gingivalis*, *Bacteroides forsythus (Tannerella forsythia)*, and *A. actinomycetemcomitans* (currently named *Aggregatibacter actinomycetemcomitans*).[21] Moderate evidence also exists that other species are etiologic factors in periodontitis (Box 5-1).[21]

Concerns with the specific plaque hypothesis exist among researchers. First, all of the potentially pathogenic organisms listed in Box 5-1 can be isolated from not only diseased individuals, but from those with a healthy periodontium.[22-24] This finding suggests that variability may exist in the pathogenic potential of different strains of the same bacterial species. Molecular examination of various strains of *A. actinomycetemcomitans*, demonstrated that strains associated with localized aggressive periodontitis differ from those found in other forms of periodontal disease or in health.[25-27] These data provide evidence that certain pathogenic strains or clones of bacterial species are associated with the initiation and progression of certain periodontal diseases.[28] Therefore, the presence of

PUTATIVE PERIODONTAL PATHOGENS

Actinobacillus actinomycetemcomitans
  (currently named *Aggregatibacter
  actinomycetemcomitans*)
Porphyromonas gingivalis
Bacteroides forsythus
  (currently named *Tannerella forsythia*)
Fusobacterium nucleatum
Campylobacter rectus
Prevotella intermedia/nigrescens
Peptostreptococcus micros
  (currently named *Micromonas micros*)
Eubacterium nodatum
Treponema denticola
Selemonas noxia
Eikenella corrodens

these clones in the oral flora would increase the risk of developing disease.

The second concern focuses on emerging evidence for the extreme microbial diversity of dental plaque. In the past, determining the extent of this diversity was limited by difficulties in culturing techniques. Recent advances in molecular biology have enabled investigators to determine that uncultivated species do appear to be associated with disease.[29-32] As a result, the evidence of increasing numbers of putative periodontal pathogens that place an individual at risk for developing periodontal disease is likely to expand well beyond those listed currently.

The presence of calculus, which serves as a reservoir for bacterial plaque, has been suggested as a risk factor for periodontitis. The presence of some calculus in healthy individuals receiving routine dental care does not result in significant loss of attachment. Calculus in other groups of patients, such as those not receiving regular care and patients with poorly controlled diabetes, can have a negative impact on periodontal health.[33] Several anatomical factors predispose the periodontium to disease as a result of their potential to harbor the pathogenic microorganisms found in bacterial plaque. These factors can include furcations, root concavities, developmental grooves, cervical enamel projections, enamel pearls, and bifurcation ridges. In addition to harboring bacterial plaque, these factors present a challenge to the clinician during instrumentation. Similarly, the presence of subgingival or overhanging margins, or both, can contribute to increased plaque accumulation, increased inflammation, and increased bone loss. Therefore, anatomical and restorative factors that promote plaque accumulation can play a role in specific teeth being at risk for periodontal disease.[34]

Although the accumulation of the bacterial plaque biofilm is the primary etiological factor in periodontal

diseases, the host response to this microbial challenge is primarily responsible for the inflammation and tissue destruction that are the hallmarks of these diseases. The accumulation of plaque in the gingival sulcus results in the release of bacterial products, such as lipopolysaccharide and bacterial antigens, that elicit an inflammatory host response. Fluid and host cells accumulate in the tissue leading to the erythema and edema that are synonymous with gingivitis. When the inflammatory response continues, neutrophils, macrophages, and lymphocytes migrate into the area, releasing destructive enzymes and inflammatory mediators. These mediators, which include cytokines, prostanoids, and matrix metalloproteinases, are responsible for the breakdown of the hard and soft tissues of the periodontium that characterize periodontitis.[35]

Environmental Factors

Cigarette smoking is an established risk factor for periodontal disease.[36,37] Assessment of the relationship between cigarette smoking and periodontitis in the National Health and Nutrition Examination Survey (NHANES III) revealed that on average, smokers were 4 times more likely to have periodontitis than those who had never smoked.[38] This increased risk was true after adjusting for age, gender, race/ethnicity, education, and income/poverty ratio. Former smokers were 1.68 times more likely to have periodontitis than persons who had never smoked. In addition, results from multiple cross-sectional and longitudinal studies have demonstrated that pocket depth, attachment loss, and alveolar bone loss are more prevalent and severe in patients who smoke compared with nonsmokers.[39-42]

The NHANES III study demonstrated a dose-response relationship between cigarettes smoked per day and the odds of having periodontitis. In participants who smoked less than 9 cigarettes per day, the odds for having periodontitis were 2.79 times higher than in nonsmokers, whereas participants who smoked more than 31 cigarettes per day were nearly 6 times more likely to have periodontitis. In former smokers, the odds of having periodontitis declined with the number of years since quitting.[38]

Although few studies have been conducted on the effects of cigar and pipe smoking on periodontal disease, there is a similar deleterious effect of those products on the periodontium.[37,43-45] The prevalence of moderate and severe periodontitis and the percentage of teeth with more than 5 mm of attachment loss was most severe in current cigarette smokers. Cigar and pipe smokers expressed a severity of disease between the current cigarette smokers and nonsmokers.[37] Cigar and pipe smokers also demonstrated increased tooth loss when compared with nonsmokers.[45]

Evidence of benefits of smoking cessation relative to disease severity and response to periodontal treatment has been clearly documented. In a comparison of the periodontal destruction in current smokers, former smokers, and those who have never smoked, the level of destruction in former smokers was between the level of destruction found in current and never smokers.[46-48] Smoking has an impact on the outcome of periodontal treatment, including nonsurgical, surgical, and regenerative therapy. Numerous studies have noted that current smokers demonstrate poorer responses than former or never smokers to treatment.[49-52] The intervention/cessation strategies described in Chapter 17 can have a positive impact on a patient's response to therapy.

Smokeless tobacco use is associated with oral leukoplakia and carcinoma.[53,54] Use of these substances does not appear to result in any generalized effects on periodontal disease progression, however, other than localized attachment loss and recession at the site of tobacco product placement.[55]

Systemic Factors

Age can be classified as a nonmodifiable factor for periodontal disease.[56] Both the prevalence and severity of periodontal disease increase with age.[57-59] However, aging alone will not increase periodontal disease risk. Increased loss of attachment and alveolar bone seen in older individuals results from consistent exposure to other risk factors during a person's life span, and a cumulative effect is created with time. In support of this, studies have shown minimal loss of attachment in aging subjects enrolled in lifelong preventive programs.[60,61] Although it is possible that degenerative changes related to aging may increase susceptibility to periodontitis, it appears that periodontal disease is not an inevitable consequence of the aging process and that aging alone does not increase the risk for developing disease. Factors associated with the aging process, such as systemic disease, physical and mental impairment, polypharmacy, decreased immune function, and altered nutritional status interact synergistically with other well-defined risk factors to increase susceptibility to periodontal disease.

The age at which an individual develops disease must be considered. Young individuals with periodontal disease are at greater risk for continued disease as they age. The younger the patient, the longer the exposure to etiologic factors throughout the life span. In addition, aggressive periodontitis in young individuals often is associated with a nonmodifiable risk factor such as a genetic predisposition to disease.[59] Evidence of loss of attachment may be of greater consequence in younger patients.

Gender can be classified as a nonmodifiable factor that plays a role in periodontal disease risk and progression.[56,62] National surveys conducted since 1960 demonstrate that males have greater loss of attachment[63,64] and poorer oral hygiene than females, as evidenced by higher levels of plaque and calculus.[64-66] In addition, women use health care services more frequently than men.[67] Gender differences in the risk for periodontitis are related to health

behaviors and decreased access to care, although gender-specific differences in the response to these factors can not be ruled out as potential contributors to an increased risk for disease.[56]

Earlier paradigms of the pathogenesis of periodontal disease state that environmental factors are primarily responsible for the variability in disease severity and progression seen in individuals. It is now widely accepted, however, that environmental factors alone can account for differences in disease in only a small proportion of individuals. The remainder of these differences can be attributed to the host's susceptibility to disease. Genetic variability among individuals may be classified as a nonmodifiable factor.[56] Studies conducted in twins have shown that similarities in the periodontal condition in pairs of identical (monozygous) twins were greater than the similarities found in fraternal (dizygous) twins. These studies support the concept of inheritance of risk for disease and provide evidence that genetic factors influence clinical measures of gingivitis, probing pocket depth, attachment loss, and interproximal bone height.[68-70] A population-based study that used data from 10,000 Swedish twin pairs revealed that genetic factors accounted for approximately one third of periodontal disease risk for women and men, and nonshared environmental factors accounted for the remaining variation.[71]

The familial aggregation seen in localized and generalized aggressive periodontitis is indicative of genetic involvement in these diseases.[9,72-74] A single/major locus autosomal dominant gene may be involved in the etiology of aggressive disease in a U.S. population,[74] and autosomal recessive inheritance has been seen in certain northern European and South American populations.[9,75] No specific genetic test has been developed that can accurately identify those at risk for periodontal disease. On the basis of the strong evidence for the familial nature of aggressive periodontitis, children and siblings of those diagnosed with aggressive disease may be at increased risk, and should be encouraged to receive regular periodontal evaluations and preventive care.

Results of a study by Kornman et al.[76] demonstrate that alterations in specific genes encoding the inflammatory cytokines, interleukin 1 alpha and interleukin 1 beta (IL-1α and IL-1β), were associated with severe chronic periodontitis in nonsmoking participants. These results led to the development of the Periodontal Susceptibility Test (PST), the only commercially available genetic susceptibility test for severe chronic periodontitis. The test is used to identify patients positive for the occurrence of allele 2 at the IL-1α +4845 and IL-1β +3954 loci. Persons with these combined alleles are hypothesized to produce more IL-1 in response to a microbial challenge, potentially leading to increased inflammation and destruction of the periodontal tissues. Results of other studies have shown limited association between this composite genotype and the presence of periodontitis.[77-79] Changes in the IL-1 genes may be only one of several genetic changes involved in the risk for chronic periodontitis. Although alterations in the IL-1 genes may be a valid marker for periodontitis in defined populations, the usefulness of these alterations as genetic markers in the general population may be limited.[80]

Genetic alterations can result in abnormalities in the host response. These alterations may include neutrophil abnormalities,[81] monocytic hyperresponsiveness to lipopolysaccharide stimulation,[82] and changes in the monocyte/macrophage receptors for the Fc portion of antibody.[80,83] These alterations can result in individuals exhibiting hyporesponsiveness or hyperresponsiveness to microbial challenge. Both groups of individuals would likely be at greater risk for developing periodontitis than normal responders. Genetics plays a role in regulating the titer of the protective IgG2 antibody response to *A. actinomycetemcomitans* in patients with aggressive periodontitis.[84] Commercially available tests for these alterations are currently not available.

The associations among periodontal infection, inflammation, and pregnancy have been well documented. "Pregnancy gingivitis" characterized by erythema, edema, hyperplasia, and increased bleeding, occurs in approximately 30% to 100% of pregnant women.[85,86] Increased tissue edema may lead to increased pocket depths and subsequent increased tooth mobility.[87] Changes occur in the subgingival microflora during pregnancy, with increases in anaerobic to aerobic ratios occurring in addition to *Bacteroides melaninogenicus* (currently named *Prevotella melaninogica)* and *Prevotella intermedia* proportions.[88] These increases may be related to hormonal modifications, specifically elevated levels of estradiol or progesterone. Pyogenic granulomas ("pregnancy tumors") frequently occur in pregnant women, most commonly during the second or third month of pregnancy.

Emotional stress can interfere with normal immune function,[89,90] resulting in increased levels of circulating hormones and inflammatory markers that can have an impact on the periodontium.[91] Stressful life events such as bereavement and divorce, in addition to financial strain, distress, and depression can lead to a higher prevalence and increased severity of periodontal disease.[92,93] Studies reveal that although stress may not be directly correlated with periodontal disease, the inability to cope with stress can be correlated to the incidence and severity of disease.[93,94] Altered coping mechanisms can result in behavioral changes that lead to smoking and poor oral hygiene, factors with a known impact on periodontal health.[56] Therefore, the effects of stress on the periodontium can be moderated by working with individuals to develop adequate coping mechanisms.

Nutritional status can be an underlying factor that determines the immune response to a microbial challenge. Additionally, diet influences dental plaque biofilm development and composition.[95-97] The change to the biofilm can alter the nature of the biological challenge faced by the host. Protein energy malnutrition can impair the acute-phase response to infection, impact the ability of neutrophils to kill bacteria, and decrease the antimicrobial properties of saliva. Studies conducted in animal models demonstrate that deficiencies of specific micronutrients alter immune responses. For example, experimental animals with vitamin A deficiency have increased susceptibility to infection, and vitamin-E–deficient animals have reduced adaptive immune responses and a subsequent decrease in antibody production. Water-soluble vitamins are involved in nucleic acid synthesis and cellular metabolism. Deficiencies in nutrients can affect neutrophil function and cytotoxic function of T cells. For example, immune cell function can be impacted by deficiencies in minerals such as iron and zinc. Iron deficiency diminishes the bactericidal activity of neutrophils and lymphocyte proliferation, and zinc deficiency is associated with impaired T-cell and B-cell formation in the bone marrow.[98]

Supplementation with nutrients known to have anti-inflammatory activity can have a positive impact on an individual's periodontal status. Dietary supplementation with n-3 polyunsaturated fatty acids (PUFA) may inhibit the synthesis of lipid mediators of inflammation and modulate cellular functions of neutrophils.[99] Rats given n-3 PUFA show an increase in bone formation, bone strength, bone-specific alkaline phosphatase activity, reduced mineral loss, and decreased *ex vivo* prostaglandin E2 production, suggesting a role for this dietary supplement in skeletal biology and bone health.[100-102] Results of two pilot studies have suggested a potential role for fatty acid supplementation in the management of periodontal disease. In the first, lower levels of inflammation were found when human experimental gingivitis was modified by n-3 PUFA administration.[103] In the second, borage oil supplementation in patients with adult periodontitis resulted in improved gingival inflammation as assessed by the Modified Gingival Index.[104] Although both studies did not include sufficient numbers of subjects to reach statistical significance, a trend existed toward decreased inflammation in the supplemented subjects. Vitamins C and E and carotenoids are extracellular antioxidants that can inhibit tissue damage by oxygen radicals released during an inflammatory response. An epidemiological study of vitamin C intake identified an association between periodontal disease and low dietary intake of vitamin C.[105,106] Studies of gingival tissues from animal models reported that lower gingival levels of vitamin E were found in those with periodontal disease compared with healthy controls.[107,108]

Body fat can serve as a promoter of inflammation. The possible links between obesity and a hyperinflammatory state, and aberrant lipid metabolism was explored relative to periodontitis.[109] Studies suggest a link between increased body mass index (BMI) and an increased risk for periodontitis.[110,111] Gingival bleeding and periodontal disease were associated with weight gain. Evidence exists that adipose tissue secretes a variety of molecules that contribute to low-grade inflammation. Therefore, increased body fat may modulate the host's inflammatory and immune response, leading to increased risk for periodontal disease.[112]

Immune dysfunction associated with human immunodeficiency virus (HIV) infection and acquired immunodeficiency syndrome (AIDS) increases the risk of periodontal disease. Epidemiological studies reveal that HIV-infected individuals have a higher prevalence of bone loss and attachment loss, with increased gingival recession, than control subjects.[113,114] More recent reports have failed to demonstrate significant differences between the periodontal status of individuals with HIV infection and that of healthy controls.[115,116] The apparent discrepancy in these reports may be the result of the inclusion of patients with AIDS (as opposed to patients who were exclusively HIV-seropositive) in some studies.[40] Reports about the periodontal status of patients who were either HIV-seropositive or who had AIDS stated that these patients often had severe periodontal destruction characteristic of necrotizing ulcerative periodontitis.[117] Newer therapies, however, exemplified by highly active antiretroviral therapy (HAART), decreased the incidence of these aggressive forms of periodontal disease in HIV-positive subjects.[118] AIDS-affected individuals, who practice good preventive oral health measures, including effective home care, and seek appropriate professional therapy, can maintain periodontal health.[119] It seems reasonable to hypothesize that HIV infection and immunosuppression are risk factors for periodontal disease.[40,62]

Both type 1 diabetes and type 2 diabetes are major risk factors for the development of periodontal disease in certain populations.[120-126] Potter et al.[127] demonstrated that Hispanic Americans with type 2 diabetes have more supragingival and subgingival calculus, increased extent and severity of periodontal destruction, and an increased frequency of tooth loss because of periodontitis. The role of diabetes as a risk factor for periodontal disease has been clearly established. Along with the relationship between periodontal disease and diabetes, prolonged hyperglycemia is responsible for diabetic complications such as retinopathy, nephropathy, and neuropathy. Infections are known to disturb the metabolic control of diabetes. Glycemic control is the hallmark of good metabolic management. In addition to the negative effects of diabetes on periodontal disease, periodontitis can impact the medical management of diabetes.[128-131] Grossi and Genco[132] proposed the following theory to explain why diabetics have more severe periodontitis. Nonenzymatic advanced glycation end products (AGEs) are the irreversible, glucose-derived compounds that form as a result of an elevated blood glucose concentration. AGE accumulation affects migration and phagocytic activities of mononuclear and polymorphonuclear cells, leading to a more pathogenic subgingival flora. AGE proteins upregulate cytokine production, including secretions of TNFα and IL1-β that may promulgate collagenase secretions

and connective tissue degradation. The interplay between the pathogenic microbiota and the host response is the hallmark of periodontal disease.

Periodontal inflammation occurs in approximately 30% to 100% of pregnant women,[85,86] and is related to plaque bacteria and hormonal changes.[87,88] Preterm labor (PTL) is associated with ascending intrauterine infection[133-137] accompanied by leukocyte infiltration, enhanced local production of cytokines and other inflammatory mediators, in addition to degradation of the extracellular matrix (ECM) in fetal membranes. Various microorganisms, such as *Prevotella* spp., *Porphyromonas* spp., and *Bacteroides* spp., normally associated with the oral biofilm, have been associated with bacterial vaginosis. Intraamniotic infections with *Fusobacterium* spp.,[138-140] viridans streptococci,[141] and at least 14 cases of chorioamnionitis related to *Capnocytophaga* spp.[142,143] were identified and associated with preterm labor. Studies support an association between periodontal infections and preterm birth/intrauterine growth retardation (PTB/IUGR)[144,145] in pregnant women who exhibited severe or generalized periodontal disease.[141,146] Jeffcoat et al.[147] studied 1313 pregnant women and demonstrated an increased odds ratio for preterm birth (PTB), low birth weight, or both, with increasing severity of periodontitis. Additionally, Lopez et al.[148] provided data on a randomized treatment study of periodontitis in pregnant women. A significant decrease in PTB, low birth weight infants, or both was demonstrated in the treatment group in this study. In contrast, findings of a recent multicenter intervention study demonstrated that treatment for periodontal disease does not alter the rates of preterm birth, low birth weight, or fetal growth restriction. Importantly, however, results of this study did demonstrate that periodontal treatment provided in the second and third trimesters of pregnancy is safe and that periodontal treatment does reduce the rates of spontaneous abortion and stillbirth.[149] A recent case-control study supported an association between severe maternal periodontal disease and spontaneous PTB at less than 32 weeks of gestation when compared with women with normal-term births or women with early indicated PTB at less than 32 weeks.[150] Recent evidence also exists to suggest that maternal periodontal disease not only increases the relative risk for preterm or spontaneous preterm births, but that periodontal disease progression during pregnancy is a predictor of the severe adverse outcome of very preterm birth. This finding is independent of traditional obstetric, periodontal, and social risk factors.[151] Finally, reports describe various study designs and a mixed outcome for this relationship, reflecting variations in patient populations, extent of disease, study design, and therapeutic approaches.[152,153]

Coronary heart disease and cerebrovascular disease (CVD) are attributed to atherosclerosis—a narrowing of the arteries because of deposition of cholesterol on arterial walls. Chronic inflammation associated with infection is implicated as an additional etiologic factor. Chronic infection directly interacts with the agent on the vessel wall or indirectly by modulation of the acute phase response leading to increased levels of acute phase reactants such as C-reactive protein.[154] Infectious agents implicated in CVD pathogenesis include *Chlamydia pneumoniae, Helicobacter pylori,* and cytomegalovirus. Although several studies have evaluated the impact of each of these microorganisms individually on the risk for CVD,[155-157] evidence supports a more significant role for the total bacterial burden rather than for a single microorganism. In this model, microorganisms have a cumulative burden of infection and resultant inflammatory response that contributes to atherosclerosis. In a study measuring IgG antibodies directed against a consortium of pathogens including cytomegalovirus, hepatitis A virus, herpes simplex virus 1 or 2, *C. pneumoniae* and *H. pylori,* an increasing pathogenic burden was significantly associated with increasing risk of myocardial infarction or death in a dose-dependent fashion.[158] Similarly, Espinola-Klein et al.[159] reported a significant increased risk for CVD death among participants seropositive to six to eight pathogens after adjusting for other risk factors for CVD. These studies support the relationship between chronic infections and CVD.

Epidemiologic studies reveal similar correlations between oral infections and cerebrovascular disease. Case-control studies show a positive association between indicators of poor dental health and outcomes associated with cerebrovascular disease.[160-162] Cross-sectional studies similarly support an association between periodontal disease and cerebrovascular events.[163-167] Tooth loss is related to greater carotid artery plaque prevalence.[168-169] Thicker carotid walls are associated with higher levels of *P. gingivalis, T. forsythia, A. actinomycetemcomitans,* and *T. denticola.*[170] Greater alveolar bone loss is associated with the presence of carotid artery plaque.[171] As a chronic, cyclical disease associated with a complex microbial biofilm and resultant local and systemic inflammatory response, periodontitis may present an additional microbial burden in individuals at risk for vascular disease.

Periodontal disease is a purported risk factor for dementias, including Alzheimer's disease. A study of 109 pairs of identical twins in the Swedish Twin Registry showed that the twin in each pair with dementia was 6 times more likely to have had a stroke, 4 times more likely to have periodontal disease by midlife, and 3 times more likely to have less education. Analysis of these data revealed that no one factor could account for the risk of dementia. In a separate analysis, the only factor that significantly served as a predictor for developing Alzheimer's disease was the presence of periodontal disease.[172]

Osteoporosis is another potential risk factor for periodontitis. Studies in animal models showed that osteoporosis does not initiate periodontitis, but evidence suggested that the reduced bone mass seen in animals with osteoporosis exacerbated periodontal disease progression.[173,174] Studies in humans suggest that women with low bone mineral density were more likely to have loss of attachment, gingival recession, and pronounced inflammation when compared with the control cohort.[175-177] Kribbs[178] examined pocket depth, bleeding on probing, and gingival recession in women with and without osteoporosis, and although the two groups had significant differences in bone mass, no differences in periodontal status were noted. A link may exist between loss of bone density associated with osteoporosis, heredity, and other host factors and periodontitis,[56,179,180] but additional studies are needed to clearly determine whether osteoporosis is a true risk factor for periodontal disease.

Economic Factors

Gingivitis and poor oral hygiene are related to lower socioeconomic status[62,181,182] attributable to decreased dental awareness and limited access to dental care. Individuals with more education and higher socioeconomic status (SES) are thought to practice consistent preventive behaviors and avoid more "unhealthy" behaviors such as smoking, poor diet, high alcohol consumption, and poor oral hygiene.[183] In a systematic literature review of studies that evaluated SES and risk for periodontal diseases, Kling and Norlund[184] determined that SES variables associated with periodontal diseases were of less importance than smoking. Therefore, lower SES alone does not result in increased risk for periodontal disease after adjusting for other risk factors such as smoking and poor oral hygiene.

RISK ASSESSMENT IN CLINICAL PRACTICE

Evaluation of data obtained during a routine patient visit can describe a patient's risk for developing periodontal disease. To develop a periodontal risk profile, the clinician should look at the interactions among demographic data, medical history, dental history, behavioral and social history, and results of the clinical periodontal examination. Demographic data provides information on the patient's age, gender, race/ethnicity, and socioeconomic status. The medical history of diseases such as diabetes, CVD, HIV/AIDS, pregnancy status, or osteoporosis aids in the development of a risk profile. The social/behavioral history provides details of the patient's smoking history, oral hygiene behaviors, and perceived level of stress. The dental history describes the frequency of dental care, health care beliefs and a family history of early tooth loss (suggestive of a genetic predisposition for aggressive periodontitis). The clinical examination documents the location and extent of bacterial plaque accumulation, the presence of plaque retentive factors such as overhanging restorations and subgingival margins, anatomical grooves, and furcation involvements, the presence of calculus, the extent of attachment loss, and the presence or absence of bleeding on probing.

Once collected, the information is analyzed to identify patients at risk for periodontal disease and the local, economic, environmental and systemic factors that contribute to their risk. The analysis is accomplished by evaluation of the information by the health care provider and/or through the use of computer-based information systems. An example of the latter is the Oral Health Information Suite (OHIS)™ and the Periodontal Assessment Tool (PAT) that is a component of the OHIS.[185] Twenty-three items taken from the periodontal examination generate a risk score for the patient that is used to develop a plan of prevention, adjust treatment plans, establish recall schedules, and evaluate outcomes of care. Longitudinal evaluations over time allow the health care provider and the patient to see changes in the risk and disease scores and to evaluate treatment progress. Risk-based systems engage the patient as a partner to outcomes of care.

Risk assessment is used to tailor periodontal disease prevention to the patient's profile. A patient with a history of diabetes should be informed of the relationship between diabetes and periodontitis. He or she also should be informed of the impact of poor diabetic control on the prognosis and the impact that controlling periodontal infection can have on his or her diabetic status. The treatment plan may be altered on the basis of the level of diabetic control, and a consultation with his or her physician may be indicated as part of the treatment plan. A patient diagnosed with aggressive periodontitis can be encouraged to have an immunological and microbiological assessment as part of his or her treatment plan. If alterations in the host response and specific microorganisms are identified, the treatment plan may be modified to include administration of systemic antimicrobial agents, host modifiers, or both. In all patients, once modifiable risk factors are implicated in the patient's disease profile, the patient can be instructed on reducing/controlling these factors. Reassessment of risk should become a component of the patient's care and lead to modifications on the basis of adherence to the established care program. Patient adherence to preventive programs is discussed in Chapter 11.

In summary, risk assessment identifies factors that predispose a patient to developing periodontal disease or influence the progression of disease that already exists. In either case, modification of the patient's prognosis, plan of prevention, and treatment plan are necessary both during the initial phase of therapy and during surgical or restorative care, or both. After an evaluation of the factors contributing to disease risk, patients can be educated about their risk, how to modify their risk for future disease, and, when appropriate, suitable intervention strategies can be implemented.

CONCLUSION

Periodontal diseases have a multifactorial etiology and risk for disease can be influenced by a number of nonmodifiable and modifiable factors. Additional studies that evaluate the significance of different genetic backgrounds and polymorphisms related to the host's response to a microbial challenge and which clarify the role of gender differences in the response to these local elements could lead to new diagnostic tests that would improve our ability to identify patients at risk of periodontal disease. The evaluation of intervention strategies that target modifiable elements such as smoking, stress, and nutrition also could lead to definitive information about the importance of those variables and the planned intervention.

A continuum clearly exists of both disease (ranging from health to severe disease) and the presence of risk elements (ranging from no risk factors to the entire list of factors presented in the preceding text). Further evaluation of computer-based systems designed to determine which risk elements are present, rank those elements, and use the ranking to place the patient on the disease continuum may provide the clinician with a very systematic approach to identifying patients at low, moderate, and high risk for periodontal diseases.

REFERENCES

1. Albander JM, Brunelle JA, Kingman A: Destructive periodontal disease in adults 30 years of age and older in the United States, 1988-1994, *J Periodontol* 70:13, 1999.
2. Armitage GC: Development of classification system for periodontal diseases and conditions, *Ann Periodontol* 4:1, 1999.
3. Zambon JJ, Christersson LA, Slots J: *Actinobacillus actinomycetemcomitans* in human periodontal disease. Prevalence in patient groups and distribution of biotypes and serotypes within families, *J Periodontol* 54:707, 1983.
4. Ruben MP: Periodontosis—an analysis and clarification of its status as a disease entity, *J Periodontol* 50:311, 1979.
5. Baer PN: The case for periodontosis as a clinical entity, *J Periodontol* 42:516, 1971.
6. Jorgenson RJ, Levin LS, Hutcherson ST et al.: Periodontosis in sibs, *Oral Surg* 39:396, 1975.
7. Melnick M, Shields ED, Bixler D: Periodontosis: a phenotypic and genetic analysis, *Oral Surg* 42:32, 1976.
8. Saxén L: Heredity of juvenile periodontitis, *J Clin Periodontol* 7:276, 1980.
9. Saxén L, Nevanlinna HR: Autosomal recessive inheritance of juvenile periodontitis: a test of a hypothesis, *Clin Genet* 25:332, 1984.
10. Boughman JA, Halloran SL, Roulston D et al.: An autosomal-dominant form of juvenile periodontitis: its localization to chromosome 4 and linkage to dentinogenesis imperfecta and Gc, *J Craniofac Genet* 6:341, 1986.
11. Beaty TH, Boughman JA, Yang P et al.: Genetic analysis of juvenile periodontitis in families ascertained through an affected proband, *Am J Human Genet* 40:44, 1987.
12. Hart TC, Marazita ML, Schenkein HA et al.: Re-interpretation of the evidence for X-linked dominant inheritance of juvenile periodontitis, *J Periodontol* 63:169, 1992.

13. Löe H, Theilade E, Jensen SB: Experimental gingivitis in man, *J Periodontol* 36:177, 1965.
14. Paster BJ, Boches SK, Galvin JL et al.: Bacteria diversity in human subgingival plaque, *J Bacteriol* 183:3770, 2001.
15. Loesche WJ: Chemotherapy of dental plaque infections, *Oral Sci Rev* 9:65, 1976.
16. Socransky SS: Microbiology of periodontal disease: present status and future considerations, *J Periodontol* 48:497, 1977.
17. Slots J: Subgingival microflora and periodontal disease, *J Clin Periodontol* 6:351, 1979.
18. Ranney R, Debski BF, Tew JG: Pathogenesis of gingivitis and periodontal disease in children and young adults, *Pediatr Dent* 3:89, 1981.
19. Slots J: Bacterial specificity in adult periodontitis. A summary of recent work, *J Clin Periodontol* 13:912, 1986.
20. Slots J, Listgarten MA: *Bacteroides gingivalis, Bacteroides intermedius* and *Actinobacillus actinomycetemcomitans* in human periodontal diseases, *J Clin Periodontol* 15:85, 1988.
21. Genco R, Kornman K, Williams R et al.: Consensus report: periodontal diseases: pathogenesis and microbial factors, *Ann Periodontol* 1:926, 1996.
22. Haffajee AD, Socansky SS: Microbial etiological agents of destructive periodontal diseases, *Periodontol 2000* 5:78, 1994.
23. Griffen AL, Becker MR, Lyons SR et al.: Prevalence of *Porphyromonas gingivalis* and periodontal health status, *J Clin Microbiol* 36:3239, 1998.
24. Papapanou PN, Neiderud A-M, Papadimitriou A et al.: "Checkerboard" assessments of periodontal microbiota and serum antibody responses: a case-control study, *J Periodontol* 71:885, 2000.
25. Haubek D, Poulsen K, Westergaard J et al.: Highly toxic clone of *Actinobacillus actinomycetemcomitans* in geographically widespread cases of juvenile periodontitis in adolescents of African origin, *J Clin Microbiol* 34:1576, 1996.
26. Zambon JJ, Haraszthy VI, Hariharan G et al.: The microbiology of early-onset periodontitis: association of highly toxic *Actinobacillus actinomycetemcomitans* strains with localized juvenile periodontitis, *J Periodontol* 67:282, 1996.
27. Bueno LC, Mayer MP, DiRienzo JM: Relationship between conversion of localized juvenile periodontitis-susceptible children from health to disease and *Actinobacillus actinomycetemcomitans* leukotoxin promoter structure, *J Periodontol* 69:998, 1998.
28. Guthmiller JM, Lally ET, Korostoff J: Beyond the specific plaque hypothesis: are highly leukotoxic strains of *Actinobacillus actinomycetemcomitans* a paradigm for periodontal pathogenesis, *Crit Rev Oral Biol Med* 12:116, 2001.
29. Choi BK, Paster BJ, Dewhirst FE et al.: Diversity of cultivable and uncultivable oral spirochetes from a patient with severe destructive periodontitis, *Infect Immun* 62:1889, 1994,
30. Spratt DA, Weightman AJ, Wade WG: Diversity of oral asaccharolytic *Eubacterium* species in periodontitis: identification of novel phylotypes representing uncultivated taxa, *Oral Microbiol Immunol* 14:56, 1999.
31. Kumar PS, Griffen AL, Barton JA et al.: New bacterial species associated with chronic periodontitis, *J Dent Res* 82:338, 2003.
32. Kumar PS, Griffen AL, Moeschberger ML et al.: Identification of candidate periodontal pathogens and beneficial species by quantitative 16S clonal analysis, *J Clin Microbiol* 43:3944, 2005.
33. Page RC, Beck JD: Risk assessment for periodontal diseases, *Int Den J* 47:61, 1997.
34. Blieden TM: Tooth-related issues, *Ann Periodontol* 4:91, 1999.
35. Preshaw PM, Seymour RA, Heasman PA: Current concepts in periodontal pathogenesis, *Dent Update* 31:570, 2004.
36. Ismail AI, Morrison EC, Burt BA et al.: Natural history of periodontal disease in adults: findings from the Tecumseh Periodontal Disease Study, *J Dent Res* 69:430, 1990.
37. Albandar JM, Streckfus CF, Adesanya MR et al.: Cigar, pipe, and cigarette smoking as risk factors for periodontal disease and tooth loss, *J Periodontol* 71:1874, 2000.
38. Tomar SL, Asma S: Smoking-attributable periodontitis in the United States: findings from NHANES III, *J Periodontol* 71:743, 2000.
39. Papapanou PN: Periodontal diseases: epidemiology, *Ann Periodontol* 1:1, 1996.
40. Papapanou PN: Risk assessments in the diagnosis and treatment of periodontal diseases, *J Dent Educ* 62:822, 1998.
41. Tonetti MS: Cigarette smoking and periodontal diseases: etiology and management of disease, *Ann Periodontol* 1998; 3:88.
42. Johnson GK, Hill M: Cigarette smoking and the periodontal patient, *J Periodontol* 75: 196, 2004.
43. Feldman RS, Bravacos JS, Close CL: Associations between smoking different tobacco products and periodontal disease indexes, *J Periodontol* 54:481, 1983.
44. Feldman RS, Alman JE, Chauncey HH: Periodontal disease indexes and tobacco smoking in healthy aging men, *Gerodontics* 3:43, 1987.
45. Krall EA, Garvey AJ, Garcia RI: Alveolar bone loss and tooth loss in male cigar and pipe smokers, *J Am Dent Assoc* 130:57, 1999.
46. Haber J, Kent RL: Cigarette smoking in periodontal practice, *J Periodontol* 63:100, 1992.
47. Bergström J, Eliasson S, Dock J: A 10 year prospective study of tobacco smoking and periodontal health, *J Periodontol* 71:1338, 2000.
48. Bergström J, Eliasson S, Dock J: Exposure to tobacco smoking and periodontal health, *J Clin Periodontol* 27:61, 2000.
49. Kaldahl WB, Johnson GK, Patil KD et al.: Levels of cigarette consumption and response to periodontal therapy, *J Periodontol* 67:675. 1996.
50. Scabbia A, Cho KS, Sigurdsson TJ et al.: Cigarette smoking negatively affects healing response following flap debridement surgery, *J Periodontol* 72:43, 2001.
51. Rieder C, Joss A, Lang NP: Influence of compliance and smoking habits on the outcomes of supportive periodontal therapy (SPT) in a private practice, *Oral Health Prev Dent* 2:89, 2004.
52. Sculean A, Stavropoulos A, Berakdar M et al.: Formation of human cementum following different modalities of regenerative therapy, *Clin Oral Investig* 9:58, 2005.
53. Creath CJ, Cutter G, Bradley DH et al.: Oral leukoplakia and adolescent smokeless tobacco use, *Oral Surg Oral Med Oral Pathol* 72:35, 1991.
54. Wray A, McGuirt WF: Smokeless tobacco usage associated with oral carcinoma: incidence, treatment, outcome, *Arch Otolaryngol Head Neck Surg* 119:929, 1993.
55. Robertson PB, Walsh M, Greene J et al.: Periodontal effects associated with the use of smokeless tobacco, *J Periodontol* 61:438, 1990.
56. Borrell LN, Papapanou PN: Analytical epidemiology of periodontitis, *J Clin Periodontol* 32:132, 2005.
57. Burt BA: Periodontitis and aging: reviewing recent evidence, *J Am Dent Assoc* 125:273, 1994.
58. Papapanou PN: Epidemiology and natural history of periodontal disease. In Lang NP, Karring T, editors: *Proceeding of the*

first European workshop on periodontology, London, 1994, Quintessence.

59. Papapanou PN: Risk assessments in the diagnosis and treatment of periodontal diseases, *J Den Edu* 62:822, 1998.

60. Papapanou PN, Lindhe J: Preservation of probing attachment and alveolar bone levels in two random population samples, *J Clin Periodontol* 19:583, 1992.

61. Papapanou PN, Lindhe J, Sterrett JD et al.: Considerations on the contribution of aging to loss of periodontal tissue support, *J Clin Periodontol* 18:611, 1991.

62. American Academy of Periodontology: Position paper: epidemiology of periodontal diseases, *J Periodontol* 67:935, 1996.

63. U.S. Public Health Service, National Center for Health Statistics: Basic data on dental examination findings of persons 1-74 years, United States 1971-1974, DHEW PHS Publ. No 79-1662, Series 11 No. 214, Washington, DC, 1979, Government Printing Office.

64. U.S. Public Health Service, National Institute of Dental Research: Oral health of United States adults: national findings, NIH Publ No 87-2868, Bethesda, MD, 1987, NIDR.

65. U.S. Public Health Service, National Center for Health Statistics: Oral hygiene in adults, United States 1960-1962, PHS Publ. No 1000, Series 11 No 16, Washington, DC, 1966, Government Printing Offic.

66. Abdellatif HM, Burt BA: An epidemiological investigation into the relative importance of age and oral hygiene status as determinants of periodontitis, *J Dent Res* 66:13, 1987.

67. Dunlop DD, Manheim LM, Song J et al.: 2002. Gender and ethnic/racial disparities in health care utilization among older adults, *J Gerontol Series B—Psychological Sciences and Social Sciences* 57:S221, 2002.

68. Michalowicz BS, Aeppli DP, Kuba RK et al.: A twin study of genetic variation in proportional radiographic alveolar bone height, *J Dent Res* 70:1431, 1991.

69. Michalowicz BS, Aeppli DP, Virag JG et al.: Risk findings in adult twins, *J Periodontol* 62:293, 1991.

70. Michalowicz BS, Diehl SR, Gunsolley JC et al.: Evidence for a substantial genetic basis for risk of adult periodontitis, *J Periodontol* 71:1699, 2000.

71. Mucci LA, Bjorkman L, Douglass CS et al.: Environmental and heritable factors in the etiology of oral diseases—a population-based study of Swedish twins, *J Dent Res* 34:800, 2005.

72. Benjamin SD, Baer PN: Familial patterns of advanced alveolar bone loss in adolescence (periodontosis), *Periodontics* 5:82, 1967.

73. Butler JH: A familial pattern of juvenile periodontitis (periodontosis), *J Periodontol* 40:115, 1968.

74. Marazita ML. Burmeister JA, Gunsolley JC et al.: Evidence for autosomal dominant inheritance and race-specific heterogeneity in early-onset periodontitis, *J Periodontol* 65:623, 1994.

75. Lopez NJ: Clinical, laboratory, and immunological studies of a family with a high prevanece of prepubertal and juvenile periodontitis, *J Periodontol* 63:457, 1992.

76. Kornman KS, Crane S, Wang HY et al.: The interleukin-1 genotype as a severity factor in adult periodontal disease, *J Clin Periodontol* 24:72, 1997.

77. Mark LL, Haffajee AD, Socransky SS et al.: Effect of the interleukin-1 genotype on monocyte IL-1β expressions in subjects with adult periodontitis, *J Periodont Res* 35:172, 2000.

78. Thomson WM, Edwards SJ, Dobson-Le DP et al.: Il-1 genotype and adult periodontitis among young New Zealanders, *J Dent Res* 80:1700, 2001.

79. Papapanou PN, Neiderud A-M, Sandros J et al.: Interleukin-1 gene polymorphism and periodontal status. A case-control study, *J Clin Periodontol* 28:389, 2001.

80. Kinane DF, Hart TC: Genes and gene polymorphisms associated with periodontal disease, *Crit Rev Oral Biol Med* 14:430, 2003.

81. Hart TC, Shapira L, Van Dyke TE: Neutrophil defects as risk factors for periodontal diseases, *J Periodontol* 65: 521, 1994.

82. Shapira L, Soskolone WA, Van Dyke TE et al.: Prostaglandin E2 secretion, cell maturation, and CD14 expression by monocyte-derived macrophages from localized juvenile periodontitis patients, *J Periodontol* 67:224, 1996.

83. Wilson ME, Kalmar JR: FcγIIa (CD32): a potential marker defining susceptibility to localized juvenile periodontitis, *J Periodontol* 67:323. 1996.

84. Gunsolley JC, Tew JG, Gooss CM et al.: Effects of race, smoking and immunoglobulin allotypes on IgG subclass concentrations, *J Periodont Res* 32:381, 1997.

85. Löe J, Silness J: Periodontal disease in pregnancy. Prevalence and severity, *Acta Odontol Scan* 21:533, 1984.

86. Levin RP: Pregnancy gingivitis, *Maryland State Dental Association* 30:27, 1987.

87. Raber-Durlacher JE, van Steenbergen TJM, van der Velden U: Experimental gingivitis during pregnancy and postpartum; clinical endocrinological and microbiological aspects, *J Clin Periodontol* 21:549, 1994.

88. Kornman KS, Loesche WJ: The subgingival flora during pregnancy, *J Periodontol* 15:111, 1980.

89. Ballieux RE: Impact of mental stress on the immune response, *J Clin Periodontol* 18:427, 1991.

90. Sternberg EM, Chrousos GP, Wilder RL et al.: The stress response and the regulation of inflammatory disease, *Ann Intern Med* 117:854, 1992.

91. Rose RM: Endocrine responses to stressful psychological events, *Psychiatr Clin N Am* 3:251, 1980.

92. Green LW, Tryon WW, Marks B et al.: Periodontal disease as a function of life events stress, *J Stress* 12:32, 1986.

93. Genco RJ, Ho AW, Grossi SG et al.: Relationship of stress, distress, and inadequate coping behaviors to periodontal disease, *J Periodontol* 70:711, 1999.

94. Genco RJ, Ho AW, Kopman J et al.: Models to evaluate the role of stress in periodontal disease, *Ann Periodontol* 3:288, 1998.

95. Bowden GH, Li YH: Nutritional influences on biofilm development, *Adv Dent Res* 11:81, 1997.

96. Schilling KM, Blitzer MH, Bowen WH: Adherence of *Streptococcus mutans* to glucans formed in situ in salivary pellicle, *J Dent Res* 68:1678, 1989.

97. Fletcher M: The physiological activity of bacteria attached to solid surfaces, *Adv Microb Physiol* 32:52, 1991.

98. Boyd LD, Madden TE: Nutrition, infection, and periodontal disease, *Dent Clin North Am* 47:337, 2003.

99. Sperling PI: Dietary omega-3 fatty acids: effects on lipid mediators of inflammation and rheumatoid arthritis, *Rheum Dis Clin North Am* 17:373, 1991.

100. Li Y, Watkins BA: Conjugated linoleic acids alter bone fatty acid composition and reduce ex vivo prostaglandin E2 biosynthesis in rats fed n-6 or n-3 fatty acids, *Lipids* 33:417, 1998.

101. Seifert MF, Ney DM, Grahn M et al.: Dietary conjugated linoleic acids alter serum IGF-I and IGF binding protein concentrations and reduce bone formation in rats fed (n-6) or (n-3) fatty acids, *J Bone Miner Res* 14:1153, 1999.

102. Watkins BA Allen KG, Hoffmann WE, Seifert MF: Dietary ratio of (n-6)/(n-3) polyunsaturated fatty acids alters the fatty acid composition of bone compartments and biomarkers of bone formation in rats, *J Nutr* 130:2274, 2000.

103. Campan P, Planchard PO, Duran D: Pilot study of n-3 polyunsaturated fatty acids in the treatment of human experimental gingivitis, *J Clin Periodontol* 24:907, 1997.

104. Rosenstein ED, Kushner LJ, Kramer N et al.: Pilot study of dietary fatty acid supplementation in the treatment of adult periodontitis, *Prostaglandins Leukot Essent Fatty Acids* 68:213, 2003.

105. Nishida M, Grossi SG, Dunford RG et al.: Dietary vitamin C and the risk for periodontal disease, *J Periodontol* 71:1215, 2000.

106. Leggott PJ, Robertson PB, Jacob RA et al.: Effects of ascorbic acid depletion and supplementation on periodontal health and subgingival microflora in humans, *J Dent Res* 70:1531, 1991.

107. Offenbacher S, Odle BM, Green MD et al.: Inhibition of human periodontal prostaglandin E2 synthesis with selected agents, *Agents Actions* 29:232, 1990.

108. Cohen ME, Meyer DM: Effect of dietary vitamin E supplementation and rotational stress on alveolar bone loss in rats, *Arch Oral Biol* 38:601, 1993.

109. Saito T, Shimazaki Y, Sakamoto M: Obesity and periodontitis, *N Engl J Med* 339:482, 1998.

110. Saito T, Shimazaki Y, Koga T et al.: Relationship between upper body obesity and periodontitis, *J Dent Res* 80:1631, 2001.

111. Wood N, Johnson RB, Streckfus CF: Comparison of body composition and periodontal disease using nutritional assessment techniques: Third National Health and Nutrition Examination Survey (NHANES III), *J Clin Periodontol* 30:321, 2003.

112. Ritchie CS, Kinane DF: Nutrition, inflammation, and periodontal disease, *Nutrition* 19:475, 2003.

113. Barr C, Lopez MR, Rua-Dobles A: Periodontal changes by HIV serostatus in a cohort of homosexual and bisexual men, *J Clin Periodontol* 19:794, 1992.

114. Yeung SCH, Stewart GJ, Cooper DA et al.: Progression of periodontal disease in HIV seropositive patients, *J Periodontol* 64:651, 1993.

115. Swango PA, Kleinman DV, Konzelman JL: HIV and periodontal health: a study of military personnel with HIV, *J Am Dent Assoc* 122:49, 1991.

116. Lamster IB, Begg MD, Mitchell L et al.: Oral manifestations of HIV infection in homosexual men and intravenous drug users: study design and relationship of epidemiologic, clinical, and immunologic parameter to oral lesions, *Oral Surg Oral Med Oral Pathol* 78:163, 1994.

117. Winkler JR, Herrera C, Westenhouse J et al.: Periodontal disease in HIV-infected and uninfected homosexual and bisexual men [letter], *AIDS* 6:1041, 1992.

118. McCaig RG, Thomas JC, Patton LL et al.: Prevalence of HIV-associated periodontitis and chronic periodontitis in a southeastern US study group, *J Public Health Dent* 58:294, 1998.

119. Stanford TW, Rees TD: Acquired immune suppression and other risk factors/indicators for periodontal disease progression, *Periodontol 2000* 32:118, 2003.

120. Ervasti T, Knuuttila M, Pohjamo L et al.: Relationship between control of diabetes and gingival bleeding, *J Periodontol* 56:154, 1985.

121. Tervonen T, Knuuttila M: Relation of diabetes control to periodontal pocketing and alveolar bone level, *Oral Surg Oral Med Oral Pathol* 61:346, 1986.

122. Emrich LJ, Schlossman M, Genco RJ: Periodontal disease in non-insulin dependent diabetes mellitus, *J Periodontol* 62:123, 1991.

123. Oliver RC, Tervonen T: Periodontitis and tooth loss: comparing diabetics with the general population, *JADA* 124:71, 1993.

124. Tervonen T, Oliver RC: Long-term control of diabetes and periodontitis, *J Clin Periodontol* 20:431, 1993.

125. Grossi SG, Zambon JJ, Ho AW et al.: Assessment of risk for periodontal disease. I. Risk indicators for attachment loss, *J Periodontol* 65:260, 1994.

126. Oliver RC, Tervonen T: Diabetes—a risk factor for periodontitis in adults?, *J Periodontol* 65:530, 1994.

127. Potter RM, Ebersole JL, Holt SC et al.: NIDDM in Hispanics: increased frequency and severity of periodontal disease, *J Dent Res* 74:(Special Issue)Abst. 927, 1995.

128. Miller LS, Manwell MA, Newbold D et al.: The relationship between reduction in periodontal inflammation and diabetes control: a report of 9 cases, *J Periodontol* 63:843, 1992.

129. Grossi SG, Skrepcinski FB, DeCaro T et al.: Treatment of periodontal disease in diabetics reduces glycated hemoglobin, *J Periodontol* 68:713, 1997.

130. Taylor GW: Bi-directional interrelationships between diabetes and periodontal diseases: and epidemiologic perspective, *Ann Periodontol* 6:99, 2001.

131. Taylor GW: The effects of periodontal treatment on diabetes, *JADA* 134:41S, 2003.

132. Grossi SG, Genco RJ: Periodontal disease and diabetes mellitus: a two-way relationship, *Ann Periodontol* 3:151, 1998.

133. Gibbs RS, Romero R, Hillier SI et al.: A review of premature birth and subclinical infection, *Am J Obstet Gynecol* 166:1515, 1992.

134. Brocklehurst P, Hannah M, McDonald H: Interventions for treating bacterial vaginosis in pregnancy, *Cochrane Database Syst Rev* 2:CD000262, 2003.

135. Goldenberg R, Hauth J, Andrews WW: Intrauterine infection and preterm delivery, *N Engl J Med* 342:1500, 2000.

136. King J, Flenady V: Antibiotics for preterm labour with intact membranes, *Cochrane Database Syst Rev* 2:CD000246, 2000.

137. McGregor J, French J: Bacterial vaginosis in pregnancy, *Obstet Gynecol Surv* 55: S1, 2000.

138. Hillier SL, Nugent RP, Eschenbach DA et al.: Association between bacterial vaginosis and preterm delivery of a low birthweight infant, *N Engl J Med* 333:1737, 1995.

139. Dezoete J, MacArthur B: Some influences on cognitive development in a group of very low birthweight infants at four years, *N Z Med J* 113: 207, 2000.

140. Irving R, Belton N, Elton RA et al.: Adult cardiovascular risk factors in premature babies, *Lancet* 355: 2135-2136, 2000.

141. Offenbacher S, Jared HL, O'Reilly PG et al.: Potential pathogenic mechanisms of periodontitis-associated pregnancy complications, *Ann Periodontol* 3:233, 1998.

142. Douvier S, Neuwirth C, Filipuzzi L et al.: Chorioamnionitis with intact membranes caused by *Capnocytophaga sputigena*, *Eur J Obstet Gynecol Reprod Biol* 83:109.1999.

143. Hill GB: Preterm birth: associations with genital and possibly oral microflora, *Ann Periodontol* 3:222, 1998.

144. Offenbacher S: Periodontal diseases: pathogenesis, *Ann Periodontol* 1:821, 1996.

145. Dasanayake AP: Periodontal disease as a risk factor in pregnancy, *Ann Periodontol* 3:206, 1998.

146. Mitchell-Lewis D, Engebretson SP, Chen J et al.: Periodontal infections and pre-term birth: early findings from a cohort of young minority women in New York, *J Oral Sci* 109:34, 2001.

147. Jeffcoat MJ, Geurs NC, Reddy MS et al.: Periodontal infection and preterm birth: results of a prospective study, *J Am Dent Assoc* 132:875, 2001.

148. Lopez NJ, Smith PC, Gutierrez J: Higher risk of preterm birth and low birth weight in women with periodontal disease, *J Dent Res* 81:58, 2002.

149. Michalowicz BS, Hodges JS, DiAngelis AJ et al.: Treatment of periodontal disease and the risk of preterm birth, *N Engl J Med* 355:1885, 2007.

150. Goepfert AR, Jeffcoat MK, Andrews WW et al.: Periodontal disease and upper genital tract inflammation in early spontaneous preterm birth, *Obstet Gynecol* 104:777, 2004.

151. Offenbacher S, Boggess KA, Murtha AP et al.: Progressive periodontal disease and risk for very preterm delivery, *Obstet Gynecol* 107:29, 2006.

152. Moore M, Ide E, Wilson M et al.: Periodontal disease and adverse pregnancy outcome. A prospective study, *J Dent Res* (Special Issue A) Abstract 1750, 81:A230, 2002.

153. Jarjoura P, Devine A, Perez-Delboy M: Periodontal disease and preterm birth: A case control study, *J Dent Res* (Special Issue A) Abstract 1754, 81:A231, 2002.

154. Offenbacher S, Beck JD: A perspective on the potential cardioprotective benefits of periodontal therapy, *Am Heart J* 149:950, 2005.

155. Gupta S, Leathan EW, Carrington D et al.: Elevated *Chlamydia pneumoniae* antibodies, cardiovascular events, and azithromycin in male survivors of myocardial infarction, *Circulation* 96:404, 1997.

156. Danesh J: Coronary heart disease, *Helicobacter pylori*, dental disease, *Chlamydia pneumoniae*, and cytomegalovirus: meta-analyses of prospective studies, *Am Heart J* 138:S434, 1999.

157. Higgins JP: *Chlamydia pneumoniae* and coronary artery disease: the antibiotic trials, *Mayo Clin Proc* 78:321, 2003.

158. Zhu J, Nieto FJ, Horne BD et al.: Prospective study of pathogen burden and risk of myocardial infraction or death, *Circulation* 103:45, 2001.

159. Espinola-Klein C, Rupprecht JH, Blankenberg S et al.: Impact of infectious burden on extent and long-term prognosis of atherosclerosis, *Circulation* 105:15, 2002.

160. Mattila KJ, Valle MS, Nieminen MS et al.: Dental infections and coronary atherosclerosis, *Atherosclerosis* 103:205, 1993.

161. Mattila KJ, Nieminem MS, Valtonen VV et al.: Association between dental health and acute myocardial infarction, *BMJ* 298:779, 1999.

162. Mattila KJ, Asikainen S, Wolf J et al.: Age, dental infections, and coronary heart disease, *J Dent Res* 79:756, 2000.

163. Emingil G, Buduneli E, Aliyev A et al.: Association between periodontal disease and acute myocardial infarction, *J Periodontol* 71:1882, 2000.

164. DeStefano F, Anda RF, Kahn HS et al.: Dental disease and risk of coronary heart disease and mortality, *BMJ* 306:688, 1993.

165. Paunio K, Impivaara O, Tiesko J et al.: Missing teeth and ischaemic heart disease in men aged 45-64 years, *Eur Heart J* 14:54, 1993.

166. Joshipura KJ, Rimm EB, Douglass CW et al.: Poor oral health and coronary heart disease, *J Dent Res* 75:1631, 1996.

167. Beck J, Garcia R, Heiss G et al.: Periodontal disease and cardiovascular disease, *J Periodontol* 67:1123, 1996.

168. Desvarieux M, Demmer RT, Rundek T et al.: Relationship between periodontal disease, tooth loss, and carotid artery plaque: the Oral Infections and Vascular Disease Epidemiology Study (INVEST), *Stroke* 34:2120, 2003.

169. Desvariuex M, Schwahn C, Volzke H et al.: Gender differences in the relationship between periodontal disease, tooth loss and atherosclerosis, *Stroke* 35:2029, 2004.

170. Desvarieux M, Demmer RT, Rundek T et al.: Periodontal microbiota and carotid intima-media thickness: the Oral Infections and Vascular Disease Epidemiology Study (INVEST), *Circulation* 111:576, 2005.

171. Engebretson SP, Lamster IB, Elkind MS et al.: Radiographic measures of chronic periodontitis and carotid artery plaque, *Stroke* 36:561, 2005.

172. Gatz M, Mortimer JA, Fratiglioni L et al.: Potentially modifiable risk factors for dementia in identical twins, *Alzheimer's Dementia* 2:110-117, 2006.

173. Aufdemorte TB, Boyan BD, Fox WC et al.: Diagnostic tools and biologic markers: animal models in the study of osteoporosis and oral bone loss, *J Bone Miner Res* 8:S529, 1993.

174. Krook L, Whalen JP, Lesser GV et al.: Experimental studies on osteoporosis, *Methods Achiev Exp Pathol* 7:72, 1975.

175. Van Wowern J, Klausen B, Kollerup G: Osteoporosis: a risk factor in periodontal disease, *J Periodontol* 65:134, 1994.

176. Mohammad AR, Brunsvold M, Bauer R: The strength of association between systemic postmenopausal osteoporosis and periodontal disease, *Int J Prosthodont* 9:47, 1996.

177. Tezal M, Wactawski-Wende J, Grossi SG et al.: The relationship between bone mineral density and periodontitis in postmenopausal women, *J Periodontol* 71:1492, 2000.

178. Kribbs PJ: Comparison of mandibular bone in normal and osteoporotic women, *J Prosthet Dent* 63:218, 1990.

179. Kinane DF: Periodontitis modified by systemic factors, *Ann Periodontol* 4:55, 1999.

180. Guers NC, Lewis CE, Jeffcoat MJ: Osteoporosis and periodontal disease progression, *Periodontol 2000* 32:105, 2003.

181. U.S. Public Health Service, National Center for Health Statistics: Periodontal Disease in Adults, United States 1960-1962, PHS Publ. No 1000, Series 11 No 12, Washington, DC, 1965, Government Printing Office.

182. U.S. Public Health Service, National Center for Health Statistics: Basic data on dental examination findings of persons 1-74 years; United States 1971-1974, DHEW PHS Publ No 79-1662, Series 11 No. 214, Washington, DC, 1979, Government Printing Office.

183. Sheiham A, Nicolau B: Evaluation of social and psychological factors in periodontal disease, *Periodontol 2000* 39:118, 2005.

184. Kling B, Norlund A: A social-economic perspective on periodontal diseases—a systematic review, *J Clin Periodontol* 32:314, 2005.

185. Page RC, Martin JA, Loeb CF: The oral health information suite (OHIS): its use in the management of periodontal disease, *J Dent Educ* 69:509, 2005.

Chapter 6

Oral Cancer and Associated Risk Factors

DANIEL L. JONES AND K. VENDRELL RANKIN

RISK FACTORS

Nonmodifiable Risk Factors
Modifiable Risk Factors
    Smoking
    Tobacco Use in Other Forms
    Alcohol
    Sunlight (Actinic Radiation)
    Immune System Deficiencies
    Infections
    Nutritional Deficiencies
    Other Oral Conditions

DETECTION AND DIAGNOSIS

Clinical Examination
Biopsy
Diagnostic Aids

SUMMARY

LEARNING OBJECTIVES

Upon completion of this chapter, the learner will be able to:
- Outline the risk factors for oral cancer.
- Differentiate between modifiable and nonmodifiable risk factors.
- Discuss the strength of the evidence associated with each of the putative risk factors.
- Know current techniques to detect and diagnose oral cancer.
- Describe the evidence for the efficacy and appropriate use of current diagnostic techniques.

KEY TERMS

Initiator
Promoter
Leukoplakia
Erythroplakia
Erythroleukoplakia
Risk factor (modifiable and nonmodifiable)
Relative risk
Pack-year
Bidi
Kretek
Hookah
Biopsy
Brush biopsy
Toluidine blue

Almost 30,000 new cases and more than 7000 deaths from cancers of the oral cavity and pharynx are expected to occur each year in the United States.[1] These statistics have remained constant during the past decade. These statistics fail to underscore disparities in the extent of oral cancer in the population. Incidence rates are more than twice as high in men when compared with women, and are highest among black men.[2] Although the 5-year survival rate may be as high as 80% for lesions diagnosed at the localized stage, the overall rate for survival for all stages is only 50%, and for primary lesions with distant metastases, survival may be as low as 15%. More than half of all oral cancer cases are not diagnosed until regional spread has occurred. A fundamental understanding of the disease, including risk factors and strategies for prevention and early detection, is a vital component of all dental professional education.

Current evidence underscores the multifactorial nature of carcinogenesis in oral cancer. An individual's genotype can influence cancer risk, but genetic predisposition is responsible for only a fraction of all cancers. The factor that most strongly influences susceptibility to oral cancer, as with other neoplasms, is age. If an individual lives long enough, he or she will develop some form of cancer. Carcinogenesis is theorized to have at least two stages, or intracellular transitions. Carcinogenic agents are **initiators** if they act in the early stages and **promoters** if they act in later stages of the disease. Differences in exposure to various carcinogenic initiators or promoters result in incidence rates that vary among specific groups or populations. A body of evidence has identified certain exposures as risk factors for oral cancer. Tobacco and alcohol are significant risk factors for oral cancer, in addition to actinic radiation (sunlight exposure), immune system deficiencies, viral infections, nutritional deficiencies, and certain oral conditions. A previous history of oral cancer places an individual at greater risk for the future development of oral cancer.[3]

Cancers of the oral cavity and pharynx arise primarily from epithelial cells, and almost all (90%) are squamous cell carcinomas (OSCC).[3] Typically, premalignant changes and dysplasia precede malignant oral lesions. **Leukoplakia** (a raised white patch on the mucosa that cannot be scraped off), **erythroplakia** (a reddened, erythematous area), and **erythroleukoplakia** (a white patch with a red component) are the most common clinical manifestations in the oral cavity. These manifestations are described in Chapter 3. The transformation of healthy oral epithelium to invasive and metastatic carcinoma is characterized by accumulation of genetic mutations that disrupt normal cell growth.[4] The most common change seen in oral cancer is chromosomal loss at *9p21*.[5] Inactivation of the tumor suppressor gene at *9p21* (p14^{ARF}) decreases *p53* degradation and increases *p53* levels. Approximately half of all primary OSCC lesions exhibit *p53* mutations and diminished *p53* tumor suppressor activity. Malignant progression in leukoplakia is strongly associated with heterozygosity at 3p14-21 or 9p21.[6-9] Mutations of the *p53* gene commonly occur in leukoplakias among tobacco users, but are not observed in premalignant oral lesions in nontobacco users.[10] Mutations of *p53* increase with the number of cigarettes smoked and are augmented by alcohol intake.[11] Chromosomal losses associated with the progression of head and neck cancers are more common in the tumors of smokers than nonsmokers.[11,12]

RISK FACTORS

A **risk factor** for any disease is defined as something that increases the likelihood of developing that disease. Risk factors may be **modifiable** or **nonmodifiable**. A modifiable risk factor is one that the individual may be able to control. Modifiable risk factors are primarily associated with environmental and behavioral choices. These include, for example, tobacco and alcohol use. A nonmodifiable risk factor is a factor that is considered outside of one's control, including heredity and demographic variables such as age and gender. Similar to other oral diseases, oral cancer is multifactorial and risk factors associated with oral cancer include behavioral, biological, and economic variables. A risk model for oral cancer that contains modifiable and nonmodifiable factors is provided in Figure 6-1.

Nonmodifiable Risk Factors

Gender plays a significant role in the distribution of oral cancer in the general population. Males have significantly higher incidence rates for all oral cancers compared with females, and more than twice the lifetime probability of developing oral cancer.[13] The overall male-to-female ratio is currently 2.4:1, but varies by site from 1.5:1 for salivary gland, gingival, and oropharyngeal tumors to as high as 4.3:1 for hypopharyngeal sites.[14] Although males are at a significantly greater risk for oral cancer, the 5-year survival rates for males and females do not differ significantly.[15]

Racial/ethnic background is also a significant risk factor for oral cancer. Blacks have higher incidence rates than whites for some oral cancers (hypopharynx, oropharynx, tonsil, and floor of the mouth), but lower rates for developing oral cancer at other sites (lip, tongue, and salivary glands).[13] Asian-Pacific Islanders have lower incidence rates than whites or blacks for all oral cancers. Blacks are more frequently diagnosed with oral cancer at an advanced stage and 5-year survival rates for blacks are consistently lower than those of whites and Asian-Pacific Islanders, for all sites except the lip.[13] Mortality rates for blacks are almost one third higher than for whites and are more than twice that of Asian-Pacific Islanders, American Indians, and Hispanics. In general, black males

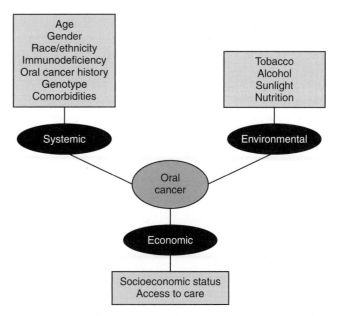

Figure 6-1 Risk model for oral cancer. Oral cancer is a multifactorial disease process that includes systemic, environmental, and economic effects. The interplay of these variables ultimately lead to the incidence of this disease. The multifactorial nature of oral cancer should be addressed in the assessment of a patient's risk.

have the highest probability of developing oral cancer and experience an associated increased rate of mortality.

As with all forms of cancer, the incidence of oral cancer increases markedly with age. In 2002, approximately 20% of oral cancers were diagnosed in individuals younger than 50 years, and more than half were diagnosed before the age of 70 years. The relationship of cancer to age is considered to be related to duration (length of time) of exposure.

A previous history of oral cancer is associated with a higher risk of recurrence. Overall, 18% of patients develop second primary oral or pharyngeal cancers in an average of 5 years after diagnosis of the initial lesion. Patients who continue their tobacco use habits may increase their risk of a second primary cancer by as much as 30%.

Modifiable Risk Factors

Smoking. Tobacco use is currently the leading preventable cause of death in the United States.[16] Cigarette smoking causes an estimated 440,000 deaths, about 1 of every 5 deaths, each year.[17,18] More deaths are caused each year by tobacco use than from human immunodeficiency virus (HIV), illegal drug use, alcohol use, motor vehicle injuries, suicides, and murders combined.[17,19] Cigarettes, cigar, and pipe smoking as well as smokeless (spit) tobacco use are all associated with an increased risk for oral cancer.[16-20] Furthermore, the risk of oral cancer associated with tobacco use is dose-dependent.

Since 1964, the Surgeon General's Reports on smoking and health have implicated the use of smoking and smokeless tobacco as a cause of cancers of the oral cavity and pharynx.[21] The most recent report concludes that all forms of tobacco use cause oral cancers, and that all sites in the oral cavity and pharynx except the salivary glands are at increased risk.[22] Epidemiological studies provide consistent evidence that cigarette smokers have higher incidence and mortality from oral cancer than do lifetime nonsmokers. The average risk for current cigarette smokers is approximately 10 times higher in men and 5 times greater in women compared with lifetime nonsmokers of the same gender.

Relative risk (RR) is a measure of the degree to which the exposure to a certain factor increases a person's risk of experiencing a specific disease when compared with someone without the exposure. Relative risk is calculated as a ratio between the magnitude of the incidence of a disease among the exposed group compared with the nonexposed group. Therefore, a RR estimate of 1.0 would indicate that no relationship exists between the exposure and the disease, and that both the exposed and nonexposed group have an equal risk of getting the disease. Any RR estimate greater than 1.0 would indicate that a relationship exists between the disease and the exposure such that the larger the RR estimate, the greater the risk for disease. Relative risk estimates among males who are current smokers compared with lifetime nonsmokers range from 3.6 to 11.8[23] for cancers within the oral cavity, to as high as 14.1[24] for cancers of the pharynx. The RR of death from any cancer of the oral cavity or pharynx was 9.3 among male current smokers and 4.9 among female current smokers in a study population followed from 1982 to 1996.[25] In general, risk is strongly associated with the number of cigarettes smoked daily by current smokers. This daily exposure appears to have a stronger influence on risk than the cumulative tar exposure or **pack-years**. The number of years of smoking multiplied by the number of packs of cigarettes smoked per day are expressed as pack-years.[26] By calculating the exposure in pack-years, one can estimate both the length of the exposure (time) and the extent of the exposure (amount). Most studies indicate the risk of cancer of the oral cavity and pharynx among former smokers decreases rapidly after smoking cessation compared with the risk among continuing smokers,[27,28] with a substantial decrease in risk occurring within the first 10 years after quitting.

The use of various forms of tobacco differs according to cultures. Figure 6-2 provides a world map indicating the derivation of some tobacco products. As the United States becomes more diverse, the use of these different forms of tobacco is becoming more prevalent in the U.S. **Bidis** ("bee-dees") are small hand-rolled cigarettes imported from India and other Southeast Asian countries. They can be flavored (e.g., chocolate, cherry, and mango) or unflavored.[29,30] Bidis have significantly higher concentrations of nicotine, tar, and carbon monoxide than conventional cigarettes sold in the United States.[31] Meta-analysis data has demonstrated a threefold increased risk for oral cancer among bidi smokers compared with nonsmokers.[32]

Kretek ("cree-tech") or clove cigarettes are a tobacco alternative popular for a unique smell, taste, and appearance. They typically contain a mixture of tobacco, cloves, and other additives.[33] As with bidis, kreteks deliver more nicotine, carbon monoxide, and tar than conventional cigarettes,[34] and no evidence exists to indicate that either are safe alternatives to conventional cigarettes. Beyond the usual risks associated with smoking, the eugenol oil in kretek cigarettes contributes to laryngeal anesthesia and increases the risk for aspiration pneumonia and hemorrhagic pulmonary edema. No research studies have been conducted in the United States on the health effects of bidis or kreteks. Studies from India indicate that bidi smoking is associated with an increased risk for oral cancer.[35] As the population in the United States becomes increasingly multicultural, the potential exists that these alternate forms of tobacco will contribute to an increased incidence of oral cancer.

Tobacco use in other forms. Carcinogenic agents have been isolated from pipe, cigar, and smokeless tobacco. The available data show a strong association between these forms and sources of tobacco and oral cancer, although not studied as extensively as cigarettes.

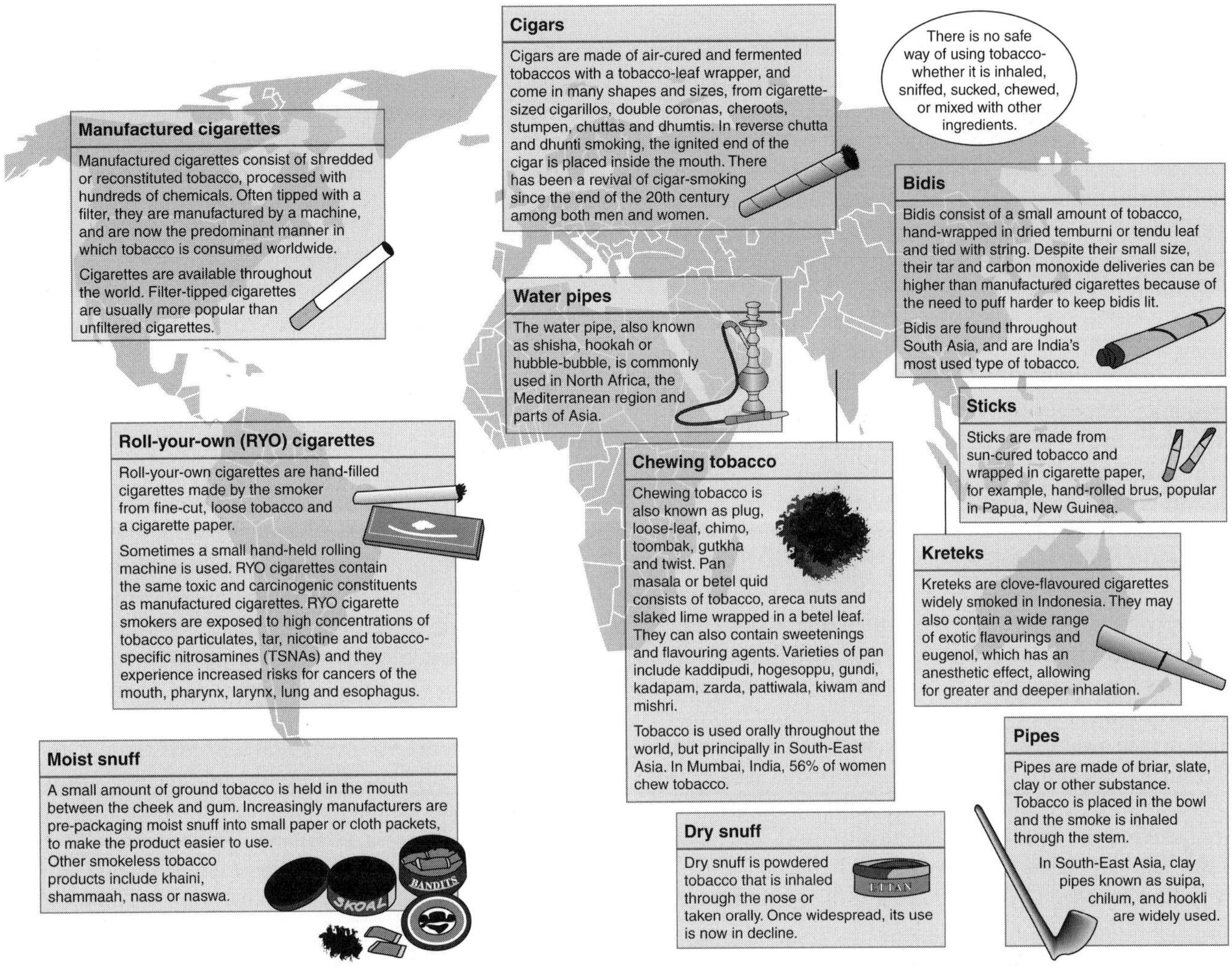

Cigars

Cigars are made of air-cured and fermented tobaccos with a tobacco-leaf wrapper, and come in many shapes and sizes, from cigarette-sized cigarillos, double coronas, cheroots, stumpen, chuttas and dhumtis. In reverse chutta and dhunti smoking, the ignited end of the cigar is placed inside the mouth. There has been a revival of cigar-smoking since the end of the 20th century among both men and women.

There is no safe way of using tobacco-whether it is inhaled, sniffed, sucked, chewed, or mixed with other ingredients.

Manufactured cigarettes

Manufactured cigarettes consist of shredded or reconstituted tobacco, processed with hundreds of chemicals. Often tipped with a filter, they are manufactured by a machine, and are now the predominant manner in which tobacco is consumed worldwide.

Cigarettes are available throughout the world. Filter-tipped cigarettes are usually more popular than unfiltered cigarettes.

Bidis

Bidis consist of a small amount of tobacco, hand-wrapped in dried temburni or tendu leaf and tied with string. Despite their small size, their tar and carbon monoxide deliveries can be higher than manufactured cigarettes because of the need to puff harder to keep bidis lit.

Bidis are found throughout South Asia, and are India's most used type of tobacco.

Water pipes

The water pipe, also known as shisha, hookah or hubble-bubble, is commonly used in North Africa, the Mediterranean region and parts of Asia.

Roll-your-own (RYO) cigarettes

Roll-your-own cigarettes are hand-filled cigarettes made by the smoker from fine-cut, loose tobacco and a cigarette paper.

Sometimes a small hand-held rolling machine is used. RYO cigarettes contain the same toxic and carcinogenic constituents as manufactured cigarettes. RYO cigarette smokers are exposed to high concentrations of tobacco particulates, tar, nicotine and tobacco-specific nitrosamines (TSNAs) and they experience increased risks for cancers of the mouth, pharynx, larynx, lung and esophagus.

Sticks

Sticks are made from sun-cured tobacco and wrapped in cigarette paper, for example, hand-rolled brus, popular in Papua, New Guinea.

Chewing tobacco

Chewing tobacco is also known as plug, loose-leaf, chimo, toombak, gutkha and twist. Pan masala or betel quid consists of tobacco, areca nuts and slaked lime wrapped in a betel leaf. They can also contain sweetenings and flavouring agents. Varieties of pan include kaddipudi, hogesoppu, gundi, kadapam, zarda, pattiwala, kiwam and mishri.

Tobacco is used orally throughout the world, but principally in South-East Asia. In Mumbai, India, 56% of women chew tobacco.

Kreteks

Kreteks are clove-flavoured cigarettes widely smoked in Indonesia. They may also contain a wide range of exotic flavourings and eugenol, which has an anesthetic effect, allowing for greater and deeper inhalation.

Moist snuff

A small amount of ground tobacco is held in the mouth between the cheek and gum. Increasingly manufacturers are pre-packaging moist snuff into small paper or cloth packets, to make the product easier to use. Other smokeless tobacco products include khaini, shammaah, nass or naswa.

Pipes

Pipes are made of briar, slate, clay or other substance. Tobacco is placed in the bowl and the smoke is inhaled through the stem.

In South-East Asia, clay pipes known as suipa, chilum, and hookli are widely used.

Dry snuff

Dry snuff is powdered tobacco that is inhaled through the nose or taken orally. Once widespread, its use is now in decline.

Figure 6-2 World map of the derivation of tobacco products. Although some tobacco products are indigenous to the United States, more and more types of tobacco products are being introduced to the U.S. as the population becomes more multicultural. (Adapted from Mackey J, Eriksen M: *The tobacco atlas*, 2002, World Health Organization.)

The causal relationship between pipe smoking and cancer of the lip was noted in the Surgeon General's Report on Smoking and Health in 1964.[21] Since then, both epidemiological and experimental studies have continued to demonstrate that pipe smoking, alone or in combination with other forms of tobacco use, is causally related to cancer of the lip. Clemmesen[36] was one of the earliest investigators to support a causal role between pipe smoking and cancer of the lip. The findings of Levin et al.[37] and Wynder et al.[38] added strength to this association. Spitzer et al.[39] reported that although the use of tobacco in general (cigarette, pipe, or chewing tobacco) was not an important risk factor for cancer of the lip, the risk ratio for pipe smoking taken alone was 1.5:1. Fortunately, the incidence of lip cancer has been declining slowly. The relative risk for cancer of the oropharynx for a pipe smoker however, can be almost 4 times higher than that

of a lifetime nonsmoker and the risk for laryngeal cancer 13 times higher.[40]

Hookah or waterpipe smoking has been practiced extensively in different cultures for 400 years. In recent years, this practice has been revived, notably among youth. Hookah smoking is known by a number of different names, including waterpipe, narghile, argileh, goza, hubblebubble, and shisha. A study of 14 healthy, young, male, habitual waterpipe users who abstained from use for 84 hours before the study had plasma levels of nicotine at baseline of 1.11 ng/ml ±0.62, and a maximum of 60.31 ng/ml ±7.58 ($p < 0.0001$) after 45 minutes of smoking.[41] In comparison, a peak plasma level of nicotine for a cigarette smoker is 30 to 40 ng/ml. This observation suggested that plasma levels of nicotine may be twice as high after using a waterpipe than after smoking cigarettes. Only a small number of studies have examined the composition of the smoke associated with hookah use. Studies that have examined hookah smokers and the aerosol of the smoke have reported high concentrations of carbon monoxide, nicotine, tar, and heavy metals. These concentrations were found at levels that were high or higher than among cigarette smokers. The available data regarding the adverse health consequences of water-pipe smoking point to dangers similar to those associated with cigarette smoking: malignancy, impaired pulmonary function, low birth weight, and others.[42-44]

Cigar use in the United States increased substantially during the 1990s,[45, 46] reaching a peak of 3.7 million new users in 1998.[47] Cigars contain the same toxic and carcinogenic compounds found in cigarettes and are not a safe alternative to cigarettes. Comparisons between cigarettes and cigars demonstrate that the amount of nicotine and tars in one cigar is equivalent to that in a full pack of cigarettes. Current data show that regular cigar smoking is associated with increased risk for cancers of the larynx, oral cavity, and esophagus.[48] The results of a large, 12-year, prospective study[49] strongly supported a causal relationship between cigar smoking and mortality from cancers of the larynx, esophagus, and oral cavity/pharynx, independent of the use of alcohol or other tobacco products. Current cigar smoking is associated with a fourfold increase in risk of death from cancers of the oral cavity and pharynx when compared with never smoking.

The two main types of smokeless tobacco (ST) available in the United States are chewing tobacco and snuff.[50,51] Smokeless tobacco is a significant health risk and is not a safe substitute for smoking cigarettes,[52] because it increases the risk of cancer of the oral cavity[53] and contributes to gingival recession. Smokeless tobacco use can lead to nicotine addiction and dependence. Adolescents who use smokeless tobacco are more likely to become cigarette smokers. Although the nicotine is delivered over a longer period of time, the total nicotine dose can be approximately three times higher than the nicotine dose delivered by a single cigarette. Determining the absolute health risks associated with ST use is confounded by the lack of homogeneity of the products, and cofactors for diseases in the study populations. In the United States approximately three quarters of the ST market is snuff and one fourth is chewing tobacco. The International Agency for Research on Cancer concluded that oral use of snuff is carcinogenic and that some evidence exists that chewing tobacco is also carcinogenic."[54]

All forms of tobacco use (cigarettes, pipes, cigars, snuff, chewing tobacco, betel, and other smoked and smokeless products) increase the occurrence of premalignant lesions and malignant transformation of oral epithelium. Elimination of exposure causes most premalignant lesions to regress and reduces the incidence and recurrence of and mortality from invasive cancers of the oral cavity and pharynx. Among tobacco users, premalignant lesions may regress after the discontinued use of cigarettes or smokeless tobacco[55] but may become more dysplastic with continued exposure to tobacco. Smoking cessation decreases the risk of second or multiple primary tumors in patients with a previous cancer of the oral cavity or pharynx.[56] Leukoplakia observed in cigarette smokers differs morphologically from the keratoses caused by smokeless tobacco. Although less common, the leukoplakia induced by cigarettes is more susceptible to malignant transformation.[57] Quitting smoking has substantial and immediate health benefits for smokers of all ages. Former smokers live longer than continuing smokers, no matter when they stop smoking.[58] The increased risk of death from smoking begins to decrease shortly after cessation and continues to diminish for at least 10 to 15 years.[59] Smokers who quit before age 50 years have half the risk of dying within the next 15 years compared with those who continue to smoke.[60]

Alcohol. Alcohol intake has long been known to increase oral cancer risk and mortality.[61,62] In one study, alcoholics diagnosed with oropharyngeal cancer suffered a mortality rate three times that which would be expected in nondrinkers. Studies have shown a clear correlation between alcohol-related cirrhosis of the liver and cancer of the floor of the mouth, palate, and tonsillar fossa. The risk for oral cancer is independent of tobacco use, but the combination of cigarette smoking and alcohol consumption substantially and synergistically increases the risk of oropharyngeal cancer compared with the risk of either alone. Blot[63] found that men who smoked two or more packs of cigarettes daily for 20 or more years but drank less than one alcoholic beverage per week experienced a risk approximately 7 times higher than nonsmokers who were light drinkers. The combination of prolonged smoking of at least two packs daily and drinking 30 or more alcoholic drinks per week is associated with a RR of almost 38 in men and nearly 108 in women. Despite these findings, data from one study reported that 6 months after the diagnosis of malignancy, 47% of study patients still smoked and 36% of the diagnosed patients drank alcohol to excess.[64] This observation is testimony to the addictive power of both of these substances. Only one third of these patients were aware that their behavior was important in the development of oral cancer. These results also indicated that the population as a whole is uninformed about the causes of oral cancer and that education about the causes of oral cancer is required, particularly among those with the disease.

Sunlight (actinic radiation). Chronic exposure to sunlight is the predominant risk factor for cancer of the lip, especially the lower lip. Geographically, the risk of lip cancer approximately doubles with exposure that is associated with an increase in every 10 degrees latitude approaching the equator. Persons working outdoors for extended periods of time are at greater risk of developing cancer of the lip, and the risk is related to the duration of exposure to the sunlight.[65]

Immune system deficiencies.   The risk of malignant disease is increased in individuals with immune systems compromised by genetics, disease, or treatment sequelae. The incidence rate of malignancies for patients with a primary immunodeficiency is more than 100 times that of the population in general.[66,67] Further, immunocompetence and immune cell surveillance diminish with age, contributing to the association between age and malignancy. Both smoking and alcohol use, in addition to iron deficiency, are known to reduce cell-mediated reactivity. Although changes in immune status are associated with the course of malignant disease, it is not clear whether these changes cause the malignancy or result from it. Immune system deficiencies can contribute to an increased risk for infections. Certain viral infections have been shown to contribute to an increased risk for oral cancer. Immune system deficiencies, in conjunction with other factors, may contribute to a greater probability of infection that can lead to a greater risk for oral cancer.

Infections.   Human papilloma virus (HPV) has been shown to be a risk factor for oral cancer in several studies. More than 90 different human papilloma viruses have been identified, and several types of HPV are known to be oncogenic (HPV 16, 18, 30s, 50s). HPVs cause malignancies by altering epithelial cell growth and replication or disrupting the cell cycle.[68,69] An increase in HPV titer was observed in oral cancer and precancerous lesions, but the significance of this finding is not clear, because not all oral cancers contain HPVs. HPV DNA can be found in the tumor cells of up to two thirds of oral cancer cases, however. HPV is often present in proliferative verrucous leukoplakia, and the presence of HPV is positively correlated with dysplastic changes of oral mucosa. Verrucous leukoplakia is a variant that results from use of smokeless tobacco (snuff or chewing tobacco). Although HPV DNA is present in these cancers, the significance is not completely understood. Although HPV DNA is found in the oral mucosa of many patients, only a small percentage of these patients actually develop oral cancer. Studies suggest that two types of HPV, HPV-16 and HPV-18, may play a role in the malignant transformation of oral pre-cancerous lesions and are considered risk factors for oral cancer.

Herpes simplex viruses 1 and 2 (HSV-1 and 2) were originally thought to be associated with increased risk of oral malignancies in a manner similar to the association of HSV-2 and cervical cancer. These viruses are now thought to be a cofactor, potentiating the effects of alcohol and tobacco. HSV-1 interacts with oral carcinogens to produce tumors,[70] and both HSV-1 and HSV-2 can cause malignant transformation of cells *in vitro*, although HSV-2 does not usually infect oral tissues.

Epstein-Barr virus (EBV) is found in the lymphocytes and frequently in the saliva of healthy persons. EBV infection of human lymphocytes can produce malignant changes, and EBV is associated with certain head and neck cancers. EBV can infect oral epithelial cells and is present in hairy leukoplakia, but is rarely found in oral cancers. Because hairy leukoplakia is not associated with development of oral cancer, EBV is not considered a risk factor.

Human herpesvirus 8 (HHV-8) is found in AIDS-associated Kaposi's sarcoma (KS). Because most KS patients have antibodies to HHV-8, and the virus has been shown to produce KS-like lesions in animals, HHV-8 is considered the etiological agent of KS. Like many of the herpes viruses, HHV-8 is widespread in the healthy population. Impaired immune function and the presence of HHV-8 may influence the development of KS in AIDS patients.

Nutritional deficiencies.   Currently, no deficiencies or excesses of dietary proteins, fats, or carbohydrates are linked conclusively as etiological factors for oral cancer. Cancers of the mouth, larynx, and esophagus may be related to low intake of fruits and carotene-rich vegetables. Other antioxidants in fruits and vegetables may help in controlling cell growth, and vegetable fiber is associated with a reduced risk of oral cancer. High rates of oral cancer have been reported in countries where vitamin A intake is low. The correlation between vitamin A deficiencies and hyperkeratosis indicate an association between deficiency of this vitamin and oral precancerous lesions and cancer.[71] No studies to date have confirmed that either vitamin C or E deficiencies increase the risk of oral cancer, or that supplementation with these vitamins reduces the risk. Plummer-Vinson syndrome, a complex of symptoms that includes low serum iron levels, is associated with an increased risk of carcinoma of the buccal mucosa and tongue, hinting at a relationship between chronic iron deficiency and malignant transformation of epithelium. Iron deficiency has not been a common finding in patients presenting with oral cancer, although high iron storage has been indicated as one possible risk factor in cancer.[72] Deficiencies of other minerals (zinc, copper, calcium selenium) are implicated by some studies as causative factors, but to date there is no conclusive evidence linking any of them to increased incidence of oral cancer.

Other oral conditions.   Chronic hyperplastic candidiasis is linked to an increased risk for oral cancer. Candidiasis is a fungal infection that is found most often on the tongue and buccal mucosa. Often associated with an altered immune response, candidal infection appears as white, elevated plaques. Approximately 10% of leukoplakias are infected with *Candida albicans*. These candidal leukoplakias exhibit dysplasia associated with invasion of candidal hyphae. Subsequent development of malignancy is more likely to occur with this form of leukoplakia than with other types of leukoplakia. One hypothesized mechanism of action implies that the candidal infection disturbs epithelial cellular activity in a manner that is more likely to induce neoplastic changes. The evidence in this instance is circumstantial, but it is clear that candidal infections are not simply superimposed infections, because no evidence exists of another, preexisting lesion.

Oral lichen planus is one of the most common diseases to manifest in the oral cavity. The lesions appear as linear white or grey streaks across the buccal mucosa. Rates of malignant transformation in patients with oral lichen planus (OLP) range from 1.2% to 3.27%, when measured over a period of 6 to 12 years.[73-75] The prevalence of oral cancer in these patients was greater than would be expected in the general population. Thus, a risk of associated malignancy appears to exist in patients with OLP, particularly in the erosive form and in erythematous areas, but the evidence to date is not conclusive.

Chronic irritation has been linked with oral cancer because many oral cancers develop in areas covered by or adjacent to a prosthetic appliance. A possible association between chronic irritation from the denture and oral malignancies was postulated; however, at present no sufficient data exist to demonstrate conclusively whether this is an active or passive relationship. Denture material has not been shown to be carcinogenic. Chronic irritation in combination with other risk factors may promote neoplastic activity, but does not appear to promote carcinogenesis. A simple explanation of the association between dentures and oral cancer may be that most denture patients tend to be older, and thus at greater risk for the development of oral cancer because of prolonged exposure to other risk factors.

DETECTION AND DIAGNOSIS
Clinical Examination

Regular, thorough intraoral and extraoral examination by a dental professional is the most effective technique for early detection and prevention of oral cancer. All patients should be examined annually, and those at higher risk should be given even closer, more frequent scrutiny. The profile of a high-risk patient includes age of 50 years or older, and/or a positive history for any of the risk factors listed above, especially tobacco or alcohol use, either singly or in combination. In female patients younger than 50 years, with no history of alcohol or tobacco use, suspect lesions have a greater risk of malignant potential and may be more aggressive. Lesions observed in this group of patients must be treated quickly and aggressively.

All areas of the oral cavity and vermillion border of the lip, the floor of the mouth, and the lateral border of the tongue should be examined thoroughly. This examination should be done both visually and by using palpation (see Figure 3-7). Suspect lesions should be biopsied and sent for histological analysis.

Biopsy

Regular examination, sound clinical judgment, and experience are enough to detect suspicious lesions, but biopsy is the only method to definitively diagnose oral cancer. Treatment for an oral lesion suspected of being malignant should not be initiated until the diagnosis is confirmed by a histological examination.

Diagnostic Aids

Both **brush biopsy** and **toluidine blue** staining techniques provide the dental professional with an in-office technique to assess the malignant potential of oral lesions. Brush biopsy uses a specially designed brush that obtains cells from all epithelial layers that are assessed by microscopic screening.[76] Histologic examination of the cells can be made by a computerized image analysis system and certified by a pathologist. The technique does not require anesthesia and is a simple procedure that is easily performed in the dental office. One important advantage of brush biopsy is that the ease of the procedure may lead to an early diagnosis of suspicious lesions. Because the vast majority of oral cancers are squamous (epithelial) cell carcinomas, this technique provides accurate sampling of lesions. The brush biopsy technique allows quick evaluation of questionable lesions that clinically do not appear to be malignant, and may thus increase the likelihood of biopsy in these cases and hasten the diagnosis of malignancies that might otherwise remain undiscovered until a later time. Brush biopsies should be accompanied by a traditional surgical biopsy to confirm the presence or absence of malignant cells.

Vital staining with toluidine blue can assist in early recognition and accelerate biopsy and subsequent diagnosis in the same manner as brush biopsy.[77-79] Aqueous toluidine blue (1%) is applied to the lesion, which is then rinsed with 1% acetic acid. The dye binds selectively to dysplastic and malignant cells with a high degree of accuracy and can also indicate the best site for biopsy. The dye used is neither mutagenic nor carcinogenic, and thus the technique can be a safe and useful adjunct to examination of a suspicious lesion. Similar to brush biopsy, this technique, which can be applied in the scope of routine practice, can lead to an early diagnosis of suspicious lesions.

SUMMARY

The incidence of oral cancer in the United States has remained fairly constant during the last decade with approximately 30,000 new cases and 7000 deaths per year.[1] Oral health care professionals are the first line for both prevention and diagnosis of this disease. Oral cancer examinations are a standard of practice exercised by most oral health care providers, but follow-up, including referral for cancer prevention services, such as counseling regarding cessation of tobacco use and alcohol abuse, are often lacking.

In a national survey conducted from 1994 to 1995, only 33% of dentists determined the smoking status of most or nearly all of their patients. Less than one third of the dental practitioners who responded to the survey reported providing tobacco cessation counseling to patients using tobacco products.[80]

In a study comparing the smoking cessation counseling activities of six different health care professionals (primary care physicians, dentists, dental hygienists, family planning clinic practitioners, mental health, and nutritional counselors), Secker-Walker and colleagues[81] found that dental professionals ranked lowest among the providers surveyed with respect to overall smoking cessation counseling activities.

More recently, Albert et al.[82] surveyed dentists in a managed care setting and found that fewer than one fifth of the providers had inquired about tobacco use during the previous month with more than 80% of their patients. Only 13% of the respondents reported they used a specific cessation counseling strategy with patients who smoked, and routine documentation of counseling activities in the dental record occurred infrequently (12%). Notably, only 9% of the dentists surveyed had received previous training in tobacco cessation.

These findings provide a clear explanation for the stable rate in oral cancer incidence and mortality despite the fact that tobacco use among adults has declined during the past decade. Knowledge of the principles of effective risk reduction and prevention strategies (Chapter 17) can empower the dental professional to more effectively engage patients and help to reduce their risk for oral cancer.

REFERENCES

1. Jemal A, Murray T, Ward E et al.: Cancer statistics, 2005, *CA Cancer J Clin* 55:1, 11-30, 2005.
2. Ries LAG, Eisner MP, Kosary CL et al., editors: SEER Cancer Statistics Review, 1975-2000.
3. Silverman S Jr: Leukoplakia and erythroplasia. In *Oral cancer*, Hamilton (Canada), 1998, B. C. Decker.
4. Califano J, van der Reit P, Westra W et al.: Genetic progression model for head and neck cancer: implications for field cancerization, *Cancer Res* 56:2488-2492, 1996.
5. Reed AL, Califano J, Cairns P et al.: High frequency of p16 (CDKN2/MTS-1/INK4A) inactivation in head and neck squamous cell carcinoma, *Cancer Res* 56:3630-3633, 1996.
6. Mao L, Lee JS, Fan YH et al.: Frequent microsatellite alterations at chromosomes 9p21 and 3p14 in oral premalignant lesions and their value in cancer risk assessment, *Nat Med* 2:682-685, 1996.
7. Lee JJ, Hong WK, Hittelman WN et al.: Predicting cancer development in oral leukoplakia: ten years of translational research, *Clin Cancer Res* 6:1702-1710, 2000.
8. Partridge M, Pateromichelakis S, Phillips E et al.: A case-control study confirms that microsatellite assay can identify patients at risk of developing oral squamous cell carcinoma within a field of cancerization, *Cancer Res* 60:3893-3898, 2000.
9. Rosin MP, Cheng X, Poh C et al.: Use of allelic loss to predict malignant risk for low-grade oral epithelial dysplasia, *Clin Cancer Res* 6:357-362, 2000.
10. Lazarus P, Garewal HS, Sciubba J et al.: A low incidence of p53 mutations in pre-malignant lesions of the oral cavity from non-tobacco users, *Int J Cancer* 60:458-463, 1995.
11. Brennan JA, Boyle JO, Koch WM et al.: Association between cigarette smoking and mutation of the p53 gene in squamous-cell carcinoma of the head and neck, *N Engl J Med* 332:712-717.
12. Koch WM, Lango M, Sewell D et al.: Head and neck cancer in nonsmokers: a distinct clinical and molecular entity, *Laryngoscope* 109:1544-1551, 1999.
13. National Cancer Institute, DCCPS, Surveillance Research Program, Cancer Statistics Branch: Surveillance, Epidemiology, and End Results (SEER) Program SEER*Stat Database Incidence-SEER 13 Regs Public-Use, Nov 2004 Sub (1973-2002 varying) (website): http://www.seer.cancer.gov, released April 2005, based on the November 2004 submission.
14. National Cancer Institute, DCCPS, Surveillance Research Program, Cancer Statistics Branch: Surveillance, Epidemiology, and End Results (SEER) Program DevCan database: "SEER 12 Incidence and Mortality, 1997-2001, Follow-back year=1992" (website): http://www.seer.cancer.gov, released October 2004, based on the November 2003 submission. Underlying mortality data provided by NCHS (http://www.cdc.gov/nchs).
15. U.S. Department of Health and Human Services: Women and smoking: a report of the Surgeon General, Atlanta, GA., 2001, U.S. Department of Health and Human Services, Centers for Disease Control and Prevention, National Center for Chronic Disease Prevention and Health Promotion, Office on Smoking and Health.
16. Centers for Disease Control and Prevention: Annual smoking-attributable mortality, years of potential life lost, and economic costs—United States, 1995-1999, *MMWR Morb Mortal Wkly Rep* 51:300-303, 2002.
17. Centers for Disease Control and Prevention: Health United States, 2003 with chartbook on trends in the health of Americans, Hyattsville, MD, 2003, U.S. Department of Health and Human Services, Centers for Disease Control and Prevention, National Center for Health Statistics.
18. McGinnis J, Foege WH: Actual causes of death in United States, *JAMA* 270:2207-2212, 1993.
19. U.S. Department of Health and Human Services: Reducing the health consequences of smoking—25 years of progress: a report of the Surgeon General, Atlanta, GA, U.S. Department of Health and Human Services, Centers for Disease Control and Prevention, 1989, DHHS Pub. No. (CDC) 89-8411.
20. U.S. Department of Health and Human Services: The health consequences of using smokeless tobacco: a report of the Advisory Committee to the Surgeon General, Bethesda, MD, 1986, U.S. Department of Health and Human Services, Public Health Service, NIH Pub. No. 86-2874.
21. U.S. Department of Health, Education, and Welfare: Smoking and Health: Report of the Advisory Committee to the Surgeon General of the Public Health Service. Washington, DC, 1964, U.S. Department of Health, Education, and Welfare. Public Health Service, PHS Publication 1103.
22. U.S. Department of Health and Human Services: The health consequences of smoking: a report of the Surgeon General, Atlanta, GA, Centers for Disease Control and Prevention, National Center for Chronic Disease Prevention and Health Promotion, Office on Smoking and Health; Washington, DC, 2004.
23. Franceschi S, Barra S, La Vecchia C et al.: Risk factors for cancer of the tongue and the mouth: a case-control study from northern Italy, *Cancer* 70:2227-2233, 1992.
24. McLaughlin JK, Hrubec Z, Blot WJ et al.: Smoking and cancer mortality among U.S. veterans: a 26-year follow-up, *Int J Cancer* 60:190-193, 1995.

25. Muscat JE, Richie JP Jr, Thompson S et al.: Gender differences in smoking and risk for oral cancer, *Cancer Res* 56:5192-5197, 1996.

26. Risks associated with smoking cigarettes with low machine-measured yields of tar and nicotine, Smoking and Tobacco Control Monograph 13, Bethesda, MD, 2001, U.S. Department of Health and Human Services, National Institutes of Health, National Cancer Institute, NIH Pub. No. 02-5974.

27. U.S. Department of Health and Human Services: Reducing tobacco use: a report of the Surgeon General, Atlanta, GA, 2000, U.S. Department of Health and Human Services, Centers for Disease Control and Prevention, National Center for Chronic Disease Prevention and Health Promotion, Office on Smoking and Health.

28. Institute of Medicine: Clearing the smoke: assessing the science base for tobacco harm prevention, Washington, DC, 2001, National Academy Press.

29. Centers for Disease Control and Prevention: Bidi use among urban youth—Massachusetts, March-April 1999, *MMWR Morb Mortal Wkly Rep* 48:796-799, 1999.

30. Yen KL, Hechavarria E, Bostwick SB: Bidi cigarettes: an emerging threat to adolescent health, *Arch Pediatr Adolesc Med* 154:1187-1189, 2000.

31. Watson CH, Polzin GM, Calafat AM et al.: Determination of the tar, nicotine, and carbon monoxide yields in the smoke of bidi cigarettes, *Nicotine Tob Res* 5:747-753, 2003.

32. Rahman M, Sakamoto J, Fukui T: Bidi smoking and oral cancer: a meta-analysis, *Int J Cancer* 106:600-604, 2003.

33. Malson JL, Lee EM, Murty R et al.: Clove cigarette smoking: biochemical, physiological, and subjective effects, *Pharmacol Biochem Behav* 74:739-745, 2003.

34. Council on Scientific Affairs: Evaluation of the health hazard of clove cigarettes, *JAMA* 260:3641-3644, 1988.

35. Rahman M, Fukui T: Bidi smoking and health, *Public Health* 114:123-127, 2000.

36. Clemmesen, JC: *Statistical studies in the aetiology of malignant neoplasms*, vol 1, Munksgaard, 1965, Copenhagen.

37. Levin ML, Goldstein H, Gerhardt PR: Cancer and tobacco smoking, *JAMA* 143:336, 1950.

38. Wynder EL, Bross IJ, Feldman RM: A study of the etiological factors in cancer of the mouth, *Cancer* 10:1300, 1957.

39. Spitzer WO, Hill GB, Chambers LW et al.: The occupation of fishing as a risk factor in cancer of the lip, *N Engl J Med* 293:419, 1975.

40. Henley SJ, Thun MJ, Chao A et al.: Association between exclusive pipe smoking and mortality from cancer and other diseases, *J Natl Cancer Inst* 96:853-861, 2004.

41. Shafagoj YA, Mohammed FI, Hadidi K: Hubble-bubble (water pipe) smoking: levels of nicotine and cotinine in plasma, saliva and urine, *Int J Clin Pharmacol Ther* 40:249-255, 2002.

42. Knishkowy B, Amitai Y: Water-pipe (narghile) smoking: an emerging health risk behavior, *Pediatrics* 116;113-119, 2005.

43. Maziak W, Ward KD, Afifi Soweid RA et al.: Tobacco smoking using a waterpipe: a re-emerging strain in a global epidemic, *Tob Control* 13:327-333, 2004.

44. Kulwicki A, Rice VH: Arab American adolescent perceptions and experiences with smoking, *Public Health Nurs*, 20:177-183, 2003.

45. National Cancer Institute: Cigars: health effects and trends, Smoking and Tobacco Control Monograph No. 9, Bethesda, MD, 1998, National Institutes of Health, National Cancer Institute, NIH Pub. No. 98-4302.

46. Baker F, Ainsworth SR, Dye J et al.: Health risks associated with cigar smoking, *JAMA* 284:735-740, 2000.

47. Substance Abuse and Mental Health Services Administration: Results from 2003 national survey on drug use and health: national findings, Rockville, MD, 2004, Substance Abuse and Mental Health Services Administration, Office of Applied Studies.

48. U.S. Department of Health and Human Services: The health consequences of smoking: cancer. A report of the Surgeon General, Rockville, MD, 1982, U.S. Department of Health and Human Services, Public Health Service.

49. Shapiro JA, Jacobs EJ, Thun MJ: Cigar smoking in men and risk of death from tobacco-related cancers, *J Natl Cancer Inst* 92:333-337, 2000.

50. Hatsukami DK, Severson HH: Oral spit tobacco: addiction, prevention and treatment, *Nicotine Tob Res* 1:21-44, 1991.

51. Centers for Disease Control and Prevention: Determination of nicotine, pH, and moisture content of six U.S. commercial moist snuff products—Florida, January-February 1999, *MMWR Morb Mortal Wkly Rep* 48:398-401, 1999.

52. National Institutes of Health: Health implications of smokeless tobacco use (1986), NIH consensus statement online: http://consensus.nih.gov/cons/053/053_statement.htm.

53. Winn DM, Blot WJ, Shy CM et al.: Snuff dipping and oral cancer among women in the southern United States, *N Engl J Med* 304:745-749, 1981.

54. International Agency for Research on Cancer (IARC): Summaries & Evaluations Tobacco habits other than smoking, Vol 37, 1985.

55. Martin GC, Brown JP, Eifler CW et al.: Oral leukoplakia status six weeks after cessation of smokeless tobacco use, *J Am Dent Assoc* 130:945-954, 1999.

56. Moore C: Smoking and cancer of the mouth, pharynx, and larynx, *JAMA* 25:191:283-286, 1965.

57. Bouquot JE: Oral leukoplakia and erythroplakia: a review and update, *Pract Periodont Aesthet Dent* 6:9-17, 1994.

58. Doll R, Peto R, Wheatley K et al.: Mortality in relation to smoking: 40 years: observations on male British doctors, *BMJ* 309:901-911, 1994.

59. Peto R, Darby S, Deo H et al.: Smoking, smoking cessation, and lung cancer in the UK since 1950: combination of national statistics with two case-control studies, *BMJ* 321:323-329, 2000.

60. U.S. Department of Health and Human Services: The health benefits of smoking cessation: report of the Surgeon General, Rockville, MD, 1990, U.S. Department for Health and Human Services.

61. Mashberg A, Garfinkel L, Harris S: Alcohol as a primary risk factor in oral squamous cell carcinoma, *CA Cancer J Clin* 31:146-155, 1981.

62. Thun MJ, Peto R, Lopez AD et al.: Alcohol consumption and mortality among middle-aged and elderly U.S. adults, *N Engl J Med* 337:1705-1714, 1997.

63. Blot WJ, McLaughlin JK, Winn DM et al.: Smoking and drinking in relation to oral and pharyngeal cancer, *Cancer Res* 48:3282-3287, 1988.

64. Thomson PJ, Potten CS, Appleton DR: Characterization of epithelial cell activity in patients with oral cancer, *Br J Oral Maxillofac Surg* 37:384-390, 1999.

65. Huber MA, Terezhalmy GT: The patient with actinic cheilosis, *Gen Dent* 54:274-282, 2006.

66. Gatti RA, Good RA: Occurrence of malignancy in immunodeficiency disease, *Cancer* 28:89, 1971.

67. Kersey JH, Spector BD, Good RA: Primary immunodeficiency diseases and cancer: the immunodeficiency-cancer registry, *Int J Cancer* 12:333, 1973.

68. Gillison ML, Koch WM, Capone RB et al.: Evidence for a causal association between human papillomavirus and a subset of head and neck cancers, *J Natl Cancer Inst* 92:709-720, 2000.

69. Miller CS, Johnstone BM: Human papillomavirus as a risk factor for oral squamous cell carcinoma: a meta-analysis, 1982-1997, *Oral Surg Oral Med Oral Pathol Oral Radiol Endod* 91:622-635, 2001.

70. Park K, Cherrick HM, Min BM et al.: Active HSV-1 immunization prevents the cocarcinogenic activity of HSV-1 in the oral cavity of hamsters, *Oral Surg Oral Med Oral Pathol* 70:186-191, 1990.

71. Maserejian NN, Giovannucci E, Rosner B et al.: Prospective study of vitamins C, E, and A and carotenoids and risk of oral premalignant lesions in men, *Int J Cancer* 120:970-977, 2006.

72. Stevens RG, Jones DY, Micozzi MS et al.: Body iron stores and the risk of cancer, *N Engl J Med* 319:1047-1052, 1988.

73. Silverman S Jr, Gorsky M, Lozada-Nur F et al.: A prospective study of findings and management in 214 patients with oral lichen planus, *Oral Surg Oral Med Oral Pathol* 72:665-670, 1991.

74. Chainani-Wu N, Silverman S Jr, Lozada-Nur F et al.: Oral lichen planus: patient profile, disease progression and treatment responses, *J Am Dent Assoc* 132:901-909, 2001.

75. Barnard NA, Scully C, Everson JAW: Oral cancer development in patients with oral lichen planus, *J Oral Pathol Med* 22:421-424, 1993.

76. Christian DC: Computer-assisted analysis of oral brush biopsies at an oral cancer screening program, *J Am Dent Assoc* 133:357-362, 2002.

77. Mashberg A, Samit A: Early diagnosis of asymptomatic oral and oropharyngeal squamous cancers, *CA Cancer J Clin* 45:328-351, 1995.

78. Portugal LC, Wilson KM, Biddinger PW et al.: The role of toluidine blue in assessing margin status after resection of squamous cell carcinomas of the upper aerodigestive tract, *Arch Otolaryngol Head Neck Surg* 122:517-519, 1996.

79. Warnakulasuriya KAAS, John NW: Sensitivity and specificity of Orascan toluidine blue mouthrinse in the detection of oral cancer and precancer, *J Oral Pathol Med* 25:91-110, 1996.

80. Dolan TA, McGorray SP, Grinstead-Skigen CL et al.: Tobacco control activities in U.S. dental practices, *J Am Dent Assoc* 128:1669-1679, 1997.

81. Secker-Walker RH, Solomon LJ, Flynn BS et al.: Comparisons of the smoking cessation counseling activities of six types of health professionals, *Prev Med* 23:800-808, 1994.

82. Albert D, Ward A, Ahluwalia K et al.: Addressing tobacco in managed care: a survey of dentists' knowledge, attitudes, and behaviors, *Am J Public Health* 92:997-1001, 2002.

Synergism Between Pharmacology and Oral Health

ARTHUR H. JESKE

ADVERSE EFFECTS OF DRUGS ON THE ORAL CAVITY

Drugs Affecting the Central Nervous System and Oral Health
Candidiasis
Dysgeusia (Taste Alterations)
Drug-Associated Xerostomia
Drugs Associated with Gingival Enlargement
Intraoral Allergic and Allergic-Type Reactions
Osteonecrosis (Osteochemonecrosis)
Adverse Effects of Drugs on Teeth
Adverse Oral Effects of Herbal Supplements

SUMMARY

LEARNING OBJECTIVES

Upon completion of this chapter, the learner will be able to:
- Examine the relationship between chemotherapeutics used to treat systemic diseases and the potential effects of these drugs on oral health.
- Identify specific drugs and groups of drugs associated with various adverse effects on oral health.
- Characterize the clinical presentation of the adverse oral effects of drugs for systemic disease.
- Identify strategies to prevent or minimize the adverse oral effects of drugs used to treat systemic diseases.

KEY TERMS

Candidiasis
Central nervous system
Dysgeusia
Erythema multiforme
Gingival enlargement
Herbal supplements
Lichenoid reactions
Osteonecrosis
Staining
Stevens-Johnson syndrome
Taste alterations
Tetracycline antibiotics
Xerostomia

The increasing availability of sophisticated, target-directed drugs and biologicals has led to the expectation that the number of adverse ("side") effects of medical therapy will be reduced. Modern medical and dental therapies rely on drugs most of which were developed before the twentieth century. These pharmacotherapies precede the era of modern proteomics and recombinant DNA techniques for identification of receptor molecules known to modulate disease processes. Their relative lack of specificity for disease targets, coupled with the widespread tissue distribution of common biological receptors for a variety of exogenous drugs, results in a wide spectrum of effects. These effects frequently involve oral tissues and oral physiological processes, produce systemic adverse effects with oral manifestations, and have potentially serious implications for dental treatment. This chapter highlights specific drugs or entire groups of drugs that may alter oral health. The term "synergism," as used in the title of this chapter, refers to adverse dental conditions resulting from medical drug therapy that can alter various preventive oral health care strategies. Over-the-counter (OTC) products, including **herbal** and dietary supplements, are capable of producing adverse conditions in the oral cavity and altering systemic physiology. These products and their effect on oral health are also described.[1,2,3]

ADVERSE EFFECTS OF DRUGS ON THE ORAL CAVITY

Drugs Affecting the Central Nervous System and Oral Health

Drugs used to treat neurological and psychiatric illnesses are best identified in the patient's health history. The clinician should confirm the presence of adverse oral effects, including any of the following conditions: **xerostomia** and associated problems with caries, chewing, swallowing, and speaking; hypersalivation; abnormal muscular movements (e.g., tardive dyskinesias), and enhanced intraoral pain sensation.[4] Other adverse effects of dental importance include sedation and associated problems of lethargy and memory lapses. These effects can significantly interfere with patients' understanding of dental treatment plans and adherence to preventive strategies. During the diagnostic process, the clinician should note whether these same problems result from the disease or the medications. Major groups of neurological drugs associated with these effects are shown in Table 7-1.

The most common adverse oral effect of drugs in this class is xerostomia and the associated problems of caries, **dysgeusia**, stomatitis, and glossitis.[5] Because the dentist should not change or discontinue a patient's medical therapy, preventive approaches must be used to reduce these adverse effects through reinforcement of oral hygiene, prescription of topical fluoride agents, avoidance of adverse drug interactions, and dental home care instructions to the caregivers of patients when appropriate.[6] In cases that require surgical intervention, deep sedation or general anesthesia with hospitalization may be required when neuromuscular complications or mental disease preclude routine, outpatient dental care.

Candidiasis

Intraoral **candidiasis** is readily recognized by the presence of white, irregular patches or pseudomembranes that can be easily wiped off, and fungal hyphae confirmed by routine microscopy (Figure 7-1). Drug-related candidiasis is seen as atrophy of the oral mucosa, or generalized stomatitis and glossitis.

Drug-related candidiasis is typically associated with drugs that disrupt the normal oral flora (e.g., antibiotics), drugs that suppress the immune system, and drugs that cause xerostomia. Broad-spectrum antibiotics, including **tetracyclines** and aminoglycosides (e.g., streptomycin), contribute to candidiasis. Long-term corticosteroid therapy results in a progressive impairment of immune function. Cancer chemotherapeutic agents and antirejection drugs (e.g., cyclosporine) produce an even greater and more rapid-onset immune suppression that can precipitate the development of oral candidiasis.[7]

Oropharyngeal candidiasis occurs in any patient taking immunosuppressive drugs and is aggravated by agents that cause xerostomia. Oral candidiasis is linked to human immunodeficiency viral (HIV) disease and drug-resistant candidal infections. One potential benefit of Highly Active Antiretroviral Therapy (HAART) is reduction of the burden of oral candidiasis in HIV patients. A recent systematic review highlighted the importance of various factors in determining the treatment outcomes

TABLE 7-1

CLASSES OF NEUROLOGICAL AND PSYCHOTROPIC DRUGS ASSOCIATED WITH ADVERSE ORAL EFFECTS

ADVERSE EFFECT	CAUSATIVE DRUG CLASS
Xerostomia/ anticholinergic actions	Monoamine oxidase inhibitors (MAOIs) Selective serotonin reuptake inhibitors (SSRIs) Tricyclic antidepressants Phenothiazine Sedatives, hypnotics
Tardive dyskinesia	Phenothiazine
Sedation (impaired memory and thought processes, motor incoordination)	Barbiturates (e.g., phenobarbital) Benzodiazepines (e.g., diazepam) Butyrophenones (e.g., haloperidol) Phenothiazine Pimozide (e.g., Orap) Lithium carbonate Anticonvulsants (e.g., phenobarbital)

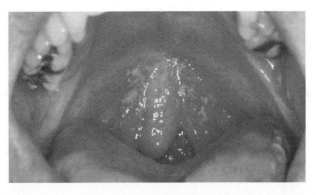

Figure 7-1 Intraoral candidiasis of the posterior palatal and oropharynx. (From Gage T, Pickett F: *Mosby's dental drug reference 2005,* ed 7, St Louis, 2006, Mosby.)

for oral candidiasis. The factors included immune system status, severity of infection, mutations, compliance issues, and the drug regimen used in a given patient.[8] The review noted the probable prophylactic effect of HAART, which produced general improvement of immune function.

Topical therapy with nystatin (available in a variety of doses and dose forms) is useful to treat patients with non–drug-resistant candidal infections. When used in a 2-week course of therapy, evidence exists that some azole antifungal drugs (fluconazole and itraconazole) are more effective in producing clinical improvement in HIV-infected patients than other members of the azole class (e.g., clotrimazole).

Patients taking antirejection and cancer chemotherapeutic drugs are at risk for a variety of opportunistic infections and adverse drug effects and interactions. Their dental care must be carefully coordinated with their physicians. Similarly, patients may be taking broad-spectrum antibiotics for serious systemic infections that may prohibit routine dental care. The dentist must document these medications and medical conditions by taking a detailed medical/health history and carefully evaluating the oral cavity. Azole antifungal drugs can precipitate serious adverse pharmacokinetic drug interactions with some sedative agents used in dentistry (e.g., midazolam and triazolam).

Dysgeusia (Taste Alterations)

Changes in the sensation of taste can take several forms, from ageusia (loss of the sensation of taste) to dysgeusia (altered taste sensation) and hypogeusia (diminished sensation of taste). Dysgeusia is the most common type of **taste alteration** associated with drug use. Most cases involve a bitter or metallic taste. The change in taste sensation should be differentiated from the persistent taste of oral dose forms of various drugs and from dentally applied agents and dental restorative materials.[9]

As shown in Table 7-2, a variety of drugs are associated with taste alterations. Angiotensin-converting enzyme inhibitors (e.g., captopril) and dihydropyridine-type calcium channel blockers (e.g., nifedipine) are among the agents most frequently associated with taste alterations. The precise incidence of this adverse effect is unknown.[9] Dysgeusia may also accompany xerostomia, which can precipitate or aggravate taste alterations.

text continued on p.84

TABLE 7-2

DRUGS ASSOCIATED WITH TASTE ALTERATIONS (DYSGEUSIA)

DRUG CLASS	OFFICIAL NAME	TRADE NAME
Alcohol detoxification	Disulfiram	Antabuse
Alzheimer's	Donepezil	Aricept
Analgesics (nonsteroidal anti-inflammatory drugs)	Diclofenac	Voltaren
	Etodolac	Lodine
	Ketoprofen	Orudis
	Meclofenamate	Meclofen
	Sulindac	Clinoril
Anesthetics (general)	Midazolam	Versed
	Propofol	Diprivan
Anesthetics (local)	Lidocaine transoral	DentiPatch
Anorexiants	Diethylpropion	Tenuate
	Mazindol	Mazanor
	Phendimetrazine	Adipost
	Phentermine	Lonamin
Antacids	Aluminum hydroxide	Amphojel
	Calcium carbonate	Tums
	Lansoprazole	Prevacid
	Magaldrate	Riopan
	Omeprazole	Prilosec
	Sucralfate	Carafate
Antianxiety	Buspirone	BuSpar
Antiarthritic	Leflunomide	Arava
Anticholinergics	Clidinium	Quarzan
	Mepenzolate	Cantil
	Propantheline	Pro-Banthine

TABLE 7-2

DRUGS ASSOCIATED WITH TASTE ALTERATIONS (DYSGEUSIA)—cont'd

DRUG CLASS	OFFICIAL NAME	TRADE NAME
Anticonvulsants	Fosphenytoin	Cerebyx
	Phenytoin	Dilantin
	Topiramate	Topamax
Antidepressants	Amitriptyline	Elavil
	Clomipramine	Anafranil
	Desipramine	Norpramin
	Doxepin	Sinequan
	Fluoxetine	Prozac
	Imipramine	Tofranil
	Nefazodone	Serzone
	Nortriptyline	Pamelor
	Protriptyline	Vivactil
	Sertraline	Zoloft
Antidiabetics	Metformin	Glucophage
	Tolbutamide	Orinase
Antidiarrheals	Bismuth subsalicylate	Pepto Bismol
Antiemetics	Aprepitant	Emend
	Dolasetron mesylate	Anzemet
Antifungals	Terbinafine	Lamisil
Antigout	Allopurinol	Zyloprim
	Colchicine	
Antihistamine (H$_1$) antagonists	Azelastine	Astelin
	Cetirizine	Zyrtec
Antihistamine (H$_2$) antagonists	Famotidine	Pepcid
Antihyperlipidemics	Clofibrate	Atromid-S
	Fluvastatin	Lescol
Antiinfectives	Ciprofloxacin	Ciloxan
	Daptomycin	Cubicin
	Ethionamide	Trecator-SC
	Gatifloxacin	Zymar
	Gemifloxacin	Factiv
	Levofloxacin	Levaquin
	Lincomycin	Lincocin
	Metronidazole	Flagyl
	Ofloxacin	Floxin
Antiinflammatory/antiarthritic	Auranofin	Ridaura
	Aurothioglucose	Solganal
	Celecoxib	Celebrex
	Rofecoxib	Vioxx
	Sulfasalazine	Azulfidine
Antimigraine	Almotriptan	Axert
	Frovatriptan	Froval
Antiparkinson	Entacapone	Comtan
	Levodopa	Larodopa
	Levodopa-carbidopa	Sinemet
	Pergolide	Permax
	Pramipexole dihydrochloride	Mirapex
Antipsychotics	Lithium	Eskalith
	Pimozide	Orap
	Prochlorperazine	Compazine

Continued

DRUGS ASSOCIATED WITH TASTE ALTERATIONS (DYSGEUSIA)—cont'd

DRUG CLASS	OFFICIAL NAME	TRADE NAME
	Quetiapine fumarate	Seroquel
	Risperidone	Risperdal
Antithyroid	Methimazole	Tapazole
	Propylthiouracil	
Antivirals	Acyclovir	Zovirax
	Amprenavir	Agenerase
	Atazanavir	Reyataz
	Delavirdine mesylate	Rescriptor
	Didanosine	Videx
	Efavirenz	Sustiva
	Foscarnet	Foscavir
	Indinavir	Crixivan
	Penciclovir	Denavir
	Ribavirin	Copegus
	Rimantadine	Flumadine
	Ritonavir	Norvir
	Saquinavir	Invirase
	Valacyclovir	Valtrex
	Zidovudine	Retrovir
Anxiolytic/sedatives	Chloral hydrate	
	Estazolam	Prosom
	Quazepam	Doral
	Zolpidem	Ambien
Asthma preventives	Cromolyn	Intal
	Nedocromil	Tilade
Bronchodilators	Albuterol	Proventil
	Bitolterol	Tornalate
	Formoterol fumarate	Foradil
	Ipratropium	Atrovent
	Isoproterenol	Isuprel
	Metaproterenol	Alupent
	Pirbuterol	Maxair
	Terbutaline	Brethine
Calcium-affecting drugs	Alendronate	Fosamax
	Calcitonin	Calcimar
	Etidronate	Didronel
Cancer chemotherapeutics	Capecitabine	Xeloda
	Fluorouracil	Efudex
	Levamisole	Ergamisol
	Tamoxifen	Nolvadex
Cardiovascular	Amiodarone	Cordarone
	Amlodipine	Norvasc
	Bepridil	Vascor
	Captopril	Capoten
	Clonidine	Catapres
	Diltiazem	Cardizem
	Enalapril	Vasotec
	Flecainide	Tambocor
	Fosinopril	Monopril
	Guanfacine	Tenex
	Labetalol	Trandate

TABLE 7-2

DRUGS ASSOCIATED WITH TASTE ALTERATIONS (DYSGEUSIA)—cont'd

DRUG CLASS	OFFICIAL NAME	TRADE NAME
	Losartan	Cozaar
	Mecamylamine	Inversine
	Mexiletine	Mexitil
	Moricizine	Ethmozine
	Nadolol	Corgard
	Nifedipine	Procardia XL
	Penbutolol	Levatol
	Perindopril	Aceon
	Propafenone	Rythmol
	Quinidine	Cardioquin
	Valsartan	Diovan
CNS stimulants	Dextroamphetamine	Dexedrine
	Methamphetamine	Desoxyn
Decongestant	Phenylephrine	Neo-Synephrine
Diuretics	Acetazolamide	Diamox
	Methazolamide	Naptazine
	Polythiazide	Renese
Glucocorticoid	Budesonide	Rhinocort
	Flunisolide	AeroBid
	Rimexolone	Vexol
Gallstone solubilization	Ursodiol	Actigall
Hemorheologic immunomodulators	Pentoxifylline	Trental
	Interferon alfa	Roferon-A
	Levamisole	Ergamisol
	Tacrolimus	Protopic
Immunosuppressants	Azathioprine	Imuran
Irritable bowel syndrome	Alosetron	Lotronex
Methylxanthine	Aminophylline	Somophyllin
	Dyphylline	Dilor
	Oxtriphylline	Choledyl
	Theophylline	Theo-Dur
Nicotine cessation	Nicotine polacrilex	Nicorette
Ophthalmics	Apraclonidine	Iopidine
	Brimonidine	Alphagan
	Brinzolamide	Azopt
	Dorzolamide	Trusopt
	Olopatadine	Patanol
Proton pump inhibitors	Esomeprazole	Nexium
	Lansoprazole	Prevacid
	Omeprazole	Prilosec
Retinoid, systemic	Acitretin	Soriatane
Salivary stimulant	Pilocarpine	Salagen
Skeletal muscle relaxants	Baclofen	Lioresal
	Cyclobenzaprine	Flexeril
	Methocarbamol	Robaxin
Vitamins	Calcifediol	Vitamin D
	Calcitriol	Vitamin D
	Dihydrotachysterol	Vitamin D
	Phytonadione	Vitamin K

(Modified from Gage T, Pickett F: *Mosby's dental drug reference 2005*, ed 7, St Louis, 2006, Mosby.)

The occurrence of dysgeusia and other alterations of taste cannot be prevented. Symptoms can be relieved or even completely reversed by certain strategies. These strategies include the reduction of xerostomia with saliva substitutes or intraoral mechanical stimulation (lozenges), use of topical anesthetic agents for short-term relief (e.g., dyclonine-containing lozenges), and avoidance of irritants (e.g., smoking). The dental professional should consult with the patient's physician to discuss alternate drugs to treat the medical condition. Consultation with the treating physician should occur when patients are taking drugs that may contribute to xerostomia. Although studies indicate a beneficial effect of zinc supplementation for idiopathic (non–drug-related) dysgeusia, results in patients with drug-related taste alterations are equivocal.[10] These preventive and interventional strategies can result

in recovery of taste sensation, but in some cases the condition is irreversible.

Drug-Associated Xerostomia

Xerostomia is the subjective complaint of dry mouth, which can be accompanied by significant salivary gland dysfunction. Medication use is the most common cause of xerostomia in the elderly.[11] The agents associated with xerostomia and its related problems are summarized in Table 7-3. Quality-of-life issues such as chewing and swallowing are affected by inadequate salivary flow and poor saliva consistency, which can lead to an increased risk for dental caries and oral fungal infections. Intraoral hard- and soft-tissue examinations may reveal salivary gland pathology, mucositis, cervical and root-surface

TABLE 7-3

PRESCRIPTION AND OVER-THE-COUNTER DRUGS ASSOCIATED WITH DRY MOUTH

DRUG CLASS	OFFICIAL NAME	TRADE NAME
Anorexiants	Phentermine	Adipex-P, Fastin, Ionamin
	Phendimetrazine	Anorex
	Mazindol	Mazanor, Sanorex
	Diethylpropion	Tenuate, Tepanil
Antacid	Esomeprazole	Nexium
	Rabeprazole	AcipHex
Antiacne	Isotretinoin	Accutane
Antianxiety	Hydroxyzine	Atarax, Vistaril
	Lorazepam	Ativan
	Buspirone	BuSpar
	Meprobamate	Equanil, Miltown
	Chlordiazepoxide	Librium
	Halazepam	Paxipam
	Oxazepam	Serax
	Zaleplon	Sonata
	Diazepam	Valium
	Alprazolam	Xanax
Antiarthritic	Leflunomide	Arava
Anticholinergic/antispasmodic	Atropine	Sal-Tropine
	Belladonna alkaloids	Bellergal
	Dyclonine	Bentyl
	Oxybutynin	Ditropan
	Hyoscyamine, atropine, phenobarbital, scopolamine	Donnatal, Kinesed
	Chlordiazepoxide, clidinium	Librax
	Propantheline	Pro-Banthine
	Scopolamine	Transderm-Scop
	Tolterodine	Detrol
Anticonvulsant	Felbamate	Felbatol
	Lamotrigine	Lamictal

TABLE 7-3

PRESCRIPTION AND OVER-THE-COUNTER DRUGS ASSOCIATED WITH DRY MOUTH—cont'd

DRUG CLASS	OFFICIAL NAME	TRADE NAME
Antidepressant	Gabapentin	Neurontin
	Carbamazepine	Tegretol
	Clomipramine	Anafranil
	Amoxapine	Asendin
	Citalopram	Celexa
	Venlafaxine	Effexor
	Amitriptyline	Elavil
	Fluxoamine	Luvox
	Isocarboxazid	Marplan
	Phenelzine	Nardil
	Desipramine	Norpramin
	Tranylcypromine	Parnate
	Paroxetine	Paxil
	Fluoxetine	Prozac
	Eletriptan	Relpax
	Doxepin	Sinequan
	Imipramine	Tofranil
	Bupropion	Wellbutrin, Zyban
	Sertraline	Zoloft
Antidiarrheals	Loperamide	Imodium AD
	Diphenoxylate, atropine	Lomotil
	Difenoxin	Motofen
Antihistamines	Triprolidine, pseudoephedrine	Actifed
	Hydroxyzine	Atarax, Vistaril
	Diphenhydramine	Benadryl
	Chlorpheniramine	Chlor-Trimeton
	Loratadine	Claritin
	Promethazine	Phenergan
Antihypertensive	Captopril	Capoten
	Clonidine	Catapres
	Carvedilol	Coreg
	Guanethidine	Ismelin
	Perindopril	Aceon
	Prazosin	Minipress
	Reserpine	Serpasil
	Guanabenz	Wytensin
	Enalapril	Vasotec
Nonsteroidal antiinflammatory	Diflunisal	Dolobid
	Celecoxib	Celebrex
	Piroxicam	Feldene
	Ibuprofen	Motrin
	Fenoprofen	Nalfon
	Naproxen	Naprosyn, Anaprox
	Balsalazide	Colazal
Antinausea	Aprepitant	Emend
	Cyclizine	Marezine
	Dimenhydrinate	Dramamine
	Meclizine	Antivert
Antiparkinson	Benztropine	Cogentin
	Biperiden	Akineton

Continued

TABLE 7-3

PRESCRIPTION AND OVER-THE-COUNTER DRUGS ASSOCIATED WITH DRY MOUTH—cont'd

DRUG CLASS	OFFICIAL NAME	TRADE NAME
	Carbidopa, levodopa	Sinemet
	Ethopropazine	Parsidol
	Tolcapone	Tasmar
	Trihexyphenidyl	Artane
Antipsychotic	Amitriptyline, perphenazine	Triavil
	Aripiprazole	Abilify
	Chlorpromazine	Thorazine
	Clozapine	Clozaril
	Haloperidol	Haldol
	Lithium	Eskality
	Olanzapine	Zyprexa
	Pimozide	Orap
	Prochlorperazine	Compazine
	Promazine	Sparine
	Risperidone	Risperdal
Antiviral	Efavirenz	Sustiva
	Ribavirin	Copegus
Bronchodilator	Albuterol	Proventil, Ventolin
	Ephedrine	
	Isoproterenol	Inderal
	Levalbuterol	Xopenex
Central nervous system stimulant	Dextroamphetamine	Dexedrine, Adderall
	Methamphetamine	Desoxyn
	Methylphenidate	Ritalin
Decongestant	Pseudoephedrine	Sudafed
Diuretic	Spironolactone	Aldactone
	Chlorothiazide	Diuril
	Triamterene	Triamterene, Maxzide
	Hydrochlorothiazide	Esidrix, HydroDIURIL
	Furosemide	Lasix
	Amiloride	Midamor
Migraine	Naratriptan	Amerge
	Almotriptan	Axert
	Frovatriptan	Frova
	Rizatriptan	Maxalt
	Eletriptan	Relpax
Muscle relaxant	Cyclobenzaprine	Flexeril
	Baclofen	Lioresal
	Orphenadrine	Norflex
Narcolepsy	Modafinil	Provigil
Opioid analgesic	Buprenorphine	Buprenex
	Meperidine	Demerol
	Morphine	MS Contin
	Dihydrocodeine combinations	Synalgos-DC
Ophthalmic sedative	Brinzolamide	Azopt
	Flurazepam	Dalmane
	Triazolam	Halcion
	Temazepam	Restoril

(Modified from Gage T, Pickett F: *Mosby's dental drug reference 2005*, ed 7, St Louis, 2006, Mosby.)

caries, and frank dryness of the oral soft tissues. These symptoms should be noted in the patient's record. The clinician can confirm hyposalivation by direct measurement of both resting and stimulated saliva flow rates.[11] Chapter 9 outlines methods and indications for measuring flow rates. The clinician can assist the patient with strategies to alleviate symptoms and obtain relief. In some cases, referral to a physician or oral medicine specialist is warranted.

Dental patients diagnosed with xerostomia or salivary gland dysfunction should be instructed in daily oral hygiene measures and placed on a frequent recall schedule. Fluoride therapy is an important preventive therapy for patients with xerostomia who are also at risk for future caries.[12] Patient counseling that addresses strategies for management of symptoms can be an adjunct to these therapies. In a recent systematic review, therapies for xerostomia were generally nonspecific, and included parasympathomimetic agents (pilocarpine and cevimeline), oral stimulants/lozenges, saliva substitutes, chewing gums, acupuncture, and even electrostimulation. Only pilocarpine, prescribed as systemic therapy for xerostomia related to Sjögren's syndrome and head-and-neck irradiation therapy for cancer, is supported with strong scientific evidence.[13]

Drugs Associated with Gingival Enlargement

Gingival enlargement (also referred to as gingival overgrowth, and previously known as gingival hyperplasia) is a swelling of the attached gingivae that obliterates the gingival contours. This condition frequently begins at the interdental papillae and is found at the labial surfaces of both anterior and posterior teeth (Figure 7-2). The enlargement is fibrotic and involves large tissue lobulation,

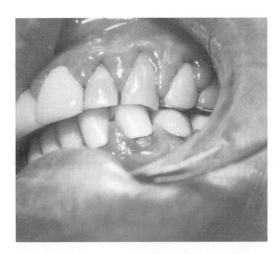

Figure 7-2 Gingival enlargement and upper right posterior teeth in a patient taking nifedipine for hypertension. (From Gage T, Pickett F: *Mosby's dental drug reference 2005*, ed 7, St Louis, 2006, Mosby.)

which typically occur after 1 to 3 months of therapy with causative agents. The clinical appearance does not depend on the various drugs that cause it.[14] Gingival inflammation is associated with this condition, and poor oral hygiene exacerbates it. Bleeding on probing occurs, especially in individuals taking immunosuppressants.

Several drugs are consistently associated with gingival enlargement. They include the anticonvulsant medication phenytoin (Dilantin), the calcium channel blockers (nifedipine, diltiazem, and verapamil), and the immunosuppressant/antirejection agent cyclosporine A (Sandimmune). Prevalence rates of gingival enlargement associated with phenytoin is approximately 50%, 5% to 20% with calcium channel blockers, and 25% to 30% with the immunosuppressant agents.[15,16] The mechanism by which these drugs cause gingival enlargement is unknown, but likely involves release of inflammatory mediators, altered enzyme activities and shifts in ion permeabilities.[17] Dosage does not correlate with the severity of gingival enlargement clinically, but increased incidence is associated with male gender, younger age, and poor oral hygiene.[17] Deficiency of vitamin A or magnesium have also been implicated as causes of gingival enlargement.[18]

The severity of this gingival condition and coexisting inflammation are reduced by providing oral hygiene instruction, scheduling frequent (3-month) periodontal recall visits, and use of adjunctive chemotherapeutic measures (e.g., chlorhexidine gluconate mouth rinses). Gingivectomy may be the preferred therapy for severe cases, medical condition permitting. Physicians should consider substituting the offending drug with another medication, although it is unlikely that more severe cases would resolve from this measure alone. The use of phenytoin, calcium channel blockers, and immunosuppressants indicate the presence of serious medical conditions, and physicians treating patients stabilized on such therapy may be unable to alter the drug regimen. Excellent oral hygiene and frequent professional recall represents the best nonsurgical dental therapy for gingival enlargement.

Intraoral Allergic and Allergic-Type Reactions

Lichenoid reactions are seen as ulceration and desquamation of the oral mucosa, frequently associated with lichen planus-like white striae on the buccal mucosa. A link between oral lichen planus and drugs that reduce saliva flow is suggested, but the most recent study of such patients found that only 6.5% of the participants with oral lichen planus were taking such medications.[19] **Stevens-Johnson syndrome (erythema multiforme)** is characterized by the occurrence of target-type lesions of the skin and multiple areas of intraoral necrosis (Figure 7-3).

Erythema multiforme is a rare condition associated with prolonged (more than 1 week) therapy with some antibiotics (clindamycin and tetracycline), anticonvulsants (carbamazepine and phenytoin), certain barbiturates

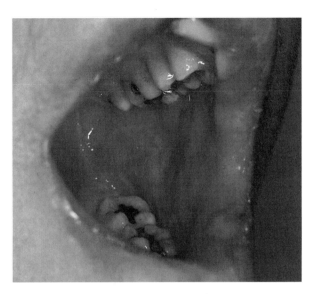

Figure 7-3   Bullous erythema multiforme (Stevens-Johnson syndrome) in a patient taking a sulfonamide antimicrobial drug. (From Gage T, Pickett F: *Mosby's dental drug reference 2005,* ed 7, St Louis, 2006, Mosby.)

(pentobarbital, phenobarbital, and secobarbital), the AIDS drug acyclovir, and the oral antidiabetic agent chlorpropamide.[1] Lichenoid reactions accompany therapy with the ACE inhibitor captopril, the oral antidiabetic drug chlorpropamine, the antihypertensive agents methyldopa and furosemide, and some nonsteroidal antiinflammatory agents (e.g., diflunisal, flurbiprofen, and ibuprofen).[1]

Therapy is mostly palliative and consists of avoidance of irritating substances, administration of corticosteroids to treat the inflammatory lesions, and analgesic drugs for associated pain. Both conditions resolve when the precipitating drugs are withdrawn. Because of the potentially life-threatening nature of severe erythema multiforme, the patient should be referred to appropriate medical personnel.

Osteonecrosis (Osteochemonecrosis)

Drug-associated **osteonecrosis** is caused by therapy with bisphosphonates, corticosteroids, or antineoplastic agents. Radiation therapy and immunotherapy are also associated. Diagnosis is accomplished by assessment of clinical appearance, symptoms, and a history of tooth extraction, intraoral infection, or other jaw trauma. Other markers associated with osteonecrosis are cagulopathies, exostoses-tori, smoking, alcohol abuse, malnutrition, or arthritis. Drug-associated osteonecrosis is more frequently observed among females. Clinical signs and symptoms of osteonecrosis can include pain, swelling, purulence, denuded bone, mobility, and complaints of dysesthesia.[20]

Bisphosphonate drugs (Table 7-4) were introduced and developed for the treatment of osteoporosis and osteolytic lesions caused by a variety of disorders, including hypercalcemia of malignancy, Paget's disease, breast cancer, and multiple myeloma. Most cases of osteonecrosis are related to use of intravenous bisphoshonates. Oral agents used to treat osteoporosis have also been implicated.[21] The manufacturer of two intravenous agents (Aredia and Zometa, Novartis Pharmaceutical Corporation) has issued recommendations for the prevention, diagnosis, and management of osteonecrosis of the jaws of cancer patients taking these medications.[22] Drug-associated osteonecrosis is best prevented by avoiding tooth extractions or other invasive dental procedures in patients who are at risk, and by performing thorough dental examinations on patients before bisphosphonate therapy is initiated. No evidence exists at present to confirm whether cessation of bisphosphonate treatment reduces the risk, and no evidence-based guidelines exist for the management of bisphosphonate-related osteonecrosis of the jaw.[22,23] The dentist must undertake dental treatment of such patients very carefully, and make treatment decisions in consultation with the patient's oncologist and, if appropriate, an oral surgeon, particularly if signs and

TABLE 7-4

SUMMARY OF BISPHOSPHONATE DRUGS CURRENTLY AVAILABLE IN THE UNITED STATES

OFFICIAL NAME	TRADE NAME	ADMINISTRATION ROUTE	FOOD AND DRUG ADMINISTRATION APPROVAL DATE
Alendronate	Fosamax	Oral	1995
Etidronate	Didronel	Oral, intravenous	1977
Ibandronate	Boniva	Oral	2005
Pamidronate	Aredia	Intravenous	1991
Risedronate	Actonel	Oral	1998
Tiludronate	Skelid	Oral	1997
Zoledronic acid	Zometa	Intravenous	2001

symptoms of osteonecrosis occur. In any event, conservative treatment is mandatory and may include antibiotic therapy, protective stents, and locally applied chemotherapeutic agents (e.g., chlorhexidine). When the osteonecrosis does not respond to conservative measures, conservative surgery may be necessary. Dental implants are strictly contraindicated in such patients.[20,21] In all cases involving intravenous bisphosphonates, a preventive approach should be adhered to and, when dental procedures are indicated, it is suggested that minimally traumatic procedures be done in a stepwise manner (e.g., by sextant) using topical antimicrobial therapy and other local measures to reduce the possibility of osteonecrosis.[24]

Adverse Effects of Drugs on Teeth

The effects of drugs on teeth include extrinsic and intrinsic **staining**, physical alteration of tooth structure, and changes in tooth sensation.[25] Tooth discoloration can range from white spots to yellow, to dark brown, to gray generalized discoloration. The most common form of alteration of tooth structure related to drug use is to the result of carious destruction of enamel and dentin associated with reduced salivary flow or the use of oral medications or nutritional supplements with high sucrose content. Acidic drugs (e.g., powdered antiasthmatic drugs) can cause enamel erosion, although the incidence and significance of this type of tooth damage are not known.[25] Similarly, certain oral vitamin supplements are acidic and can cause similar damage.

Extrinsic tooth staining has been associated with the use of the antimicrobial mouth rinse chlorhexidine gluconate, liquid preparations of iron salts, some antibiotics in liquid form, and some essential oils.[25] Fluoride is a known source of intrinsic tooth staining, particularly in regional areas where the fluoride content of the drinking water greatly exceeds the recommended limits of 1.0 ppm. By avoiding the offending drug and by initiating routine dental prophylaxis, some extrinsic stains can be removed. Medical agents such as antibiotics and cancer chemotherapeutic agents known to cause discoloration and distorted development of teeth should be avoided in pregnant females or in infants and children, unless the medical benefits of these agents are deemed to outweigh the risk of permanent damage to the dentition. Lightening ("bleaching") agents may be of benefit in reducing the severity of dark, drug-related intrinsic staining, such as that produced by tetracycline antibiotics. Additionally, stained tooth structures can be masked by the placement of esthetic restorative materials on the labial surfaces of stained teeth. Caution should be exercised in choosing to place esthetic restorative materials in patients with less-than-optimal oral hygiene practices.

Adverse Oral Effects of Herbal Supplements

Herbal medications and nutritional supplements manifest a variety of intraoral effects on soft tissues, teeth, or both. Presentation of signs and symptoms may be quite variable from patient to patient because of differences in the frequency of use, the concentration of active ingredients, or both, in the various proprietary products on the market.

Several herbs and nutritional supplements are associated with adverse intraoral effects, although no systematic scientific evidence exists to firmly establish a cause-and-effect relationship in most cases.[18,26] Reports indicate that several agents (Table 7-5) are strongly implicated in producing adverse intraoral effects.

TABLE 7-5

HERBAL MEDICATIONS AND DIETARY SUPPLEMENTS ASSOCIATED WITH ADVERSE ORAL EFFECTS

COMMON NAME	SCIENTIFIC NAME	ADVERSE ORAL EFFECT	COMMENTS
Gingko	Gingko biloba	Gingival bleeding	Enhanced by anticoagulant drugs
Garlic	Allium sativum	Gingival bleeding	Enhanced by anticoagulant drugs
Feverfew	Chrysanthemum parthenium	Gingival bleeding, aphthae, mucositis	
Betel nut	Areca catechu	Tooth staining, submucous fibrositis, leukoplakia	Linked to oral and esophageal cancer
St. John's wort	Hypericum perforatum	Xerostomia	
Echinacea	Echinacea angustifolia	Tongue numbness	
Kava	Piper methysticum	Lingual/Oral dyskinesia	
Vitamin C	Ascorbic acid	Dental enamel erosion	When used as a lozenge
Vitamin D	Calciferol, other forms	Pulp calcification, enamel hypoplasia	Clinical significance unknown

Use of herbal medications, nutritional supplements, or both must be included in the patient's health history. A thorough intraoral examination should screen for any adverse intraoral effects. Because few scientific studies exist of these agents and their intraoral effects, the dentist must exercise clinical judgment in caring for patients who report using supplements. Discontinuation of use or reduction in the dose of the herb or nutritional supplement may provide partial or complete reversal of the adverse intraoral condition.

SUMMARY

The oral cavity is affected by many drugs used to treat medical conditions, and most intraoral effects are adverse to the overall oral health of the patient. No alternative medical agent may exist that can be used to reduce adverse drug-related oral effects. It is, therefore, incumbent on the dental care team to recognize these effects and proactively provide preventive and interventional measures to reduce their severity. No single treatment paradigm exists to address the multiple drug-related effects described in this chapter. If appropriate, the possibility of altering medical therapy should be discussed with the patient's physician to achieve the best outcomes. In these cases, coordination between medical and dental professionals is key to a successful patient outcome. Careful evaluation, including a detailed medical history, engaging the patient as a partner in their home care and frequent professional recall will help to minimize adverse oral effects of medications.

REFERENCES

1. Byrne JE: Oral manifestations of systemic agents. In Ciancio SE, editor: *ADA guide to dental therapeutics*, ed 2, Chicago, 2003, ADA Publishing.
2. Ciancio SJ: Medications' impact on oral health, *JADA* 135: 1440-1447, 2004.
3. Guggenheimer J: Oral manifestations of drug therapy, *Dent Clin North Am* 46:857-868, 2002.
4. Friedlander A et al.: Dental management of the child and adolescent patients with schizophrenia, *J Dent Child*, Special Issue July-October:281-287, 1993.
5. Smith R, Burtner P: Oral side effects of the most frequently prescribed drugs, *Spec Care Dentist* 14:96-102, 1994.
6. Clark DB: Dental care for the patient with bipolar disorder, *J Can Dent Assoc* 69:20-24, 2004.
7. Rossie K, Guggenheimer J: Oral candidiasis: clinical manifestations, diagnosis and treatment, *Pract Periodont Aesthet* 9:635-642, 1997.
8. Patton LL, Bonito AJ, Shugars DA: A systematic review of the effectiveness of anti-fungal drugs for the prevention and treatment of oropharyngeal candidiasis in HIV-positive patients, *Oral Surg Oral Med Oral Pathol Oral Radiol Endodont* 92:170-179, 2001.
9. Ackermann BH, Kasbekar N: Disturbances of taste and smell induced by drugs, *Pharmacotherapy* 17:482-496, 1997.
10. Heckman SM, Hujoel P, Habiger S et al.: Zinc gluconate in the treatment of dysgeusia—a randomized clinical trial, *J Dent Res* 84:35-38, 2005.
11. Navazesh M: How can oral health care providers determine if patients have dry mouth? *JADA* 134:613-620, 2003.
12. Eichmiller FC, Eidelman N, Carey CM: Controlling the fluoride dosage in a patient with compromised salivary function, *JADA* 136:67-70, 2005.
13. Brennan MT, Shariff G, Lockhart PB et al.: Treatment of xerostomia: a systematic review of therapeutic trials, *Dent Clin North Am* 46:847-856, 2002.
14. Dongari-Batzoglou A: Research, Science and Therapy Committee, American Academy of Periodontology Report: drug-associated gingival enlargement, *J Periodontol* 75:1424-1431, 2004.
15. Nery E, Edson R, Lee K et al.: Prevalence of nifedipine-induced gingival hyperplasia, *J Periodontol* 66:572-578, 1995.
16. Boltchi FE, Rees TD, Iacopino AM: Cyclosporine A-induced gingival overgrowth. A comprehensive review, *Quintessence Int* 30:775-783, 1999.
17. Hallman WW, Rossmann JA: The role of drugs in the pathogenesis of gingival overgrowth, *Oral Surg Oral Med Oral Pathol* 543-548, 1993.
18. Fugh-Berman A: Herbs and dietary supplements. In Ciancio SE, editor: *ADA guide to dental therapeutics*, ed 2, Chicago, 2003, ADA Publishing.
19. Colqhoun AN, Ferguson MM: An association between oral lichen planus and a persistently dry mouth, *Oral Surg Oral Med Oral Pathol Oral Radiol Endodont* 98:60-68, 2004.
20. Marx RE: Pamindronate (Aredia) and zoledronate (Zometa) induced asvascular necrosis of the jaws: a growing epidemic, *J Oral Maxillofac Surg* 61:1115-1117, 2003.
21. Ruggiero SL, Mehrotra B, Rosenberg TJ et al.: Osteonecrosis of the jaws: associated with the use of bisphosphonates: a review of 63 cases, *J Oral Maxillofac Surg* 62:527-534, 2004.
22. Updated recommendations for the prevention, diagnosis, and treatment of osteonecrosis of the jaws in cancer patients. East Hanover, NJ, 2006, Novartis Pharmaceutical Corp.
23. Migliorati CA, Casiglia J, Epstein J et al.: Managing the care of patients with bisphosphonate-associated osteonecrosis, *J Am Dent Assoc* 136:1658-1668, 2005.
24. Hellstein JW, Marek CL: Bisphosphonate-induced osteochemonecrosis of the jaws: an ounce of prevention may be worth a pound of cure, *Spec Care Dentist* 26:8-12, 2006.
25. Tredwin CJ, Scully C, Bagan-Sebastian J-V: Drug-induced disorders of teeth, *J Dent Res* 84:596-602, 2005.
26. Abebe W: An overview of herbal supplement utilization with particular emphasis on possible interactions with dental drugs and oral manifestations, *J Dent Hyg* 77:37-46, 2003.

Part *III*

Assessment Strategies to Tailor Your Patient Care Plan

Chapter 8

Nutritional Risk Assessment

CONNIE C. MOBLEY

NUTRITIONAL SCREENING AND ASSESSMENT IN RISK REDUCTION

SCREENING AND ASSESSMENT COMPONENTS

> **Historical Survey Measures**
> **Dietary Measures**
> **Physical Measures**
> Anthropometrics
> Physical Findings
> **Biochemical Data**

INTERPRETATION OF FINDINGS

SUMMARY

LEARNING OBJECTIVES

Upon completion of this chapter, the learner will be able to:
- Examine the rationale for nutritional screening and assessment activities in dental settings.
- Differentiate elements associated with nutrition and dietary assessment.
- Describe alternative approaches to aspects of nutritional screening and assessment.
- Review examples of interpretation and translation of nutritional/dietary findings.

KEY TERMS

Anthropometrics
Dietary assessment
Malnutrition
Nutritional assessment
Nutritional screening

Nutritional screening and assessment is a dynamic, evolving, and timely process used to determine the nutritional needs of clients and patients in health care and health promotion settings. The World Health Organization (WHO), in an expert review of evidence of the effects of diet and nutrition on chronic disease, identified the following five life stages: fetal development and maternal environment, infancy, childhood and adolescence, adulthood, and aging and older people.[1] Obesity, diabetes, cardiovascular disease, cancer, osteoporosis, and dental diseases are related to diet and nutrition and present the greatest public health burden to the world.[2] A decrease in the risk factors for development of these diseases is paramount in the effort to improve the quality of life of dental patients and, ultimately, in delaying or preventing the onset of dental disease. Descriptions of the strength of the evidence linking diet to dental diseases are presented in Table 8-1.[3] Knowledge of the synergy between diet/nutrition and oral health will continue to evolve with increasing research. Consumption of a balanced and varied diet to support health is dependent on oral health at every stage of the life course. Similarly, limitations in mastication, digestion, and use of nutrients can affect overall oral and systemic health. As shown in Figure 8-1, the integrity and function of oral tissues are dependent on an adequate nutrient intake and an adequate nutrient intake will determine the integrity and function of the oral anatomy.[4] Thus, an unequivocal rationale exists for conducting nutrition screening and, possibly, nutritional assessment in dental settings.

When pediatricians and pediatric dentists were surveyed about their nutritional counseling practices, dentists were found to make slightly better behavioral recommendations to patients, particularly about cariogenic foods. Both types of providers indicated a significant need for effective skills in nutritional screening and patient education/counseling.[5] Surveys of dental and medical students confirm inconsistent interpretations of dietary practices to promote oral and general health status.[6] Understanding the techniques, advantages, limitations, and interpretations associated with the procedures used in conducting nutritional assessment augments the dental practitioner's diagnostic,

TABLE 8-1

SUMMARY ACCORDING TO THE WORLD HEALTH ORGANIZATION'S EXPERT PANEL OF STRENGTHS AND WEAKNESSES FOR CONVINCING AND PROBABLE EVIDENCE LINKING DIETARY FACTORS TO DENTAL DISEASES

	INCREASED RISK	DECREASED RISK	NO RELATIONSHIP	POSSIBLE OR INSUFFICIENT EVIDENCE*
CARIES	Frequent intake of free, simple sugars Total amount of free, simple sugars consumed	Fluoride exposure Hard cheese Use of sugar-free chewing gum	Starch intake from cooked and raw starch foods, such as rice, potatoes and bread.	Dried or whole fresh fruit Xylitol Milk Dietary fiber
DENTAL EROSION	Intake of sugar-sweetened carbonated beverages Intake of fruit juices	N/A	N/A	Fresh whole fruit Hard cheese Fluoride
ENAMEL DEVELOPMENTAL DEFECTS	Excessive fluoride Inadequate calcium intake	Adequate vitamin D	N/A	N/A
PERIODONTAL DISEASE	Deficiency of vitamin C	Absence of dental plaque	N/A	Sucrose Vitamin E supplementation Fibrous foods Antioxidant nutrients

*Insufficient evidence because of lack of availability and documentation of well-designed, controlled studies to support the role of these factors.
(Adapted from Moynihan P, Petersen PE: Diet, nutrition and the prevention of dental diseases, *Public Health Nutr* 7:201-226, 2003.)

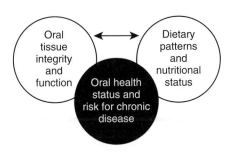

Figure 8-1 The interaction between oral health and diet and nutrition.

treatment planning, and patient education activities. This chapter identifies nutrition screening elements and differentiates the components of a comprehensive nutritional assessment. This chapter discusses alternative approaches to identification and interpretation of elements appropriate for oral health care delivery and is organized to provide a framework for decision making on the application of nutritional assessment components.

NUTRITIONAL SCREENING AND ASSESSMENT IN RISK REDUCTION

Nutrition screening and assessment is an attempt to identify a patient's current nutritional status and related nutrient recommendations and requirements. Screening is a simple process used to discover those who are at risk of being malnourished and are therefore susceptible to diseases. In general, subjective data related to diet and associated lifestyle behaviors, body weight history, medical history, and **anthropometric** measures are included in the screening process. These findings can be quickly correlated with observed oral health conditions, and a global determination can be stated. The risk for oral diseases and conditions can be identified, and the dental professional can take action on the basis of the evaluation of the data within this limited scope. The purpose of a **nutritional screening** is to provide a snap shot of the dietary factors of interest, define germane nutritional education goals, guide recommendations for dietary supplements, and identify the need to refer a patient either to social services for resources or a registered dietitian for consultation.[7]

If a complete **nutritional assessment** is needed, additional comprehensive and systematic methods of gathering patient data and, possibly, of categorizing degrees of malnutrition are necessary. This type of assessment is unlikely to occur in typical dental practice settings. However, dental practitioners located in hospitals, critical acute care settings, and long-term care facilities should use nutritional assessment measures when indicated.

Malnutrition results from alterations in dietary intake, digestion absorption, metabolism, or excretion of metabolic requirements for dietary energy, protein, and other nutrients.[8] A definition of malnutrition can encompass states of undernutrition (intake of insufficient nutrients to meet requirements), overnutrition (intake of nutrients in excess of requirements), nutrient insufficiency, and nutrient imbalances.[8] The identified incidence of a specific degree of malnutrition can be higher than anticipated, can jeopardize health outcomes, can delay positive outcomes of treatment, and determines appropriate interventions that can be implemented. Ultimately, a comprehensive nutritional assessment should lead to prevention or correction of an identified related problem and to a plan for evaluation, follow-up, or referral. In some cases, an initial nutritional assessment provides baseline data for patient monitoring and for evaluation of the quality of care provided over time.

SCREENING AND ASSESSMENT COMPONENTS

Essential data for assessment of nutritional status generally includes interpretation of clinical information from four main categories described as historical medical/social survey, dietary, physical/clinical or anthropometric, and biochemical data. Screening can involve one or more of these components, depending on the objective and intent of the screening process. Specific methodological approaches have been developed to address each component of nutritional assessment and are based on indices derived from previous population-based assessment programs as well as clinical and evidence-based research.[9]

The National Health Examination Surveys (NHES) in the United States were first conducted in 1956, and are currently continued as the National Health and Nutrition Examination Surveys (NHANES).[10] These cross-sectional surveys, designed to provide national health statistics, are based on representative population samples. NHES I, II, and III were followed by NHANES beginning in 1970 when survey methods were modified to include nutritional assessment data, because the link between dietary habits and disease was becoming increasingly important.[10] Protocols for these surveys provide a template for nutritional assessment activities that can be used once or repeatedly to provide longitudinal measures of individual markers of nutritional status.

Historical Survey Measures

Psychosocial and medical history variables can indicate risk factors that require an assessment of the patient's dietary intake. Medical, psychosocial, and socioeconomic histories are routinely gathered by dental professionals during an initial patient visit. A review of the patient's medical and physical findings can provide information that can be associated with a patient's dietary intake and nutrient use. Health and socioeconomic status noted in a medical history can be linked to physical activity, food selection, and eating patterns. Similarly, diseases, medication, and dietary supplement use (see Chapter 7), addictions associated with tobacco use, and alcohol abuse are factors that influence how nutrients are used by the body. General meal and snacking patterns and meal skipping, use of nutrient and nonnutrient supplements, food allergies and intolerances, alcohol consumption, and special dietary practices (i.e., vegetarianism and chronic dieting or fasting) can be addressed within history-taking activities. Table 8-2 lists risk factors identified in histories that reflect potential nutritional risks.[11,12] Responses to survey questionnaires serve as screening data for decisions about the need for further assessment.[7] Table 8-3 provides sample questions that can be used by dental professionals to probe for details that could assist the clinician in determining whether more in-depth nutritional assessment is needed.

The paucity of validated nutritional screening tools has contributed to the limited use of these approaches in dental settings. Caries risk assessment models rarely include **dietary assessment**. A set of screening questions has been validated in a study by Mendoza and Mobley, and is presented in Table 8-4.[13] Retrospective data were used to identify caries risk, caries status, and salivary bacterial counts in 155 patients, aged 19 to 81 years (39% male, 95% female).[4] Caries risk and status were defined by previously established protocols, and 3-day dietary intake records were used to identify correlations between dietary screening scores derived from the validated questionnaire and measures of caries. The specificity (74%) and sensitivity (77%) values indicate that the questionnaire meets the minimum criteria for a predictive test of caries risk attributable to dietary factors. Figure 8-2 presents an algorithm for using the dietary screening results to make decisions about further nutritional assessment.

The Nutrition Screening Initiative (NSI) developed for older adults has been useful as a screening tool in dental settings.[14] Figure 8-3 includes a copy of the Determine Your Nutritional Health Checklist. Although this instrument was developed in the early nineties on the basis of a review of Medicare patients 70 years old and

TABLE 8-2

RISK FACTORS IN PATIENT HISTORIES THAT REFLECT POTENTIAL NUTRITIONAL RISK

PSYCHOSOCIAL FACTORS	PHYSICAL COMPLAINTS	EVIDENCE OF DISEASES
Poverty	Difficulty biting, chewing, and swallowing	Extensive caries
Age and gender	Altered taste	Oral lesions/ulcerations
Education and literacy	Unintentional weight changes	Oral infection
Access to care	Xerostomia	Arthritis
Polypharmacy	Orofacial pain	Cancer
Food insecurity	Outcome of previous care	Cardiovascular disease
Substance abuse		Diabetes mellitus
Tobacco use		HIV infection/AIDS
		Inflammatory bowel disease
		Anemia
		Bone diseases
		Sjögren's syndrome

TABLE 8-3

SAMPLE FOLLOW-UP QUESTIONS TO EXTEND THE NUTRITION SCREENING PROCESS

RISK FACTOR	QUESTIONS
Body weight	Has your weight changed in the past 6 months? If yes, how? What contributed to your change in weight?
Diabetes	How do you monitor your diabetes? What do you do that contributes to the best control you have over your diabetes? What instructions have you received about managing your diabetes?
Xerostomia	Do you have difficulty chewing or swallowing any foods or beverages? If yes, can you describe those foods? Can you describe foods that prevent a severe degree of difficulty? Can you eat a food without needing liquids? Can you describe any changes in your medications or dietary supplements that might be contributing to your problem?
Taste	Can you describe how your taste of foods and beverages has changed? Have you changed medications, dietary supplements, or dietary practices that might be associated with your change in taste?
Biting and chewing	Can you describe the foods and beverages that cause difficulty biting and or chewing? How often do you eat during the day?
Food insecurity	Where do you shop or buy foods? Are you familiar with programs to assist others with access to food?

older, and has never been validated as a true measure of nutritional intake, it can accurately identify persons at risk for low nutrient intake and related health problems.[14] Thus, the checklist meets the definition of a screening approach that can help to target issues of concern. The list can be self-administered and quickly reviewed.

Dietary Measures

Dietary data are essential to understanding the metabolic energy equation. Dietary intake and physical activity (or energy output) together explain metabolism, which supports the efficient function of all organ systems.

TABLE 8-4

DIETARY SCREENING QUESTIONS FOR CARIES RISK

QUESTION	POINTS*
1. Do you eat food or drink beverages five or more times a day?	1 point if yes
2. Do you chew regular (non-sugar-free) gum?	1 point if yes
3. Do you drink any sweetened beverages between meals?	2 points if yes
4. Do you eat mints, candies, pastries, chips, crackers, etc., between meals?	2 points if yes
5. Do you drink milk or eat cheese every day?	1 point if no
TOTAL (If the total number of points is equal to or greater than 4, the diet is considered to be a major contributor to categorizing the individual at high caries risk.)	

*Circle the score based on the response to the question. Total all circled scores for a final number.
(Courtesy of Connie C. Mobley.)

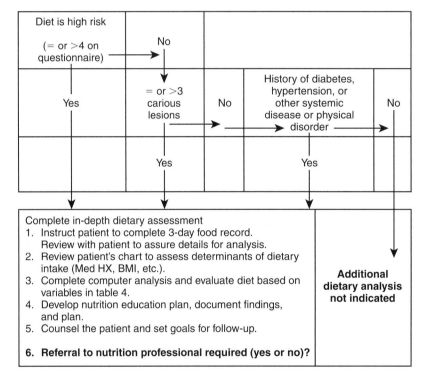

Figure 8-2 Algorithm for use of a dietary screening, assessment, and analysis model in dental settings. (From Mobley C: Dietary analysis in a restorative practice. In Duke S, editor: *The Changing Practice of Restorative Dentistry*. Indianapolis, IN, 2002, Indiana University School of Dentistry, pp. 139-156.)

The assumption that evaluation of dietary intake alone is sufficient to make nutritional status interpretations is erroneous. Dietary intake is only one piece of the nutrition assessment puzzle. Thus, a dietary assessment does not equal a nutritional assessment. All foods are organic substances designed to replace and replenish nutrients and their metabolites in the maintenance of life. Within the human body are dynamic systems of nutrient storage and turnover that cannot be accounted for with dietary assessment alone. Nutrient status is also dependent on nutrient storage capacity, rate of absorption and metabolism, and the degree and extent of nutrient losses that can vary with climate, health status, physical activity, and age. The human body is a dynamic organism that seeks to maintain equilibrium between dietary intake and nutrient losses, while maintaining health status. This fact limits the isolated and singular interpretation of dietary data.

The warning signs of poor nutritional health are often overlooked. Use this checklist to find out if you or someone you know is at nutritional risk.

Read the statements below. Circle the number in the "yes" column for those that apply to you or someone you know. For each "yes" answer, score the number in the box. Total your nutritional score.

DETERMINE YOUR NUTRITIONAL HEALTH

	YES
I have an illness or condition that made me change the kind and/or amount of food I eat.	2
I eat fewer than 2 meals per day.	3
I eat few fruits or vegetables or milk products.	2
I have 3 or more drinks of beer, liquor, or wine almost every day.	2
I have tooth or mouth problems that make it hard for me to eat.	2
I don't always have enough money to buy the food I need.	4
I eat alone most of the time.	1
I take 3 or more different prescribed or over-the-counter drugs a day.	1
Without wanting to, I have lost or gained 10 pounds in the last 6 months.	2
I am not always physically able to shop, cook, and/or feed myself.	2
TOTAL	

Total your nutritional score. If it's –

0-2   **Good!** Recheck your nutritional score in 6 months.

3-5   **You are at moderate nutritional risk.** See what can be done to improve your eating habits and lifestyle. Your office on aging, senior nutrition program, senior citizens center, or health department can help. Recheck your nutritional score in 3 months.

6 or more   **You are at high nutritional risk.** Bring this checklist the next time you see your doctor, dietitian, or other qualified health or social service professional. Talk with them about any problems you may have. Ask for help to improve your nutritional health.

Remember that warning signs suggest risk but do not represent a diagnosis of any condition. Turn the page to learn more about the warnings signs of poor nutritional health.

These materials are developed and distributed by the Nutrition Screening Initiative, a project of:

 AMERICAN ACADEMY OF FAMILY PHYSICIANS
 THE AMERICAN DIETETIC ASSOCIATION
 THE NATIONAL COUNCIL ON THE AGING, INC.

 The Nutrition Screening Initiative • 1010 Wisconsin Avenue, NW • Suite 800 • Washington, DC 20007
The Nutrition Screening Initiative is funded in part by a grant from Ross Products Division of Abbott Laboratories, Inc.

Figure 8-3   Form for the Nutrition Screening Initiative. (Courtesy of the Nutrition Screening Initiative, a project of the American Academy of Family Physicians, the American Dietetic Association, and the National Council on the Aging, Inc.)

The nutrition checklist is based on the warning signs described below.
Use the word <u>DETERMINE</u> to remind you of the warning signs.

DISEASE

Any disease, illness, or chronic condition that causes you to change the way you eat or makes it hard for you to eat puts your nutritional health at risk. Four out of five adults have chronic diseases that are affected by diet. Confusion or memory loss that keeps getting worse is estimated to affect one out of five or more of older adults. This can make it hard to remember what, when, or if you've eaten. Feeling sad or depressed, which happens to about one in eight older adults, can cause big changes in appetite, digestion, energy level, weight, and well-being.

EATING POORLY

Eating too little and eating too much both lead to poor health. Eating the same foods day after day or not eating fruit, vegetables, and milk products daily will also cause poor nutritional health. One in five adults skip meals daily. Only 13% of adults eat the minimum amount of fruit and vegetables needed. One in four older adults drink too much alcohol. Many health problems become worse if you drink more than one or two alcoholic beverages per day.

TOOTH LOSS/MOUTH PAIN

A healthy mouth, teeth, and gums are needed to eat. Missing, loose, or rotten teeth or dentures that don't fit well or cause mouth sores make it hard to eat.

ECONOMIC HARDSHIP

As many as 40% of older Americans have incomes of less than $6,000 per year. Having less -- or choosing to spend less -- than $25-30 per week for food makes it very hard to get the foods you need to stay healthy.

REDUCED SOCIAL CONTACT

One-third of all older people live alone. Being with people daily has a positive effect on morale, well-being, and eating.

MULTIPLE MEDICINES

Many older Americans must take medicines for health problems. Almost half of older Americans take multiple medicines daily. Growing old may change the way we respond to drugs. The more medicines you take, the greater the chance for side effects such as increased or decreased appetite, change in taste, constipation, weakness, drowsiness, diarrhea, nausea, and others. Vitamins or minerals, when taken in large doses, act like drugs and can cause harm. Alert your doctor to everything you take.

INVOLUNTARY WEIGHT LOSS/GAIN

Losing or gaining a lot of weight when you are not trying to do so is an important warning sign that must not be ignored. Being overweight or underweight also increases your chance of poor health.

NEEDS ASSISTANCE IN SELF CARE

Although most older people are able to eat, one of every five have trouble walking and shopping, buying, and cooking food, especially as they get older.

ELDER YEARS ABOVE AGE 80

Most older people lead full and productive lives. But as age increases, risk of frailty and health problems increase. Checking your nutritional health regularly makes good sense.

The Nutrition Screening Initiative • 1010 Wisconsin Avenue, NW • Suite 800 • Washington, DC 20007
The Nutrition Screening Initiative is funded in part by a grant from Ross Products Division of Abbott Laboratories, Inc.

Figure 8-3, (Continued)

Assessment of dietary intake involves the identification of foods, beverages, and dietary supplements consumed, in addition to the associated specific consumption patterns of patients. These data can be used to estimate the dietary prevalence of a particular food or food components, study time trends in dietary intake patterns, and design dietary education and counseling programs.

In a dental setting, a dental professional can estimate the frequency and quantity of excessive intake of sugar-sweetened beverages, assess the daily repetitiveness of the behavior, and develop a patient education message tailored to the patient's need if he or she has completed a dietary intake assessment. Dietary deficiencies cannot be inferred, however.

Methods of dietary assessment include 24-hour food recalls, food records or diaries, diet histories, food frequency recalls, and simple brief dietary screeners. The NSI discussed previously is a prime example of a dietary screener.[14] No single method is generally accepted as appropriate for all purposes. Some methods are retrospective, and others are prospective in nature. Table 8-5 provides a descriptive explanation of each method.

Selection of an appropriate method should be based on the degree of detail sought, the interviewee's characteristics, and the complexity and expense that is tolerable.

Food and beverage recall intake for any period of time can be obtained by a self-administered questionnaire or by a process that can involve a face-to-face or telephone or computer-initiated interview. The choice depends on literacy issues, personnel, and time needed for completion.

The single-day recall is frequently used to get a snap shot of a typical 1-day dietary intake. Estimates of the prevalence of low nutrient intakes based on raw 24-hour survey data are invariably misleading, and should always be interpreted in light of relevant biochemical and physiological measures of nutritional status.[15] The goal is to identify all foods eaten in one 24-hour period and to estimate the quantities eaten by using props or pictures of shapes, dimensions, or measures, as shown in Table 8-6. To ascertain intake for a 1-day period, approximately 15 to 20 minutes are needed for completion. Examples of forms useful in a 24-hour data collection are shown in Figure 8-4. The time and place of consumption of foods

TABLE 8-5

COMPARATIVE CHARACTERISTICS OF DIETARY ASSESSMENT METHODS

	FOOD DIARY	24-HOUR TYPICAL RECALL	FOOD FREQUENCY	DIETARY HISTORY	BRIEF DIETARY SCREENER
CHARACTERISTICS	A written account of food and beverage intake during a given time period.	Recall of the past diet during a given time period and attained through interview.	List of foods selected during a period of time.	Descriptive data of past eating habits.	Short list of foods oriented to a single nutrient or food group.
ADVANTAGES	Accurate; does not rely on patient's memory; is quantifiable.	Saves time; is quantifiable; low burden.	Can be self-administered; inexpensive to collect; low bias; low burden; can be analyzed.	Literacy not required; can obtain details as needed.	Low burden; quick; inexpensive; can be self-administered.
DISADVANTAGES	Requires literacy; burden is on the respondent; interpretation of data can be expensive and time-consuming.	Relies on memory; difficult to estimate portions; trained interviewer is required; interpretation of data can be expensive and time consuming.	Least accurate; quantification is imprecise; food list may not be culturally sensitive.	Relies on memory and lacks accuracy; may require excessive interview time.	Dietary information is limited in scope.

TABLE 8-6

VISUAL MODELS FOR ASSESSING PORTION SIZES OF FOODS EATEN

A SERVING OF—	MEASURES—	AND IS ABOUT AS BIG AS—
Vegetable or fruit	1 cup	Your fist
Cheese	1 oz	Four dice
Cooked vegetables or cooked rice	1/2 cup	A rounded handful or half a baseball
Meat	3 oz	A deck of cards
Peanut butter	2 tablespoons	A ping pong ball
Pasta	1 cup	A tennis ball
Baked potato	1 small	Computer mouse
Pancake or waffle	1 serving	Compact disc
Fish	3 oz	Check book
Mayonnaise/margarine	1 teaspoon	Thumb tip

Please answer or complete the following:
Enter today's date: _____

Which day of the week does this record represent?
Sunday ____ Monday ____ Tuesday ____ Wednesday ____ Thursday ____ Friday ____ Saturday ____

Is this a typical day?   ____ Yes   ____ No
If not, fill in the following with a typical day that happened before today.

Time	Quantity eaten	Details about food and drink
7:15 a.m.	1 cup	Hot tea
	2 tablespoons	Skim milk
	4 teaspoons	White sugar
	2 cups	Rice cereal and sliced bananas
10:00 a.m.	1 cup	Instant coffee
	2 teaspoons	White sugar
	1 large piece	Pound cake
12:30 p.m.	1 frozen	Individual pot pie
	1 cup	Squash
	12 ounces	Cola
3:00 p.m.	1 cup	Ice cream
	2 small	Sugar cookies
6:30 p.m.	1/2	Chicken breast, fried
	1 cup	Hash brown potatoes
	1 cup	String beans
	2 slices	White bread
	2 teaspoons	Butter
	1 cup	Fruity gelatin
9:00 p.m.	12 cups	Microwave popcorn
	1 cup	Hot tea
	2 teaspoons	White sugar

Figure 8-4   Sample form for 24-hour recall.

and beverages are useful for the interpretation of dietary patterns. Because the frequency of dietary intake of cariogenic foods is a contributing factor to oral disease, time and place data are valuable. The major criticism of this method is the accuracy of data recorded. Some people may have distorted perceptions of portion sizes, or may selectively forget what might be interpreted as "bad" foods (e.g., fats, alcohol, sugar).[16] Men have been reported to underestimate energy intake when compared with women.[17] Individuals with a high body mass index (BMI) tend to report diets that are higher in energy content and reflect frequent eating patterns and diets high in fat and low in dietary fiber content.[18] Most experts agree that one 24-hour dietary recall does not provide reliable estimates of "usual" or "typical" dietary intake but is useful when time is an issue for the health care professional.[19] If precision in assessment is the goal, researchers recommend using multiple and varied dietary assessment methods to reduce potential errors in data.[5] Usually, the 24-hour recall is useful for interpretation in the assessment of groups rather than individuals. If the goal is to identify typical behaviors, however, this method can be effective when the "typical" nature of the data is stressed to the interviewee. Collection of recalls for multiple days, including both weekdays and weekend days, can improve estimates of both the variety of food choices and the food consumption patterns of an individual. The advantages of the 24-hour dietary recall method are that it minimizes patient burden, can be administered quickly, and can be used to assess daily intake patterns.

Food frequency questionnaires (FFQs) are considered to be more qualitative than quantitative in nature. When information about dietary patterns of specific foods is of interest, this method proves to be the best choice.[20] The FFQ involves identification of a defined list of foods that may represent sources of specific food groups or nutrients. The patient/respondent is asked to identify frequency of intake of these foods for a given period of time that may be described as daily, weekly, monthly, or yearly. In some instances, semiquantitative FFQs will ask about typical portions or serving sizes. Figure 8-5 illustrates an FFQ designed to identify frequency of intake of beverages and fruits. These questionnaires can be self-administered or interviewer administered in formats similar to 24-hour dietary recalls. The advantage to this method is that it is cost-effective and time-efficient, but it does require both memory and mathematical skills of the patient/respondent.

Food records or diaries are necessary when detailed, accurate information is required about a patient's dietary intake. Use of electronic diaries or personal digital assistants (PDAs) have proved to be useful for recording and self-monitoring daily dietary intake.[21] Usually, these are maintained for a specified time period and are kept for a number of days. Shorter time periods are less likely to reveal usual eating patterns. Longer periods can be burdensome for the client/respondent and can result

in inaccuracies. A decision to use this method would be dependent on the client/respondent's literacy level, interest, and willingness to adhere to detailed record keeping. This approach is most useful in follow-up and evaluation of progress rather than as an initial screening activity for patients.

The methods used should be tailored to meet the individual patient's needs, literacy level, and tolerance for detail. They should be compatible with the purpose of the assessment and the method of analysis used in interpretation of the data collected. Numerous computer programs and websites offer access to software that provides the practitioner with opportunity to complete dietary analyses if they so desire. Table 8-7 lists several options that not only provide interpretation of data but also compare outputs to standard references. Note that the Healthy Eating Index (HEI) is free and electronically accessible on a home computer. It can be recommended to patients interested in monitoring their dietary intake over time.[22]

Physical Measures

Both anthropometric and clinical findings identified in patient assessment and in screening are significant determinants of nutritional status. These objective measures allow the dental practitioner to discriminate meaningful data from the subjective data derived in histories and dietary queries.

Anthropometrics. Measures of body composition are key components of health and can influence health outcomes. The size and weight of patients are important anthropometric indications of growth, risk for disease and malnutrition, and general well-being. Measurement techniques and interpretations of the outcomes vary with age. Note that a single measurement technique is unlikely to be optimal in all circumstances.

Techniques for measuring body composition may include skin fold thickness, BMI, waist circumference, and waist-to-hip ratio. Other more complex measures include bioelectric impedance analysis (BIA), dual energy x-ray absorptometry (DXA), and magnetic resonance imaging (MRI). Table 8-8 lists each of these techniques with advantages and disadvantages of each.[23]

Nutrition screening should include accurate measurements of height and weight and a calculation of BMI.[24] Other simple techniques that are quick and highly informative assessments for adult patients include waist and hip circumferences. These anthropometric measures are useful indicators of risk for a number of chronic diseases. BMI, calculated from a person's weight and height as shown in Table 8-9, does not measure body fat directly, but can be considered an alternative to direct measures. BMI is an inexpensive and easy-to-perform technique for screening for weight categories associated with health problems.[24] Research has shown that BMI

PLEASE PUT A TICK (✓) ON EVERY LINE

FOODS AND AMOUNTS	AVERAGE USE LAST YEAR								
DRINKS	Never or less than once/month	1-3 per month	Once a week	2-4 per week	5-6 per week	Once a day	2-3 per day	4-5 per day	6+ per day
Tea (cup)								✓	
Coffee, instant or ground (cup)						✓			
Coffee, decaffeinated (cup)	✓								
Coffee whitener (e.g., Coffee-mate [teaspoon])	✓								
Cocoa, hot chocolate (cup)						✓			
Horlicks, Ovaltine (cup)	✓								
Wine (glass)	✓								
Beer, lager or cider (half pint)	✓								
Port, sherry, vermouth, liqueurs (glass)	✓								
Spirits (e.g., gin, brandy, whisky, vodka [single])	✓								
Low-calorie or diet fizzy soft drinks (glass)	✓								
Fizzy soft drinks (e.g., Coca cola, lemonade [glass])						✓			
Pure fruit juice (100%) (e.g., orange, apple [glass])	✓								
Fruit squash or cordial (glass)							✓		
FRUIT (1 fruit or medium serving) **For very seasonal fruits such as strawberries, please estimate your average use when the fruit is in season**									
Apples				✓					
Pears				✓					
Oranges, satsumas, mandarins		✓							
Grapefruit	✓								
Bananas			✓						
Grapes			✓						
Melon	✓								
Peaches, plums, apricots				✓					
Strawberries, raspberries, kiwi fruit						✓			
Tinned fruit		✓							
Dried fruit (e.g., raisins, prunes)	✓								
	Never or less than once/month	1-3 per month	Once a week	2-4 per week	5-6 per week	Once a day	2-3 per day	4-5 per day	6+ per day

Please check that you have a tick (✓) on EVERY line

Figure 8-5   Food frequency collection form.

correlates to direct measures of body fat derived from underwater weighing and DXA.[25] BMI has also been shown to overestimate chronic disease risk in older adults. Waist-to-hip ratio appears to be a better measure of risk in those 75 years of age or older.[26] Among those diagnosed with type 2 diabetes, waist-to-hip ratio is considered to be a better measure of central obesity than a calculated BMI of less than or equal to 27 kg/m^2, but when BMI exceeds 27 kg/m^2, the BMI is a better indicator.[27] Simple measures of waist circumference as shown in Table 8-10 have been highly correlated and

recommended to identify the role of body weight in some metabolic disorders such as metabolic syndrome and diabetes.[28]

In infants and children, growth and development are defined by repeated measures of height, weight, head circumference, and BMI and are expressed as percentiles. The growth charts published by the Centers for Disease Control and Prevention present a series of percentile curves that illustrate the distribution of specific body measurements in U.S. children.[29] As a general rule, an appropriate state of health and nutritional status is

TABLE 8-7

DIETARY ASSESSMENT INSTRUMENTS, NUTRIENT ANALYSIS SOFTWARE, AND WEBSITES FOR CONDUCTING ANALYSES

INSTRUMENTS	WEBSITES
Block Food Frequency Questionnaire (A brief screener with versions suitable for use with adults and children.)	http://www.nutritionquest.com/index.htm
National Cancer Institute Dietary Questionnaire (A food frequency questionnaire with a dietary analysis component.)	http://riskfactor.cancer.gov/DHQ/
Harvard Food Frequency Questionnaire (A screener suitable for adults, and one for children.)	http://regepi.bwh.harvard.edu/health/nutrition.html
NUTRIENT ANALYSIS SOFTWARE	WEBSITES
ESHA Food Processor	http://www.esha.com/products/foodpro
Nutritionist Pro	http://ww/nutritionistpro.com/
Food Intake Analysis System	http://www.sph.uth.tmc.edu/hnc/FIAS/software.htm
Nutrition Data System	http://www.ncc.umn.edu/swmenu.htm
USDA Healthy Eating Index	http://www.mypyramidtracker.gov/login.aspx

TABLE 8-8

ADVANTAGES AND DISADVANTAGES OF DIFFERENT TECHNIQUES FOR MEASURING BODY COMPOSITION

TECHNIQUE	ADVANTAGES	DISADVANTAGES
Skinfold thickness	Index of regional fatness	Poor accuracy in obese individuals; requires technician skill.
Body mass index (BMI) (weight/height^2)	Simple measure of relative weight; a global index of nutritional status.	Does not assess changes in fat and lean muscle mass that may vary in special groups such as trained athletes or the elderly.
Waist circumference	Simple measure of central body fatness that is of greater relevance to metabolic risk (lipid profile, insulin resistance); highly correlated with magnetic resonance imaging (MRI) measures of intraabdominal fat.	
Waist-to-hip ratio	Gives a better measure of morbidity than either measure alone.	
Bioelectrical impedance analysis (BIA)	Provides measure of changes in lean body mass.	Poor accuracy; changes in body weight will introduce error; has limited use for measuring fat mass.
Dual energy x-ray absorptiometry (DXA)	Used to measure regional lean mass (limb) to determine nutritional requirements.	

TABLE 8-9

BODY MASS INDEX

BMI	19	20	21	22	23	24	25	26	27	28	29	30	31	32	33	34	35
HEIGHT (INCHES)								Body Weight (pounds)									
58	91	96	100	105	110	115	119	124	129	134	138	143	148	153	158	162	167
59	94	99	104	109	114	119	124	128	133	138	143	148	153	158	163	168	173
60	97	102	107	112	118	123	128	133	138	143	148	153	158	163	168	174	179
61	100	106	111	116	122	127	132	137	143	148	153	158	164	169	174	180	185
62	104	109	115	120	126	131	136	142	147	153	158	164	169	175	180	186	191
63	107	113	118	124	130	135	141	146	152	158	163	169	175	180	186	191	197
64	110	116	122	128	134	140	145	151	157	163	169	174	180	186	192	197	204
65	114	120	126	132	138	144	150	156	162	168	174	180	186	192	198	204	210
66	118	124	130	136	142	148	155	161	167	173	179	186	192	198	204	210	216
67	121	127	134	140	146	153	159	166	172	178	185	191	198	204	211	217	223
68	125	131	138	144	151	158	164	171	177	184	190	197	203	210	216	223	230
69	128	135	142	149	155	162	169	176	182	189	196	203	209	216	223	230	236
70	132	139	146	153	160	167	174	181	188	195	202	209	216	222	229	236	243
71	136	143	150	157	165	172	179	186	193	200	208	215	222	229	236	243	250
72	140	147	154	162	169	177	184	191	199	206	213	221	228	235	242	250	258
73	144	151	159	166	174	182	189	197	204	212	219	227	235	242	250	257	265
74	148	155	163	171	179	186	194	202	210	218	225	233	241	249	256	264	272
75	152	160	168	176	184	192	200	208	216	224	232	240	248	256	264	272	279
76	156	164	172	180	189	197	205	213	221	230	238	246	254	263	271	279	287

BMI	36	37	38	39	40	41	42	43	44	45	46	47	48	49	50	51	52	53	54
HEIGHT (INCHES)										Body Weight (pounds)									
58	172	177	181	186	191	196	201	205	210	215	220	224	229	234	239	244	248	253	258
59	178	183	188	193	198	203	208	212	217	222	227	232	237	242	247	252	257	262	267
60	184	189	194	199	204	209	215	220	225	230	235	240	245	250	255	261	266	271	276
61	190	195	201	206	211	217	222	227	232	238	243	248	254	259	264	269	275	280	285
62	196	202	207	213	218	224	229	235	240	246	251	256	262	267	273	278	284	289	295
63	203	208	214	220	225	231	237	242	248	254	259	265	270	278	282	287	293	299	304
64	209	215	221	227	232	238	244	250	256	262	267	273	279	285	291	296	302	308	314
65	216	222	228	234	240	246	252	258	264	270	276	282	288	294	300	306	312	318	324
66	223	229	235	241	247	253	260	266	272	278	284	291	297	303	309	315	322	328	334
67	230	236	242	249	255	261	268	274	280	287	293	299	306	312	319	325	331	338	344
68	236	243	249	256	262	269	276	282	289	295	302	308	315	322	328	335	341	348	354
69	243	250	257	263	270	277	284	291	297	304	311	318	324	331	338	345	351	358	365
70	250	257	264	271	278	285	292	299	306	313	320	327	334	341	348	355	362	369	376
71	257	265	272	279	286	293	301	308	315	322	329	338	343	351	358	365	372	379	386
72	265	272	279	288	294	302	309	316	324	331	338	346	353	361	368	375	383	390	397
73	272	280	288	295	303	310	318	325	333	340	348	355	363	371	378	386	393	401	408
74	280	287	295	303	311	319	326	334	342	350	358	365	373	381	389	396	404	412	420
75	287	295	303	311	319	327	335	343	351	359	367	375	383	391	399	407	415	423	431
76	295	304	312	320	328	336	344	353	361	369	377	385	394	402	410	418	426	435	443

(From National Heart, Lung, and Blood Institute. Obesity Education Initiative (website): http://www.nhlbi.nih.gov/guidelines/obesity/bmi_tbl.htm. Accessed October 18, 2006.)

TABLE 8-10

CLASSIFICATION OF OVERWEIGHT/OBESITY BY BMI, WAIST CIRCUMFERENCE, AND DISEASE RISK

	BMI (kg/m²)	OBESITY CLASS	Disease risk* relative to normal weight and waist circumference	
			MEN 102 CM (40 IN) OR LESS WOMEN 88 CM (35 IN) OR LESS	MEN >102 CM (40 IN) WOMEN >88 CM (35 IN)
Underweight	<18.5		—	—
Normal	18.5-24.9		—	—
Overweight	25.0-29.9		Increased	High
Obesity	30.0-34.9	I	High	Very high
	35.0-39.9	II	Very high	Very high
Extreme obesity	40.0†	III	Extremely high†	Extremely high†

* Disease risk for type 2 diabetes, hypertension, and cardiovascular disease.
†Increased waist circumference can also be a marker for increased risk even in persons of normal weight.
(From National Heart, Lung, and Blood Institute, Obesity Education Initiative (website): http://www.nhlbi.nih.gov/health/public/heart/obesity/lose_wt/bmi_dis.htm. Accessed October 18, 2006.)

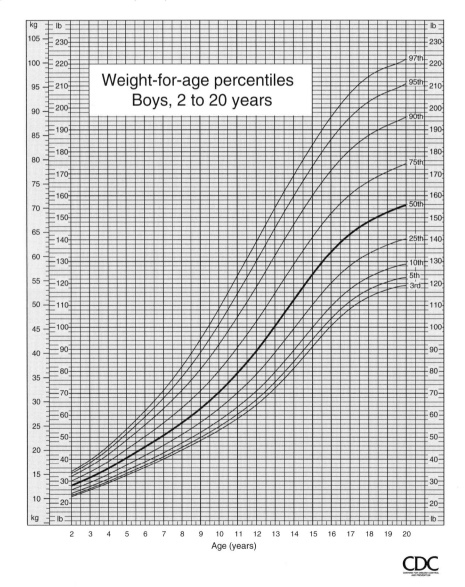

Figure 8-6 Sample growth chart for boys. (Courtesy of the National Center for Health Statistics, in collaboration with the National Center for Chronic Disease Prevention and Health Promotion, 2000.)

associated with expected rates of growth. Rates of growth as plotted on growth charts are intended to contribute to impressions of health but are not intended to be diagnostic. Representative growth charts for BMI for boys and girls older than 2 years are shown in Figure 8-6 and Figure 8-7, respectively.

Physical findings.   The oral mucosal cells act as a barrier to invasion of underlying collagenous connective tissue by oral microbes. Because the turnover rate of oral mucosal cells occurs within 3 to 7 days, these tissues are highly susceptible to changes associated with nutritional inadequacies. Physical changes in the lips, tongue, gingival

and oral mucosa mirror changes in other body tissue that occur in response to nutritional anomalies.[8] Anatomical lesions, changes in color or texture, complaints of burning mouth or tongue, and evidence of inflammation can be associated with inadequate dietary intake. Table 8-11 relates evidence of physical findings in the head and neck region with possible associated changes in nutritional adequacy.

The dental professional must exercise caution in the interpretation of clinical signs relative to nutritional status. Just as no single measure of dietary intake or body composition can be definitely interpreted into a true determinant of nutritional status, no single clinical

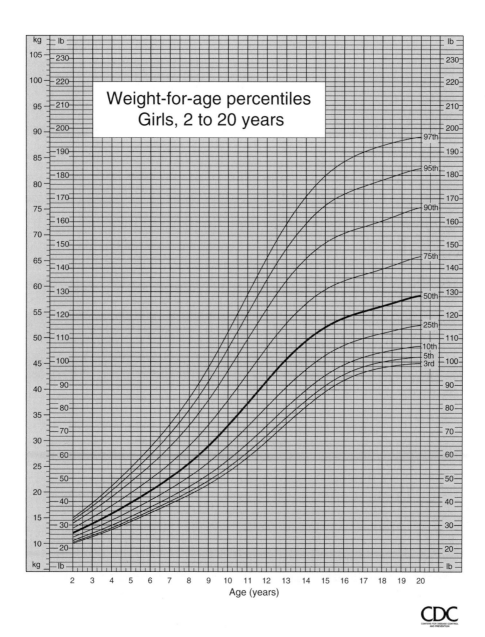

Figure 8-7   Sample growth chart for girls. (Courtesy of the National Center for Health Statistics, in collaboration with the National Center for Chronic Disease Prevention and Health Promotion, 2000.)

TABLE 8-11

EXTRAORAL, INTRAORAL, AND OTHER PHYSICAL FINDINGS ASSOCIATED WITH CHANGES IN DIETARY NUTRIENT ADEQUACY

PHYSICAL FINDINGS	NUTRIENT INFERENCE
Dental caries	Excessive dietary intake of fermentable carbohydrate and frequent consumption of cariogenic foods and beverages. Inadequate dietary intake of vitamin D, calcium, and/or phosphorus.
Alveolar bone loss	Inadequate dietary intake of vitamin D, calcium, and/or phosphorus.
Glossitis (raw, fissured, red tongue)	Inadequate dietary sources of B vitamins, including niacin (B_3), pyridoxine (B_6), folic acid, biotin, riboflavin (B_2), cobalamin (B_{12}) and/or iron.
Atrophy of filiform papillae of the tongue	Inadequate dietary sources of B vitamins including riboflavin (B_2), cobalamin (B_{12}), niacin (B_3), folic acid, biotin, and/or iron.
Burning tongue	Inadequate dietary sources of B vitamins, including thiamin (B_1), riboflavin (B_2), cobalamin (B_{12}), niacin (B_3), pyridoxine (B_6), and/or iron.
Magenta tongue	Inadequate dietary sources of riboflavin (B_2).
Thickening of the tongue with atrophy in supporting muscles	Inadequate dietary sources of zinc.
Smooth edematous tongue	Inadequate dietary sources of protein.
Spongy, bleeding, red gingivae	Inadequate dietary sources of vitamins C and/or K.
Stomatitis	Inadequate dietary sources of B vitamins, including niacin (B_3), pyridoxine (B_6), cobalamin (B_{12}), and/or iron.
Angular cheilosis of lips	Inadequate dietary sources of B vitamins including niacin (B_3), pyridoxine (B_6), riboflavin (B_2), and/or iron, and/or protein.
Altered taste and loss of appetite	Inadequate dietary sources of B vitamins, including thiamin (B_1), niacin (B_3), and cobalamin (B_{12}).
Changes in oral mucosa (ulceration, necrosis, erosion)	Inadequate dietary sources of B vitamins, including folic acid, biotin, cobalamin (B_{12}), and/or vitamin C and/or iron.
Xerostomia	Inadequate dietary sources of vitamin C, vitamin A, and/or protein.
Pale eye membranes	Inadequate dietary sources of iron.
Dull, pluckable hair	Inadequate dietary intake of protein and calories.

physical finding can be translated into a specific nutrient inadequacy. These add to a differential assessment of the role of diet and nutrition in decreasing risk for oral diseases and disorders (see Chapters 7 and 18).[30]

Biochemical Data

Laboratory test and analyses can illuminate suspected physical findings thought to be related to nutritional status. In dental settings, routine comprehensive laboratory data analyses of body fluids like blood and urine are not always available. Referral to a laboratory may be indicated when dietary data and physical findings suggest a nutrient abnormality. Techniques used to measure nutritional status include the possible assessment of nutrient levels in body fluids, excretion rate of nutrients, abnormal metabolic products in the blood, or changes in enzyme activity in response to nutrient intakes. Note that tests may vary in their diagnostic value, accuracy, and precision. Chapter 9 provides a list of routine and specific tests used to evaluate nutrient status.

TABLE 8-12

RATIONALE FOR TARGETED DIETARY AND NUTRITION EDUCATION MESSAGES FOR PATIENT EDUCATION

FINDINGS	RATIONALE
Excessive and frequent consumption of sugar-sweetened beverages.	Beverages other than water may contain added sugars that increase caries risk and caloric intake. Carbonated beverages are acidic and can cause tooth erosion. Water promotes oral clearance without increasing oral acidity.
Frequently skipped breakfasts.	Sleep diminishes salivary flow rate and breakfast stimulates flow and energy levels.
Eats and/or drinks beverages other than water more than 5 times per day.	Spacing eating and drinking occasions more than 2 hours apart allows the oral pH levels to return to normal and enhances weight management behaviors.
Snacks on fermentable carbohydrates frequently throughout the day.	Snacks should be limited to twice a day and chosen from foods that are cariostatic. Cheese and crackers, cottage cheese and fruit, nuts and apple slices, yogurt and granola, skim milk and cookies, and peanut butter and celery are neutral rather than acidic combinations.
Drinks less than 2 cups of low-fat or fat-free milk per day and does not eat cheese.	Calcium, phosphorus, and the protein, casein, in dairy products are thought to increase salivary production, decrease dental caries, and help to maintain bone health.
Eats less than four cups of fruits and vegetables daily.	Fresh fruits and vegetables increase salivary flow rate, provide an excellent source of antioxidants important for oral soft tissue health, and decrease risk for constipation.
Eats less than three servings of whole-grain breads/cereals daily.	Whole-grain foods are a primary source of B vitamins and other minerals important in maintaining the health of oral soft tissue. Dietary fiber increases mastication and salivary output to decrease oral pH and improve digestion.
Eats less than one serving per day of high-quality protein food such as meat, poultry, fish, eggs, dry beans, or nuts.	Protein foods, rich in vitamin and minerals, buffer acidic oral environments, promote the health of oral tissue, and strengthen the immune system's defenses against oral infection.
Uses tobacco routinely.	A daily intake of five to nine fruits and vegetables decreases risk of oral cancer among habitual tobacco users.
Drinks more than two servings of alcohol daily, if a man, and more than one daily if a woman.	Excessive alcohol intake, especially combined with tobacco use, increases risk for oral cancer.
Avoids use of sugar-free chewing gum.	Sugar-free chewing gums sweetened with sugar alcohols and high-intensity sweeteners do not promote caries or breakdown of tooth enamel and increase salivary flow.

INTERPRETATION OF FINDINGS

Screening activities ultimately lead to conclusions about nutritional status that can guide the dental practitioner in the selection of patient education messages leading to decreased risk of oral diseases. Table 8-12 provides the rationale for messages that can be tailored to the patient's needs and motivations (see Chapters 10 and 11).

SUMMARY

In summary, psychosocial and medical history variables are the first predisposing factors that indicate a need to further assess dietary intake, physical status, and possible biochemical indices. Dietary intake alone may provide a snapshot for determining patterns of eating associated with risk for dental disease, particularly those that affect hard tissue. Soft tissue disorders can be associated with nutritional status, but cannot be definitively identified without more extensive biochemical data. When inadequate intakes are accompanied by changes in absorption, use, or loss of nutrients, changes occur in body stores that are best identified with biochemical or laboratory data. When abnormal laboratory values are accompanied by wasting or delayed growth and physical or clinical manifestations of a nutritional inadequacy, the clinician should provide corrective dietary and nutritional counseling. Finally, repeated measures of interest in those patients identified at risk of oral diseases can be a beneficial preventive approach.

REFERENCES

1. Diet, nutrition and the prevention of chronic diseases. Report of a Joint WHO/FAO Expert Consultation, WHO Technical Report 916, Geneva, World Health Organization, 2003.
2. Watt RG: New WHO diet and nutrition review: implications for dental disease prevention. *Nutrition* 19:1028-1029, 2003.
3. Moynihan P, Petersen PE: Diet, nutrition and the prevention of dental diseases, *Public Health Nutr* 7:201-226, 2003.
4. Mobley CC: Dietary analysis in a restorative practice. In Duke SE, editor: *The changing practice of restorative dentistry*, Indianapolis, IN 2002, Indiana University School of Dentistry.
5. Sajnani-Oommen G, Perez-Spiess S, Julliard K: Comparison of nutritional counseling between provider types, *Pediatr Dent* 28:369-374, 2006.
6. Chung MH, Kaste LM, Loerber A et al.: Dental and medical students' knowledge and opinions of infant oral health, *J Dent Educ* 70:511-517, 2006.
7. Touger-Decker R: Clinical and laboratory assessment of nutrition status in dental practice. *Dent Clin North Am* 47:259-278, 2003.
8. Shils ME, Shike M, Ross AC et al, editors: *Modern nutrition in health and disease*, ed 10, Philadelphia, 2006, Lippincott, Williams & Wilkins.
9. Morrison G, Hark L: *Medical nutrition and disease*, ed 2, Malder, MA, 2003, Blackwell Science.
10. Centers for Disease Control and Prevention (CDC), National Center for Health Statistics (NCHS): National health and nutrition examination survey data, 1999-2000 (website): http://www.cdc.gov/nchs/about/major/nhanes/questexam.htm. Accessed September 4, 2006.
11. Touger-Decker R, Mobley CC: Oral health and nutrition: position of the American Dietetic Assoc. *J Am Diet Assoc* 103:615-625, 2003.
12. McMahon K, Brown J: Nutritional screening and assessment. *Seminars in Oncology Nursing* 16:106-112, 2003.
13. Mendoza M, Mobley CC, Hattaway KK: Caries risk management and the role of dietary assessment, *J Dent Res* 74 (abstract 33):16, 1995.
14. Posner BM, Jette AM, Smith KW et al.: Nutrition and health risks in the elderly. the nutrition screening initiative. *Am J Public Health* 83:972-978, 1993.
15. Mackerras D, Rutishauser I: 24-hour national dietary survey data: how do we interpret them most effectively? *Public Health Nutr* 8:657-665, 2005.
16. Schwartz J, Byrd-Bredbenner C: Portion distortion: typical portion sizes selected by young adults, *J Am Diet Assoc* 106:1412-1418, 2006.
17. Jonnalagadda SS, Mitchell DC, Smiciklas-Wright H et al.: Accuracy of energy intake data estimated by a multiple-pass, 24-hour dietary recall technique, *J Am Diet Assoc* 100:309-311, 2000.
18. Howarth NC, Huang TT, Robert SB et al.: Eating patterns and dietary composition in relation to BMI in younger and older adults, *Int J Obes* (Epub): (http://www.nature.com.ezproxy.library.unlv.edu/ijo/journal/vaop/ncurrent/full/0803456a.html), 2006.
19. Natarajan L, Rock CL, Thomson CA et al.: On the importance of using multiple methods of dietary assessment, *Epidemiology* 15:738-745, 2004.
20. Vatanparast H, Whiting SJ: Early milk intake, later bone health: result from using the milk history questionnaire, *Nut Rev* 62:256-260, 2004.
21. Burke LE, Warziski M, Starrett T et al.: Self-monitoring dietary intake: current and future practices, *J Ren Nut* 15:281-290, 2005.
22. Weinstein SJ, Vogt TM, Gerrior SA: Healthy Eating Index scores are associated with blood nutrient concentrations in the third National Health And Nutrition Examination Survey, *J Am Diet Assoc* 104:576-584, 2004.
23. Wells JCK, Fewtrell MS: Measuring body composition, *Arch Dis Child* 91:612-617, 2006.
24. Bray GA: Obesity: the disease, *J Med Chem* 49:4001-4007, 2006.
25. National Heart, Lung, and Blood Institute and the North American Association for the Study of Obesity: The practical guide: identification, evaluation, and treatment of overweight and obesity in adults, Bethesda, MD, 2000, NIH publication 00-4084. (http://www.nhlbi.nih.gov/guidelines/obesity/prctgd_c.pdf) Accessed September 16, 2005.
26. Price GM, Uauy R, Breeze E et al.: Weight, shape, and mortality risk in older persons: elevated waist-hip ratio, not high body mass index, is associated with a greater risk of death, *Am J Clin Nutr* 84:449-460, 2006.
27. Hadaegh F, Zabetian A, Harati H et al.: Waist/height ratio as a better predictor of type 2 diabetes compared to body mass index in Tehranian adult men—a 3.6-year prospective study, *Exp Clin Endocrinol Diabetes* 114:310-315, 2006.
28. U.S. Public Health Service, National Institutes of Health, NHLBI: National Cholesterol Education Program. Third Report of the Expert Panel on Detection, Evaluation and Treatment of High Blood Cholesterol in Adults, NIH Publication No. 01-3305, 2001. Accessed September 16, 2005.
29. Kuczmarski RJ, Ogden CL, Guo SS et al.: CDC growth charts for the United States: methods and development, *Vital Health Stat 11* 246:1-190. 2002.
30. Mahan LK, Escott-Stump SE, editors: *Food, nutrition, and diet therapy*, ed 11, Philadelphia, 2004, Saunders.

Chapter 9

Biological and Chemical Indicators of Disease Risk

DAVID P. CAPPELLI AND CONNIE C. MOBLEY

CARIES

Microbiological Testing for Caries
Testing the Salivary Flow Rate

PERIODONTAL DISEASE

Analysis of Subgingival Plaque
Subgingival Temperature
Genetic Testing for Periodontal Disease Risk
Gingival Crevicular Fluid

ORAL CANCER

SYSTEMIC DISEASE

SUMMARY

LEARNING OBJECTIVES

Upon completion of this chapter, the learner will be able to:
- Describe the assessment components that can be used to measure biological and chemical variables that are associated with a patient's risk for oral diseases, including dental caries, periodontal disease, and oral cancer.
- Outline the strengths and limitations of independent assessment methods.
- Explain which assessment components are appropriate to determine the patient's risk profile for a given oral condition.
- Review how and when to initiate ancillary risk assessment activities.
- Apply identified outcomes of disparate assessment components to the development of a plan of prevention tailored to a patient's individual risk for oral disease.

KEY TERMS

Assessment modalities
Bacteria
Culture method
Diabetes mellitus
Facultative anaerobic species
Gene polymorphism
Genetics
Gingival crevicular fluid
Microorganisms
Salivary components
Salivary diagnostics
Salivary gland hypofunction
Subgingival plaque
Subgingival temperature
Xerostomia

A comprehensive profile is necessary for the oral health care practitioner to apply prevention-based initiatives to oral conditions. Information gathered from the patient about his or her risk factors and behaviors help to create the most effective preventive and treatment care plan that will, ultimately, reduce the future burden of oral disease. Because oral diseases are biobehavioral, the etiology of oral diseases can be explained by certain exposures that increase the risk for disease. Understanding the links among risk, disease, and prevention depends on dental practitioner skills. Quantification of risk factors as a measure of disease requires the appropriate selection, administration, and interpretation of measures of a patient's risk and the effect on the patient's disease.

Obtaining a complete medical and social history is important in any patient care setting, but this history is especially important when the dental practitioner is developing a plan to prevent future disease. Laboratory tests of biological functions, exposures, or health outcomes are often affected by both treatment and medication histories, in addition to specific adopted individual behaviors. A comprehensive, detailed history ensures accurate information that is critical to determining the patient's risk status. When related to health behaviors, history taking should obtain the information needed to adequately develop individual risk profiles, motivate the patient to change his or her behavior, or guide the dental practitioner in selecting preventive interventions to improve health status. Motivating a patient to change behavior requires an assessment of both current behavior and willingness to change or adopt a new specific behavior. This assessment is a key component in designing and providing overall patient care. Motivational interviewing techniques are reviewed in Chapter 11.

The global objective of data gathering and assessment is to compile appropriate information that will allow the dental professional to develop a plan of prevention to the needs of the patient. In Chapters 4, 5, and 6, risk factors associated with oral diseases are discussed. Knowledge of these risk factors provides the basis for selection of **assessment modalities** to address these risks. Once the patient's risk is understood, the goal is to continue to tailor a plan of prevention on the basis of changes in that risk. Additional information is often needed to accomplish this, thus more comprehensive and targeted measures are needed. This chapter addresses the intermediate additional steps needed to best develop a sound individualized preventive plan.

CARIES

On the basis of the etiology of this disease (see Figure 4-2), testing for risk for dental caries examines the concentration of putative pathogenic **bacteria**, the adequacy of salivary flow, and additional contributing factors, including diet. Dietary assessment in oral health is described in Chapter 8. Specific modalities for addressing bacteria, **salivary components**, and **genetics** are reviewed in this chapter.

Microbiological Testing for Caries

Two species of **microorganisms** are primarily implicated in caries development: *Streptococcus* spp.[1] and *Lactobacillus* spp.[2] Although other species of bacteria (e.g., *Actinomyces* spp. in root caries) are hypothesized to play a role in caries development, these two species of bacteria are of greatest interest in disease formation.[3] Furthermore, only the organisms identified as mutans streptococci are implicated in the formation of the initial carious lesion and therefore are of greatest interest in risk for caries.[4] Microbiological testing for caries risk involves testing for the presence of the consortium of indicator organisms identified as mutans streptococci and lactobacilli. Bacterial testing can be used to assess adherence to dietary recommendations for caries risk management.

Bacterial testing can be accomplished by using three different strategies. Each strategy has individual strengths and weaknesses, so the application of each depends on the information needed for each patient. The first method is to directly examine the plaque microscopically.[5] With a dental instrument or toothpick,[6] a sample of the biofilm is removed from the tooth surface and placed on the pad of a plastic test strip. The instrument is moved over the pad by using a circular motion with gentle pressure to distribute the sample. The plaque strip is placed in a culture medium and incubated for 48 hours at 37° C. After drying, the strips are examined and the bacterial species are identified at 10× microscopic magnification.[5] The strength of this method is its high specificity. In other words, the microorganisms identified in the sample can be translated into the risk for a tooth to become cavitated. The limitation of this method is that the information cannot be generalized to describe the biological ecology of the entire oral cavity. Another limitation is that the method is cumbersome when one is seeking to identify colonization of organisms from multiple sites.

The other two methods rely on saliva as the vehicle for the microorganism. These tests are based on the premise that the biological milieu of the oral cavity is reflected in the microbiological composition in the saliva. Methods that use saliva as a vehicle, therefore, are considered to be representative and can be used to describe the environment of the entire oral cavity. The problem with these methods is the reverse of the problem with the plaque strip application. In this case results are not specific, and cannot be related to individual sites or teeth. In addition, bacterial salivary testing is influenced by the number of active untreated lesions where these organisms are harbored.

The **culture method** relies on saliva as the vehicle for bacteriological testing.[7] This method requires that 1.5 to 2 mL of a stimulated saliva sample is obtained from the patient. Before sample collection, the dental professional should record all medications and pertinent medical history. A saliva sample should not be obtained if the patient is currently taking medications that might alter the oral microbiological burden or affect the results, especially if he or she is consuming systemic antibiotics or temporarily using antihistamines. The patient should not have had food, drink, or disclosing tablets within the past hour before a sample collection. Also, a dental prophylaxis should not have been performed before a sample collection.

The patient is first asked to expectorate into a graduated, plastic tube with a conical base graduated to 0.1 mL. In the mouth of the tube, a small plastic funnel is inserted to facilitate collection of the saliva. Either stimulated or unstimulated saliva can be used to test for the presence of oral microorganisms. To collect an unstimulated saliva sample, request that the patient expectorate directly into the calibrated collection tube and funnel. To collect a stimulated saliva sample, the patient is asked to chew a piece of wax to stimulate salivary flow. Once the wax is the consistency of chewing gum, the patient is asked to swallow the pooled saliva and then spit into the tube. At this point one can begin to collect the patient sample by having the patient expectorate directly into the collection tube and funnel. After 1.0 to 2.0 mL of saliva has been collected in the tube, and within 1 hour of collection, the saliva should be transported to the laboratory. If delivery to the laboratory is delayed, the sample should be kept cold for as long as 4 hours until the sample can be delivered. Transport of the sample as soon as possible is critical to avoid degradation of the bacteria.[7]

Once delivered to the laboratory, the sample is cultured on an SB20 agar for mutans streptococci identification, or a Rogosa agar for culture of Lactobacilli species. The saliva is serially diluted onto the agar plates and incubated for 48 hours. Because mutans are **facultative anaerobic species**, these organisms are best cultured in an anaerobic environment for identification. The sensitivity of this method ranges from 62% to 83%, and the specificity ranges from 82% to 84%,[8] suggesting that microbiological identification is more accurate at detecting individuals at a lower caries risk than those who are at greater risk for developing disease.

Once in the laboratory, 3 mL of transport media is added to the sample to stabilize the bacteria. Serial dilutions are created by adding increasing volumes of saliva to sterile saline. Approximately 25 mL of each dilution is added to the SB20 agar plate, which is incubated under anaerobic conditions at 37° C for 48 hours. An antibiotic, bacitracin, is added to the agar to suppress growth of competing bacteria (especially gram-negative spp.).[7]

After 48 hours, the colonies are counted under a microscope. Colonies appear as yellow or white with a "cauliflower" formation. Mutans streptococci have a glucan "ring" or coat and grow into the agar. Glucan, produced by these organisms, allows them to adhere to the tooth in the oral environment. Plates with different dilutions are counted, and results are stated as colony-forming units per mL of whole saliva (CFU/mL). Table 9-1 outlines the relationship between colony counts of mutans streptococci and caries risk.[7]

A series of analytical methods use saliva as a vehicle, but rely on changes to the salivary pH resulting from acid production as a measure of potential caries risk.[9] Since the pH is directly linked to both acidogenicity or the oral environment and an increase in the sucrose challenge in the diet, one can assume that it can be used to describe the microbiological activity in the oral cavity. Direct measures of pH are not used routinely in the dental setting.

TABLE 9-1

CARIES RISK CATEGORIES ASSOCIATED WITH MUTANS STREPTOCOCCI LEVEL IN WHOLE SALIVA

CARIES RISK CATEGORY	MUTANS STREPTOCOCCI (CFU/ML)
High	$\geq 5.5 \times 10^5$
Moderate	$\geq 1 \times 10^5 - <5.5 \times 10^5$
Low	$<1 \times 10^5$

Commercial test kits rely on bacterial culture techniques to assess the potential caries risk. Chair side methods are available to measure the levels of mutans streptococci in saliva. Dentocult-SM is one such method that uses saliva to measure the level of bacteria.[10] The kit contains a mitis salivarius broth for culture. Before sample collection, a 5-μg bacitracin tablet is added to the broth to inhibit growth of competing organisms. A stimulated saliva sample is collected by asking the patient to chew a paraffin sample that is included in the kit. After two minutes of chewing, a plastic strip that is provided in the kit is inserted between the lips and rotated to obtain an adequate sample. The strip is smooth on one side and rough on the other to promote bacterial adherence. The strip is removed through closed lips and attached to the cap. The cap is closed onto the vial and incubated for 48 hours at 37° C (Orion Diagnostica, Espoo, Finland).[10]

Testing the Salivary Flow Rate

The role of **salivary diagnostics** in risk assessment for caries is described in this chapter and others, so the use of saliva to assess risk for disease is well founded.[11] Although the role of saliva in quality of life is recognized by numerous health care professionals, the dental provider often lacks a clear understanding of the role of saliva in risk assessment. This section addresses the role of saliva in caries risk assessment, and oral cancer and salivary diagnostics are discussed later in the chapter.

Hyposalivation is a symptom that reflects that the mouth is too dry most of the time. Patients verbally express symptoms of dry mouth that can be related to chronic disease, medications, or other factors. **Xerostomia** and **salivary gland hypofunction** are associated with an increased incidence of dental caries. To understand the clinical impact of salivary gland hypofunction on oral disease, the dental practitioner must assess the extent of the hyposalivation. Answers to questions to ascertain existing xerostomia may contribute to the patient's known risk factors, and should be included as a part of the overall risk assessment (see Chapter 4, Box 4-2). If the screening reflects dry mouth, further testing is warranted. This testing is accomplished by measuring unstimulated saliva flow.

A series of analytical methods use saliva as a vehicle, but rely on changes of the salivary pH resulting from acid production as a measure of potential caries risk.[9] Buffering capacity of saliva can be determined by measuring the pH of the saliva.[12] Because the pH of unstimulated saliva varies during the day, a more generalizable measure can be determined by using stimulated saliva. Salivary flow rates can be measured by using an unstimulated or stimulated saliva collection procedure. Significant correlations have been observed between unstimulated and stimulated flow rates.[12] The unstimulated flow rate represents the resting oral status, and is better to assess hyposalivation.

Before measuring the unstimulated salivary flow rate, the patient should be asked to refrain from eating or drinking for at least 2 hours before the collection period, and also to refrain from mouth rinsing, especially with rinses containing alcohol. These directions should be included in the patient instructions. The patient's medication and health history should be reviewed. If the patient is currently taking antihistamines or cold medications, it is prudent to postpone testing for salivary flow. A graduated tube and funnel should be used to collect the saliva sample. Immediately before collection, the patient should be asked to swallow to remove residual pooled saliva. The patient will collect saliva in their mouth and expectorate into the tube for 6 minutes. During this time, the practitioner should minimize conversation with the patient to avoid stimulating the production of saliva. After the 6-minute collection, the practitioner should measure and record the amount of saliva in the tube. The total volume should be divided by 6 to provide an average unstimulated flow rate in milliliter per minute (mL/min).[7]

An average unstimulated salivary flow rate is considered to be 0.4 mL/min. Salivary gland hypofunction is diagnosed if an unstimulated salivary flow rate is less than 0.2 mL/min.[7] Although the evidence is not clear whether this level of salivary flow is associated with an increased risk for dental caries, this flow rate has been consistent with patient reported symptoms of dry mouth. If the patient salivary flow rate is less than 0.2 mL/min, the dental professional should intervene, through counseling and behavior change strategies, to assist with management of the condition.

Salivary flow rates of less than 0.1 mL/min is abnormally low and indicates a more severe medical problem that warrants additional attention. Referral to a physician or a specialist in oral medicine is recommended. Medications, such as pilocarpine, are available to assist with the management of salivary gland hypofunction. See Chapter 18 for additional measures to consider in addressing xerostomia.

Commercial systems measure the buffering capacity of saliva. These systems use the pH to ascertain the capability of the saliva to buffer acid. Studies show a correlation between salivary flow rate and buffering capacity. Dentobuff (Orion Diagnostica, Espoo, Finland) and Saliva-Check (GC America, Alsip, Ill.) requires the patient to collect a volume of whole saliva. The pipette that comes in the kit is used to apply one drop of saliva to the test strip. After an incubation time of 5 minutes, the color on the test strip is compared with a card that describes the buffer capability. The colormetric analysis indicates whether the saliva has a low buffering capacity (acidic), moderate capacity (neutral pH), or high buffering capacity (basic). The color changes vary with the system used.[13]

PERIODONTAL DISEASE

Biological indicators for periodontal disease risk examine four major areas: physical markers, microbiological markers, host response markers, and genetic markers. Tests to assess risk for periodontal disease use currently understood etiologic pathways.

Early testing methods for periodontal disease risk focused on the identification of putative pathogenic bacteria that colonized the subgingival niche. Several approaches were used to quantify the presence of the microbiota including anaerobic culture with microscopic examination and determination and DNA/RNA probes. The best justification for bacterial analysis is in the case of early onset disease, where an association has been demonstrated between *Aggregatibacter actinomycetemcomitans* (formerly *Actinobacillus actinomycetemcomitans*) and localized juvenile periodontitis.[14] In these cases, bacterial identification provides a foundation to prescribe antimicrobial therapy. Although several other bacterial species have been linked with the progression of destructive disease, these organisms have not been proven to be causal, either in isolation or as a consortium. Therefore, their presence in the subgingival pocket does not provide the dental practitioner with a clear indication of their role in disease. The provider may assume a relationship only if longitudinal assessment is available and the dental provider can demonstrate an increase in organisms associated with destructive disease. Although the presence of these organisms can guide the dental provider to choose the appropriate antimicrobial regimen, the removal of these organisms in the pocket by using conventional treatment methods may control progression of the disease.

Analysis of Subgingival Plaque

Subgingival plaque collection can be accomplished by using two somewhat similar techniques. Before sample collection, the medical history should be reviewed and sample collection delayed if the patient is taking antimicrobial medications, including systemic antibiotics, which could interfere with the test results. The paper point technique requires the insertion of three sterile paper points into the gingival sulcus after removal of heavy deposits of supragingival plaque with an instrument or gauze. The paper points are inserted to the depth of the pocket by using sterile forceps and placing the paper points in an apicolingual direction.[15] After 10 seconds, the paper points are removed simultaneously and placed in a vial containing buffer for transport to the laboratory for analysis.

Subgingival plaque can be collected directly by using a curette. Again, the supragingival pellicle can be removed by using gauze or a plastic instrument. A sterile curette is inserted at the angle of the tooth at the gingival margin and directed subgingivally to the base of the pocket. After the curette is extricated from the pocket, the plaque can be placed on a slide for direct examination, or in an Eppendorf vial for transport to the laboratory. The size of the vial can dictate the curette used.

Again, multiple techniques exist to examine plaque to identify and quantify the microorganisms. Direct examination can be accomplished using microscopic techniques. This technique can be accomplished in the office, but has limited value, because it is best used to assess motile organisms and spirochetes, which are easily visualized. Culture of the organisms and sensitivity testing can be accomplished, but preservation of the sample is critical for the success of this particular technique. More sophisticated microbiological approaches can be used, including polymerase chain reaction (PCR) and DNA probes.[16]

Perioscan (Oral-B Laboratories) is an in-office test that indicates the presence of several periodontopathogens that hydrolyze the enzyme BANA (*N*-benzoyl-DL-arginine-2-naphthylamide), an enzyme unique to periodontal pathogens. Organisms that are capable of this activity include *Treponema denticola*, *Bacteroides forsythus*, and *Porphyromonas gingivalis*.[17]

Subgingival Temperature

The **subgingival temperature** is measured as a correlate for inflammation.[18] An increase in temperature is thought to reflect an ongoing inflammatory response to the infection. Ultimately, this increase results in loss of attachment and clinical manifestation of disease. Measurement of subgingival temperature is accomplished by using a commercial instrument (Periotemp, Abiomed, Danvers, Mass.) similar to a periodontal probe that is inserted to the base of the periodontal pocket. Before sample collection, the sublingual temperature or core temperature is collected by using the Periotemp to "calibrate" the instrument to the individual patient. After collection of the core temperature, the subgingival temperature can be collected at six sites per tooth. The instrument will account for variations in the core temperature. The instrument uses a light indicator system to identify normal (green), slightly elevated (yellow), and elevated (red) temperatures. The green indicator light identifies a subgingival temperature equal to or less than the mean temperature for healthy patients. The red light corresponds to values that are higher than temperatures observed with healthy teeth and teeth with marked periodontal inflammation. The yellow light indicates a temperature value between these two measures.[18] Very precise, the device measures temperature of the pocket to 0.1° C.

Genetic Testing for Periodontal Disease Risk

A commercial test (PST, Interleukin Genetics, Boston, MA) is available to test for the presence of two interleukin-1 genes, which have been associated with an increased risk for periodontal disease in some patients. Although still inconclusive, reports have suggested an increased risk for tooth loss in patients who express this genotype[19] and an increased risk for expression of a more severe chronic periodontal disease presentation in patients with this

genotype.[20] Other studies do not report an increased risk in patients with this genotype for 2 years after periodontal therapy.[21]

A finger stick blood sample can be collected to measure the **gene polymorphism**. Before collection, the finger is cleaned with an antiseptic wipe, and the skin is punctured on the fleshy pad of the finger with a sterile lancet. A drop of the finger stick blood is collected on a DNAase-free blotting paper and analyzed in the laboratory by using PCR-based techniques.[19] Samples should be stored and transported according to the manufacturer's instruction.

Gingival Crevicular Fluid

Another strategy to assess risk for periodontitis is to examine markers that would indicate bacterial presence in the subgingival pocket. These methods include identification of specific antigens, antibodies and mediators, measurement of enzymatic activity or the presence of the host-bacterial interaction products, and determination of products of tissue destruction. **Gingival crevicular fluid** (GCF) provides a vehicle to measure these events in the local environment.

Gingival crevicular fluid is a serous transudate that, in periodontal health, provides an active mechanism to maintain homeostasis in the gingival sulcus. During gingival inflammation, the fluid becomes an inflammatory exudate, delivering immune cells and cytokines to the local environment. The vasculature of the gingival tissue provides a vehicle for an entire immune process to occur in response to a bacterial challenge in the local subgingival environment. Immunological analysis of this fluid can provide one mechanism to measure changes in the host response to periodontitis.

Several host inflammatory mediators have been suggested as possible biomarkers for periodontal disease risk and progression. These include a prostaglandin E_2, ß-glucuronidase, interleukin-1ß, interleukin-6, interleukin-8, tumor necrosis factor-α, cytokines, specific bacterial antibodies, and acute phase proteins.[22] These cellular products have been shown to have a relationship with disease primarily in cross-sectional studies; however, no conclusive evidence indicates that these markers can predict risk for future disease.

Enzymatic activity in the local periodontal environment has been explored as a potential measure of risk for future disease.[23] Studies have examined several enzymes (e.g., neutral proteases,[24] lactate dehydrogenases, β-glucuronidase, and alkaline phosphatase)[23,25,26] and their role as markers for inflammation and future disease. Commercial test kits are available for chair side use (Periocheck, CollaGenex Pharmaceuticals, Newtown, PA). To date, the focus on GCF is as a diagnostic fluid; however, the presence of inflammatory mediators in the local subgingival environment as measured in GCF suggests some promise for prognostic activity.

Gingival crevicular fluid is collected on a filter paper strip (Periopaper, OraFlow Inc., Plainview, N.Y.). The strip is composed of a treated filter paper strip with an area defined on the strip that allows for manipulation. Moisture control is critical for the collection of GCF. The tooth/teeth should be isolated with cotton rolls before collection.[27] After isolation, careful removal of existing debris from the tooth at the gingival margin is accomplished and the tooth is further dried with air or gauze. The strip is gently inserted into the gingival sulcus with sterile forceps and directed apically until resistance is felt. Multiple strips (three or more) should be obtained per tooth to obtain sufficient volume of GCF. The paper is left in place until it appears saturated or is no longer absorbing additional fluid. The strips are then removed individually and measured in a precalibrated Periotron (OraFlow, Inc., Plainview, N.Y.). The fluid volume is recorded and the Periopaper is inserted into a buffer solution for transport and storage. GCF samples should be stored on ice or frozen as soon as possible after collection. Laboratories use enzyme-linked immunosorbent assay (ELISA) techniques to analyze the samples for the presence of antibody.[27]

ORAL CANCER

Saliva is ideal for diagnostic purposes for several reasons. Saliva is readily available and easy to collect. In addition, the presence of many diagnostic markers, including oral pathogens,[28] steroid hormones,[29] and HIV antibody provide valuable sources of information.[30] Brush biopsy and toluidine blue staining techniques for oral cancer detection are discussed in Chapter 6.

Salivary diagnostics is the most promising area in the detection of oral cancer. The role of saliva in caries risk assessment was discussed previously. Because saliva is easily obtained, its use in both diagnostics and risk assessment is obvious. The breakthrough in using saliva as a diagnostic biofluid has been linked to genomic advances in oral disease diagnostics. The further links between oral and systemic diseases, including diabetes, has enhanced the possibility that saliva could be used as a predictor for future disease.

During the past 30 years, dental professionals have been relatively unsuccessful in changing morbidity and mortality rates associated with oral cancer. Studies suggest that dental professionals do not routinely provide their patients with an oral cancer screening examination. In one study, only 20% of adults reported receiving an oral cancer examination in the past year.[31] In a study of both dentists and dental hygienists who reported providing patients with an oral cancer screening examination, the majority of providers did not palpate the oral cavity and did not provide an examination to their edentulous patients. An unrelated study indicated that oral cancers were diagnosed at a late stage and most patients reported not having had an oral cancer screening.[32] These observations suggest the need for a chair side protocol for assessment of oral cancer risk.

Saliva as a diagnostic fluid has a long-standing interest among the scientific community, primarily because it is relatively noninvasive and involves inexpensive sampling methods. Studies demonstrate that markers for disease are present in saliva, including HIV antibody.[28] The major reason for not using saliva as the preeminent diagnostic fluid is that the concentration of biomarkers in saliva is less than that of other fluids, especially serum.

Renewed interest in the use of saliva as a diagnostic fluid has emerged with increasing sensitivity of testing methods. Wong and his colleagues at the University of California, Los Angeles, developed a test that uses saliva to measure markers for oral cancer. This group identified 309 proteins in the human saliva and identified the salivary transcriptome markers for patients with oral cancer. Four genes (*IL-8*, *IL-1β*, *spermidine acetyltransferase*, and *ornithine decarboxylase*) were used to distinguish patients with oral cancer from those who were healthy at a sensitivity and specificity of 91%.[33,34] This group developed an instrument called the Oral Fluid NanoSensor Test (OFNASET), which allows for the detection of multiple salivary proteins and nucleic acid targets.[27] This emerging technology appears to be promising for chair side applications, and it may improve early detection of oral cancers.

SYSTEMIC DISEASE

Interactions between oral and systemic health have been described as both complex and bidirectional.[35] The evidence to support these links are considered weak, however, because of the paucity of well designed and executed research protocols addressing this issue. Both longitudinal and outcomes studies are needed to delineate the nature of the interactions and the clinical implications for health promotion.

The mouth is considered to be a source of fungal, bacterial, and viral pathogens. These oral pathogens and their toxins can be transmitted to other human organs and tissues. Bacteria from oral plaque can enter the blood stream through soft tissue in the mouth. For example, increasing evidence indicates periodontitis as a risk factor for cardiovascular diseases, **diabetes mellitus**, low-birth-weight infants, and pulmonary diseases. Associations between dental caries and obesity have also been suggested,[36] and osteoporosis has been indicated as a risk factor for periodontitis progression.[37] Additional studies are needed to determine the mechanisms by which such associations exist. Research demonstrates that oral diseases are important determinants that influence the development and management of adverse chronic health conditions. Physicians and dental professionals should address this link in their care plans, and provide respective preventive and treatment interventions

TABLE 9-2

LABORATORY CRITERIA FOR PREVENTION DIAGNOSIS AND MANAGEMENT OF DIABETES

TEST	DEFINITION	NORMS	IMPAIRED GLUCOSE TOLERANCE	DIABETES
Casual blood glucose concentration	Any time of day without regard to time of last meal	<100 mg/dl		≥200 mg/dl
Fasting plasma glucose (FPG)	No caloric intake for at least 8 hours before	<100 mg/dl	100-125 mg/dl	≥126 mg/dl
Oral glucose tolerance test (OGTT)	2-hour postload glucose after glucose load containing the equivalent of 75 g anhydrous glucose dissolved in water	<140 mg/dl	>140-<200 mg/dl	≥200 mg/dl
Glycated hemoglobin (A1C)	Measures average blood glucose level during the past 2-3 months	<6.0%		

(Adapted from American Diabetes Association: Diagnosis and classification of diabetes mellitus, *Diabetes Care* 29(Suppl 1):S43-S48, 2006.)

to address interactions rather than single health-related factors.[38]

Some have suggested that triggers of inflammation, including oral infection, are associated with insulin resistance and diabetes mellitus (DM), a metabolic disorder. Conversely, diabetes increases risk for periodontal disease. Measures of blood glucose concentration and glycated hemoglobin are indicative of the management status of a person with diabetes mellitus. It has been reported that glycated hemoglobin is second to tobacco use as a prime indicator of risk for periodontal disease among patients with type 2 diabetes.[39] Table 9-2 lists criteria to interpret markers of diabetes status. Dental health care providers can anticipate a greater number of diabetics in their practices, because of the increasing number of diagnosed and undiagnosed diabetics in the general population. Familiarity with the systemic and oral signs and symptoms of DM can facilitate its diagnosis and foster positive individual overall health care and promotion.

DM is a major risk factor for cardiovascular disease (CVD). Similarly, CVD and periodontal disease are both inflammatory disorders. Data from the National Health and Nutrition Examination Survey (NHANES) were used to report significant relationships between existing periodontal disease and heart disease in the general population.[40] Conversely, other investigators who examined data gleaned from health care professionals failed to substantiate this association, implying an indirect rather than direct link between CVD and periodontal disease.[41] Although more study is needed, the dental professional should be knowledgeable about laboratory determinations of CVD risk. Table 9-3 provides a list of biological markers that delineate risk of CVD.

Ultimately, the associations among inflammation, systemic diseases, and oral disease are modulated by nutritional status. Nutritional factors have a direct effect on the development and maintenance of oral tissue. Compromised status includes oral conditions that reflect protein energy malnutrition, alterations in immunological/hematological factors, and deficiencies of vitamins and minerals. Table 9-4 provides a quick reference for interpretation of laboratory indices of these variables. Nutrient deficiencies are best confirmed with biological data of this nature. See Chapter 7 for a description of clinical oral manifestations of some of these nutritional disorders.

SUMMARY

Information gathering and the application of information to create an individual plan of prevention are not readily embraced as components of dental practice. Often, patients come to dental practices with a cycle of disease, usually caries or periodontal disease. Care from the dental provider focuses primarily on treating the disease, but

TABLE 9-3

LABORATORY CRITERIA FOR PREVENTION, DIAGNOSIS, AND MANAGEMENT OF CARDIOVASCULAR DISEASE

TEST	DEFINITION	NORMS	INCREASED RISK OF CARDIOVASCULAR DISEASE
Total serum cholesterol	A fatty substance that occurs in all animal tissues. Produced in the liver, and ingested in the diet. It is a component of bile, carried in the blood by lipoproteins.	<200 mg/dl	200-239 mg/dl, borderline high ≥240 mg/dl, high
Low-density lipoprotein cholesterol (LDL)	Provides cholesterol for necessary body functions, but in excessive amounts it tends to accumulate in artery walls.	<100 mg/dl	100-129 mg/dl, above optimal 130-159 mg/dl, borderline high 160-189 mg/dl, high ≥190 mg/dl, very high
High-density lipoprotein cholesterol (HDL)	Transports cholesterol out of the arteries and back to the liver for reprocessing or excretion. The higher the HDL level, the lower the risk of heart disease.	≥60 mg/dl, high	<40 mg/dl, low
C-reactive protein	Assesses inflammatory response associated with coronary heart disease.	<1.0 mg/dl	1.5-3.0 mg/dl, moderate risk >3 mg/dl, high risk

(Adapted from U.S. Public Health Service, NIH, NHLBI: National Cholesterol Education Program. Third Report of the Expert Panel on Detection, Evaluation and Treatment of High Blood Cholesterol in Adults, NIH Publication No. 01-3305, National Institutes of Health, 2000, Bethesda, MD)

TABLE 9-4

LABORATORY DATA FOR ASSESSMENT OF POTENTIAL NUTRITION-RELATED DISORDERS OR DEFICIENCIES

CONSTITUENT PROTEIN-ENERGY STATUS	RATIONAL	NORMAL RANGE	INTERPRETATION
Albumin	Serum protein with half-life of 3 weeks; reflects visceral protein stores.	3.5-5.0 g/dl (35-50 g/l)	Confounded by stress, pregnancy, strenuous exercise, and liver and kidney disease. <3.0 g/dl associated with edema
Transferrin	Iron transport protein calculated from total iron- binding capacity (TIBC); reflects visceral protein stores; half-life varies within 8 days	200-400 mg/dl	Confounded by stress, pregnancy, strenuous exercise, and liver and kidney disease.

(Adapted from Mahan K, Escott-Stump S: *Food, nutrition, and diet therapy*, ed 11, Philadelphia, 2004, Saunders.)

TABLE 9-4

LABORATORY DATA FOR ASSESSMENT OF POTENTIAL NUTRITION-RELATED DISORDERS OR DEFICIENCIES—CONT'D

CONSTITUENT PROTEIN-ENERGY STATUS	RATIONAL	NORMAL RANGE	INTERPRETATION
Total protein (TP)	Serum protein concentration; reflects visceral protein stores; is 50%-60% albumin.	6.4-8.3 g/dl (64-83 g/l)	Does not reflect visceral protein status during acute-phase inflammatory response.
Immunological/ hematological markers			
Total lymphocyte count (TLC)	Decreased in malnutrition and immunocompromised state.	Normal, >2700 Severe depletion, 900-1500	Increased by tissue necrosis and infection. Decreased by viral infection and some drugs.
COMPLETE BLOOD COUNT			
White blood cell count (WBC) Leukocyte count	Produced in bone marrow; fights infection and removes harmful substances from blood.	Total 3.5-10.5 × 109/1 (includes neutrophils, monocytes, lympho-cytes, basophils, and eosinophils)	Can be found in large numbers in other body tissue (lymphatic system).
Red blood cell count (RBC)	Bring oxygen from the lungs to the various tissues in the body and carries carbon dioxide back to the lungs.	Female, 4.1-5.1 × 10^{12}/l Male, 4.5-5.3 × 10^{12}/l	
Hemoglobin (Hb)	A protein in RBCs that transports oxygen to tissues.	Female, 12-16 g/dl Male, 14-18 g/dl	High in smokers, in high altitudes, and dehydration. Low values reflect anemia.
Hematocrit (HCT)	Reflects proportion of blood volume occupied by RBCs.	Female, 37%-47% Male, 42%-52%	Lower levels associated with hemorrhaging and sensitive to hydration status.
Mean corpuscular volume blood (MCV)	Measure of the average RBC volume that is reported as part of a standard CBC.	80-99 g fL	Increases in pernicious anemia and alcoholism and decreases in iron-deficiency anemia and lead poisoning.
MICRONUTRIENT STATUS SELECT VITAMINS			
Folate	Essential in RNA/DNA synthesis and regulation of RBC function.	MCV<100 Serum: 2-10 µg/L	Laboratory assays are confounded by vitamin B_{12}, drugs, and pregnancy.
Cobalamin (B_{12})	Essential in RNA/DNA synthesis and regulation of RBC function; dependent on intrinsic factor for absorption in GI tract.	MCV<100 Serum: 200-1000 ng/L	Schilling test for intrinsic factor assesses absorption.

Continued

TABLE 9-4

LABORATORY DATA FOR ASSESSMENT OF POTENTIAL NUTRITION-RELATED DISORDERS OR DEFICIENCIES—CONT'D

CONSTITUENT PROTEIN-ENERGY STATUS	RATIONAL	NORMAL RANGE	INTERPRETATION
Ascorbic acid (C)	Essential for numerous functions ranging from scar tissue repair to bone formation; major antioxidant.	Plasma: 0.50-1.40 mg/dl	Recent intakes can mask a deficiency.
SELECT MINERALS			
Potassium (K)	Serum electrolytes in maintenance	3.5-5.1 mEq/L	Minimally effected by
Sodium (Na)	of fluid homeostasis.	135-145 mEq/L	diet and can change rapidly in response to physiological changes.
Calcium (Ca)	Serum Ca may be bound to albumin or complexed with other molecules.	8.8-10 mg/dl	Status is related to vitamin D, phosphate, parathyroid, and renal function.
Serum Iron (Fe)	Serum levels are considered insensitive to total Fe stores.	50-175 μg/L	May be higher in males and reflect recent Fe intake.

little time is spent on exploring the patient's individual risk or understanding the related oral and systemic factors that lead to repetitive cycles of disease. If the goal is to maintain a patient's oral health, it is critical that factors causing the disease are understood, and that efforts to effectively mitigate the exposure to these factors are facilitated. Most important, the role of the dental practitioner is to inform and educate the patient about the cause of his or her disease and provide strategies that the patient can use to reduce the disease burden. The primary step in this process involves data identification and interpretation to establish a baseline for complete and sustainable activity targeted at decreasing the patient's disease burden.

REFERENCES

1. Loesche WJ: Role of *Streptococcus mutans* in human dental decay, *Microbiol Rev* 50:353-380, 1986.
2. Crossner CG: Salivary lactobacillus counts in the prediction of dental caries, *Commun Dent Oral Epidemiol* 9:182-190, 1981.
3. Firestone AR, Graves CN, Feagin FF: The effects of different levels of dietary sucrose on root caries subsequent to gingivectomy in conventional rats infected with *Actinomyces viscosus* M-100, *J Dent Res* 67:1342-1345, 1988.
4. Caufield PW, Dasanayake AP, Li Y et al.: Natural history of *Streptococcus sanguinis* in the oral cavity of infants: evidence for a discrete window of infectivity, *Infect Immun* 68:4018-4023, 2000.
5. Seki M, Karakama F, Terajima T et al.: Evaluation of mutans streptococci in plaque and saliva: correlation with caries development in preschool children, *J Dent* 31:283-290, 2003.
6. Tenovuo J, Häkkinen P, Paunio P et al.: Effects of chlorhexidine-fluoride gel treatments in mothers on the establishment of mutans streptococci in primary teeth and the development of dental caries in children, *Caries Res* 26:275-280, 1992.
7. Dodds MWJ: Salivary testing. In Cappelli D, editor: *Clinical preventive dentistry manual*, Department of Community Dentistry, University of Texas Health Science Center at San Antonio, 2003.
8. Twetman S, Garcia-Godoy F: Caries risk assessment and caries activity testing. In Harris NO, Garcia-Godoy F, eds: *Primary Preventive Dentistry*, 6th ed. Pearson, Prentice Hall, New Jersey, 2004.
9. Neff D: Acid production from different carbohydrate sources in human plaque in situ, *Caries Res* 1:78-87, 1967.
10. Jensen B, Bratthall D: A new method for the estimation of mutans streptococci in saliva, *J Dent Res* 68:468-471, 1989.
11. Dodds MWJ, Johnson DA, Yeh C-K: Health benefits of saliva: a review, *J Dent* 33:223-233, 2005.
12. Moritsuka M, Kitasako Y, Burrow MF et al.: The pH change after HCl titration into resting and stimulated saliva for a buffering capacity test, *Aust Dent J* 51:170-174, 2006.
13. Ericsson D, Bratthall DP: A simplified method to estimate the salivary buffer capacity, *Scand J Dent Res* 97:405-407, 1989.
14. Zambon JJ: Actinobacilllus actinomycetemcomitans in human periodontal disease, *J Clin Periodontol* 12:1-20, 1985.
15. Kornman KS, Robertson PB: Clinical and microbiological therapy for juvenile periodontitis, *J Periodontol* 56:443-448, 1985.
16. Tran SD, Rudney JD: Improved multiplex PCR using conserved and species-specific 16S rRNA gene primers for simultaneous detection of *Actinobacillus actinomycetemcomitans*, *Bacteroides forsythus*, and *Porphyromonas gingivalis*, *J Clin Microbiol* 37: 3504-3508, 1999.

17. Loesche WJ, Bretz WA, Kerschensteiner D et al.: Development of a diagnostic test for anaerobic periodontal infections based on plaque hydrolysis of benzoyl-DL-arginine-naphthylamide, *J Clin Microbiol* 28:1551-1559, 1990.

18. Haffajee AD, Socransky SS, Goodson JM: Subgingival temperature. I. Relation to baseline clinical parameters, *J Clin Periodontol*, 19:401-408, 1992.

19. Kornman KS, Crane A, Wang HY et al.: The interleukin-1 genotype as a severity factor in adult periodontal disease, *J Clin Periodontol* 24:72-77, 1997.

20. Gore EA, Sanders JJ, Pandey JP et al.: Interleukin-1 beta + 3953 allele 2: association with disease status in adult periodontitis, *J Clin Periodontol* 25:781-785, 1998.

21. Ehmke B, Kress W, Karch H et al.: Interleukin-1 haplotype and periodontal disease progression following therapy, *J Clin Periodontol* 26:810-813, 1999.

22. Ebersole JL, Cappelli D: Acute phase reactants in infections and inflammatory diseases, *Periodontol 2000* 23:19-49, 2000.

23. Lamster IB: Evaluation of components of gingival crevicular fluid or diagnostic tests, *Ann Periodontol* 2:123-127, 1997.

24. Bowers JE, Zahrandek RT: Evaluation of a chairside gingival prolease test for use in periodontal diagnosis, *J Clin Dent* 1: 106-109, 1989.

25. Lamster IB, Grbic JT: Diagnosis of periodontal disease based on analysis of host response. *Periodontol 2000* 7:83-89, 1995.

26. Papapanou PN: Periodontal diseases: epidemiology, *Ann Periodontol* 1:1-36, 1996.

27. Ebersole JL, Cappelli D: Gingival crevicular fluid antibody to *Actinobacillus actinomycetemcomitans* in periodontal disease, *Oral Microbiol Immunol* 9:335-344, 1994.

28. Wong DT: Salivary diagnostics powered by nanotechnologies, proteomics and genomics, *JADA* 137:313-321, 2006.

29. Forde M, Koka S, Eckert S et al.: Systematic assessments utilizing saliva. Part 1: general considerations and current assessments, *J Prosthodontics* 19:43-52, 2006.

30. Reynolds SJ, Munonga J: OraQuick ADVANCE Rapid HIV-1/2 antibody test, *Expert Rev Molecular Diag* 4:587-591, 2004.

31. Alfano MC, Horwitz AM: Professional and community efforts to prevent morbidity and mortality from oral cancer, *JADA* 132:24S-29S, 2001.

32. McDowell JD: An overview of epidemiology and common risk factors for oral squamous cell carcinoma, *Otolaryngol Clin North Am* 39:277-294, 2006.

33. Li Y, Elashoff D, Oh M et al.: Serum circulating human mRNA profiling and its utility for oral cancer detection, *J Clin Oncol* 24:1754-1760, 2006.

34. Li Y, St John MAR, Zhou X et al.: Salivary transcriptome diagnostics for oral cancer detection, *Clin Cancer Res* 10:8442-8450, 2004.

35. Johnson NW, Glick M, Mbuguye TNI: Oral health and general health, *Adv Dent Res* 19:118-121, 2006.

36. Kantovitz KR, Pascon FM, Pontain RMP et al.: Obesity and dental caries-a systematic review, *Oral Health Prev Dent* 4:137-144, 2006.

37. Dervis E: Oral implications of osteoporosis, *Oral Surg Oral Med Oral Pathol Oral Radiol Endod* 100:349-356, 2005.

38. Anil S, Al-Ghamdi HS: The impact of periodontal infections on systemic diseases. An update for medical practitioners, *Saudi Med J* 27:767-776, 2006.

39. Jansson H, Lindholm E, Lindh C et al.: Type 2 diabetes and risk for periodontal disease: a role for dental health awareness, *J Clin Periodontol* 33:408-414, 2006.

40. Arbes SJ Jr, Slade GD, Beck JD: Association between extent of periodontal attachment loss and self-reported history of heart attack: an analysis of NHANES III data, *J Dent Res* 78: 1777-1782, 1999.

41. Joshipura KJ, Pitiphat W, Hung HC et al.: Pulpal inflammation and incidence of coronary heart disease, *J Endodont* 32:99-103, 2006.

Chapter 10

Integrating Risk and Health-Promotion Counseling

CONNIE C. MOBLEY AND VICTOR A. SANDOVAL

LEARNING OBJECTIVES

Upon completion of this chapter, the learner will be able to:
- Define patient education and counseling strategies appropriate for risk reduction and health promotion.
- Review theoretical models for understanding patient education and counseling approaches.
- Examine communication techniques for oral health education and promotion.
- Describe a framework for communicating patient instructions and educational activities in dental health environments.
- Discuss issues in selecting patient education materials and methods.
- List necessary sequential steps in delivering effective patient education.

KEY TERMS

Andragogy
Behaviorism
Cognitivism
Epigenetics
Health education
Health promotion
Humanism

In developed countries the major causes of death and chronic diseases, including oral diseases, are associated with behavioral factors.[1] Infectious diseases, such as antibiotic-resistant infections, tuberculosis and others, are also largely affected by human behavior. The concept of **health promotion** implies that health can be enhanced by enabling people to assume control over their environment and choices. In addition, organizational, economic, and environmental support in communities can assist individuals in their quest for health.

Health education, promotion, behavior, and counseling are terms that are frequently used interchangeably in health care settings to describe or explain the role of health care professionals as patient educators and counselors. Dental health is regarded as one of many disciplines uniquely positioned to address health and preventive health behaviors with individual patients. Dental health practitioners see their patients routinely for preventive oral health care and have periodic follow-up appointments with the same patients. Thus, they are able to provide education and counseling and use tailored strategies in an atmosphere that supports the concepts of health promotion and risk reduction.

Personal risk for caries, periodontal disease, oral cancer, and oral injury is dependent on the absence or presence of modifiable and nonmodifiable risk factors. The field of **epigenetics** studies the effect of interactions of genes and environment on an individual's risk for some diseases. Genetics determine potential risk but environment can activate genetic expression. Empirical findings have been reported on the demonstrated and replicated biological interactions between identified common single genetic variants and the operation of environmentally mediated risks.[2] The behaviors subsumed in environmental exposure can be addressed with education and counseling. The purpose of this chapter is to differentiate elements of health promotion and to present **health education** and counseling strategies appropriate for oral health promotion in the dental care setting.

PATIENT EDUCATION

Patient education is part of total, comprehensive patient care and includes teaching the specifics of a disease state. It is considered an integral part of most chronic disease prevention and management programs.[3] Assumptions inherent in health and patient education are based primarily on epidemiological studies. Dental practitioners assume that health behaviors are mediators of health status, that behaviors result from knowledge combined with attitudes, and that if behavior changes, health will improve.[4] Outcomes anticipated in response to patient education include a patient's choice to modify behavior and achieve compliance with a prescribed regimen designed to enhance self-care.[5] Compliance is an issue of power and control. Adherence suggests choice and a relationship between the dental care provider and the patient that is based on trust and respect. Chapter 11 discusses these issues and provides strategies to enhance patient adherence once education and counseling have commenced. In all patient education settings, the goal of interpretation and integration of information is to inspire attitude or behavior changes that can benefit the patient's health status. This goal is central to all practitioner-patient interactions.

Patient education includes four tenets that underpin the importance of this activity. First, patient education is a necessity for quality health care. Second, it is a patient's right to receive education and possibly counseling. Furthermore, patient education has the potential to increase the efficacy of the health care delivery system. Finally, dental health care providers have a legal responsibility to ensure that they have imparted knowledge and resources to the patient that can bring about optimum outcomes of patient care.[6] Unfortunately, a paucity of patient education theory that is grounded in health professional practice exists, and this is particularly true for oral health promotion.

Theories of Learning

Educational approaches are based on a composite of theories derived from social science disciplines in communication, development, and personality. Theoretical approaches to learning, **behaviorism** and **cognitivism** have been used to describe patient learning concepts.[7] Learning theory is organized around four orientations that each reflect a distinct school of thought. As shown in Table 10-1, these include the behaviorists and the cognitive, humanist, and social learning orientations.[8]

Behaviorism. In simple terms, behaviorists believe learning results from reinforcements that activate desired behaviors. In 1938, Skinner developed the widely accepted hypothesis that the frequency of a behavior hinges on the consequences.[9] His operant conditioning or "behaviorist" approach encouraged a technique focused on developing goals and setting up a punishment-reward system that supports desired behavior.

TABLE 10-1

THEORETICAL APPROACHES TO PATIENT EDUCATION AND COUNSELING

ORIENTATION	TENETS	APPLICATION
Behaviorism	Learning results from reinforcement and can lead to behavioral changes.	Behavior modification
Cognitivism	Learning results from reasoning based on subjective values and associated identified action leading to desired outcomes.	Gestaltism Relativism
Humanism	Learning is continuous because of human potential and desire for growth.	Patient-centered models Motivational interviewing
Social learning theory	Learning occurs in response to modeling and observation of normative social environments.	Social cognitive theory Self-efficacy

In patient education, behavior modification is based on a cause-and-effect explanation of behavior that stems from this philosophy. By focusing on cues, the behavior itself, or consequences of the behavior, the patient educator attempts to change maladaptive behavior.

Cognitivism. In the cognitive orientation, the belief exists that behavior is determined more as a function of the subjective value of an outcome and the expectation that a specific action will achieve that outcome. Thus, reasoning is required to explain the behavior.

In 1974, Gagne, a cognitive theorist influenced by behaviorists, delineated a specific sequence of steps in learning and remembering thought to result in behavioral responses.[10] Internal and external conditions can be arranged to produce eight sets of circumstances which produce eight types of learning, listed in Box 10-1. When teaching is sensitive to the sequence of steps, it can be effective in patient education. In fact, patient education outcomes are frequently stated as behavioral objectives, and demonstrate a level of patient competency that reflects Gagne's eight types of learning.[10]

GESTALTISM. Other patient educators choose to base their practice on models considered to be more holistic. Gestaltists broaden the meaning of learning to include a problem-solving approach that includes insight coupled with motivation.[11] Reorganizing experiences into a meaningful pattern, enlightens perspectives and creates a system for learning. Thus, the realization of the dynamic interaction of a physiological orientation with one's environment results in a unique learning experience. In patient education, gestalt theory is most frequently used to guide a patient's experiences by promoting an awareness of the present. Metaphors are often used to demonstrate the relationship between what the patient is thinking and the behavior that the thought leads to in a given situation. For example, intervention focuses on the "shoulds" versus the "wants" of life. This focus leads to discussions of personal options that can open up the patient's thinking to provide insight into a wide range of behaviors. Learning is facilitated by using strategies that present the problem, evaluate alternative behaviors, and lead the patient to not only select a behavior but also verbalize the possible outcome of that choice.

RELATIVISM. Relativism is a central theme in education that emphasizes the present and perceptual realities as a motivator for learning. Kurt Lewin, a cognitive-field theorist, created the concept of "life space" which is everything within a person's psychological and physical environment at a given time.[12] Interactions between a person and his environment can provide the individual with new insights, or can change old ones. Once realized, changes in behavior, attitude, value, or perception can then occur and lead to a change in a person's subsequent outlook on how a health behavior can deter or improve oral health status.

BOX 10-1

GAGNE'S EIGHT TYPES OF LEARNING

TYPE	DESCRIPTION
Signal learning	The individual learns to make a general, diffuse response to a signal, as in the classic conditioned response of Pavlov's test subjects.
Stimulus-response learning	The learner acquires a precise response to a discriminated stimulus.
Chaining	A chain of two or more stimulus-response connections is acquired.
Verbal association	The learning of chains that are verbal.
Discrimination learning	The individual learns to make different identifying responses to many different stimuli that may resemble each other in physical appearance.
Concept learning	The learner acquires the capacity to make a common response to a class of stimuli.
Rule learning	A rule is a chain of two or more concepts.
Problem solving	A kind of learning that requires the internal events usually called thinking.

(Adapted from Gagne RM: *Essentials of learning for instruction*, Hinsdale, IL, 1974, Dryden Press.)

Humanism. The humanist orientation considers learning from the perspective of human potential for growth. Maslow's hierarchy of needs as shown in Figure 10-1 and Carl Rogers' patient-centered approach reflect this thinking.[13,14] Maslow's theory suggests that all the needs in the hierarchy are always present, but each individual's needs must be satisfied at the lower levels before they can progress to the higher, more complex levels. He also suggested that when individuals progress to higher levels, higher-level motivators are needed. The motivational interviewing discussed in Chapter 11 and illustrated in

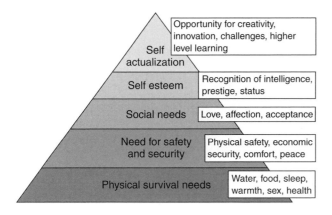

Figure 10-1   Maslow's hierarchy of needs.

Figure 11-2 is considered to be compatible with Carl Rogers' patient-centered approach to learning. Rogers maintained that all human beings have a natural desire to learn. He defined two categories of learning: cognitive (e.g., memorizing facts) and significant, or experiential (applied knowledge, which addresses the needs and wants of the learner).[14] According to Rogers, the role of the educator is to facilitate experiential learning by creating a positive climate for learning and clarifying the individual learner's motivation for learning. **Andragogy**, a theory of adult learning defined by Knowles as an art and a science, is grounded in humanistic learning theory.[15]

Social learning theory (SLT).   Bandura's social learning theory emphasizes the importance of observing and modeling the behaviors, attitudes, and emotional reactions of others.[16] This theory supposes that most human behavior is learned observationally through modeling. Social learning theory explains human behavior in terms of continuous reciprocal interaction between cognitive, behavioral, and environmental influences.

Derived from SLT, social cognitive theory (SCT) is relevant to health communication primarily because it deals with cognitive and emotional events, environmental factors, and aspects of behavior as shown in Figure 10-2. It is based on the learning principles and motivational ideas of Hull, who attempted to explain behavior relative to internal states known as "drives."[17] According to SCT, behavior is a function of what one would expect to happen as reinforcement for a particular behavior. The eleven main concepts shown in Box 10-2 provide the

cognitive basis for SCT. Individuals who value the outcome of a situation will attempt to learn behaviors appropriate to the situation when they believe they are capable of acceptable performance, and the performance and outcome are connected. SCT is relevant to patient education for three reasons. First, this theoretical approach brings elements of knowing, feeling, and behaving into a synergistic complex. Second, it suggests that there are varying avenues for explaining behavior. Third, it provides an opportunity to bring the fields of psychology and health behavior together in a synergistic fashion. The concepts of goal setting, skill training, and other self-care skills that are important in patient education and in a patient's adherence to a new behavior are embedded in SCT.

Other theoretical approaches.   Other client-centered models (CCM) taken from the social sciences have been used to explain learning in patient education. For example, the theory of reasoned action (TRA) explains how an attitude founded on a belief is formed and a decision is made to perform a health behavior.[18] Identification of individual beliefs can help to determine how a person will translate knowledge acquired in patient education. The patient educator often plans for learning without assessing a patient's belief system or his/her knowledge of a concept or behavior. Written materials are often provided with no explanation or opportunity to tailor the messages to the patient's needs. This approach needs patient interactions that bridge the gap between the written or packaged education program and the individual needs of the learner. The transtheoretical model (TTM) that supports the stages of change model discussed in Chapter 11 and shown in Figure 11-1 is another model frequently used to explain health behaviors.[19] A more recent and evolving model, the precaution adoption process model (PAPM), questions whether changes in health-relevant behaviors can be described by a single prediction equation.[20] PAPM illustrates six stages of important issues that are considered in the decision to adopt a behavior and accounts for other issues that are peripheral to the decision. Thus, it explains factors beyond those that describe just one stage in the process.

Despite a large empirical body of literature to support models of health behavior, no consensus exists that one is more accurate, more influential, or results in better understanding than another.[21] In the patient education setting, two learning/behavior change models are routinely used in patient education. These are the self-efficacy model (SCT) and the health belief model, based on expectancy theory.[16,22] Table 10-2 illustrates the differences and similarities of these two approaches.

Compared with medical-centered models (MCM), patient-centered models (PCMs) for patient education have proved to be philosophically quite different (Table 10-3). MCMs are thought to be objective, value-free, bias-free, valid, reliable, and transferable and generalizable.[23]

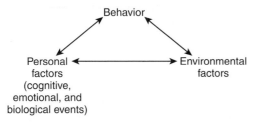

Figure 10-2   Conceptual model of social cognitive theory and self-efficacy.

BOX 10-2

Major Operant Concepts in Social Cognitive Theory Models

CONCEPT	DESCRIPTION
Environment	Factors physically external to the person that provide opportunities and social support.
Situation	Perception of the environment that corrects misperceptions and promote healthful forms.
Behavioral capability	Knowledge and skill to perform a given behavior.
Expectations	Anticipatory outcomes of a behavior.
Expectancies	The values that the person places on a given outcome.
Self-control	Personal regulation of goal-directed behavior or performance that provides opportunities for self-monitoring, goal setting, problem solving, and self-reward.
Observational learning	Behavioral acquisition that occurs by watching the actions and outcomes of others' behavior. Includes credible role models.
Reinforcements	Responses to a person's behavior that increase or decrease the likelihood of recurrence. Promotes self-initiated rewards and incentives.
Self-efficacy	The person's confidence in performing a particular behavior.
Emotional coping responses	Strategies or tactics that are used by a person to deal with emotional stimuli. This concept provides training in problem solving and stress management.
Reciprocal determinism	The dynamic interaction of a person, a behavior, and an environment.

(Adapted from Bandura A: *Social learning theory*, Englewood Cliffs, NJ, 1977, Prentice-Hall.)

TABLE 10-2

COMPARISON OF BELIEFS IN TWO MODELS USED IN PATIENT EDUCATION TO DESIGN AND DELIVER PROGRAMS

	SOCIAL COGNITIVE MODEL	HEALTH BELIEF MODEL
Attitudes and key elements	Outcomes and expectations. Perception of one's ability to perform a behavior is a predictor of a future behavior.	Benefits, barriers, and threats. Health behaviors depend on the simultaneous occurrence of sufficient motivation, belief in a perceived threat, and belief that a recommended health practice would reduce threats and increase benefits.
Self-efficacy	Self-efficacy comes from mastery of experience, observations, verbal persuasion, and physiological states in response to perception of capability to perform a behavior.	Self-efficacy comes from belief in ability to perform the behavior.
Norms about activities	Social support Modeling Reinforcement	Cues to action come from the media and friends who portray similar behaviors.

(Adapted from Bandura A: *Social learning theory*, Englewood Cliffs, NJ, 1977, Prentice-Hall; and Becker MH: The health belief model and personal health behavior, *Health Educ Monogr* 2:324–473, 1974.)

TABLE 10-3

COMPARATIVE ASPECTS OF TWO MODELS OF PATIENT EDUCATION

	MEDICAL MODEL	PATIENT-CENTERED MODEL
Interest	Eliminating uncertainty Evidence-based practice	Acknowledging uncertainty Promoting health
Outcome/aim	Increase patient's technical knowledge	Build on patient's existing knowledge
Content	Technical and factual	Social and realistic
Strategies	Identifying the best options	Identifying choices
Evaluation	Technical knowledge	Holistic knowledge
Driving forces	Economics Efficiency Empowering clinicians	Socialism Effectiveness Empowering patients

(From McEwen C, Flowers R, Tracie F: Learner-centered and culturally responsive patient education: drawing on traditions of cultural development and popular education, *AMIA Annu Symp Proc* 892, 2005.)

This approach aims to predict and control the patient's natural world. This model assumes that only the physical aspects of patients are of concern and interest and that the relationship should be founded on a clinician-patient interaction that is equal to that of an expert-layman relationship. Information is a one-way dissemination that uses traditional teaching and learning approaches such as brochures and posters. The emphasis is on content, and the health care provider assumes that behavior change is a linear process. Presentation of medical knowledge will automatically be followed by attitudinal and then behavioral changes.[23]

Adult Learning

In the health care setting the trauma of disease, the press of time, the freedom to choose not to participate in a new behavior, the requirement to actively participate in the act of learning, and the social/psychological setting all require consideration in planning and choosing patient education materials and models. Health care professionals assume that if they provide health education, behavioral change will follow. Adults change behavior only after they have made a conscious decision to change, made plans to change, and have had an opportunity to consistently implement the change over an extended period of time.[15]

Intentional change is a term used to describe a choice to change. Individuals may accept new information and guidance from a health professional but usually independently manage their change process. Because health education is often rudimentary and prescriptive rather than elective, the individual choice to change is not always immediate. Adaptive behaviors suggested in health education may vary. Studies show that adults try to adapt to change events in several ways. They may react by frantically and compulsively changing a behavior, or they

may seek additional education or advice before acting. Alternatively, they may extend the time spent contemplating an action, or they may totally withdraw from any consideration. This reflects the stages of change model discussed in Chapter 11.[19]

In 1984, Houle stated "Whether the requirement to learn is lax or stringent, those on whom it is imposed think of education as compulsory."[24] When patients are given instructive education as though it were a mandated or prescriptive directive, it will be rejected at the outset. Health educators should be facilitators who assist adults in becoming self-directed learners through the technology of learning referred to as andragogy.[15] "Fact-giving" approaches have proved to be the least effective in achieving positive outcomes in health education.

In 1970, Knowles defined andragogy as "an emerging technology for adult learning."[15] His four andragogical assumptions are that adults generally move from dependency to self-directedness, constantly draw on their past learning experiences, are most ready to learn when they assume new roles, and want to solve problems and apply new knowledge when an immediate need exists. The principles of adult learning listed in Box 10-3 have been used to guide the development of patient education programs based on this philosophical orientation. In essence, patient education is a process that occurs throughout the span of time that defines the dental professional-patient interaction and therefore is a unique venue for implementing this approach. The professional comes to know the individual patient's needs and motivation.

COMMUNICATION

Communication includes all methods used to convey thoughts, feelings, and attitudes among people. It has also been described as a process of sending and receiving

BOX 10-3

PRINCIPLES OF ADULT LEARNING

1. People learn when they perceive a need to learn.

2. Learning takes place when the learner is able to relate a previous experience to the present experience. The health educator should build on this sequencing by identifying what the learner already knows, what is going to be introduced, and what the individual needs.

3. Patients learn most effectively when they are actively involved in the learning. Listening does not imply understanding. Most people need to become minimally engaged in conversation to learn.

4. People learn more when their senses are stimulated. Audio-visuals, animation, and practice are examples of effective learning tools.

5. People learn best when they know the goals of learning and perceive they are realistic and attainable. Sometimes intermediate goals must be set before the final goal can be achieved.

6. Learning takes place when there is an optimal stress level. Too much or too little stress results in ineffective learning. The internal stress level of the learner needs to be coupled with that established by the educator for learning to occur.

7. Patients learn best when they are encouraged to take responsibility for their own learning and are able to independently solve their own problems. Supportive feedback becomes the function of the educator.

(Adapted from Knowles MS: *The modern practice of adult education*, New York, 1980, Associated Press.)

messages or transmissions of ideas to achieve mutual understanding between a communicator and a listener.[25] Communication involves processes of encoding, transmission, decoding, and synthesis of information.[26,27] A person selects specific information from all possible sources of information to engender a specific message. The message is then prepared in several ways so that if one way of saying it fails, another way can succeed. Thus, an effective message is one that includes a sender, a receiver, and a mechanism for feedback. On the basis of sources of information, the sender speaks the message and initiates communication. The receiver is the listener, who interprets and may transmit the message back to the sender. Feedback is the process of responding to messages after the receiver interprets them. Once this process is initiated, interference from psychological, social, or physical elements can distort the message. Figure 10-3 illustrates the dynamics of this process.

Patients may not feel they can communicate with a dental professional who restricts his/her interest to a very narrow set of clinical concerns and directives. Several advantages are associated with achieving good communication skills in the patient care setting. A clinician with good communication skills can provide comprehensive assessments that lead to improved diagnosis and patient satisfaction. This leads to a decreased potential for complaints and misunderstood self-care instructions. Similarly, the patient is more likely to exhibit improved self-efficacy in practicing routine preventive behaviors.

How can communication skills be tailored to meet the needs of dental clinical settings? The key to good communication is to practice and use good listening skills. A major problem with successful patient education occurs when the dental professional gives either insufficient, poorly understood information or far more information than is appropriate. Discussion of risk for dental disease, options for supportive clinical care and self-management, and longitudinal preventive behaviors associated with optimum health status require professional skills based on education, communication, and counseling principles.

Verbal and nonverbal communication are equally important in patient education and can occur simultaneously. Verbal communication includes the actual words

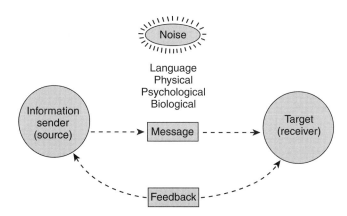

Figure 10-3 Model of communication. (Adapted from Shannon CE, Warren W: *A mathematical model of communication*, Urbana, Ill., 1949, University of Illinois Press.)

crafted by the sender in message transfer. Nonverbal communication includes the manner and style of delivery, the immediate environment in which the message is delivered, and the inherent qualities of the sender and the receiver that can influence the interpretation of any external stimuli in the environment.[25] A supportive climate is an important element of good communication. When one person speaks, the other listens, attending to the discussion rather than their own internal thoughts and feelings.[28] Supportive climates are those that encourage descriptive rather than evaluative discussions of an issue or problem, problem solving versus manipulative discussion, provisional alternatives rather than dogma, an egalitarian rather than authoritative atmosphere, and an empathetic rather than neutral or self-centered attitude. Table 10-4 suggests examples of each of these approaches.

Nonverbal Communication

Nonverbal communication broadens the education or counseling interaction, or both, between patient and dental professional. Nonverbal communication functions to augment words and express emotion through face and body movements. Curry states that it is noticed more by the sender when it reinforces verbalization and by the receiver when it is inconsistent with verbalization.[29] Nonverbal communication, such as the smile, is universal, whereas other forms, such as eye contact, may be cultural. Some experts believe that all nonverbal behavior imparts cultural meaning and that it is more representative of communication than words.[30]

A person's use of space and control of body movements constitute nonverbal factors that influence communication. Specifically, these factors can be categorized as follows: (1) posture, including standing, sitting, and lying down; (2) the angle of the shoulder relative to the other person; (3) closeness of bodies and body parts; (4) touching behaviors; (5) visual contact; (6) perceived heat from another communicator; (7) kind and degree of odor perceived in a conversation; and (8) voice loudness.[31] In addition, paralanguage, the use of vocal signs other than words, is considered a nonverbal form of communication.[29] Paralanguage includes the following vocal descriptors: the quality (range and rhythm), characterizers

TABLE 10-4

VERBAL STRATEGIES FOR USE IN A SUPPORTIVE CLIMATE FOR PATIENT EDUCATION AND COUNSELING

VERBAL STRATEGIES	OUTCOMES	VERBAL EXAMPLES
Description rather than evaluation of the problem.	Judgmental statements evoke resistance and defensiveness. Describing the facts provide a reasonable explanation.	It is really hard to floss everyday when you get to bed so late. (Evaluative) Finding time to floss is important for everyone. (Descriptive)
Problem-solving rather than manipulation.	Preplanning solutions to problems are interpreted as manipulative.	Tell me what you can do to find the time to floss.
Provisional alternative rather than dogmatic ones.	Possibilities rather than parental directives open the door to explore solutions to a problem.	You must floss every night right before bedtime. (Dogmatic) There are several ways you might include flossing in your evening routine. (Provisional)
Egalitarian rather than authoritarian.	Those who perceive they are equals are more open to discussion and understanding.	You probably don't understand the importance of flossing. (Authoritarian) Many of my patients have problems making time for flossing, but you probably have some ideas about how to accomplish this in your daily routine. (Egalitarian)
Empathetic rather than being neutral.	Lack of empathy is considered an undesirable trait in a health care professional.	The rule is that you must floss daily before bedtime. (Netural) I realize that after a long day flossing is another chore, but it is important. (Empathetic)

(laughing, yawning, and belching), qualifiers (manner in which words are spoken), and segregates (use of "ah") of language.

When nonverbal and verbal behaviors reflect inconsistency, explanations are needed. The dental practitioner engaged in patient education and counseling can develop skills in observing and understanding nonverbal behavior in self as well as in others.

COUNSELING

Skills in communication, techniques in listening, and establishing rapport are essential to effective counseling. Three strategies, known as confirmation, confrontation, and commitment, hinge on listening skills. Confirmation of a patient's ability to make a behavioral change, confrontation of barriers to change, and the patient's commitment to change are essential to effective counseling.[29]

Listening has been identified as the most important skill in counseling practices. Listening requires an alert, aware ability to focus attention on an immediate situation by engaging all the senses and a comprehension of the meaning of the communication as it is occurring. One must listen with one's ears and eyes and be aware of one's immediate life space. Listening is synonymous with openness, concentration, and comprehension. Openness implies allowing others to influence your perception of the world with a nonjudgmental attitude. Intuitive skills, perception of nuances, and physical openness (body language) implies full attention. Concentration paired with openness shuts out irrelevant issues. Finally, comprehension of language, paralanguage, and the patient's frame of reference is the result of careful listening. Those who are uncomfortable with silence usually have difficulty practicing good listening skills, and must overcome this orientation. Barriers to ineffectual listening include being defensive, planning rebuttals or questions rather than listening, placing too much emphasis on words and data, ignoring the emotional content being divulged, and selectively listening because one feels one is more important than the messenger.

Verbal interventions can be effective in an education/counseling situation. Probing for additional information should convey to the listener that any answer given will be accepted. Clarifying a statement helps to diffuse misunderstanding, confront issues, and confirm strategies. Reflecting, interpreting, and paraphrasing are all techniques that can enrich the communication and ultimately the arrival at a commitment to practice a new behavior.[29]

Commitment results in a contract between the counselor and the patient. Thus, a statement of what is to be accomplished within a specific time period, with the positive results of the change, is the expected outcome. This expected outcome can be expressed verbally by the patient and paraphrased by the dental practitioner for confirmation. Goal setting can be a simple statement. Likewise, if it entails major behavioral changes, it may be

appropriate to consider setting interim objectives leading to goal achievement. This type of counseling is not successful unless it includes plans for longitudinal follow-up. In the dental setting, a brief review of progress can be paired with follow-up routine dental clinic visits.

EDUCATIONAL METHODS FOR PATIENT INSTRUCTION

In health care settings, patients generally receive individualized instruction. Other modalities exist, however, including group lectures or talks, live demonstrations or audiovisual technology, guided practice, and media delivery systems such as print or computer-based channels.

In general, materials and methods are designed to address a level of learning that occurs sequentially. The first level of learning is recall, followed by understanding, application, analysis, synthesis, and finally evaluation.[32] Education in patient settings is designed to address recall and understanding. In some situations, such as the use of oral hygiene products or dental appliances, application is the goal. The dental practitioner may elect to instruct the patient in application techniques without first orienting the patient to his/her understanding of the value and beliefs associated with the practice or experimentation. This fact illustrates the need to initiate effective communication techniques before educational materials or demonstration techniques are introduced.

Group lectures or talks are appropriate when there is little time, but less learning takes place in this format than in any other method. People remember approximately 20% of what they hear, 10% of what they read, and 30% of what they see.[25] Learners usually remain passive unless they are asked to participate by speaking about or doing something with materials in the educational setting. Demonstrations are most effective when the learner is asked to participate or repeat the skill being taught. Guided practice is an example of an activity that combines demonstration with practice. The following are general guidelines for selecting a format or materials for patient education, counseling, or both.

1. The more senses that are stimulated the more learning will take place.
2. The learner will retain more information when he or she participates in the learning process.
3. Time restrictions guide the type of method that can best be used in any given situation.

Selection of print, audio-visual, or computer-based learning requires the use of "plain" language. Furthermore, the language should be that of the patient's preferred language if English is not their first language. Thus, information should be easily read, understood, and acted on the first time it is read.[33] Simple, short sentences written in large simple type are appropriate for the majority of audiences. White space on brochures and other print material have a calming effect and convey an attitude "in sync" with openness that is important in counseling. Most dental professionals choose materials from those that are available from professional organizations and the dental industry. These should be reviewed for readability and fit for the intended audience. Age, cultural background, educational level, and special needs should be considered when selecting materials for an individual patient.

A review of websites in oral health was conducted to identify content and design features. Fifty-six oral health Web sites originating from nongovernmental organizations and associations (28.6%), regional/state agencies (21.4%), federal government (19.6%), academia (19.6%), and commercial (10.7%) sources were reviewed using a 52-item evaluation instrument that included use of visual resources, procedural skills, and assessment. Commercial sites incorporated the highest number of content areas and web design features. The majority of sites covered content areas in anticipatory guidance, caries, and fluorides. Materials in risk assessment, oral screening, cultural issues, and dental/medical interface were lacking. This review identified a major gap in the use of visual resources for posting didactic information, demonstrating procedural skills, and assessing user knowledge related to oral health education.[34] There is a paucity of risk assessment and oral screening materials accessible to dental professionals that can be used in patient education and counseling.

Health literacy is a composite term used to describe a range of outcomes associated with health education and communication activities (see Chapter 13). It encompasses not just the transfer of information, but the bidirectional relationship between health and social, economic, and environmental variables.[35] According to the World Health Organization (WHO) it represents the cognitive and social skills which determine the motivation and ability of individuals to gain access to, understand, and use information to promote and maintain good health.[36] Health literacy means more than being able to read brochures and make dental appointments. By improving people's access to health information, health literacy is considered critical to empowerment. Health education is directed toward improving health literacy. Past educational programs have failed to address social and economic determinants of health. These perceptions may have led to a significant underestimation of the potential role of health education in addressing health outcome. Table 10-5 highlights educational goals as a function of achieving health literacy.

ORAL HEALTH EDUCATION IN PRACTICE

In the year 2000, the Surgeon General's Report on Oral Health called for improved education about oral health, and an interdisciplinary approach to oral health involving primary care providers.[37] A paucity of documented evidence exists to indicate that this directive has been successfully addressed.

Anticipatory guidance, defined as a process of providing practical, developmentally appropriate health information about children to their parents in anticipation of significant physical, emotional, and psychological milestones, has been promoted in pediatric practices as a venue to oral health education.[38] This process is based on guidelines and topics identified by The Maternal and

---

TABLE 10-5

LEVELS OF HEALTH LITERACY, EDUCATIONAL GOALS, INDIVIDUAL BENEFITS, AND EXAMPLES OF ACTIVITY

HEALTH LITERACY (HL) LEVEL/EDUCATIONAL GOAL	CONTENT	INDIVIDUAL PATIENT OUTCOMES	EXAMPLE OF EDUCATIONAL ACTIVITY
Functional HL communication	Transmission of factual information on health risks and health services use.	Improved knowledge of risks and health services and compliance with prescribed actions.	Transmit information through existing channels, interpersonal contact, and available media.
Interactive HL personal skills	Functional HL and opportunities to develop skills in a supportive environment.	Capacity to act independently on knowledge, improved motivation, and self-confidence.	Tailor communication to specific need; identify community self-help and social support groups.
Critical HL empowerment	Functional and interactive HL and provision of information on social and economic determinants of health.	Individual resilience to social and economic adversity.	Provide technical advice to support community advocacy.

(Adapted from Nutbeam D: Health promotion glossary, *Health Promot Int* 13:349–364, 1998.)

Child Health Bureau's Bright Futures and the American Academy of Pediatrics (AAP).[39,40] Data are lacking, however, on what parents recall when health care professionals present concise and targeted information to patients and their parents. In a study designed to evaluate the relationship between parental recall after an encounter with a practitioner, recall dwindled as an increasing number of topics were discussed.[41]

Time constraints limit the attention the practitioner can devote to the family, and not all parents value information on the same topics. Evidence suggests that parents fail to raise questions that concern them and the clinician fails to use good communication techniques in patient-clinician interactions.[42] Other investigators have reported findings that suggest that the "topic" approach is satisfactory for the practitioner but less satisfactory for the patient.[43] These findings reinforce the need for clinicians to develop skills in communication and patient education to support the development of anticipatory guidance programs addressing oral health in children and in other population cohorts.

A longstanding history exists of providing oral hygiene education in dental care settings. When adult dental patients were surveyed about oral hygiene instruction in private dental practices, they recall being given a toothbrush but had low frequencies of recall about the specifics of the oral health education.[44] Dental providers reported spending less than 10 minutes per patient in completing oral hygiene instruction on flossing and brushing techniques. Lack of time and patient resistance to oral health education were identified as major deterrents to perceived patient education. It was suggested that more emphasis should be placed on the psychological approach to behavioral change than on techniques in oral hygiene and that more time should be spent in follow-up appointments to provide patient support for suggested behavioral changes.[45]

Tobacco use accounts for 75% of oral cancer deaths in the United States.[46] One objective of *Healthy People 2010* is to increase the percentage of dentists who provide smoking cessation counseling.[47] Studies of dentists have shown that the majority feel inadequately prepared to do so. In 2002, 163 dental students enrolled in an east coast dental school were given a written questionnaire that included questions about tobacco use interventions. Although 89% of students agreed that dentists should be trained to provide tobacco cessation education, only 39% thought that they themselves were adequately trained. Only a small percentage of the students were confident in their ability to help patients stop smoking. This study indicated that dental professionals require training in effective education programs and in related communication and counseling skills to meet the 2010 objectives.[48]

Models for oral health education to reduce risk and prevent oral diseases should include four major elements. Risk assessment, including an inventory of social, environmental, and perceived needs, is the cornerstone for addressing behavioral changes associated with prevention or oral disease and risk reduction. This assessment should be followed by attention to a tailored education or counseling plan that is derived from effective communication with patients. Once a plan evolves and patient rapport and motivation is acknowledged, the educational or counseling program can be implemented. Continuous evaluation and follow-up based on periodic reassessment and attention to feedback mechanisms will ensure patient success.

SUMMARY

Although health education programs have been documented in the public health sector, very few definitive conclusions about the effectiveness of oral health promotion can be drawn from the currently available evidence.[49] Chairside oral health promotion has been shown to be effective more consistently than some other methods of health promotion. It is well known that caries and periodontal disease can be controlled by regular tooth brushing with a fluoride toothpaste, but a cost-effective method for reliably promoting such behaviors has not yet been established. In addition, as science continues to examine the associations between oral and systemic health, it will become more important than ever for the dental professional to take a proactive role in health promotion. This health care profession routinely cares for patients who are not in an immediate health crisis. Dental professionals are in an ideal position to assume leadership in health promotion and disease prevention, using workable education, communication, and counseling techniques to reduce risk. Knowledge levels can almost always be improved by oral health promotion initiatives, but whether these shifts in knowledge and attitudes can be causally related to changes in behavior or clinical indices of disease has not been extensively studied. Therefore, the profession needs to continue to pursue and improve the quality of oral health promotion evaluation research.

References

1. McGuire LC, Strine TW, Okoro CA et al.: Healthy lifestyle behaviors among older U.S. adults with and without disabilities, behavioral risk factor surveillance system, 2003, *Prev Chronic Dis* 4:A09, 2006.
2. Rutter M: Gene-environment interdependence, *Dev Sci* 10:12-18, 2007.
3. Weingarten S, Henning JM, Adamgarav E et al.: Interventions used in disease management programmes for patients with chronic illness—which one works? *Br Med J* 325:925-933, 2002.
4. Lorig K, Laurin J: Some notions about assumptions underlying health education, *Health Educ Q* 12:231-243, 1985.
5. Rankin SH, Stallings KD: *Patient education: principles and practice*, Philadelphia, 2001, Lippincott.
6. Mobley C: *Interactions between diabetes educators and clients of low socioeconomic status: a naturalistic study*, College Station, TX, 1993, Texas A & M University.

7. Bigge ML: *Learning theories for teachers*, New York, 1982, Harper & Row.

8. Merriam SB, Caffarella RS: *Learning in adulthood*, ed 2, San Francisco, 1999, Jossey-Bass.

9. Skinner BF: *The behavior of organisms*, New York, Appleton-Century Crofts, 1938.

10. Gagne RM: *Essentials of learning for instruction*, Hinsdale, IL, 1974, Dryden Press.

11. Abbatiello G: Integrative perspectives. Cognitive-behavioral therapy and metaphor, *Perspect Psychiatr Care* 42:208-210, 2006.

12. Lewin K: *Field theory in social science*, New York, 1951, Harper & Row.

13. Maslow A: *Motivation and personality*, New York, 1954, Harper & Row.

14. Rogers CR: *On becoming a person*, Boston, 1989, Houghton-Mifflin.

15. Knowles MS: *The modern practice of adult education*, New York, 1980, Associated Press.

16. Bandura A: *Social learning theory*, Englewood Cliffs, NJ, 1977, Prentice-Hall.

17. Hull CL: *Principles of behavior*, East Norwalk, CT, 1943, Appleton & Lange.

18. Fishbein M, Ajzen I: *Belief, attitude intention, and behavior: an introduction to theory and research*, Reading, MA, 1975, Addison-Wesley Publishing Company.

19. Prochaska JO, Redding CA, Evers KE: The transtheoretical model and stages of change. In Glanz K, Rimer BK, Lewis FM, editors: *Health behavior and health education theory, research, and practice*, ed 3, San Francisco, CA, 2002, Jossey-Bass.

20. Weinstein ND, Sandman PM: The precaution adoption process model. In Glanz K, Rimer BK, Lewis FM, editors: *Health behavior and health education theory, research, and practice, ed 3*, San Francisco, CA, 2002, Jossey-Bass.

21. Noar SM, Zimmerman RS: Health behavior theory and cumulative knowledge regarding health behaviors: are we moving in the right direction? *Health Educ Res* 20:275-290, 2004.

22. Becker MH: The health belief model and personal health behavior, *Health Educ Monog*r 2:324-473, 1974.

23. McEwen C, Flowers R, Tracie F: Learner-centered and culturally responsive patient education: drawing on traditions of cultural development and popular education, *AMIA Annu Symp Proc* 892, 2005.

24. Houle CO: *Patterns of learning, new perspectives on life-span education*, San Francisco, CA, 1984, Jossey-Bass.

25. Holli BB, Calabrese RJ, Maillet JO: *Communication and education skills for dietetic professionals*, ed 4, Baltimore, MD, 2003, Lippincott Williams & Wilkins.

26. Glanz K, Rimer BK, Lewis FM, editors: *Health behavior and health education theory, research, and practice*, ed 3, San Francisco, CA, 2002, Jossey-Bass.

27. Shannon CE, Warren W: *A mathematical model of communication*, Urbana, IL, 1949, University of Illinois Press.

28. Gibb J: Defensive communication, *J Commun* 11:141, 1961.

29. Bartley KC: *Dietetic practitioner skills*, New York, 1987, Macmillan Publishing Company.

30. Ekman P, Friesen WV: *Unmasking the face: a guide to recognizing oral communication*, Englewoods Cliffs, NJ, 1967, Prentice-Hall.

31. Littlejohn SW: *From theories of human communication*, ed 2, Belmont, CA, 1983, Wadsworth.

32. Woodruff AD: *Basic concepts of teaching*, San Francisco, CA, 1961, Chandler Publishing.

33. Michie S, Lester K: Words matter: increasing the implementation of clinical guidelines, *Qual Saf Health Care* 14:367-370, 2005.

34. Kim S, Mouradian WE, Leggott PJ et al.: Implications for designing online oral health resources: a review of fifty-six websites, *J Dent Educ* 68:633-643, 2004.

35. Nutbeam D: Health promotion glossary, *Health Promot Int* 13:349-364, 1998.

36. Nutbeam D: Health literacy as a public health goal: a challenge for contemporary health education and communication strategies into the 21st century, *Health Promot Int* 15:259-267, 2000.

37. U.S. Department of Health and Human Services: *Oral Health in America. A Report of the Surgeon General*, Rockville, MD, 2000, U. S. Department of Health and Human Services, National Institute of Health, National Institute of Dental and Craniofacial Research.

38. Nowak AJ, Casmassimo PS: Using anticipatory guidance to provide early dental intervention, *JADA* 126:1156-1163, 1995.

39. Green M, Palfrey JS, Clark EM et al., editors: *Bright futures: guidelines for health supervision of infants, children, and adolescent*, ed 2, Arlington, VA, 2002, National Center for Education In Maternal and Child Health.

40. American Academy of Pediatrics Committee on Psychosocial Aspects of Child and Family Health: *Guidelines for health supervision III*, ed 3, Elk Grove Village, IL, 2002, American Academy of Pediatrics.

41. Barkin SLA, Scheindlin BB, Brown CA et al.: Anticipatory guidance topics: are more better? *Ambul Pediatr* 5:372-376, 2005.

42. Nelson CS, Wissow LS, Cheng TL: Effectiveness of anticipatory guidance: recent developments, *Curr Opin Pediatr* 15:630-635, 2003.

43. Magar NA, Dabova-Missova S, Gjerdingen DK: Effectiveness of targeted anticipatory guidance during well-child visits: a pilot trial, *J Am Board Fam Med* 19:450-458, 2006.

44. McConaughy FL, Toevs SE, Lukken KM: Adult clients' recall of oral health education services received in private practice, *J Dent Hyg* 69:202-211, 1995.

45. Basson WJ: Oral health education provided by oral hygienists in private practice, *SADJ* 54: 53-57, 1999.

46. Bartecchi CE, MacKenzie TD, Schrier RW: The human cost of tobacco use-first of two parts, *N Engl J Med* 13:907-912, 1994.

47. U.S. Department of Health and Human Services: *Healthy People 2010: Understanding and Improving Health*, ed 2, Washington, DC, 2000, U.S. Government Printing Office.

48. Cannick GF, Horowitz A, Drury TF et al.: Opinions of South Carolina dental students toward tobacco use interventions, *J Public Health Dent* 66:44-48, 2006.

49. Kay E, Locker D: A systematic review of the effectiveness of health promotion aimed at improving oral health, *Community Dent Health* 15:132-144, 1998.

Chapter 11

*E*nhancing Patient Adherence to Preventive Programs

CONNIE C. MOBLEY, JOHN RUGH, JOHN WESLEY KAROTKIN, AND AVNI
ADHVARYU BHATT

**TERMINOLOGY AND HISTORICAL
PERSPECTIVE**

**DETERMINANTS OF PATIENT
ADHERENCE**

**PATIENT ADHERENCE ASSESSMENT
PROTOCOLS**

MONITORING PATIENT ADHERENCE

**STRATEGIES TO ENHANCE PATIENT
ADHERENCE**

SUMMARY

Patient/provider relationship
Predictive factors
Stage-based models
Technological advances

LEARNING OBJECTIVES

Upon completion of this chapter, the learner will be able to:
- Define terminology and historical issues used to describe concepts in individual adherence to health practices.
- Review the personal, environmental, and predictive factors associated with varying degrees of patient adherence to recommended health behaviors.
- Examine assessment and management protocols to facilitate patient adherence.
- Identify strategies to promote patient adherence to recommended oral health behaviors.

KEY TERMS

Comprehensive patient-centered counseling programs
Motivational interviewing
Patient characteristics
Patient/parent relationship

Advances have been made in preventive regimens and treatment modalities associated with health promotion. Evolving knowledge of preventive lifestyle behaviors has led to a better understanding of how personal choices can modulate the risk factors for major life-threatening diseases and disorders such as stroke, heart disease, and certain cancers. Patient adherence to recommended practices has continued to be problematic. Patient noncompliance with oral hygiene and treatment protocols has been particularly frustrating for the dentist, because the two most common oral health problems, caries and periodontal disease, are almost entirely preventable with appropriate behaviors. Unfortunately, long-term patient adherence to oral health preventive strategies and programs is perceived to be difficult to achieve. Reports indicate that individual adherence to preventive oral health behaviors ranges from 10% to 60%, depending on the specific behavior.[1-3] Even when faced with life threatening-conditions, personal adherence to diet and prescription medicines is estimated to be no higher than 50%.[4] Adherence to oral preventive measures and long-term treatments, such as that associated with orthodontics and periodontics and chronic medical illnesses is also likely to be only 50%.[3-7] Unsuccessful outcomes of some treatment modalities, such as orthodontic intervention, has been questioned in the context of patient adherence. Is the outcome the result of the dental professional's ineffective treatment, or was the patient nonadherent with the recommended oral health practices protocol?

Adherence rates to preventive and treatment regimens are considered serious and costly public health problems. Nonadherence to treatment regimens is the greatest single reason for hospital readmissions.[8] The cost of nonadherence to medication regimens is estimated to be as much as 300 billion dollars annually,[9] and the cost of treating preventable oral disease in the United States is expected to exceed 60 billion dollars in the coming millennium.[10] Assisting patients in achieving sustained behavioral changes to support oral health and live healthier lives is a responsibility of the dental professional that transcends individual life course events.

This chapter identifies patient characteristics and environmental factors related to patient nonadherence to recommended health practices. Because no methods exist to accurately predict which patients will be adherent, establishing long-term assessment and monitoring programs for patient adherence is an essential first step. An individually tailored, comprehensive program for long-term behavioral change is suggested. Any program designed to increase adherence must recognize patient differences and be tailored to each patient's personal and environmental situation. Strategies to enhance individual long-term patient adherence discussed in this chapter complement the patient education programs discussed in Chapter 10.

TERMINOLOGY AND HISTORICAL PERSPECTIVE

A dramatic evolution has occurred in medicine and dentistry with respect to approaches to patient adherence. Traditionally, physicians and dentists would simply prescribe and/or advise patients about measures they should adopt (e.g., "take one tablet with each meal," "begin an exercise program," or "floss daily"). Conscientious clinicians sometimes provided specific written or video instructions, or both. These instructions and advice were offered in an authoritative manner, with the assumption that the patient understood the directives and would be motivated to "comply" with the recommendations. Thus, patient compliance was the term coined to describe the expected responses.

By the mid1980s, it became increasingly clear that simple advice, education, or both, had failed to change health behaviors in patients. In response, some dental and medical practitioners implemented reinforcement programs based on behavioral psychology. Reinforcement of desired behaviors was helpful for some patients; however, patient adherence remained a significant concern for most health care providers. In the 1990s, nonadherence was noted to be a multifactorial problem, and each patient was seen to have unique impediments to adherence. Providing advice and education was necessary but not sufficient to change behavior. A number of motivational, cognitive, lifestyle, psychosocial, and socioeconomic factors needed to be addressed to increase the probability of changing health behaviors.

With this realization that each patient has a unique set of circumstances, defining the context of patients'

individual behaviors led to the development of several "patient-centered" strategies to enhance adherence. These modern strategies generally view the patient and provider as a team who discuss, negotiate, and agree on individually tailored health behavior regimens that are compatible with the patient's unique personal and environmental situation. To reflect this change in strategy, the term "compliance," which suggests obedience to authority, was replaced with the term "adherence." The "patient-centered" programs (such as "motivational interviewing") discussed later in this chapter, are consistent with this change and have proved useful to enhance short- and long-term adherence with a wide variety of preventive health behaviors and treatment regimens.

Personal responsibility for one's health status can complement existing public health initiatives in health promotion. Public efforts have supported interventions that do not require individual initiative and personal responsibility for health. For example, community water fluoridation, sealants, and topical fluoride treatment have resulted in dramatic improvements in oral health.[11-13] These efforts have been particularly effective, do not require individual behavioral change, do not reinforce the concept of personal responsibility for one's health, and require complementary programs. Critically important health behaviors such as appropriate diet, exercise, and preventive oral health care require individual decision-making and practices. The dental professional has been identified as the health care provider most likely to have frequent patient contact. Thus, he or she can play a vital role in promoting long-term personal responsibility for oral and general health behaviors.

DETERMINANTS OF PATIENT ADHERENCE

Several patient characteristics and environmental and predictive factors are associated with patient adherence and cooperation. Classification of elements is described as follows: patient characteristics, patient-provider and patient-parent relationships, the nature of the treatment/preventive regimen, and characteristics of the disease. These elements are defined in Table 11-1.

Patient characteristics related to adherence include the patient's age, gender, mood, self-esteem, lifestyle, cognitive abilities, academic performance, and socioeconomic status.

Trends indicate that female children are more cooperative and adherent to health behaviors than male children.[14-18] This trend is consistent with findings that females of all ages tend to adhere more to treatment and preventive instructions. A child's academic performance is correlated with cooperation and adherence in orthodontic treatment and this is consistent with research findings in multiple areas of health care.[14,19-22] Similarly, children of higher socioeconomic class (SES) have been reported to generally have higher levels of adherence.[15]

TABLE 11-1

FACTORS RELATED TO TRENDS IN PATIENT ADHERENCE

FACTOR	TREND
PATIENT CHARACTERISTICS	
Age	Adherence appears to decline in children after puberty and in aging adults.
Gender	Females at all ages are more adherent in general.
Academic performance	Children with higher academic performance tend to be more adherent in general.
Socioeconomic status (SES)	Children of higher SES tend to be more adherent.
Self-esteem	Patients with higher self-esteem tend to be more adherent.
Lifestyle	Busy, stressful life styles may compromise adherence.
Cognitive abilities and mood	Dementia, substance abuse, and depression frequently limit adherence.
PATIENT/PROVIDER AND PATIENT/ PARENT RELATIONSHIPS	A positive patient/provider relationship is believed to be a key factor in promoting patient adherence.
	Positive parent/patient relationships usually result in better adherence.
PREDICTIVE FACTORS	
Perceived need for care	When the perceived need for care increases, patient adherence usually improves.
Pain and discomfort	Adherence usually declines if the regimen involves pain, discomfort, or inconvenience.
Misunderstanding of instructions	Young children, the elderly, and retarded individuals may misunderstand the regimen.
Social/family support	Adherence is usually higher when supported by peer groups and family.

Thus, prepubescent females who do well in school, have high self-esteem, and come from upper middle-class families are usually somewhat more adherent to prescribed oral health practices than others who do not have these characteristics.

Standardized psychological inventories have been used to identify personal traits and characteristics of adherent and nonadherent patients. Using the Million Adolescent Personality Inventory with 104 orthodontic patients between 13 and 18 years of age, investigators were able to account for 24% of the variation in orthodontic compliance.[18] Cucalon and Smith administered three psychological inventories to 252 orthodontic patients (ages 11 to 17).[15] They reported that more adherent patients, who generally scored higher on self-esteem, were more optimistic about the future, derived self-satisfaction from personal achievement, and were less alienated from society. Other studies have examined related factors such as "need achievement," health locus of control, self-esteem, psychological mood, attitudes, self-efficacy, life stress levels, anxiety, and self-concept.[3,23-31] Some correlations with adherence were found in some studies, most were weak, some reported inconsistent results, and many compared groups of patients with varying levels of adherence. Although group means have differed significantly on psychological inventories, on a patient-by-patient basis these inventories have not been shown to predict nonadherence (i.e., no data exist on the sensitivity, specificity, positive predictive value, and negative predictive value of selected instruments). Thus, routine use of psychosocial, personality, and attitude scales to predict adherence has not been recommended. It is not possible to identify a "noncompliant personality," rather, the evidence suggests that adherence is situational and depends on multiple and complex factors.[27,32,33]

Patient/provider and **patient/parent relationships** are a reflection of perceived shared responsibility in adherent patient behaviors.[34] Patient-provider communication is a determining factor in assessing adherence. For example, patient cooperation is reported to be the single most important factor that dental professionals must assess in developing a course of treatment.[35] Numerous research efforts have specifically addressed patient cooperation and adherence during orthodontic treatment because typically it occurs during a 2-year period. In addition, implications for patient adherence to oral health promotion and disease prevention are critical to establish sustained behavioral change. Mehra et al. obtained the opinions of 420 practicing orthodontists regarding factors in assessing and promoting patient adherence.[36] Questionnaires asked orthodontists to rate 20 predictors of patient adherence and 24 methods of improving patient adherence on a five-point, Likert-type scale. The results are listed in Table 11-2. The patient's desire for treatment received the highest ranking, followed by the patient's maintenance of good oral health and the frequency of broken appointments. These factors were

TABLE 11-2

ORTHODONTISTS (N = 420) RANKING ON A SCALE OF 1-5 OF PREDICTIVE FACTORS RELATED TO PATIENT ADHERENCE

RANK	PREDICTOR	MEAN SCORE
1	Patient's desire for or interest in orthodontic treatment	4.47
2	Frequency of broken appliance	4.35
3	Maintenance of good oral health	4.27
4	Interaction between orthodontists and patient	4.10
5	Patient's perception of their malocclusion	3.94
6	Interpersonal relationship between patient and parents	3.95
7	Promptness for appointments	3.86
8	Patient's perception of his or her facial esthetics	3.72
9	Parental desire for orthodontic treatment	3.64
10	Interaction between orthodontist and patient's parents	3.51
11	Frequent delinquency in appointments	3.62
12	Parent's perception of their child's malocclusion	3.41
13	Parent's perception of child's facial esthetics	3.35
14	Severity of the malocclusion	3.34
15	Level of education of the patient	3.47
16	Girls as more adherent than boys	3.41
17	Patient's grades in school	3.34
18	Demographic background of the family	3.35
19	Socioeconomic background of the family	3.18
20	Boys are more adherent than girls	2.31

(From Mehra T, Nanda RS et al.: Orthodontists' assessment and management of patient compliance, *Angle Orthod* 68:116, 1998.)

considered to be predictors of patient cooperativeness in this setting.

Patient adherence may be a generalizable trait, however, the evidence clearly suggests that adherence is situational and specific to a behavior. For example, a patient may floss regularly but routinely miss appointments. The importance of personal relationships in adherent individual behavior has been reported in the literature since the late 1960s.[35,37,38] For example, positive interpersonal relationships between the orthodontist and the patient, between the orthodontist and the parents, and between the patient and his or her parents are all factors related to patient adherence among children. Kreit et al. reported that children who were the most nonadherent patients were those who manifested poor relationships with their parents.[16] Child and parent relationships, and thus adherence, may change dramatically in a short time period near puberty.[16,39-41] Reports suggest that parental influence and cooperation is stronger during early stages of orthodontic treatment. When the child transitions through puberty, adherence depends less on parental control and more on the patient's self-motivation.[23] A child's cooperation may be further compromised by parents who appear helpless, frustrated, tense, hysterical, demanding, or insecure in coping with the child.[42]

Additional **predictive factors** have been examined in an effort to categorize potentially adherent patients. In pursuit of evidence-based theories, numerous aspects of the patient domain have been examined. These factors include a patient's perceived need for care, awareness of pain and discomfort, cognitive understanding of instructions, and degree of social and family support. A high perceived "need for care" generally enhances adherence. As expected, adherence is compromised when a treatment or management regimen involves pain, discomfort, or inconvenience. The lack of adherence for some patients because of misunderstood instructions is associated with complex regimens, limited patient cognitive abilities, and depression. Finally, adherence in children and aging adults is generally higher in patients who have strong social and family support.[9]

In summary, several personal and environmental factors have been correlated with patients' nonadherence to oral health practices. None of these personal or environmental factors is sufficiently robust to identify the patient who may be nonadherent. Adherence is multifactorial, situational, and unique to the individual. Thus, the development of a universal predictive tool has not evolved. The dental clinician should be aware of the factors correlated with adherence and recognize that limited interpretations of associations with adherent behaviors exist. This understanding is not adequate to replace the need for routine assessment and monitoring of adherence if beneficial oral health behaviors are to be sustained.

PATIENT ADHERENCE ASSESSMENT PROTOCOLS

Implementing systems designed to assess and monitor patient adherence to treatment, preventive programs, or both should include numerous strategies and approaches that are tailored to individual patient needs. One long-standing method of evaluating patient adherence involves the clinician asking the patient questions to identify self-reported behaviors. For example, the dental professional may ask the patient about the frequency, method, and duration of brushing and flossing. Both patients and clinicians tend to overestimate levels of adherence when this method is used. The accuracy of patient reports has been typically better when the patient is asked about nonadherence rather than adherence. Table 11-3 provides examples of questions associated with adherent and nonadherent responses and suggests neutral questions for consideration.

Accurate and objective assessments of adherence can be made by using indices that measure the results of non-adherence. These additional approaches can confirm or refute self-reported data. Some of the most common indices used include Plaque Index (PlI), Plaque Control Record, Plaque-Free Score, Patient Hygiene Performance (PHP), Simplified Oral Hygiene Index (OHI-S), Gingival Bleeding Index (GBI), and Gingival Index (GI).[43] (See Chapter 2 for descriptions of some of these indices.) Thickness, accumulation, and severity of gingival plaque, debris, and calculus that result in the presence of gingival inflammation can be used to determine previous failures in patient adherence. The Periodontal Screening and Recording (PSR) index is reported to be a particularly effective tool to assess patient adherence.[43] The plaque

index can be explained to patients with the use of disclosing agents that are available in liquid or tablet form.[25] Disclosing agents can be used for initial assessment of oral hygiene behaviors and for self-monitoring programs to be practiced in the home setting. This is an example of a technique that can foster positive communication between the dental practitioner and the patient and set the tone to instill future self-evaluation and motivation in the patient.[25]

Strategies in assessment should focus on establishing rapport with the patient to achieve a communicative atmosphere. Depending on the age, educational level, and literacy level of the patient, in addition to the specific intended behavior, the dental practitioner should allow adequate time for assessment of factors most likely to be associated with successful patient adherence.

MONITORING PATIENT ADHERENCE

Collection and interpretation of assessment data should be clearly explained to the patient prior to discussion of goal setting and the development of a monitoring plan. Because participation in shared decision-making and responsibilities involve choices, it is important to establish balanced roles for both the dental professional and the patient. The professional guides the patient in making informed choices and adaptations in self-management.[44]

Once goals are set, providing a patient with a type of self-monitoring form or log can help to establish baseline assessment. In addition, it can be extended to perpetuate long-term self-monitoring which can motivate patients to sustain behavioral changes. Patients may be asked to demonstrate techniques of brushing and flossing to further validate the accuracy of self-reporting, and to assess the use of proper technique.

Technological advances in monitoring adherence allow the clinician to adjust preventive and treatment strategies to fit the patient's unique personal attributes, interests, and environmental situation. These advances

TABLE 11-3

SAMPLE QUESTIONS LIKELY TO ILLICIT RESPONSES INDICATIVE OF ADHERENT OR NONADHERENT BEHAVIOR COMPARED WITH NEUTRAL QUESTIONS

ADHERENT PROMPTS	NONADHERENT PROMPTS	NEUTRAL PROMPTS
Do you brush your teeth twice a day?	Are you having **difficulty** brushing your teeth twice a day?	Can you **describe** your tooth brushing habits?
Were you **able** to brush this morning?	Were you **unable** to brush this morning?	**When** did you last brush your teeth?
Do you **restrict** your between meal snacks to one a day?	Do you **have difficulty** eating only one snack a day?	**What** are your snacking habits like on most days?

target behavioral self-monitoring (brushing/flossing), and strategies that focus on monitoring outcomes, such as an aspect of a disease or condition that is related to the preventive behavior (such as plaque or gingival bleeding) have been used.

In recent decades, technological advances in data collection methods and adherence monitoring devices have been adapted to dental applications. The current state of microprocessor and computer technology has facilitated these developments. For example, McCracken et al. devised a data logging system integrated into a commercially produced powered toothbrush with the capability of recording brushing time at different head speeds and recharging time between uses.[2] Importantly, the device also recorded motor current to determine brushing force. This was used to determine whether a patient simply activated the toothbrush without actually brushing. Data stored in the toothbrushes could be downloaded onto a computer at the end of each 2-month test period. A limitation of this study was that a large percentage of the data loggers had failures of some type. With refinement of the electronics and methods, however, this technology could be used to collect extremely accurate data on patient adherence to in tooth brushing behavior.[2]

Other electronic monitoring devices have been designed for numerous uses. This includes removable intraoral appliances, headgears, and splints used for sleep apnea treatment. Most of these devices could be easily adapted for a wide range of applications. Sahm, Bartsch, and Witt have described a simple method to reliably monitor removable appliance wear by using a wristwatch circuit board embedded within the acrylic resin of the appliance.[45] The circuit is activated by a reed switch, which is toggled by a magnet that has been cemented to a molar tooth in the opposite arch. A memory chip in the appliance records the time and duration of wear, and the clinician can download the information at each office visit. This system consists of commercially produced components that are readily available and inexpensive.

Kyriacou and Jones described a sophisticated headgear compliance monitor that is very resistant to patient "circumvention" or cheating.[46] Headgear timers have existed since 1974, but most have been very easy for patients to activate without actually wearing the device. In this design, a timer is triggered by both body temperature and force (stretch) sensors; both sensors must be activated to turn on the timer. In addition, the patient does not know when the device is engaged, making it extremely unlikely that he or she would be able to tamper with monitoring results. Commercially produced headgear timers are currently available but may be easy for the patient to circumvent.[47]

Tjin et al. invented a device for use in splints made to treat sleep apnea, which could easily be adapted for use in occlusal splints, orthodontic appliances, and fluoride trays. The device uses fiber optics to monitor both temperature and force associated with appliance wear. Furthermore, no electrical current is involved in this system; thus, the risk of patient electrocution is eliminated.[48]

Technologically innovative solutions for monitoring and improving patient adherence with oral medication use have been conceived in recent years. For example, an electronic pill bottle lid, meant to fit on standard-sized pill bottles, and which records the time and date of each bottle-opening event, has been evaluated by numerous investigators. On the basis of a study comparing methods of assessing patient adherence with oral medication regimens, this approach was found to be more useful and reliable than questionnaire scores, tablet counts, and blood concentration measurements.[49] The increased utility of electronic pill monitors over pill counts is even greater when considering patient adherence with drugs that are to be taken multiple times per day. Adherence measured by pill count for once-a-day dosing and twice-a-day dosing were 68% and 65%, respectively, in a study involving hypertensive patients. When electronic monitoring was introduced, these same measurements were 49% and 5%, respectively.[50] Pill counts, when used alone, can be extremely misleading, especially with multiple doses per day. Some speculate that the discrepancy may be in the patients' lack of understanding of proper scheduling.[50]

Alternative devices vary in size and function. One such monitor is the size of a videotape and includes five medication drawers, a digital display, and various buttons. An alarm alerts the patient to take a specific medication and dosage. The monitor can be programmed to provide as many as 25 reminders or questions concerning symptoms, weight, blood pressure, diet, exercise, or any other parameter of health. The device records the date and time each pill is removed in addition to answering the questions displayed. Each night through a standard telephone, the device uploads stored information to a server and downloads information such as new questions and medication schedules as provided by a clinician. Patients who use this device have shown a 94% adherence rate with oral medications in addition to increased time spent in daily monitoring of blood pressure and body weight.[51]

Modern information technology, including the World Wide Web, has precipitated innovative methods of communication between patients and providers to facilitate adherence to medical protocols. The clinician can send a set of questions or reminders to the patient that he or she can answer to maintain an ongoing "dialogue." This system allows the clinician to educate and monitor the patient from a remote location, and it promotes early intervention according to daily dialogue responses. When this technique was used in a study to monitor pediatric asthma patients, results showed a decrease in symptoms, missed school days, and health services use in the experimental group as compared with a control (asthma diary) group. Children were much more likely to use this approach than writing in a diary. Importantly, even after the children's use of the system declined towards the end of the study interval, the patients' disease management skills, medication use, and treatment adherence were sustained at the targeted level.[52] Similar results were found in studies done with indigent adult diabetes and heart failure patients.[53,54]

Text paging systems have been shown to be of benefit in medication adherence and could serve to remind patients of oral preventive behaviors. Text pagers increased AIDS patients' adherence to medication regimens. Similarly, this type of system could be used to remind patients of meal schedules, clinical appointments, and timing of oral health maintenance activities.[55]

Intraoral cameras are an integral part of patient education and may also be useful in assessing adherence. At a patient's initial examination and subsequent visits, the clinician can show the progress in treatment. This is a powerful tool that is useful in making patients aware of the consequences of lack of adherence and how it adversely affects their oral health.[56]

Practitioners can explore access to several monitoring strategies for patient adherence activities. A monitoring strategy is, in fact, one of the key components of most successful interventions and very often may be the only intervention needed to ensure patient adherence.

STRATEGIES TO ENHANCE PATIENT ADHERENCE

A comprehensive patient-centered program to enhance adherence involves three major components. The first component involves specific strategies for targeted health behaviors (i.e., flossing, taking medications, or wearing a retainer). The second critical component is a patient-education module, (described and discussed in Chapter 10) and, when necessary, a third component would be an individual-patient focused counseling strategy.

Comprehensive patient-centered counseling programs to enhance patient adherence have been described within numerous frameworks.[31,37,57-67] Practical techniques and strategies useful in oral health preventive and treatment programs are summarized in Box 11-1. The common elements of modern programs typically involve one-on-one patient discussions with the following specific goals: assessing and enhancing the patient's motivation and intention to change, assessing the patient's knowledge and skills related to the targeted health behavior, identifying the patient's unique personal and environmental constraints that may serve as barriers to adherence, and negotiating an agreed on set of health-related health goals and behaviors. The patient and care provider agree on a specific set of behaviors/goals, a plan to monitor the behavior or condition, and a time frame. Finally, the program would involve mechanisms of reinforcement for appropriate behavior. As with other components, the

reinforcement strategy is unique to each individual patient.

The oral health care provider should be familiar with the various techniques and strategies described in Box 11-1 and use them in various combinations to assist patients in establishing appropriate behaviors. Highly motivated patients may only need to be educated about proper technique. Others may fully understand the skills but need motivation to initiate and maintain the behavior. The essential aspect of all modern programs to enhance adherence is the recognition that each patient has a unique situation and will require a personalized, tailored, and unique program. No one strategy will work for all patients. Because of differences in dental providers' personalities, charisma, and enthusiasm, what works in one office may not work in another. Long-term adherence to oral health preventive programs is believed to ultimately depend on patient self-management. Patient goal setting self-monitoring, periodic reassessment, and self-reinforcement strategies should be encouraged.

Stage-based models of behavioral interventions assume that change is not a continuous process but something that occurs in different stages, in which barriers to change may differ. Basically, change models all identify three broad categories of patients. The first group includes those who have not yet decided to change, the second group consists of those who have decided to change but not yet taken action, and the third group is made up of those involved in overt changes. The best and most widely used example of the stage-based approach is explained by the Transtheoretical Model (TTM). One model of this approach is illustrated in Figure 11-1.[68] A series of five sequential stages describe differences in a patient's motivation and actions and acknowledges that changes in stages require time. Processes of change are supported by the counseling approaches described in Box 11-1. Raising awareness, self-evaluation, commitment to change, and weighing pros and cons are behaviors that move the individual to achieve maintenance of the desired behavioral changes.[69] A systematic review of literature representing this approach concluded little evidence existed to support its effectiveness.[70] The investigators agreed that stage-based models were theoretically sound but required better interpretation for delivery. Elements of this model may prove useful when tailoring programs to individual needs however and should be considered.

Motivational interviewing has been widely adopted as a patient counseling approach that is closely aligned with change theory, but is uniquely defined as being patient-centered. The specific techniques and strategies used in this approach include the following: expression of empathy by the counselor, development of discrepancies among the pros and cons of a behavior, rolling with resistance so as not to exert external pressure on the patient, and support for self-efficacy as identified by the patient.[65, 71] This approach stresses the need to avoid leading

BOX 11-1

Components of a Patient-Centered Counseling Program to Enhance Long-Term Adherence

1. ASSESS
- Determine the patient's current preventive behavior patterns. Verify that these patterns are consistent with what would be expected from clinical examination of the patient's oral health status.
- Assess the patient's interest in, and skills to perform, the preventive behavior or treatment. Does evidence exist of intention, commitment, and readiness to change?
- Ask the patient about the perceived benefits of and barriers to the preventive behavior or treatment to help assess his or her interest in change. This conversation may also serve to motivate the patient and to determine solutions to perceived barriers.
- Acknowledge ambivalence and offer choices, including no action. Adherence is enhanced when patients take responsibility and make the decision to change.

2. EDUCATE
- Provide and discuss with the patient information to ensure appropriate knowledge about the disease and the preventive strategies and treatment, or both.
- Focus and limit the amount of educational information to that which is critical.
- Ensure that the patient believes the behaviors will positively impact his or her health.
- Convey empathy, avoid arguing and establish a trusting, positive patient/provider relationship.
- Avoid jargon and communicate at the patient's educational level.
- Educate the patient on the skills to perform the behavior and ensure that he or she is confident in his or her skills.
- Simplify treatment and preventive protocols as much as possible. Complex programs significantly decrease adherence.
- Provide written or video information and skill instruction. Self-paced, interactive DVDs are helpful.
- Ensure that the patient is made aware of any side effects or pain that is likely to result from the preventive or treatment protocol. Unexpected pain is a common reason for nonadherence.
- Ask questions to assess patient comprehension of knowledge and skills. With some preventive behaviors, it is useful to ask the patient to demonstrate the behavior and provide corrective feedback.

3. ESTABLISH ACTION PLAN AND OUTCOME EXPECTANCIES
- Patient-centered, preventive programs involve the clinician and patient agreeing on a behavioral action plan with specific measurable outcome expectancies. For example, "floss at least once daily, and reduce the Patient Hygiene Performance Index (PHP) score by 50% by your next 4-week appointment," versus "improve your oral hygiene."
- Target a limited number of the most important behaviors, and set obtainable goals to increase chance of success. Increase expectancies as intermediate goals are achieved.
- Discuss with patient how new behaviors can fit into daily routines, and identify cues to elicit the behavior.
- Tie new behaviors to established behaviors.

4. MOTIVATE AND REINFORCE
- Establish patient-relevant external or internal (or both) reward contingencies to motivate performance of behaviors and obtaining goals. These rewards for adherence are in addition to the expected long-range health benefits.
- Verbalize praise, because this can be a very strong reinforcer. Some offices have found monetary rewards and gifts useful to help motivate some patients. Social recognition is a powerful motivator for many children, thus a photo board of children who obtained certain goals is often useful.
- Encourage social support for the preventive behavior. Such support is important for adherence with many patients. It is helpful to ask the patient whether family and friends endorse the behavior.
- Focus on the most immediate positive outcome of a preventive behavior (e.g., fresher breath) rather than the long-term negative consequences such as periodontal disease, caries, and tooth loss. Immediate positive reinforcement is generally more effective in changing behaviors than long-term negative consequences. Avoid scolding.
- Instill self-confidence and encourage self-management and self-reward. It is often helpful to ask the patient about past success in changing his or her behaviors. Provide praise for even moderate success.

5. MONITOR
- Initiate periodic patient exams as a step in monitoring adherence to targeted behaviors and hygiene outcome goals. The interval of follow-up is unique to the patient's performance.
- Encourage self-monitoring to promote patient self-managed long-term adherence. For example, self-monitoring with disclosing tablets at home and self-charting specific behaviors by the patient are helpful.
- Increase vigilance regarding adherence when the patient's lifestyle or psycho/social conditions are changed.

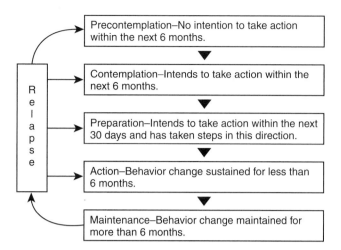

Figure 11-1   The Transtheoretical Model of the stage-based approach to behavior change. (From Prochaska JO: Staging: a revolution in helping people change, *Manag Care* 12:6-9, 2003.)

discussion and arguing, while accepting the patient's resistance and ambivalence. The counselor must recognize that even if the patient is motivated to change behavior, change does not occur unless the patient believes he or she can overcome barriers to change and can be successful in implementing new behaviors. Figure 11-2 describes how elements of motivational interviewing can be woven into patient counseling strategies.

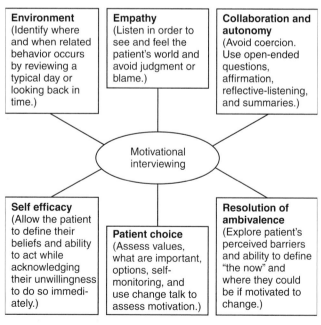

Figure 11-2   Key elements of Motivational Interviewing. (From Miller WR, Zweben A, DiClemente CC et al.: *Motivational enhancement therapy manual: a clinical research guide for therapists treating individuals with alcohol abuse dependence.* Rockville, MD, 1992, National Institute of Alcohol Abuse.)

A serious problem with patient-focused counseling strategies is that they require a significant amount of the clinician's time. Unfortunately, reimbursement mechanisms do not support time spent on prevention. To address this problem, Weinstein adapted a powerful behavioral change-counseling program based on a motivational interviewing philosophy to oral health behaviors.[72] This counseling program, which has been shown to be highly successful with changing problem behaviors such as smoking and exercise, involves a significant time commitment but can be accomplished by trained lay counselors or dental auxiliaries.[72] A published clinical trial found motivational interview counseling to be significantly more effective in preventing carious lesions than traditional health education.[73] This approach may prove to effectively modify a wide range of oral health-related behaviors in both children and adults.

SUMMARY

The dental professional can enhance patient services and treatment outcomes with attention to patient adherence to practices supporting optimum oral health status. The role of facilitator and counselor require identification of strategies uniquely tailored to the needs of the individual patient. Assessment and monitoring of a patient's adherence potential can improve dental practitioner-patient communication. Stage-based models for introducing techniques to enhance patient success can be integrated into patient visits and technology offers a menu of options to consider for additional patient support.

In many fields of medicine, information technology has been used to monitor and improve patient adherence. World Wide Web patient surveys have obvious advantages over traditional paper and pencil or face-to-face methods in facilitating behaviors. The technique reduces costs, eliminates transcription errors, reduces the need for the patient to travel, facilitates multisite studies, and allows for immediate data processing and statistical analysis. One of the major concerns is the security of the transmitted data. Security and encryption protocols are available to address this issue.[74] Given the prevalence of internet access in the United States, internet surveys also greatly increase the practicality of frequent monitoring, thus minimizing recall bias and maximizing data reliability. The patient's sense of anonymity is increased by using the internet as opposed to paper or personal methods of data collection, thereby increasing the likelihood that patients will answer questions truthfully.[75] Various groups have demonstrated that the use of cyberspace communication is effective not only for adherence monitoring but also for adherence improvement in areas as diverse as pediatric and congestive heart failure treatment.[51,52] Logically, no barrier exists to the implementation of similar methods and tools in the study and improvement of dental patient adherence. These technologies, when combined with the modern, individualized patient-centered strategies that promote personal responsibility and self-management have the potential to significantly enhance patient oral health adherence and to improve the extended relationship between a patient and his oral health care provider.

References

1. Wilson TG Jr: How patient compliance to suggested oral hygiene and maintenance affect periodontal therapy, *Dent Clin North Am* 42:389-403, 1998.

2. McCracken G, Janssen J, Heasman L et al.: Assessing adherence with toothbrushing instructions using a data logger toothbrush, *Br Dent J* 198:29-32, 2005.

3. Ojima M, Kanagawa H, Nishida N et al.: Relationship between attitudes toward oral health at initial office visit and compliance with supportive periodontal treatment, *J Clin Periodontol* 32:364-368, 2005.

4. World Health Organization: *Adherence to long-term therapies: evidence for action (WHO/M/C/03.01)* (website): http://www.who.int/chronic_conditions/adherencereport/en/print.html. Accessed July 28, 2006.

5. Morris LS, Schulz RM: Patient compliance-an overview, *J Clin Pharm Ther* 17:283-295, 1992.

6. Novaes AB Jr, Novaes AB: Compliance with supportive periodontal therapy. Part 1. Risk of non-compliance in the first 5-year period, *J Periodontol* 70:679-682, 1999.

7. Schlenk EA, Dunbar-Jacob J, Engberg S: Medication non-adherence among older adults: a review of strategies and interventions for improvement, *J Gerontol Nurs* 30:33-43, 2004.

8. Meichenbaum DC, Turk D: *Facilitating treatment adherence: a practitioner's guidebook*, New York, 1987, Plenum Press.

9. DiMatteo MR: Variations in patients' adherence to medical recommendations: a quantitative review of 50 years of research, *Med Care* 42:200-209, 2004.

10. Lawrence HP, Leake JL: The U.S. Surgeon General's Report on oral health in American: a Canadian perspective, *J Can Dent Assoc* 67:1-9, 2001.

11. Petersen PE: *The World Oral Health Report 2003, who/nmh/nph/03.2*, Geneva, Switzerland, 2003, World Health Organization.

12. Splieth CH, Nourallah AW, Konig KG: Caries prevention programs for groups: out of fashion or up to date? *Clin Oral Investig* 8:6-10, 2004.

13. U.S. Department of Health and Human Services, U.S. Public Health Services: *Oral health in America: a report of the Surgeon General*, 2000 (website): http://www.nidcr.nih.gov/sgr/oralhealth.htm. Accessed June 7, 2007.

14. Clemmer EJ, Hayes EW: Patient cooperation in wearing orthodontic headgear, *Am J Orthod* 75:517-524, 1979.

15. Cucalon A, Smith RJ: Relationship between compliance by adolescent orthodontic patients and performance on psychological tests, *Angle Orthod* 60:107-114, 1990.

16. Kreit LH, Burstone C, Delman L: Patient cooperation in orthodontic treatment, *J Am Coll Dent* 35:327-332, 1968.

17. Starnbach HK, Kaplan A: Profile of an excellent orthodontic patient, *Angle Orthod* 45:141-145, 1975.

18. Southard KA, Tolley EA, Arheart KL et al.: Application of the Millon Adolescent Personality Inventory in evaluating orthodontic compliance, *Am J Orthodont Dentofacial Orthop*, 100:553-561, 1991.

19. Herren P, Baumann-Rufer H, Demisch A et al.: The teacher's questionary-an instrument for the evaluation of psychological factors in orthodontic diagnosis, *Rep Congr Eur Orthod Soc* 41:247-266, 1965

20. Richter DD, Nanda RS, Sinha PK et al.: Effect of behavior modification on patient compliance in orthodontics, *Angle Orthodont* 68:123-132, 1998.

21. Burns KL, Green P, Chase HP: Psychosocial correlates of glycemic control as a function of age in youth with insulin-dependent diabetes, *J Adolesc Health Care* 7:311-319, 1986.

22. Jamison RN, Lewis S, Burish TG: Cooperation with treatment in adolescent cancer patients, *J Adolesc Health Care* 7:162-167, 1986.

23. Albino JE, Lawrence SD, Lopes CE et al.: Cooperation of adolescents in orthodontic treatment, *J Behav Med* 14:53-70, 1991.

24. Borkowska ED, Watts TL, Weinman J: The relationship of health beliefs and psychological mood to patient adherence to oral hygiene behaviour, *J Clin Periodontol* 25:187-193, 1998.

25. Bowen DM: Mechanical plaque control: toothbrushes and toothbrushing. In Darby ML, Walsh MM, editors: *Dental hygiene: theory and practice*, ed 2, St. Louis, 2003, Saunders.

26. Camner LG, Sandell R, Sarhed G: The role of patient involvement in oral hygiene compliance, *Br J Clin Psychol* 33:379-390, 1994.

27. El-Mangoury NH: Orthodontic cooperation, *Am J Orthod* 80:604-622, 1981.

28. Kuhner MK, Raetzke PB: The effect of health beliefs on the compliance of periodontal patients with oral hygiene instructions, *J Periodontol* 60:51-56, 1989.

29. Reisine S, Litt M: Social and psychological theories and their use for dental practice, *Int Dent J* 43(3 Suppl 1):279-287, 1993.

30. Sergl HG, Klages U, Pempera J: On the prediction of dentist-evaluated patient compliance in orthodontics, *Eur J Orthod* 14:463-468, 1992.

31. West KP, DuRant RH, Pendergrast R: An experimental test of adolescents' compliance with dental appointments, *J Adolesc Health* 14:384-389, 1993.

32. Bos A, Hoogstraten J, Prahl-Andersen B: On the use of personality characteristics in predicting compliance in orthodontic practice, *Am J Orthod Dentofacial Orthop* 123:568-570, 2003.

33. Ramsay DS, Soma M, Sarason IG: Enhancing patient adherence: the role of technology and its application to orthodontics. In JA McNamara Jr, CA Trotman, editors: *Creating the compliant patient*, vol 33, Craniofacial Growth Series, Center for Human Growth and Development, Ann Arbor, MI, 1997, University of Michigan.

34. Adams JR, Drake RE: Shared decision-making and evidence-based practice, *Commun Mental Health J* 42:87-105, 2006.

35. Nanda RS, Kierl MJ: Prediction of cooperation in orthodontic treatment, *Am J Orthod Dentofacial Orthop* 102:15-21, 1992.

36. Mehra T, Nanda RS, Sinha PK: Orhodontists' assessment and management of patient compliance, *Angle Orthod* 68:115-122, 1998.

37. Clark JR: Oral hygiene in the orthodontic practice: motivation, responsibilities, and concepts, *Am J Orthod* 69:72-82, 1976.

38. Klages U, Sergl HG, Burucker I: Relations between verbal behavior of the orthodontist and communicative cooperation of the patient in regular orthodontic visits, *Am J Orthod Dentofacial Orthop* 102:265-269, 1992.

39. Allan TK, Hodgson EW: The use of personality measurements as a determinant of patient cooperation in an orthodontic practice, *Am J Orthod* 54:433-440, 1968.

40. Bartsch A, Witt E, Sahm G et al.: Correlates of objective patient compliance with removable appliance wear, *Am J Orthod Dentofacial Orthop* 104:378-386, 1993.

41. Weiss J, Eiser HM: Psychological timing of orthodontic treatment, *Am J Orthod* 72:198-204, 1977.
42. Gershater MM: The physiological dimension in orthodontic diagnosis and treatment, *Am J Orthod* 54:327-338, 1968
43. Wilkins EM: *Clinical practice of the dental hygienist*, ed 9, Philadelphia, 1999, Lippincott, Williams & Wilkins.
44. Auerbach SM: Do patients want control over their own health care? A review of measures, findings, and research issues, *J Health Psychology* 6:191-203, 2001.
45. Sahm G, Bartsch A, Witt E: Micro-electronic monitoring of functional appliance wear, *Eur J Orthod* 12:297-301, 1990.
46. Kyriacou PA, Jones DP: Compliance monitor for use with removable orthodontic headgear appliances, *Med Biol Eng Comput* 35:57-60, 1997.
47. Cole WA: Accuracy of patient reporting as an indication of headgear compliance, *Am J Orthod Dentofacial Orthop* 121:419-423, 2002.
48. Tjin SC, Tan YK, Yow M et al.: Recording compliance of dental splint use in obstructive sleep apnea patients by force and temperature modeling, *Med Biol Eng Comput* 39:182-184, 2001.
49. George CF, Peveler RC, Heiliger S et al.: Compliance with tricyclic antidepressants: the value of four different methods of assessment, *Br J Clin Pharmacol* 50:166-171, 2000.
50. Lee JY, Kusek JW, Greene PG et al.: Assessing medication adherence by pill count and electronic monitoring in the African American Study of Kidney Disease and Hypertension (AASK) Pilot Study, *Am J Hypertens* 9:719-725, 1996.
51. Artinian NT, Harden JK, Kronenberg MW et al.: Pilot study of a Web-based compliance monitoring device for patients with congestive heart failure, *Heart Lung* 32:226-233, 2003.
52. Guendelman S, Meade K, Benson M et al.: Improving asthma outcomes and self-management behaviors of inner-city children: a randomized trial of the Health Buddy interactive device and an asthma diary, *Arch Pediatr Adolesc Med* 156:114-120, 2002.
53. Cherry JC, Moffatt TP, Rodriguez C et al.: Diabetes disease management program for an indigent population empowered by telemedicine technology, *Diabetes Technol Ther* 4:783-791, 2002.
54. LaFramboise LM, Todero CM, Zimmerman L et al.: Comparison of Health Buddy with traditional approaches to heart failure management, *Fam Commun Health* 26:275-288, 2003.
55. Safren SA, Hendriksen ES, Desousa N et al.: Use of an on-line pager system to increase adherence to antiretroviral medications, *AIDS Care* 15:787-793, 2003.
56. Willershausen B, Schlosser E, Ernst CP: The intra-oral camera, dental health communication and oral hygiene, *Int Dent J* 49:95-100, 1999.
57. Astroth DB, Cross-Poline GN, Stach DJ et al.: The transtheoretical model: an approach to behavioral change, *J Dent Hyg* 76:286-295, 2002.
58. Burke LE, Ockene IS, editors: *Compliance in healthcare and research*, Armonk, NY, 2001, Futura Publishing.
59. Chambers DW, Abrams RG: *Dental communication*, Norwalk, CT, 1986, Appleton-Century-Crofts.
60. Darby ML, editor: *Mosby's comprehensive review of dental hygiene*, ed 6, St. Louis, Mosby, 2006.
61. DiMatteo MR: Evidence-based strategies to foster adherence and improve patient outcomes, *JAAPA* 17:18-21, 2004.
62. Elder JP, Ayala GX, Harris S: Theories and intervention approaches to health-behavior change in primary care, *Am J Prev Med* 17:275-284, 1999.
63. Geboy MJ: *Communication and behavior management in dentistry*, Baltimore, MD, Williams and Wilkins, 1985.
64. Kay EJ, Millar K, Blinkhorn AS et al.: The prevention of dental disease: changing your patients' behaviour. *Dent Update* 18:245-248, 1991.
65. Miller WR, Rollnick S: *Motivational interviewing: preparing people for change*, ed 2, New York, 2002, The Guilford Press.
66. Ochene JK: Strategies to increase adherence to treatment. In Burke LE, Ockene IS, editors: *Compliance in healthcare and research*, Armonk, NY, 2001, Futura Publishing.
67. Tedesco LA, Keffer MA, Fleck-Kandath C: Self-efficacy, reasoned action, and oral health behavior reports: a social cognitive approach to compliance, *J Behav Med* 14:341-355, 1991.
68. Prochaska JO, Velicer WF, DiClemente CC et al.: Measuring processes of change: Applications to the cessation of smoking, *J Consult Clin Psychol* 56:520-528, 1988.
69. Prochaska JO: Staging: a revolution in helping people change, *Manag Care* 12:6-9, 2003.
70. Bridle C, Riemsma RP, Pattenden J et al.: Systematic review of the effectiveness of health benavior interventions based on the transtheoretical model, *Psychol and Health* 20:283-301, 2005.
71. Markland D, Ryan RM, Tobin VJ, Rollnick S: Motivational Interviewing and self-determination theory, *J Soc Clin Psychol* 24:811-831, 2005.
72. Weinstein P: *Motivate your dental patients: a workbook*, Seattle, WA, 2002, University of Washington.
73. Weinstein P, Harrison R, Benton T: Motivating parents to prevent caries in their young children: one-year findings, *JADA* 135:731-738, 2004.
74. Subramanian AK, McAfee AT, Getzinger JP: Use of the World Wide Web for multisite data collection, *Acad Emerg Med* 4:811-817, 1997.
75. Baer A, Saroiu S, Koutsky LA: Obtaining sensitive data through the Web: an example of design and methods, *Epidemiology* 13:640-645, 2002.

Chapter 12

The Fearful and Phobic Patient

JOHN P. HATCH AND ELAHEH MOHEBZAD

BACKGROUND

CLINICAL SIGNIFICANCE

STRATEGIES FOR APPLICATION IN PRACTICE

    Behavior Modification

    Medication

SUMMARY

LEARNING OBJECTIVES

Upon completion of this chapter, the learner will be able to:
- Explain the nature, clinical impact, and epidemiology of dental anxiety and its relationship to other anxiety disorders.
- Evaluate available instruments used in research and clinical settings to measure or assess dental anxiety.
- Examine the complexity of issues involved in the etiology of dental anxiety.
- Review and compare the pharmacological versus behavioral treatment of dental anxiety.
- Identify the issues in and limitations of dental anxiety research and the limitations of research findings for clinical practice.

KEY TERMS

Classical conditioning
Cognitive behavior therapy
Deep sedation
Diagnostic and Statistical Manual of Mental Disorders
Exposure therapy
Extinction
Flooding
Reinforcement
Relaxation therapy
Systematic desensitization

Anxiety has been described as a pervasive feeling of tension, dread, and apprehension associated with what may be an undefined threat.[1] The American Psychiatric Association, in its ***Diagnostic and Statistical Manual of Mental Disorders (DSM-IV)***, recognizes a broad class of anxiety disorders including panic attack, panic disorder, agoraphobia, specific phobia, social phobia, obsessive-compulsive disorder, posttraumatic stress disorder, acute stress disorder, and generalized anxiety disorder.[2] These conditions have not been widely studied in the dental context, but all of them can have important implications for dental treatment. Patients with any of these psychiatric disorders are likely to be uncomfortable in the dental treatment setting. Patients with social phobia fear embarrassment and being judged by others, and patients with agoraphobia fear situations from which they cannot easily escape. Anecdotal evidence suggests that dental treatment or an epinephrine injection can elicit panic attacks in susceptible individuals. Patients with posttraumatic stress disorder are particularly sensitive to environmental noises. Specific phobias to such things as blood, injections, or tissue damage probably are more widely recognized in the dental clinic. Other patients fear choking, gagging, vomiting, suffocating, contamination, or losing control. Because the dental literature does not address these specific anxiety disorders this discussion was limited to what is generally and generically referred to as dental anxiety. Anxiety can pose real problems for the dental professional without fulfilling specific diagnostic criteria for any psychiatric disorder. Although this review addresses primarily adult patients, children can exhibit strong dental anxiety, and much in the dental literature addresses their treatment.[3-5]

BACKGROUND

Terms encountered in the dental literature are "dental fear," "dental anxiety," "dental phobia," and, occasionally, "odontophobia," and "apprehensive patient." None of these terms has been adequately defined or clearly distinguished. Sometimes more specific terms are used, such as "dental injection phobic." Some authors link pain and anxiety, but for many patients, dental anxiety is not a fear of pain. The general term "dental anxiety" is used in this chapter to refer to all of the above except when another term is needed to make a specific distinction.

No conclusive evidence exists at this time about the prevalence of dental anxiety. Many epidemiological studies estimate the prevalence of this condition at approximately 10% of the population.[6-11] The rate varies depending on the definition used and the setting in which dental anxiety is assessed. A review of publications from 1950 to 2000 found no evidence that dental anxiety has increased or decreased appreciably.[12]

Gender differences in dental anxiety, although seemingly apparent in previous studies, have been contradicted by more recent research. Many studies show that females are more likely than males to report having dental anxiety.[6,7,9,13,14] However, one recent study indicates that men are more likely to report dental anxiety.[15] The possibility that women report dental anxiety more freely than men has been noted as a likely explanation for these differences. Therefore, no conclusive statement can be made about gender differences in dental anxiety.

Age differences in the prevalence of dental anxiety have been consistently reported. In general, dental anxiety decreases with increasing age. Age-dependent decline in prevalence is well established in the literature.[7,14,16] Dental professionals cannot assume that an older person will not have dental anxiety.

Psychological variables are also important in predicting the development of dental anxiety. Specifically, if an individual has one or more psychological disorders, such as generalized anxiety disorder, major depression, substance dependence, or specific phobia, the incidence of dental anxiety increases significantly.[16]

CLINICAL SIGNIFICANCE

Highly anxious patients exhibit greatly decreased dental clinic attendance and use of dental services. The 2000 Surgeon General's report on Oral Health in America estimates that 4.3% of the population refrains from getting dental care because of dental anxiety.[17]

Avoidance of dental care because of anxiety can perpetuate a vicious cycle. On average, fearful patients suffer pain for 17.3 days before consulting a dental professional.[18] This delay in treatment can eventually lead to additional dental complications that necessitate more extensive treatment and possibly emergency treatment. Some anxious individuals neglect their dental health to such an extent that they are in danger of losing some of their teeth.[19] High levels of anxiety, and hence avoidance of the dentist, are associated with an increased number of decayed teeth and fewer remaining teeth.[9,13] This pattern of delay in seeking care can exacerbate the anxiety. When treatment is avoided, more invasive treatments such as root canals and extractions are eventually required, which

are more traumatic and anxiety provoking than less invasive treatments.

Dental fear is cited as a reason for irregular attendance in approximately 15% of cases.[13,20] Because anxious dental patients are less likely to keep follow-up dental appointments for preventive care such as checkups and cleanings, they can compromise their future oral health status. The synergistic relationship between dental avoidance and continued pain and fear and a perception about the escalating expense associated with more invasive dental care leads to even greater irregular attendance. Preventive care is relatively inexpensive compared with more extensive dental procedures such as root canals, crowns, and restorations. There are added costs for the dentist as well.

Providing care to anxious patients can be stressful for the dental professional. Anxiety-related patient management issues require the dental staff to spend extra time and effort beyond what is expected with most patients. Anxious dental patients may break scheduled appointments and actually require more time for treatment than other patients.[15,21] Anxious patients also report more pain during dental treatment compared with nonanxious patients.[22] All of these factors place added demands on the dental professional.

Diagnosis of dental anxiety can be difficult because no standardized diagnostic criteria exist for this condition. The current lack of both a specific and widely accepted definition of dental anxiety and standardized diagnostic criteria frustrates both research and treatment. A systematic review of behavioral interventions for dental fear identified only three studies that included a formal diagnosis at entry.[23] Dental fear or phobia is often compared to the psychiatric diagnosis of specific phobia, which is defined as excessive, uncontrollable fear that exceeds the normal fear others may occasionally experience.[1] Box 12-1 lists the DSM-IV diagnostic criteria for specific phobia as an illustrative example of diagnostic criteria for one anxiety disorder.

Approximately 47% of patients seeking treatment for dental anxiety fulfill the DSM-IV criteria for specific phobia, 33% do not meet diagnostic criteria for any psychiatric disorder, and 19% meet criteria for multiple psychiatric disorders.[23] As many as 40% of dental anxiety patients meet criteria for one or more psychiatric diagnoses other than specific phobia.[24] Approximately 54% of patients with an intraoral injection phobia also have at least one other DSM-IV psychiatric disorder.[25] The most common psychiatric co-morbidities are other anxiety disorders and mood disorders. These studies demonstrate that dental anxiety patients represent a highly heterogeneous group.

Preliminary efforts have been made to develop a diagnostic classification system for subtypes of dental anxiety. Recognizing the diversity among patients, Weiner and Sheehan[26] proposed that dental anxiety should be classified as exogenous (situation-specific) versus endogenous

THE *DIAGNOSTIC AND STATISTICAL MANUAL IV* DIAGNOSTIC CRITERIA FOR SPECIFIC PHOBIA

CRITERIA
- Marked and persistent fear that is excessive or unreasonable, cued by the presence or anticipation of a specific object or situation.
- Exposure to the phobic stimulus almost invariably provokes an immediate anxiety response, which may take the form of a situationally bound or situationally predisposed panic attack.
- The person recognizes that the fear is excessive or unreasonable.
- The phobic situation(s) is avoided or else is endured with intense anxiety or distress.
- The avoidance, anxious anticipation, or distress in the feared situation(s) interferes significantly with the person's normal routine, occupational (or academic) functioning, or social activities or relationships, or there is marked distress about having the phobia.
- In individuals under age 18 years, the duration is at least 6 months.
- The anxiety, panic attacks, or phobic avoidance associated with the specific object or situation are not better accounted for by another mental disorder.

(Reprinted with permission from the *Diagnostic and Statistical Manual of Mental Disorders (DSM-IV)*, ed 4, Text Revision, Washington, DC, 2000, American Psychiatric Association.)

(spontaneous and generalized). The Seattle system, which identifies four types of dental anxiety, is described in Table 12-1.[27] No studies support the clinical value of these diagnostic schemes.

Despite difficulties with diagnosis, several instruments have been developed for scaling the severity of dental anxiety.[28,29] These assessment instruments are used in both the clinical and research settings to determine the scope and severity of the anxiety. Perhaps the simplest of these scales is the dental anxiety question, which consists of the single logical question "Are you afraid of going to the dentist?"[30] Gatchel's fear scale asks the patient to rate her/his fear on a 10-point scale where "1" indicates no

fear of dental treatment, "5" indicates moderate fear, and "10" indicates extreme fear.[31]

The most widely used scale is the Dental Anxiety Scale (DAS).[32] The Modified Dental Anxiety Scale (MDAS) was developed to address certain shortcomings of the DAS.[33] Both scales are shown in Table 12-2. The MDAS differs from the DAS, with one additional item measuring the patient's anxiety about receiving an injection of local anesthetic. It also standardizes the response categories across all items. Both the DAS and the MDAS cover a restricted range of content. Neither addresses potentially important issues such as guilt, embarrassment, fear of loss of control, feelings of helplessness, and feelings of inadequacy. These feelings can be as stressful for some patients as the more focused fears associated with dental treatment and pain. In general, available studies show the reliability, validity, sensitivity, and specificity of the DAS and MDAS to be acceptable. The positive predictive value of both instruments has been reported to be unacceptably low.[34] A rather sizable fraction of the patients (approximately 37% to 41%) who achieved high scores on the DAS or MDAS actually had visited their dentist regularly during the past 5 years, which suggests that many patients do overcome their fear and maintain regular attendance.

The Dental Fear Survey shown in Box 12-2 is an example of a scale that samples a broader range of content.[35] This scale asks patients to rate their anxiety concerning 27 dental situations. The items are grouped into three subscales covering patterns of dental avoidance and anticipatory anxiety, fear associated with specific dental stimuli and procedures, and perceived physiological arousal during dental treatment.

TABLE 12-1

THE SEATTLE CLASSIFICATION SYSTEM FOR SUBTYPING DENTAL ANXIETY

Type I	Conditioned fear of specific painful or unpleasant stimuli (drills, needles, sounds, smells)
Type II	Anxiety about some somatic reactions during treatment (allergic reactions, fainting, panic attacks)
Type III	Patients with other complicating trait anxiety or multiphobia
Type IV	Distrust of dental personnel

(Reprinted from Moore R, Brodsgaard I, Birn H: Manifestations, acquisition and diagnostic categories of dental fear in a self-referred population, *Behav Res Ther* 29:51, 1991.)

TABLE 12-2

DENTAL ANXIETY SCALE (DAS) AND MODIFIED DENTAL ANXIETY SCALE (MDAS)

DENTAL ANXIETY SCALE	MODIFIED DENTAL ANXIETY SCALE
1. If you had to go to the dentist tomorrow, how would you feel about it? a) I would look forward to it as a reasonably enjoyable experience. b) I wouldn't care one way or the other. c) I would be a little uneasy about it. d) I would be afraid that it would be unpleasant and painful. e) I would be very frightened of what the dentist might do.	1. If you went to your dentist for treatment tomorrow, how would you feel? a) Not anxious b) Slightly anxious c) Fairly anxious d) Very anxious e) Extremely anxious
2. When you are waiting in the dentist's office for your turn in the chair, how do you feel? a) Relaxed b) A little uneasy c) Tense d) Anxious e) So anxious that I sometimes break out in a sweat or almost feel physically sick.	2. If you were sitting in the waiting room (waiting for treatment), how would you feel? a – e same as for number 1
3. When you are in the dentist's chair waiting while he gets his drill ready to begin working on your teeth, how do you feel? a – e same as for number 2	3. If you were about to have a tooth drilled, how would you feel? a – e same as for number 1
4. You are in the dentist's chair to have your teeth cleaned. While you are waiting and the dentist is getting out the instruments which he will use to scrape your teeth around the gums, how do you feel? a – e same as for number 2	4. If you were about to have your teeth scaled and polished, how would you feel? a – e same as for number 1
	5. If you were about to have a local anesthetic injection in your gum, above an upper back tooth, how would you feel? a – e same as for number 1

(Dental Anxiety scale reprinted with permission from Corah NL: Development of a dental anxiety scale, *J Dent Res* 48:596, 1969; Modified Dental Anxiety Scale reprinted with permission from Humphries GM, Morison T, Lindsay SJE: The Modified Dental Anxiety Scale: Validation and United Kingdom norms, *Commun Dent Health* 12:143, 1995.)

The choice of an instrument to scale dental anxiety will depend on the particular need and setting. For screening unfamiliar patients in the clinic, the Dental Anxiety Question and Gatchel's fear scale are recommended. Follow-up questions designed to properly assess the nature and severity of any elicited report of anxiety is always necessary. Even if the level of anxiety is very low it could benefit the dental professional to be aware of it. The DAS offers the distinct advantage of being widely used, therefore comparative data are available from studies conducted in various patient populations and treatment settings. However, the MDAS is believed to be superior to the original DAS.

In the research setting the choice of an assessment instrument will depend on how dental anxiety is defined and operationalized. None of the available instruments (including those not reviewed here) possesses all the qualities needed, and more research is needed to support the existing ones. A scale to measure specific blood phobia in the dental setting will be different from one designed to measure the overall stress of a dental visit. A need exists for scales that can measure a broader array of stress eliciting factors, including financial concerns, embarrassment, guilt, fear of loss of control, and feelings of inadequacy. Research is needed to identify scales that assess dental anxiety within the context of the patient's

BOX 12-2

THE DENTAL FEAR SURVEY

AVOIDANCE OF DENTISTRY
(1 = never...5 = often)
1. Have avoided calling for an appointment
2. Have cancelled or not appeared

FELT PHYSIOLOGICAL RESPONSES
(1 = none...5 = great)
3. Muscles become tense
4. Breathing increases
5. Perspiration increases
6. Nausea
7. Heart rate increases
8. Mouth salivates

FEARFULNESS OF STIMULI
(1 = none...2 = great)
9. Making an appointment
10. Approaching office
11. Waiting room

12. Dental chair
13. Smell of office
14. Seeing dentist
15. Seeing needle
16. Feeling needle
17. Seeing drill
18. Hearing drill
19. Feeling drill
20. Feeling as if you will gag
21. Having teeth cleaned
22. Feeling pain even after anesthetic injection
23. Generally, how fearful are you of dentistry

HOW FEARFUL ARE/WERE YOUR
24. Mother
25. Father
26. Brothers and sisters
27. Childhood friends

(Reprinted from: Kleinknecht RA, Klepac RK, Alexander LD: Origins and characteristics of fear of dentistry, *JADA* 84:842-848, 1973, Table 3 with permission from the American Dental Association.)

general propensity to experience anxiety and also to assess the existence of possible independent anxiety disorders.

Direct **classical conditioning** is the theory most often advanced to explain the etiology of dental anxiety. Discovered near the end of the nineteenth century by Ivan Pavlov, classical conditioning is a type of learning in which two stimuli, one neutral and one fear-eliciting, are paired.[1] Another theory contends that anxiety is vicariously learned. According to this theory, anxiety is learned through witnessing an anxious response in someone else who serves as a model. For instance, a child might develop dental anxiety after witnessing a parent display anxiety associated with an upcoming dental appointment.

Studies using a cross-sectional, correlational design supported a possible link between experience with dental care and dental anxiety. The majority of anxious dental patients can recall a traumatic dental treatment experience, and studies using questionnaire or interview methods show an association between dental anxiety and self-reported history of painful or otherwise traumatic dental experiences.[36-39] Other studies show that the experience of a traumatic dental treatment event cannot fully explain the development of dental anxiety.[40,41] Evidence for the vicarious learning of anxiety also has been reported.[38,39] Cross-sectional studies cannot demonstrate that the onset or exacerbation of dental anxiety follows exposure to dental care. Only prospective, longitudinal studies, in which dental anxiety is measured at multiple points in time, can convincingly show that the onset of anxiety follows experience. Also, patients with dental anxiety might recall or report past experiences differently than

patients who are not anxious, and prospective designs minimize such reporting bias, which is inherent in retrospective studies.

One prospective study investigated the association between restorative dental treatment (measured by decayed, missing, and filled teeth) at ages 5 and 15 years, and dental anxiety at age 18 years.[42] Study participants who had at least one restoration (a potentially traumatic experience) before the age of 5 years were not more likely to have dental anxiety at age 18 years compared with those with no restorations. Dental patients who had one or more teeth restored at age 15 were nearly 5 times more likely to have dental anxiety at age 18 compared with those who had not had restorative dental treatment. This finding suggests that conditioning may not be the primary mechanism responsible for dental anxiety in young children, but it may play a more important role during adolescence. Another study demonstrated that although the incidence of dental anxiety increased by approximately 2.1% per year between the ages of 18 and 26 years, the incidence was greatest among patients who had not received any dental treatment during the previous 8 years.[43] Of the dental patients who were anxious at age 18 years, only 52.5% remained anxious at age 26 years, and of the patients who were not anxious at age 18 years, 16.6% became anxious by age 26 years. The authors concluded that conditioning cannot explain the onset of dental anxiety in the majority of young adults, and suggested that certain psychological traits or temperaments might indicate vulnerability to dental anxiety in young adults. Another study produced contrasting results when dental fear, which the authors distinguished from dental anxiety, was considered.[44] Patients with late onset dental fear (fear onset after age 18 years but before age 26 years) demonstrated the strongest association between potential aversive conditioning experiences such as caries and tooth loss, and dental fear. Contrary to findings for dental anxiety, the authors reported that personality traits were more strongly associated with early onset dental fear, yet the authors' distinction between dental anxiety and dental fear was not convincing.

Research into the etiology of dental anxiety is hindered by the lack of standard diagnostic criteria and by the lack of prospective study designs. At this time, conditioning and modeling remain viable theoretical models, but constitutional factors also seem to be implicated.

STRATEGIES FOR APPLICATION IN PRACTICE
Behavior Modification

Randomized controlled trials now support the effectiveness of various behavioral interventions for treating anxiety disorders.[45] Some trials are considered to have met criteria established to define empirically supported treatments for anxiety disorders, including **exposure therapy, relaxation,** and **cognitive behavior therapy.**[46-48] It is not surprising that therapies based on these methods also have been applied to the treatment of dental anxiety. Nearly all behaviorally based treatment programs described in the literature rely not on one specific technique, but rather on a combination of several behavioral techniques that are merged into a behavioral treatment package (Chapter 11). On an intuitive level, this should extend the applicability and amplify the effectiveness of treatment, but it also makes it difficult to assess the individual elements of the behavioral treatments that are commonly used to treat dental anxiety.

Exposure therapy includes various psychotherapeutic techniques designed to diminish conditioned fears by repeatedly exposing a patient, in the absence of an adverse experience, to a stimulus associated with stress.[1] Exposure therapy is theoretically based on the premise that fears are acquired through classical conditioning. In the case of dental anxiety, this premise is not universally supported by research. Classical conditioning is a form of learning in which a neutral stimulus (the dental professional or office) is paired with a stimulus that reflexively elicits anxiety (pain or social embarrassment). This pairing is known as "**reinforcement**." Classical conditioning theory further contends that the learned association between the neutral and fear-eliciting stimuli can be unlearned if the neutral stimulus is repeatedly presented without the fear-eliciting stimulus, a process known as "**extinction**." Exposure therapy seeks to break the learned association by exposing the individual to the neutral

stimulus while preventing the occurrence of the fear eliciting (reinforcing) stimulus. The objective of exposure therapy is to immerse the individual in an environment in which extinction can occur.

Exposure therapy dates back to the 1920s, but was popularized as **systematic desensitization** in the 1950s by Joseph Wolpe.[1] The first step in this behavioral therapy intervention is for the patient and therapist to collaboratively devise a graded hierarchy of fear-eliciting images. For the patient with dental anxiety, the items at the low end of the hierarchy might be thinking about calling to schedule a dental appointment, or imagining getting dressed for a dental appointment. Items at the high end of the hierarchy might be imagining receiving an injection or periodontal probing. Next, the patient is taught a series of muscle-tensing and relaxing exercises intended to generate a state of deep muscle relaxation. The final stage depends on the belief that anxiety and deep muscle relaxation are incompatible responses. It is assumed that if the patient can maintain deep muscle relaxation while imagining the scenes on the fear hierarchy, then extinction of the anxiety will occur. In this final stage, the patient is assisted to enter a state of deep muscle relaxation while the therapist verbally suggests an image from the low end of the fear hierarchy. If the patient begins to feel anxious he or she gives a signal, and the therapist withdraws the image and encourages relaxation. Once the patient remains deeply relaxed while imagining one item from the hierarchy, the therapist suggests the next higher item on the hierarchy. This process continues, perhaps during several sessions, until the patient can remain deeply relaxed while imagining the most fearful scenes within the fear hierarchy. A representative example of systematic desensitization in the treatment of dental anxiety is provided by Klepac.[49]

A variant of systematic desensitization is sometimes referred to as *in vivo* desensitization, or graded exposure therapy. In this approach, the patient is exposed to the actual events at a self-directed pace and in a nonthreatening way. First, the patient might be introduced to the dental chair and lights, encouraged to inspect or operate the chair and lights, and asked to sit in the chair until his or her anxiety passes. Next, the patient might be allowed to examine a mirror and explorer. Later, the patient might be given an injection syringe with only the cap attached, and allowed to closely examine the instrument. Finally, the dental professional might demonstrate how an injection would be given, using only the cap and applying gentle pressure to the gingiva. Depending on the patient's specific fears, graded exposure to a rubber dam or the sounds of a drill might be considered. Throughout the process every effort is made to encourage questions and to place the patient in a nonthreatening environment to facilitate extinction of the fear. An example of a detailed *in vivo* desensitization protocol can be found in Conyers et al.[50]

Flooding is another form of exposure therapy that involves exposure to a maximum-intensity, fear-producing situation for an extended time.[1] The patient is confronted with the feared object or situation either *in vivo* or through imagined scenes at full strength rather than in graded stages. The reasoning behind flooding therapy is that if the patient is allowed to escape the fearful situation, anxiety will subside and negatively reinforce the connection between the eliciting stimulus and the anxiety response. Flooding has not been widely used in treating dental fear, but it works well with other types of anxiety, including specific phobias.

Relaxation therapy focuses on promoting a deep muscle relaxation response, because it is seen as incompatible with anxiety. Many anxious patients experience increased tension when faced with dental treatment, and relaxation training equips them with a coping strategy that will help manage anxiety. Entry into a state of deep muscle relaxation is a learned skill, which later can be used to cope with any anxiety-provoking situation. Sometimes relaxation is taught using the same muscle tensing-relaxing exercises used in systematic desensitization; however, the emphasis more often is placed on mental relaxation through relaxing mental imagery. Sometimes biofeedback is added to provide patients with information about physiological changes that accompany their anxiety, and sometimes training in deep diaphragmatic breathing is added. Audiotapes containing either instructions for progressive deep muscle relaxation exercises or relaxing mental images can be provided for home practice sessions. Whatever the specific relaxation methods used, patients are encouraged to use learned relaxation skills to cope with stress or anxiety.

As opposed to the strict behavioral philosophy that only publicly observable behaviors can be measured, practitioners of cognitive behavioral therapy acknowledge that private thoughts and beliefs affect behavior. Cognitive behavior therapy is based on a set of principles and procedures that assume a synergistic interaction between cognitive mental processes and behavior without emphasizing causation.[1] Cognitive behavioral therapists use diverse psychotherapeutic techniques to alter the patient's thought process and belief system. Patients are taught to closely self-monitor their thoughts and actions, often with the aid of counters, checklists, or diaries. This will assist patients to become aware of maladaptive cognitions and actions and their context. Often patients are encouraged to self-monitor what are called self-statements—the statements people make to themselves that guide their behavior. For instance, patients may not be aware that they are engaging in irrational, catastrophic thinking. When anticipating a dental appointment, they may have the irrational idea that something catastrophic will happen, for instance, that the dental professional will slip with the drill or syringe. The therapist will explain that dental treatment is not normally or necessarily associated with anxiety, but that people can cause themselves

to become anxious by having negative and irrational beliefs about anticipated treatment. If this perception is directly confronted, patients may acknowledge that the idea is irrational, but still feel the need to use avoidance behavior. Such a patient might be instructed to self-monitor the irrational thoughts and be taught ways to reperceive their irrational self-statements or recast their destructive beliefs. They are taught to cognitively restructure the situation. The therapist typically challenges the evidence for the irrational beliefs, perhaps using information recorded by the patient during self-monitoring. Cognitive behavioral therapy often includes the use of multiple intervention techniques including self-distraction, thought stopping or substitution and the use of coping skills based on relaxation, meditation or imagery. An example of a brief cognitive behavioral protocol for treating dental anxiety is provided in De Jongh et al.[51]

Individual studies report that behavioral interventions are successful in more than 90% of dental anxiety patients and that the success rate typically ranges between 70% and 80%.[52] A recent systematic review with meta-analysis suggested that such estimates probably are inflated.[53] The reviewers identified a pool of 80 relevant studies but noted that few were of sufficient quality to be included in the meta-analysis. The studies were so heterogeneous that the authors were unable to pool them and fruitfully compare various treatment approaches. When self-reported change in dental anxiety was the measure of a treatment outcome, the majority of studies indicated that most patients who undergo behavioral treatment report a reduction in their anxiety. If the more objective criterion of actual dental treatment attendance was required as the definition of behavioral treatment success, however, the conclusions were less optimistic. A need remains for well-designed, randomized controlled trials of behavioral treatments for dental anxiety.

Patients with dental anxiety may not be willing to pay the cost of dental or behavioral treatment.[54] On entry into a 10-week dental anxiety treatment study, patients with dental anxiety were asked about their maximum willingness to pay for treatment. If a treatment package including combined dental and anxiety treatment with nitrous oxide sedation, cognitive behavioral therapy, or relaxation was offered, only 24% of patients said they would be willing to pay the actual cost of the treatment. When they were asked the same question at the completion of the study, 71% said they would be willing to pay for the treatment. This study suggests that the majority of patients who are in need of treatment for dental anxiety are not willing to pay for it.

Medication

The American Dental Association confirms the efficacy and safety of conscious sedation, deep sedation, and general anesthesia in dentistry and supports their use by dental practitioners properly trained in their administration.[55]

Pharmacological approaches to treating dental anxiety have long been a common practice. Evaluation of their efficacy and ease of applicability before adoption is important. Four basic approaches are used in dental practice: benzodiazepines, nitrous oxide conscious sedation, intravenous (IV) conscious sedation, and general anesthesia. Benzodiazepines and nitrous oxide are the more commonly used approaches for the general dental practitioner, whereas IV sedation and general anesthesia are reserved for practitioners with advanced degrees and oral and maxillofacial surgeons. Pain control needs to be distinguished from anxiety control when choosing medication. Although these techniques may have some varying degrees of analgesic effects, local/regional anesthesia is still used for pain control.

Benzodiazepines are commonly used because they are cost-effective and easy to use. Although multiple medications and routes of administration need to be considered, the most commonly used approach is oral sedation given as premedication to relieve anxiety during the period leading up to and during the dental appointment. Midazolam as a premedication has been compared with behavioral management techniques.[56,57] In this study, patients in the behavior modification group were given psychological treatment 1 week before the dental appointment. Use of audiocassettes at home, behavioral management techniques such as progressive muscle relaxation, and a 1.5-hour office intervention session teaching stress management training, relaxation training, and cognitive restructuring were included in the treatment protocol. Patients in the premedication group were given midazolam orally 30 minutes before their appointment. Although both groups experienced reduced levels of anxiety during their appointments when compared with the control group, on the day after the appointment, the midazolam group reported an increase in their fear, whereas the behavioral management group reported both short-term and more long-term reductions in anxiety. Moreover, when the patients were followed during a period of 1 year to evaluate adherence and dental attendance, it was found that only the psychologically treated group had maintained a reduced fear level and continued their dental treatment. This study suggests that although short-term results of the two techniques are equivalent, long-term results are more highly associated with a behavioral approach. A behavioral approach to managing dental anxiety addresses the problem as opposed to masking the problem by treating symptoms with medication. However, pharmaceutical approaches are invaluable and have tremendous applicability for patients in an emergency situation, for those who are mentally incapable of cooperating with the dentist, or when a behavioral approach can not be used.

One study, on the treatment of flight phobia, compared alprazolam with behavior therapy and found that the use of alprazolam was in fact counterproductive in the long term.[58] Although alprazolam acutely reduced self-reported anxiety and tension on the first flight, on a subsequent flight without the use of alprazolam, these individuals reported increased anxiety and tension compared with the placebo group. This inverse effect was obtained because the medication prevented benefits provided by the gradual exposure technique. Successful exposure therapy relies on experiencing anxiety, but with the alprazolam the patients did not experience the anxiety, and thus were unable to benefit from gradual exposure to the feared situation. Are dental professionals perpetuating the problem by not treating the anxiety with behavioral techniques before using pharmaceutical methods? Perhaps future research will investigate the long-term effects of using pharmaceutical therapy for the treatment of dental anxiety.

Nitrous oxide is an inhaled gas that can be used by trained and certified dental professionals as a method of conscious sedation. Conscious sedation is defined as a minimally depressed level of consciousness that retains the patient's ability to independently and continuously maintain an airway and respond appropriately to physical stimulation and verbal commands.[59] A study evaluating the mood-altering effects of nitrous oxide inhalation found that its use "reduced dysphoria in patients with high levels of preoperative dental anxiety and also elevates mood to the same degree as that in patients who are not anxious."[60] It was concluded that nitrous oxide use can be an effective therapy for reducing anxiety. Another study found that nitrous oxide when compared with IV sedation produces a greater degree of anxiety reduction during treatment.[61] Nitrous oxide, when administered properly, reduces anxiety but long-term effects on anxiety prevention are unknown.

A recent prospective study compared patient-controlled with clinician-controlled IV conscious sedation with propofol, specifically.[62] This technique involves the use of an infusion pump, controlled by the patient to deliver the needed dose (much like the patient-controlled morphine used in hospital settings). The study investigated whether anxiety levels can be effectively reduced depending on whether the patient or the clinician controlled the administration dosage of the medication being used. Overdosing is a major concern with giving the patient control over sedation levels. However, the results of the study concluded that patients controlling their own medication received significantly lower doses compared with patients who received clinician-controlled medication. When the patient could control their degree of sedation, the risk of excessive sedation was lower because the patient was unable to push the trigger for more medication. Although more patients preferred the patient-controlled sedation, the study failed to produce a difference in anxiety level reduction between the patient-controlled group and the clinician-controlled group. It was concluded that although the acute psychological response of dental fear can be countered using sedation, the underlying phobia does not disappear.[62]

Another study evaluating IV conscious sedation showed less anxiety reduction than behavior modification. Proportionally more patients treated with IV sedation remained dentally anxious than patients treated with a behavioral approach.[63] Future investigations should evaluate the interaction of combined psychological and pharmacological approaches to anxiety management.

The use of deep sedation and general anesthesia is limited to oral and maxillofacial surgeons and advanced degree holding practitioners because of the additional training that is required to achieve certification. The definition of **deep sedation** is an induced state of depressed consciousness accompanied by partial loss of protective reflexes, including the inability to continually maintain an airway independently, respond purposefully to verbal command, or both.[59] The definition of general anesthesia is an induced state of unconsciousness accompanied by partial or complete loss of protective reflexes, including inability to independently maintain an airway and respond purposefully to physical stimulation or verbal command.[59]

A comparison of treatment groups who received general anesthesia or behavioral therapy found that both groups had significantly reduced levels of anxiety.[64] The behavioral therapy group had significantly greater reductions of anxiety, which actually reached the level of dental patients with little to no anxiety. Moreover, the patients self-reported less tension and fewer cancellations and broken appointments when they were part of the behavioral modification group.

In summary, pharmacological therapies have been shown to be highly effective in reducing dental anxiety, especially during the short term. Their ease of use and practical application in clinical practice, have rendered them to be widely used by dental professionals. When compared with behavioral management therapy, however, pharmaceuticals tend to have fewer long-term benefits and are associated with greater relapse. Future research should evaluate the long-term advantages and disadvantages of these pharmacological treatment modalities to evaluate their applicability in effectively reducing dental anxiety.

SUMMARY

For various reasons it may be necessary to refer the highly anxious patient to another health care practitioner for treatment. A growing number of communities have dental anxiety specialty clinics, either within a dental school or as a private clinic. If this option is not available then referral to a psychologist familiar with treating anxiety disorders should be considered. Patients may be suffering from serious anxiety disorders that extend beyond the dental treatment setting and interferes with other aspects of life. Referral to a psychiatrist or psychologist for further evaluation is recommended. Finally, if the patient is receiving psychological treatment for an anxiety disorder, and an anxiety problem surfaces during dental treatment, ask permission to contact the therapist to discuss various treatment options. It is likely that the therapist will be able to make specific recommendations to the dental professional or address the patient's dental anxiety in their treatment domain.

It has been suggested that dental professionals may be somewhat reluctant to refer patients for behavioral therapy.[65] Referral letters of 115 patients who attended a dental hospital in Scotland because of high dental anxiety were reviewed. Of the referring dental professionals, 113 requested pharmacological anxiety management for their patients, and only two requested psychological techniques. Of the patients, 29% opted for psychological therapy when it was offered.

Although a substantial proportion of the population admits to being anxious about receiving dental treatment, only a small fraction of these have strong fears that lead to avoiding dental attendance. Researchers often focus on the highly anxious patient who refuses dental care, because clinic attendance can be used as an objective outcome criterion. Little attention has been given to questions about how to manage the majority of patients who routinely overcome their anxiety for the sake of maintaining their oral health. A need exists for high-quality studies to examine strategies for making dental treatment less traumatic for these patients. Although creating a relaxing atmosphere through verbal and nonverbal communication, giving the patient a sense of control over the situation, distraction techniques, avoidance of threatening language, and other approaches are often promoted, little evidence exists to guide their use. As shown in Figure 12-1, a review of both psychological and pharmacological approaches while tailoring choices for interventions to the needs of the patient and the skill level of the dental practitioner should follow assessment of anxiety levels. All successful dental treatment will depend on a cooperative relationship between the patient and the dental practitioner.

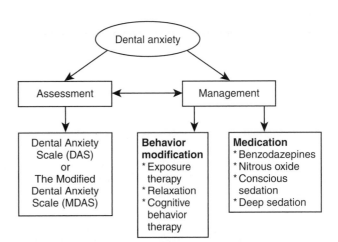

Figure 12-1 Assessment and management approaches for patients experiencing dental anxiety.

REFERENCES

1. Corsini R: *The dictionary of psychology*, New York, 2002, Brunner-Routledge.

2. American Psychiatric Association: *Diagnostic and statistical manual of mental disorders*, ed 4, Washington, DC, 1994, American Psychiatric Association.

3. Winer GA: A review and analysis of children's fearful behavior in dental settings, *Child Dev* 53:1111, 1982.

4. Matharu LM, Ashley PF: Sedation of anxious children undergoing dental treatment, *Cochrane Database of Systematic Reviews (2)*, CD003877, 2005.

5. Folayan Amo, Idehen EE, Ojo OO: The modulating effect of culture on the expression of dental anxiety in children: a literature review, *Int J Paed Dent* 14:241, 2004.

6. Doerr PA, Lang WP, Nyquist LV et al.: Factors associated with dental anxiety, *J Am Dent Assoc* 129:10, 1998.

7. Milgrom P, Fiset L, Melnick S et al.: The prevalence and practice management consequences of dental fear in a major US city, *J Am Dent Assoc* 116:6, 1988.

8. Poulton R, Thomson WM, Brown RH et al.: Dental fear with and without blood-injection fear: Implications for dental health and clinical practice, *Behav Res Ther* 36:6, 1998.

9. Schuller A, Willumsen T, Holst D: Are there differences in oral health and oral health behavior between individuals with high and low dental fear? *Commun Dent Oral Epidemiol* 31:2, 2003.

10. McGrath C, Bedi R: The association between dental anxiety and oral health-related quality of life in Britain, *Commun Dent Oral Epidemiol* 32:1, 2004.

11. Sohn W, Ismail A: Regular dental visits and dental anxiety in an adult dentate population, *J Am Dent Assoc* 136:1, 2005.

12. Smith T, Heaton L: Fear of dental care—are we making any progress? *J Am Dent Assoc* 134:8, 2003.

13. Hagglin C, Hakeberg M, Ahlqwist M et al.: Factors associated with dental anxiety and attendance in middle-aged and elderly women, *Commun Dent Oral Epidemiol* 28:6, 2000.

14. Milgrom P, Weinstein P, Getz T: *Treating fearful dental patients*, ed 2, Seattle, WA, 1995, Continuing Dental Education, University of Washington.

15. Rowe M, Moore T: Self-report measures of dental fear: gender differences, *Am J Health Behav* 22:4, 1998.

16. Locker D, Thomson WM, Poulton R: Psychological disorder, conditioning experiences, and the onset of dental anxiety in early adulthood, *J Dent Res* 80:6, 2001.

17. U.S. Department of Health and Human Services: *Oral Health in America: A Report of the Surgeon General*, Rockville, MD, 2000, U.S. Department of Health and Human Services, National Institute of Dental and Craniofacial Research, National Institutes of Health.

18. Ingersoll BD: *Behavioral aspects in dentistry*, New York, NY, 1982, Appleton-Century-Crofts Kent.

19. Kent GG, Blinkhorn AS: *The psychology of dental care*, ed 2, Oxford, 1991, Butterworth-Heineman.

20. Quteish T: Dental anxiety and regularity of dental attendance in younger adults, *J Oral Rehabil* 29:6, 2002.

21. King LJ: Treating the anxious patient, *Access* 5:8, 1991.

22. Maggirias J, Locker D: Psychological factors and perceptions of pain associated with dental treatment, *Commun Dent Oral Epidemiol* 30:2, 2002.

23. Kvale G, Raadal M, Vika M, et al.: Treatment of dental anxiety disorders. Outcome related to DSM-IV diagnoses, *Eur J Oral Sci* 110:69, 2002.

24. Roy-Byrne PP, Milgrom P, Tay K-M et al.: Psychopathology and psychiatric diagnosis in subjects with dental phobia, *J Anxiety Disord* 8:19, 1994.

25. Kaakko T, Coldwell SE, Getz T et al.: Psychiatric diagnoses among self-referred dental injection phobics, *J Anxiety Disord* 14:299, 2000.

26. Weiner AA, Sheehan DV: Etiology of dental anxiety: Psychological trauma or CNS chemical imbalance? *Gen Dent* 38:39, 1990.

27. Moore R, Brodsgaard I, Birn H: Manifestations, acquisition and diagnostic categories of dental fear in a self-referred population, *Behav Res Ther* 29:51, 1991.

28. Newton JT, Buck DJ: Anxiety and pain measures in dentistry: a guide to their quality and application, *JADA* 131:1449, 2000.

29. Schuurs A, Hoogstraten J: Appraisal of dental anxiety and fear questionnaires: a review, *Commun Dent Oral Epidemiol* 21:329, 1993.

30. Neverlien PO: Assessment of a single-item dental anxiety question, *Acta Odontol Scand* 48:365: 1990.

31. Gatchel RJ: The prevalence of dental fear and avoidance: expanded adult and recent adolescent surveys, *JADA* 118:591, 1989.

32. Corah NL, Gale EN, Illig SJ: Assessment of a dental anxiety scale, *JADA* 97:816, 1978.

33. Humphris GM, Morrison T, Lindsay SJE: The Modified Dental Anxiety Scale: validation and United Kingdom norms, *Commun Dent Health* 12:143, 1995.

34. Haugejorden O, Klock KS: Avoidance of dental visits: the predictive validity of three dental anxiety scales, *Acta Odontol Scand* 58:255, 2000.

35. Kleinknecht RA, Klepac RK, Alexander LD: Origins and characteristics of fear of dentistry, *JADA* 86:842, 1973.

36. De Jongh A, Muris P, Ter Horst G et al.: Acquisition and maintenance of dental anxiety: the role of conditioning experiences and cognitive factors, *Behav Res Ther* 33:2, 1995.

37. Davey GC: Dental phobias and anxiety: evidence for conditioning processes in the acquisition and modulation of a learned fear, *Behav Res Ther* 27:51, 1989.

38. Milgrom P, Mancl L, King B et al.: Origins of childhood dental fear, *Behav Res Ther* 33:313, 1995.

39. Rantavuori K, Zerman N, Ferro R et al.: Relationship between children's first dental visit and their dental anxiety in the Veneto region of Italy, *Acta Odontol Scand* 60:297, 2002.

40. Ten Berg M, Veerkamp JSJ, Hoogstraten J: The etiology of childhood dental fear: the role of dental and conditioning experiences, *J Anxiety Disord* 16:321, 2002.

41. De Jongh A, Aartman IHA, Brand N: Trauma-related phenomena in anxious dental patients, *Commun Dent Oral Epidemiol* 31:52, 2003.

42. Poulton R, Thomson WM, Davies S et al.: Good teeth, bad teeth and fear of the dentist, *Behav Res Ther* 35:327, 1997.

43. Thompson WM, Locker D, Poulton R: Incidence of dental anxiety in young adults in relation to treatment experience, *Commun Dent Oral Epidemiol* 28:289, 2000.

44. Poulton R, Waldie KE, Thomson WM et al.: Determinants of early- vs late-onset dental fear in a longitudinal-epidemiological study, *Behav Res Ther* 39:777, 2001.

45. Lambert MJ, Ogles BM: The efficacy and effectiveness of psychotherapy. In Lambert MJ, editor: *Bergin and Garfield's handbook of psychotherapy and behavior change*, ed 5, New York, 2004, John Wiley & Sons, pp. 139-193.

46. Chambless DL Hollon SD: Defining empirically supported therapies, *J Consult Clin Psychol* 66:7, 1998.

47. DeRubeis RJ, Crits-Christoph P: Empirically supported individual and group psychological treatments for adult mental disorders, *J Consult Clin Psychol* 66:37, 1998.

48. Chambless DL, Sanderson WC, Shoham V et al.: An update on empirically validated therapies, Task force on promotion and dissemination of psychological procedures, Washington, DC, Division 12, American Psychological Association, no date.

49. Klepac RK: Successful treatment of avoidance of dentistry by desensitization or by increasing pain tolerance, *J Behav Ther Exper Psychiatr* 6:307, 1975.

50. Conyers C, Miltenberger RG, Peterson B, et al.: An evaluation of in vivo desensitization and video modeling to increase compliance with dental procedures in persons with mental retardation, *J Appl Behav Analys* 37:233, 2004.

51. De Jongh A, Muris G, ter Horst G et al.: One-session cognitive treatment of dental phobia: preparing dental phobics for treatment by restructuring negative cognitions, *Behav Res Ther* 33:947, 1995.

52. Berggren U: Long-term management of the fearful adult patient using behavior modification and other modalities, *J Dent Educ* 65:1357, 2001.

53. Kvale G, Berggren U, Milgrom P: Dental fear in adults: a meta-analysis of behavioral interventions, *Commun Dent Oral Epidemiol* 32:250, 2004.

54. Halvorsen B, Willumsen T: Willingness to pay for dental fear treatment, *Eur J Health Econ* 49:229, 2004.

55. American Dental Association, Council on Dental Education: American Dental Association policy statement: the use of conscious sedation, deep sedation and general anesthesia in dentistry, Chicago, IL, 1999, ADA.

56. Thom A, Sartory G, Johren P: Comparison between one-session psychological treatment and benzodiazepine in dental phobia, *J Consult Clin Psychol* 68:378, 2000.

57. Johren P, Jackowski J, Ganggler P, et al.: Fear reduction in patients with dental treatment phobia, *Br J Oral Maxillofac Surg* 38:612, 2000.

58. Wilhelm FH, Roth WT: Acute and delayed effects of alprazolam on flight phobics during exposure, *Behav Res Ther* 35:831, 1997.

59. American Dental Association, Council on Dental Education: American Dental Association guidelines for the use of conscious sedation, deep sedation and general anesthesia for dentists. Chicago, IL, 2005, ADA.

60. Zacny JP, Hurst RJ, Graham L et al.: Preoperative dental anxiety and mood changes during nitrous oxide inhalation, *JADA* 133:82, 2002.

61. Goodall EM, File SE, Sanders FL et al.: Self-ratings by phobic denial patients during dental treatment: greater improvement with nitrous oxide than midazolam, *Hum Psychopharmacol* 9:203, 1994

62. Girdler NM, Rynn D, Lyne JP et al.: A prospective randomized controlled study of patient-controlled propofol sedation in phobic dental patients, *Anaesthesia* 55:327, 2000.

63. Aartman IHA, de Jongh A, Makkes PC et al.: Dental anxiety reduction and dental attendance after treatment in a dental fear clinic: a follow-up study, *Commun Dent Oral Epidemiol* 28:435, 2000.

64. Berggren U, Linde A: Dental fear and avoidance: a comparison of two modes of treatment, *J Dent Res* 63:1223, 1984.

65. McGoldrick P, Levitt J, de Jongh et al.: Referrals to a secondary care dental clinic for anxious adult patients: implications for treatment, *Br Dent J* 191:686, 2001.

Chapter 13

Culturally Effective Oral Health Care

MAGDA A. DE LA TORRE AND JANE E. M. STEFFENSEN

LEARNING OBJECTIVES

Upon completion of this chapter, the learner will be able to:

- Discuss the provision of culturally effective oral health care for patients with a wide variety of cultural attributes.
- Identify changing demographics and diversity among population groups in the United States.
- Describe conceptual models for cultural competence and transcultural health care practice.
- Discuss the cultural and social dimensions that underlie the values, beliefs, and behaviors of patients and providers.
- Explain the importance of self-awareness and self-assessment by dental professionals related to the cultural and social dimensions of their values, attitudes, skills, and behaviors that influence patient care.
- Describe strategies to understand social and cultural background of patients, their families, and the environment in which they live.
- Discuss the use of folk remedies, complementary and alternative healing practices, and health practices of traditional healers.
- Explain different concepts and explanations for health and disease.
- Describe strategies to improve patient care and enable oral health care providers to interact with patients from diverse cultural and social backgrounds.

- Identify practices to overcome communication barriers, facilitate patient-provider interactions, and enhance oral health care for socially and culturally diverse patients.
- Discuss the application of culturally competent techniques to interview and elicit a patient's values, beliefs, and behaviors during a dental visit.
- Describe legal mandates and professional standards associated with the provision of culturally effective oral health care for patients with a wide variety of cultural attributes.

KEY TERMS

Cultural competence
Culturally and Linguistically Appropriate Services (CLAS)
Health disparity
Self-assessment

IMPORTANCE OF SOCIAL AND CULTURAL DIMENSIONS IN HEALTH

A common goal for health care professionals is to provide the best care to all patients.[1-3] For this to occur, health professionals must recognize diverse cultural factors and social norms.[4,5] An ethical oral health professional values respect and is expected to care for patients accordingly; he or she has a responsibility to serve all patients without discrimination and avoid action toward any individual or group that may be interpreted as discrimination.[6]

To provide the best care, the provider should acknowledge the values, attitudes, and beliefs that patients bring to each clinical encounter. Oral health care professionals will then understand the roles that are desired by patients and provide respectful and compassionate care to patients from diverse backgrounds. Effective communication between the oral health care professional and the patient should be practiced for culturally effective oral health services.

Culturally effective health care has emerged as an important issue for three important reasons. First, the United States is becoming more diverse and providers will increasingly care for patients with a broad range of perspectives regarding health. These perspectives are often influenced by their social or cultural backgrounds. Patients may have limited English proficiency, different thresholds for seeking care or expectations about their care, and unique beliefs that influence whether or not they follow recommendations.[7] Second, research demonstrates that provider-patient communication is linked to patient satisfaction, adherence to instructions, and health outcomes.[8] Consequently, poorer health outcomes result when social and cultural factors are not considered during the clinical encounter.[9] These barriers do not only apply to minority groups but may be more pronounced when the cultural framework differs between

provider and patient. Finally, two landmark Institute of Medicine reports—*Crossing the Quality Chasm* and *Unequal Treatment*—highlight the importance of patient-centered care and cultural competence in improving quality and eliminating racial and ethnic disparities in health care.[10,11]

Patient-centeredness and cultural competence have been promoted as approaches to improving health care for individual patients, communities, and populations. This chapter discusses elements from both concepts by considering how health care providers and patients interact at the interpersonal level and how patients are cared for by the health care system as a whole.

PATIENT-CENTERED CLINICAL METHOD

Patient-centeredness originated as a way of characterizing how health care providers should interact and communicate with patients on a more personal level. The concept of patient-centered care is derived from client-centered theory which encourages practitioners to adopt a biopsychosocial model of practice. Initiatives to promote patient-centered care include efforts to improve relationships between patients and providers, as well as efforts to make systems more responsive to patients' needs and preferences.

The Patient Centered Clinical Method developed through research conducted by Stewart and colleagues is described in Figure 13-1 and includes six core features: [12]

- Exploring Both Disease and Illness Experience
  - History, physical examination, and laboratory findings
  - Dimensions of illness (e.g., feelings, ideas, effects on function and expectations)
- Understanding the Whole Person
  - The person (e.g., life history, personal, and developmental issues)
  - The proximal context (e.g., family, social support, employment)
  - The distal context (e.g., culture, community, ecosystem)
- Finding Common Ground
  - Problems and priorities
  - Goals of treatment and or management
  - Roles of patient and health professional
- Incorporating Prevention and Health Promotion
  - Health enhancement
  - Risk avoidance
  - Risk reduction
  - Early identification
  - Complication reduction
- Enhancing the Patient and Health Professional Relationship
  - Compassion
  - Power
  - Healing
  - Self-Awareness

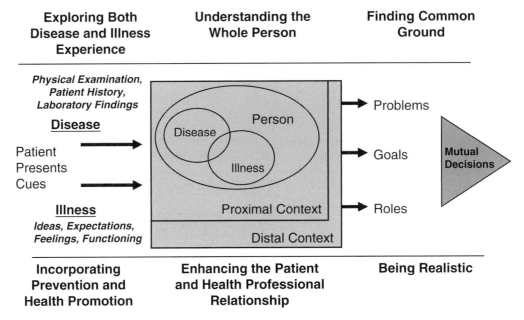

Exploring Both
Disease and Illness
Experience

Understanding the
Whole Person

Finding Common
Ground

Physical Examination,
Patient History,
Laboratory Findings

Disease

Patient
Presents
Cues

Illness

Ideas, Expectations,
Feelings, Functioning

Person

Disease

Illness

Problems

Goals

Roles

Mutual
Decisions

Proximal Context

Distal Context

Incorporating
Prevention and
Health Promotion

Enhancing the Patient
and Health Professional
Relationship

Being Realistic

Figure 13-1 The patient-centered clinical method. (Adapted from Stewart M, Brown JB, Weston WW, et al.: *Transforming the clinical method: patient-centered medicine*, Abingdon, UK, 2003, Radcliffe Medical Press.)

- Being Realistic
  - Time and timing
  - Teambuilding and teamwork
  - Wise stewardship of resources

THE FRAMEWORK FOR ORAL HEALTH ACTION

Several theories and models were developed to examine health and behavior at the individual, group, organization, community, and societal levels.[12] In addition, planning frameworks have been used to design health promotion and communication efforts at multiple levels.[12,13] These constructs can guide oral disease prevention and oral health promotion initiatives by suggesting factors to consider in formulating approaches and determining whether specific ideas are likely to work. The provision of effective oral health care should draw on models and frameworks that offer different perspectives. No single theory dominates oral health education and communication because oral health problems, populations, cultures, and contexts vary. Many oral health programs achieve the greatest impact by combining elements from different models.

Studies indicate that cultural and social factors influence values, attitudes, and beliefs and contribute to oral health behaviors, practices, and outcomes.[14,15] Therefore, the Framework for Oral Health Action (Figure 13-2) was developed to conceptualize key elements that interact and influence oral health. By better understanding the factors that shape beliefs and values, the clinician can be more

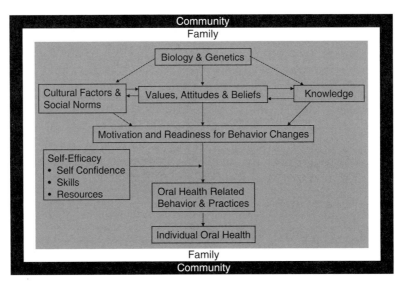

Figure 13-2 Framework for oral health action.

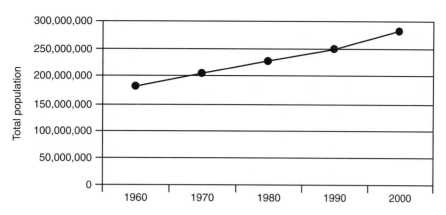

Figure 13-3 Population growth, United States, 1960-2000. (Data from www.CensusScope.org, Social Science Data Analysis Network, University of Michigan, www.ssdan.net.)

responsive to the needs of their patients and provide more effective oral health care.

POPULATION DYNAMICS

Population dynamics and demographic characteristics are changing across the globe and in the United States. This dynamic is the result of many factors, including economic, political, social, demographic, and technological changes. Communication changes, globalization, commercialization, and computerization have made the world smaller, allowed members of different cultures to interact on a more frequent basis, and provided a venue to better understand similarities and differences among cultures.

America's increasingly multicultural population creates both tremendous challenges and rich opportunities. The population of the United States as a whole has continued to expand. Altogether, 36% of the 3066 counties in the United

States reported growth that exceeded the national growth rate of approximately 13% between 1990 and 2000 (Figure 13-3).[16] Cultural attributes change between generations as values, behaviors, and customs are transformed over time. These cultural characteristics are influenced by many factors including national origin, language, race, ethnicity, religious beliefs, family relationships, gender, age, education, employment, sexual orientation, social and economic status, disabilities, and other distinct attributes of population groups.[17]

Age distribution is an important factor influencing population growth. The proportion of older persons relative to the general population is expected to increase in the coming decades.[18] This increase is the result of declining birth rates and advances in life expectancy in the second half of the twentieth century and early twenty-first century (Figure 13-4). When drawn as a "population pyramid," age distribution shows projected patterns of population growth in coming decades.

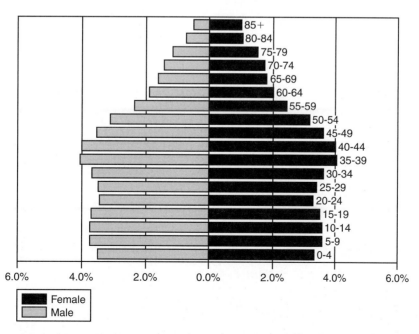

Figure 13-4 Age distribution by gender, United States, 2000. (Data from www.CensusScope.org, Social Science Data Analysis Network, University of Michigan, www.ssdan.net.)

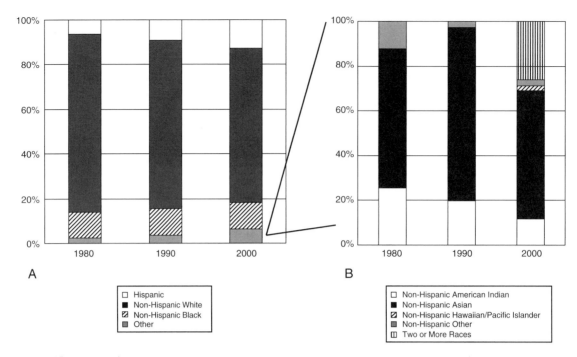

A

B

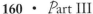

Figure 13-5   **A,** Population growth by race and ethnicity, United States, 1980-2000. **B,** Population change in racial/ethnic groups that make up less than 10% of the total population, United States 1980-2000. (Data from www.CensusScope.org, Social Science Data Analysis Network, University of Michigan, www.ssdan.net.)

An increasing number of individuals living with disabilities created a significant demographic shift in the United States. The U.S. Census in 2000 indicated that approximately 19% of the American population reported a disability of some nature.[19] This increase is partially attributed to health care advances that allow people born with disabilities to live longer lives and that allow individuals with injuries and acquired conditions to extend their life expectancy.[20] The 2000 U.S. Census reported that nearly 42% of all senior citizens (those age 65 years and older) have some form of disability, with approximately 28% having a physical disability.[18] An increased incidence of disability exists among aging cohorts.[21] According to the Centers for Disease Control and Prevention, approximately 80% of persons older than 65 years have at least one chronic condition and half have more than one such condition.[21]

The 2000 U.S. Census further confirmed that the nation's population has become more diverse and this trend is expected to continue over the next century (Figure 13-5).[22] Unique to the 2000 Census, respondents were permitted to use multiple selections to describe their racial background. Nationwide, approximately 2.4% of the population, more than 6.8 million Americans, identified with two or more races.[23] As with many racial and ethnic groups, the multiracial population is not distributed evenly across the country.

Nativity, citizenship, and migration are important factors influencing population dynamics.[16] The U.S. Census includes all residents of the United States, regardless of their citizenship status. In some areas of the country,

population dynamics are influenced by families moving between states or migrating from other countries outside the United States (Figure 13-6). Other communities have remained fairly stable and the population has not changed considerably in the past decade.[24]

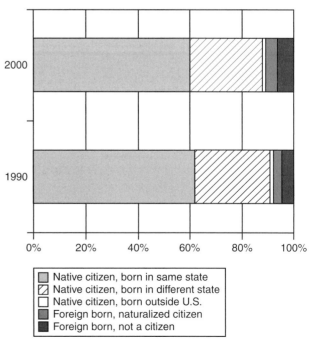

Figure 13-6   Nativity and citizenship, United States, 1990-2000. (Data from www.CensusScope.org, Social Science Data Analysis Network, University of Michigan, www.ssdan.net.)

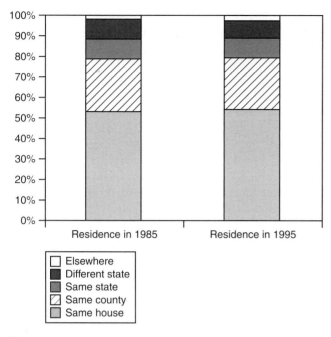

Figure 13-7   Migration: residence 5 years prior to census, United States, 1985-1995. (Data from www.CensusScope.org, Social Science Data Analysis Network, University of Michigan, www.ssdan.net.)

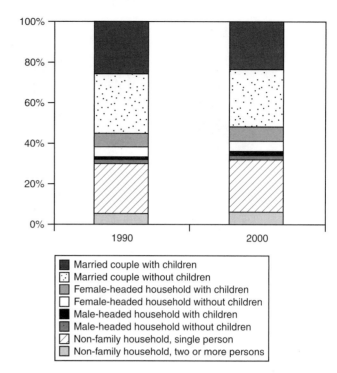

Figure 13-8   Household and family structure, United States, 1990-2000. (Data from www.CensusScope.org, Social Science Data Analysis Network, University of Michigan, www.ssdan.net.)

One important aspect of the American lifestyle is geographic mobility. For the U.S. Census, respondents identified if they lived in the same residence in the year(s) prior to completing the survey. Between 2002 and 2003, 14% of households reported moving from their previous primary residence.[24] From 1995 and 2000, only 54% of Americans remained in the same house and these rates varied among regions of the country as well as urban or rural areas (Figure 13-7).[16]

Changes in household and family structure have occurred in the last decade according to the U.S. Census (Figure 13-8).[25] A household is defined as one or more people living in a residence. A family is more than one person living together, either married or of the same bloodline. Not only has the family structure changed, but the makeup of the American workforce has evolved during the past 50 years as more women have sought paid work outside the home. Also, the type of work has changed with growth in the service sector while employment in manufacturing has declined in the United States.[26]

Oral health status is influenced by family income. The median household income in 2005 was $44,326.[27] In 2004, the poverty threshold for a family of four in the continental United States with two adults and two related children was $19,157.[28] However, poverty thresholds are misleading because they do not provide an accurate picture of life in poverty. Moreover, most families of four would have to make twice the assigned poverty threshold in order to provide their children with basic necessities, such as housing, food, and health care.[29,30] In 2005, nearly 13% of people lived in poverty in the United States.

Of related children under 18 years of age, 18% lived in families with incomes below the poverty level, compared with 10% of people 65 years and older. Approximately 10% of all families and 29% of families with a female householder had incomes below the poverty level.[27]

Language has been described as "a major tenet of anthropology" and considered the most important aspect of culture because it is the primary way that culture is transmitted.[31] Language, as a fundamental form of communication, is critical to successful health outcomes and is the cornerstone of the provider-patient relationship. The U.S. Census asks questions about language use at home to identify groups of people who speak a language other than English. The 2000 U.S. Census reported the following findings:

- 47 million people (18% of the population) in the United States aged 5 years and older spoke a language other than English at home.
- In 10 states, more than 25% of the population spoke a language other than English at home.
- 380 languages were spoken in the United States.[32]

Educational attainment and literacy levels have a profound impact on oral health outcomes. In 2005, 84% of Americans were high school graduates and 27% had bachelor's degrees or higher.[33] However, the elderly population has aged at a time when educational attainment was typically lower, and college attendance was less widespread.[18] As this population is succeeded by younger and

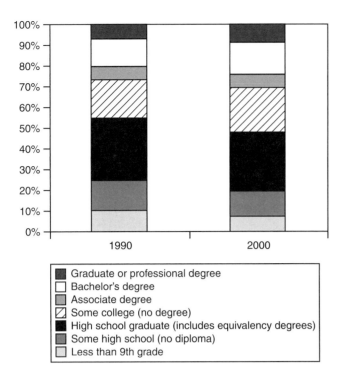

Figure 13-9   Educational attainment, United States, 1990-2000. (Data from www.CensusScope.org, Social Science Data Analysis Network, University of Michigan, www.ssdan.net.)

increasingly well-educated cohorts, the percent of the population that has attained higher levels of education will increase slowly (Figure 13-9).

The National Center for Education Statistics (NCES), 2003 National Assessment of Adult Literacy (NAAL) *A First Look at the Literacy of America's Adults in the 21(st) Century* measured the English literacy of America's adults of age 16 years or older using three

literacy scales as outlined in Table 13-1.[34] The assessment defines literacy as using printed and written information to function in society, to achieve one's goals, and to develop one's knowledge and potential.[34] The 2003 National Assessment found that 14% of the U.S. population, approximately 30 million Americans, were considered below basic literacy level and were able to perform only simple and concrete literacy tasks.[34] In addition, 63 million Americans (29%) were considered at the basic literacy level, able to perform simple and everyday literacy activities. According to the National Assessment, 57% of the U.S. population (163 million Americans) performed more challenging literacy activities.[34]

Health literacy is defined as the degree to which patients can obtain, process, and understand fundamental information and services needed to make proper decisions concerning their health.[3] Health literacy encompasses more than overall literacy. It is a measure of written, listening, speaking, arithmetic, and conceptual knowledge. Health literacy is not a new problem but research in this area demonstrated a correlation between low health literacy and the increasing complexity of the nation's health care system.[35] Health literacy is important because it impacts an individual's ability to review a prevention pamphlet, understand health insurance forms, purchase over-the-counter medications, read a label on a medicine bottle, and navigate the health care system. Box 13-1 summarizes key points about the influence of literacy on health.

An Institute of Medicine report *Health Literacy: A Prescription to End Confusion* released in April 2004 states that 90 million people in the United States have

TABLE 13-1

THREE LITERACY SCALES

Prose literacy	The knowledge and skills to search, comprehend, and use information from continuous text.
Document literacy	The knowledge and skills to search, comprehend, and use information from noncontinuous text.
Quantitative literacy	The knowledge and skills required to identify and perform computations, either alone or sequentially, using numbers embedded in printed material.

(From Kutner M, Greenberg E, Baer J: *A first look at the literacy of America's adults in the 21st century*, Washington, DC, U.S. Department of Education, National Center of Education Statistics, 2005.)

BOX 13-1

*L*ITERACY AND *H*EALTH

INDIVIDUALS WITH LIMITED LITERACY SKILLS
- Report poor overall health.
- Present in the later stages of disease.
- Are more likely to be hospitalized.
- Have a poor understanding of health care.
- Have lower adherence to health care recommendations.
- Are less likely to seek important preventive measures and screenings.
- Enter the health care system when they are sicker.
- Are more likely to have chronic conditions.

(Sources: Rudd RE: *Literacy and implications for navigating health care*, Boston, 2002, Harvard School of Public Health, Health Literacy (website). http://www.hsph.harvardstudies.edu/healthliteracy/index.html. Accessed October 5, 2006. U.S. Department of Health and Human Services, Office of Disease Prevention and Health Promotion: *Quick guide to health literacy*, Washington, DC, 2006, U.S. Department of Health and Human Services).

limited health literacy, and that nearly half of all American adults have difficulty understanding and using health information.[36] The report notes that there is a higher rate of hospitalization and use of emergency services among patients with limited health literacy. Low health literacy can affect patients' ability to read and understand instructions, health education materials, and consent forms.[36]

The 2003 National Assessment of Adult Literacy included an assessment to measure the health literacy of America's adults. The performance levels were categorized as below basic, basic, intermediate, or proficient. Findings from the National Assessment were reported in the 2006 publication, *The Health Literacy of America's Adults*.[37] The National Assessment found:

- The majority of adults (53%) had intermediate health literacy.
- Females had higher average health literacy than males; 16% of males were assessed at the below basic level compared with 12% of females.
- Adults who were age 65 years and older had lower average health literacy than adults in younger age groups. The percentage of adults in the 65 years and older age group who had intermediate and proficient health literacy levels was lower than the comparable percentage of adults in other age groups.
- Starting with adults who had graduated from high school or obtained a general equivalency diploma, average health literacy increased with each higher level of education attainment. Of adults who had never attended or did not complete high school, 49% had below basic health literacy, compared with 15% of adults who ended their education with a high school diploma, and 3% of adults with a bachelor's degree.
- Adults living below the poverty level had lower average health literacy than adults living above the poverty threshold.[37]

These alarming findings emphasize the importance for oral health professionals to become aware of the impact that literacy has on oral health outcomes and to be responsive to the literacy needs of their patients. Dental professionals need to apply effective strategies in their daily practice to assure that patients understand verbal and written communications during dental visits.[38]

DISPARITIES IN HEALTH AND ORAL HEALTH

Ethnic, racial, and low-income groups are the most frequently and directly impacted by **health disparities**. Health indicators are differentiated along other factors including gender, geographic location, sexual orientation, disability, age, English proficiency, and literacy.[3,39] The impact of these disparities is evidenced in higher mortality and morbidity rates, decreased quality of life and productivity, and overall increased health care costs.[3]

There is a risk that health disparities may increase as the population ages and becomes more diverse.[39] Not only does this affect the oral health status of culturally and linguistically diverse populations, it could also adversely affect the health of the nation as a whole. The Institute of Medicine stated that all members of a community are affected by the poor health status of its least healthy members.[11] Reduction of health disparities is one of the top priorities for the U.S. Department of Health and Human Services, as noted in *Healthy People 2010*. The second national goal is to eliminate health disparities among segments of the population.[3]

Profound and consequential oral health disparities exist within the American population.[14,40] These occur among various demographic groups in the United States and are related to age, gender, race, ethnicity, education, income, disability, and geographic location.[3,14] Dramatic disparities in oral health status among numerous cultural and ethnic groups have been described in national reports showing that some members of these groups suffer disproportionately from oral diseases and conditions such as dental caries, periodontal diseases, oral and craniofacial injuries, and oral and pharyngeal cancers.[14,41-45] Chapters 1-3 provide in-depth descriptions of disparities in oral health status among various population groups.

ACCESS TO ORAL HEALTH CARE

Although major oral health improvements have occurred during the past 50 years, many Americans lack access to oral health information and services.[41,43,44] Studies suggest that individuals from specific cultural backgrounds face greater barriers and lack access to community preventive services (e.g., community water fluoridation, school-based dental sealants, and tobacco cessation interventions) as well as clinical preventive and therapeutic services.[3,14,41-47] Regular dental visits provide opportunities for prevention, early detection, and treatment of dental problems among children and adults.

Access to the oral health system consists of many facets, including availability, accessibility, accommodation, affordability, and acceptability.[48] Measures used in surveys to assess various factors influencing access to the oral health care system include the following:

- Annual dental visit.
- Dental attendance for routine check-ups or cleanings.
- Assessment of dental insurance coverage.
- Usual source of dental care.
- Reason for not having a dental visit in the past year.
- Difficulty in obtaining needed dental care.
- Purpose of last dental visit.[49]

National surveys have reported that many vulnerable population groups face barriers accessing dental care.[3,14,41-44] Groups with limited access include low-income individuals, immigrants, homeless persons, migrant and seasonal farm workers, disabled and medically compromised individuals,

TABLE 13-2

BARRIERS TO ORAL HEALTH SERVICES

AVAILABILITY OF SERVICES	Access is limited when providers and services do not exist within a community (e.g., rural regions of the United States and poorer neighborhoods within urban areas).
GEOGRAPHIC LOCATION	Access is limited if services are located too far from patients or in places that are not easily accessible (e.g., individuals residing in rural areas and in inner cities where transportation may be limited or lacking).
TIMES AND LOGISTICS OF SERVICES	Access is limited when services are offered during the normal business day and times when patients have work, family, or other commitments.
CULTURAL COMPETENCE	Access is limited when services are provided in settings that are not welcoming and acceptable in terms of cultural diversity.
LINGUISTIC COMPETENCE	Access is limited if patients cannot communicate in the language in which they are proficient
INSURANCE	Individuals often lack adequate health insurance and/or dental insurance (e.g., for individuals enrolled in Medicaid, there are a limited number of dentists willing to accept Medicaid).

[From National Center for Cultural Competency (NCCC): *Racial and ethnic disparities in oral health, topic 3, racial and ethnic disparities,* Washington, DC, 2006, Georgetown University Center for Child and Human Development, National Center for Cultural Competency.]

rural residents, elderly and very young children.[43,44] In addition, individuals from racially and ethnically diverse populations often confront obstacles that prevent them from accessing oral health care.[3,14,41-44] Multiple factors have been analyzed to evaluate utilization of clinical oral health services. These factors have been characterized as epidemiologic, social, demographic, personal, and psychological, in addition to elements of the oral health care system. Table 13-2 summarizes key barriers to oral health services.

The percentage of people in the United States who have had at least one dental visit annually and the average number of visits vary significantly among population groups.[14] Factors that influence regular dental attendance are outlined in Box 13-2. A national oral health objective for 2010 is to have 56% of persons over the age of 2 years have a dental visit each year.[3] In 2002, only 44% of this

BOX 13-2

ANNUAL DENTAL VISITS VARY IN THE UNITED STATES BY MULTIPLE FACTORS

Age
Geographic region in the United States
Citizenship
Immigration status
Dentition status (e.g., edentulous, dentate)
Health insurance status
Disability
Nativity
Education level
Place of residence (e.g., urban, suburban, rural, frontier)
Family income
Race/ethnicity
Family structure
Residency in nursing home
Gender
Self-reported general health status

population in the United States had a dental visit in the preceding year according to the Medical Expenditure Panel Survey (MEPS).[50]

Disparities in annual dental visits were reported among persons over age 2 in 2002 according to national data from MEPS. Among racial and ethnic groups 55% Native Hawaiians or Pacific Islanders, 47% whites, 39% Asians, 31% American Indians/Alaska Natives, 28% African Americans, and 27% Hispanics or Latinos had a dental visit in the preceding year[50] (Figure 13-10). In 2002, females (48%) were more likely than males (41%) to have regular dental attendance.[50]

National reports indicate that the percentage of dental visits increases with income and educational level.[14,43,44] Differences were found for persons aged 25 years and older based on educational attainment according to the MEPS in 2002.[50] Adults with at least some college (59%) and high school graduates (43%) were more likely to have an annual dental visit than adults with less than a high school education (20%) in 2002[50] (Figure 13-11). Studies demonstrate similar trends linked to income levels.[14,43,44] Individuals living in families with higher incomes were more likely to have a dental visit during the past year compared to their peers living in families with lower incomes.[14,43,44] Also, persons with disabilities (37%) were less apt to have regular dental visits than persons without disabilities (46%) in 2002[50] (see Figure 13-11).

According to the MEPS in 2002, 50% of children 5 years of age who entered school and 55% of third-grade children had an annual dental visit[50] (Figure 13-12). Overall, 49% of children aged 2 to 17 years had a dental

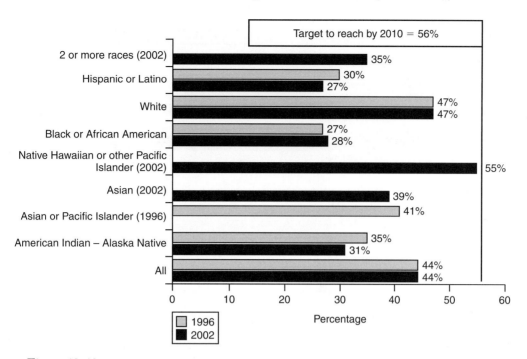

Figure 13-10   Percentage of population with annual dental visit by race/ethnicity (ages 2 years and over, age adjusted). (Data2010, *Healthy People 2010* database, January 2006 edition. Data from Medical Expenditure Panel Survey (MEPS), Agency for Healthcare Research and Quality.)

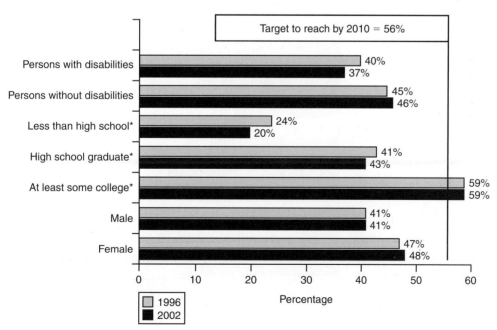

* Education level for persons aged 25 years and over

Figure 13-11   Percentage of population with annual dental visit by gender, education level, and disability status (ages 2 years and over, age adjusted). (Data2010, *Healthy People 2010* database, January 2006 edition. Data from Medical Expenditure Panel Survey (MEPS), Agency for Healthcare Research and Quality.)

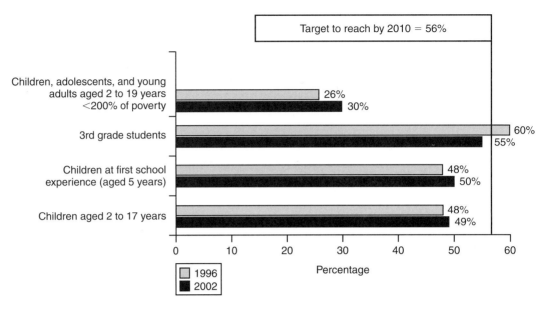

Figure 13-12 Percentage with annual dental visit for selected populations of children. (Data2010, *Healthy People 2010* database, January 2006 edition. Data from Medical Expenditure Panel Survey (MEPS), Agency for Healthcare Research and Quality.)

visit in the past year.[50] Among children, adolescents, and young adults (2 to 19 years) from families with low incomes (e.g., living in families with income less than 200% of poverty level) this proportion was only 30%.[50] This national survey found that 29% of low-income children and adolescents (under 19 years of age) received preventive dental service(s) during the preceding year compared with 25% in 1996.[50] Figure 13-13 shows disparities experienced by youth from different race and ethnic backgrounds in accessing preventive services.[50] One of the *Healthy People 2010* oral health objectives is to increase the number of children from families with low-incomes who receive preventive oral health care during a given year to 66%.[3]

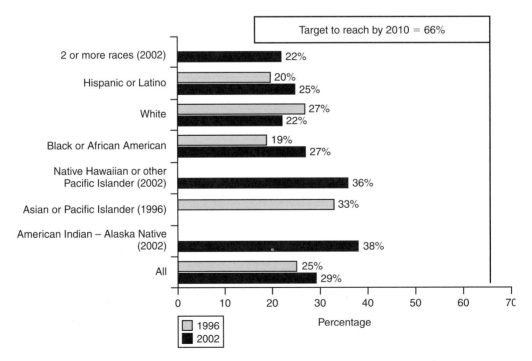

Figure 13-13 Percentage of youth with annual preventive dental services (for low-income youth, aged under 19 years) by race/ethnicity. (Data2010, *Healthy People 2010* database, January 2006 edition. Data from Medical Expenditure Panel Survey (MEPS), Agency for Healthcare Research and Quality.)

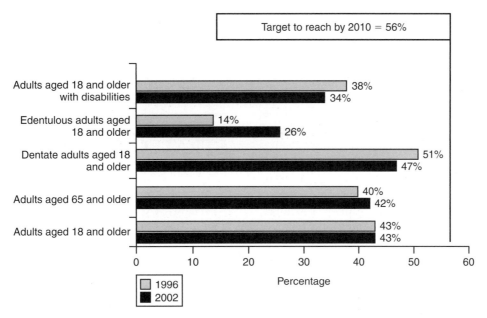

Figure 13-14   Percentage with annual dental visits for selected populations of adults. (Data2010, *Healthy People 2010* database, January 2006 edition. Data from Medical Expenditure Panel Survey (MEPS), Agency for Healthcare Research and Quality.)

In 2002, 43% of adults 18 years and older reported having an annual dental visit.[50] Older adults were less likely to schedule dental visits on a regular basis. Of people 65 years of age and older, 42% reported a dental visit in 2002[50] (Figure 13-14). Among dentate adults, 47% had a dental visit in the past year, compared with edentulous adults, 26% of whom reported an annual visit.[50] Only 19% of residents in long-term care facilities received dental care during the last 30 days in 1997[50] (see Figure 13-15). The national oral health objective is to increase this rate to 25% for nursing home residents by

2010.[3] Among residents of long-term care facilities, those who were younger, male, and African-American were more likely to have received dental care in the past month[50] (Figure 13-15).

IMPLICATIONS OF CULTURALLY EFFECTIVE ORAL HEALTH CARE

As a result of demographic changes, cultural competence has gained the attention of health professionals, policymakers, and educators as a means to improve the quality

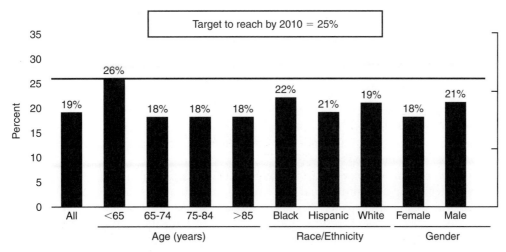

Figure 13-15   Percentage of residents in nursing homes receiving dental care during the last 30 days, 1997. (Data2010, *Healthy People 2010* database, January 2006 edition. Data from National Nursing Home Survey (NNHS), National Center for Health Statistics (NCHS), Centers for Disease Control and Prevention [CDC].)

of health care and to alleviate health disparities. **Cultural competence** is a set of congruent behaviors, knowledge, attitudes, and policies that come together in a system, organization, or among professionals that enables effective work in cross-cultural situations.[2]

Eliminating oral health disparities and increasing access to oral health care for all individuals, including those from culturally diverse populations within the United States, will require a transformation in the way oral services are currently provided within the oral health care system. Cultural competence is one tool that can be applied to eliminate disparities through the infusion of culturally competent principles into the practices of oral health professionals, the policies of the workplace and into professional organizations associated with the oral health care system.

There is a link between cultural competence and eliminating racial and ethnic disparities in oral and general health care.[14] Cultural competence alone does not address the entire problem; however, the **Culturally and Linguistically Appropriate Services** (CLAS) standards have often been referred to as an effective blueprint for improving the cultural competence of the health care system. The collective set of CLAS standards are guidelines issued by the Department of Health and Human Services, Office of Minority Health.[51] CLAS consists of three themes with fourteen standards shown in Box 13-3. The standards are intended to guide recommended practices by targeting actions of individual practitioners as well as support mechanisms that are necessary within organizations to assure access to health services that are culturally and linguistically appropriate.

STRATEGIES FOR APPLICATION IN PRACTICE

Self-Assessment: Evaluation of Knowledge, Skills, and Attitudes for Cultural and Linguistic Competence

Increasingly, both educational institutions and service organizations realize the need to better prepare students, staff, and professionals to provide culturally competent care to individuals and families living in multicultural communities. Health organizations and education institutions assessed current practices.[22,52-56] Also, health professional groups and government agencies developed guidelines and educational programs to promote the integration of culturally effective health care.[52-56]

BOX 13-3

CULTURALLY AND LINGUISTICALLY APPROPRIATE SERVICES (CLAS)

CULTURALLY COMPETENT CARE (STANDARDS 1-3)
1. Patients and consumers receive effective, understandable, and respectful health care.
2. Recruitment, retention, and promotion of diverse staff and leadership.
3. All staff receives ongoing education and training.

LANGUAGE ACCESS SERVICES (STANDARDS 4-7)
Mandated by current federal requirements for all recipients of federal funds.
4. Language assistance services, including bilingual staff and interpreters, must be offered at no cost to the patient.
5. Patients and consumers must be informed of their right to language assistance services.
6. Health organizations must assure the competence of language assistance provided by interpreters/bilingual staff.
7. Availability of easily understood patient materials and applicable signage posted.

ORGANIZATIONAL SUPPORT FOR CULTURAL COMPETENCE (STANDARDS 8-14)
8. Written strategic plan with clear goals, policies, and accountability mechanisms.
9. Conduct initial and ongoing organizational self-assessments, and integrate cultural and linguistic competence measures into overall program activities.
10. Patient data collection to include race, ethnicity, and spoken and written language.
11. Maintain current demographic, cultural, and epidemiological community profiles, and conduct needs assessment on cultural and linguistic characteristics of the service area.
12. Participatory, collaborative partnerships to facilitate community and patient/consumer involvement.
13. Ensure that conflict and grievance resolution processes are culturally and linguistically sensitive.
14. Keep the public informed about progress and successful innovations in implementing the CLAS standards.

(Source: U.S. Department of Health and Human Services, Office of Minority Health: *National standards for culturally and linguistically appropriate services in health care*, Rockville, MD, 2001, U.S. Department of Health and Human Services.)

Many programs indicate that self-evaluation is a critical first step. Evaluation techniques have been developed to evaluate the cultural competency skills of health professionals through self-assessment and professional development. Additional models were developed to assess elements within organizations that support the application of culturally competent practices and community outreach.

Providers should evaluate their knowledge and perceptions of their own culture by examining personal values and beliefs in light of their own cultural background and experiences.[60] It is important for providers to understand how their cultural background influences their view on health, and only then can they effectively develop their skills in providing effective patient-centered care. Cultural **self-assessment** is crucial because it affects daily interactions and professional relationships with patients from various cultures. Providing culturally competent oral health care increases the understanding of the diversity in the world in which we live.

The National Center for Cultural Competence (NCCC) developed the Cultural Competence Health Practitioners Assessment (CCHPA) intended to promote cultural and linguistic competence as an essential approach for practitioners in the elimination of health disparities among racial and ethnic groups.[61] The CCHPA is based on the following three assumptions: (a) cultural competence is a development process at both individual and organizational levels; (b) with appropriate support, individuals can enhance their cultural awareness, knowledge, and skills with time; and (c) cultural strengths exist within organizations or networks of professionals but often go unnoticed and untapped.[61] Oral health professionals experience daily encounters with patients that help refine the practices and skills necessary for cultural competence. Oral health professionals can enhance their care of patients by reflecting on the key points outlined in Box 13-4 and using it as a guide. The CCHPA can be adapted by dental professionals to evaluate communication, values, attitudes, and environmental factors related to promoting culturally effective oral health care. Also, a self-assessment can provide guidance to improve knowledge, enhance skills, and modify values.

EFFECTIVE HEALTH CARE

The self-assessment process allows dental professionals to consider their potential biases. Oral health care professionals may have cultural biases that affect the health care provided to patients. Dental professionals should recognize these biases so that they can become more respectful and caring oral health care professionals. Biases may arise when care is provided to people of whom one or more of the following is true:

• Do not speak the same language or do not speak it well.
• Are accompanied by family members that help make decisions and are relied on.

• Do not tell about other treatments being used.
• Do not follow the dental care that is prescribed or recommended.
• Wait too long to come in for dental care.
• Require additional provider time.[62]

When these situations are encountered, dental professionals should ask themselves: Do I provide care to the patient with respect? Do I do everything possible to meet the needs of the patient? Do I integrate the patient's values and beliefs when recommending dental care? Do I promote and make sure that the patient feels at ease during the dental visit?[62] Oral health professionals can become life-long learners as they continue to understand social and cultural dimensions of health through daily encounters with diverse patients.

CULTURAL COMPETENCY MODELS, FRAMEWORKS, AND STRATEGIES
The Purnell Model for Cultural Competence

Several models were developed to provide guidance for culturally effective health care. These models can analyze multiple factors that influence a situation or experience. The models can guide solutions to resolve key issues and apply practices that are effective in similar circumstances. The Purnell Model for Cultural Competence organizes multiple factors into a single framework.[60,63] The model can guide the practice of health professionals across settings and this approach is desirable in interdisciplinary teams.[64]

The Purnell Model for Cultural Competence consists of a circle surrounded by spheres representing macro level factors.[60,63] The first sphere represents the global society, the second represents community, the third family, and the fourth sphere represents the person. Twelve cultural domains of the model are portrayed by a pie-shaped diagram (Figure 13-16), which outline the key components of this framework.[60,63] The cultural domains are further described in Table 13-3.

CULTURAL AND SOCIAL INFLUENCES ON HEALTH

Perceptions of health and illness differ among individuals from diverse cultural backgrounds (Table 13-4). Some individuals maintain that health is purely the result of good luck and that a person loses their health if that luck changes.[65,66] Some people describe health as a reward for good behavior. Seen in this context, health is a gift from a higher being and should not be taken for granted by the individual. People are expected to maintain their own equilibrium in the universe by behaving in the proper way, eating healthy foods, and working the right amount of time. The protection of health is an accepted practice

BOX 13-4

Knowledge, Skills, and Attitudes for Provision of Culturally Effective Health Care

KNOWLEDGE
- Knowledge of patients' culture (history, traditions, values, and family systems).
- Knowledge of the impact of racism and poverty on behavior, attitudes, values and disabilities.
- Knowledge of the help-seeking behaviors of culturally diverse patients.
- Knowledge of the roles of language, speech patterns, and communication styles in different communities.
- Knowledge of the impact of the social service policies on culturally diverse patients.
- Knowledge of the resources (e.g., agencies, persons, informal helping networks, research) available for culturally diverse patients and communities.
- Recognition of how professional values may either conflict with or accommodate the needs of patients from different cultures.
- Knowledge of how power relationships within communities or institutions impact different cultures.
- Knowledge that cultural beliefs impact patient's oral health beliefs, help-seeking behaviors, interactions with oral health care professionals, oral health care practices, and oral health care outcomes, including adherence to prescribed regimens.

SKILLS
- Techniques for learning the cultures of diverse patient groups.
- Ability to communicate accurate information on behalf of culturally diverse patients and their communities.
- Ability to openly discuss cultural differences/issues and to respond to culturally based cues.
- Ability to assess the meaning that culture has for individual clients.
- Interviewing techniques that help the interviewer understand and accommodate the role of language in the patient's culture.
- Ability to use the concepts of empowerment on behalf of culturally diverse patients and communities.
- Ability to use resources on behalf of culturally diverse patients and their communities.
- Ability to recognize and combat racism, racial stereotypes, and myths among individuals and institutions.
- Ability to recognize that people of different cultures have different ways of communicating, behaving, interpreting, and problem solving.
- Ability to adapt care to be congruent with the patient's expectations and preferences.
- Ability to evaluate new techniques, research, and knowledge as to their validity and applicability in working with culturally diverse patients and communities.

ATTITUDES
- Personal qualities that reflect "genuineness, empathy, and warmth in caring" and a capacity to respond flexibly to a range of possible solutions.
- Awareness and acceptance of ethnic, social, and cultural differences between people.
- A willingness to work with culturally diverse patients and communities.
- Recognizing ways that these views may accommodate or conflict with the needs of patients from different cultures.
- Awareness of one's own cultural values.
- Willingness to adapt the way one works to fit the patient's cultural background in order to provide optimal care for the patient.

(Adapted from Salana D: *Cultural competency: a practical guide for mental health service providers*, Austin, TX, 2001, Hogg Foundation for Mental Health, University of Texas at Austin.)

that is accomplished with prayer, the wearing of religious medals or amulets, and keeping relics at home. Herbs and spices can be used to enhance this form of prevention, as can exemplary behavior. The provider should consider various perspectives of health when seeking to engage a patient as a partner in their oral health care.[65,66]

Beliefs about health and wellness and the causes of diseases and illnesses are numerous and can vary among cultural groups.[66] These beliefs can be influenced by cultural and social factors. One or more of the following

factors may be perceived as contributing to diseases or illnesses:

- Biological, anatomical, or physiological malfunction.
- Dislocation of parts of the body, magic or supernatural causes outside the body, or strong emotional states.
- Imbalance in an individual's body.
- Punishment for some wrongdoing.[66]

Given the diversity within cultural groups, it is impossible to describe all perspectives or attributes of every

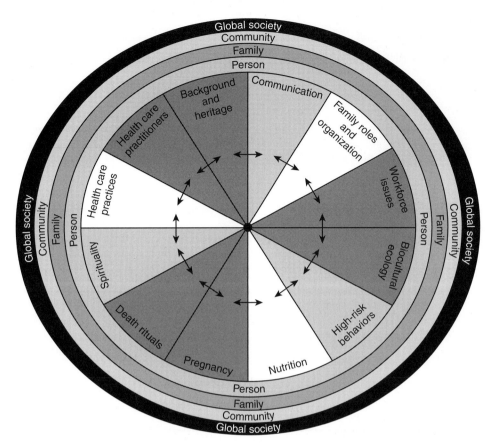

Figure 13-16 The Purnell Model for Cultural Competence. (Adapted from Purnell D, Paulanka J, editors: *Guide to culturally competent healthcare*, Philadelphia, 2005, F. A. Davis.)

individual within a cultural group. The descriptions in Table 13-5 are general considerations and cannot or should not be uniformly applied to all members of a group.

CULTURAL CONTEXT AND ORAL HEALTH CARE PROCESS

It is unrealistic and impossible to know everything about every culture. Therefore, approaches that focus on skills that can be adapted to meet the individual needs of patients are more useful for oral health care providers.

Models can be implemented in various settings and cross cultural situations can ensure that culturally competent attitudes, knowledge, and behaviors are applied when providing oral health care either in a clinical or community setting.[67] Cross-cultural approaches to oral health care and healing can be combined with the application of Western medicine and a biomedical model. Approaches to caring can be broadened by acknowledging the impact of social, environmental, cultural, psychological, behavioral, and biological factors on health.[64]

It is important for clinicians to explore ways to incorporate cultural and social dimensions into the oral health care process. Table 13-6 outlines points to consider when integrating cultural and social contexts into communication, assessment, examination, diagnosis, care planning, and provision of oral health care. Some basic attributes such as curiosity, empathy, respect, humility, and dignity

can enhance the clinical relationship to generate useful information about the patient's individual oral health beliefs and preferences.

It is recognized that provider-patient communication is a multidimensional phenomenon that has an impact on all aspects of oral health care. Core dimensions of positive interactions between patients and health care providers include listening carefully, explaining information well, showing respect, and spending sufficient time with patients.[68] Communication involves the transmission of information, thoughts, and feelings so that they are satisfactorily received or understood. An effective understanding of the interrelationship and dynamics between a provider and patient allows for optimal oral health care.

Positive patient communication involves recognizing and responding to the patient as a whole person, an approach termed "patient-centered health care."[68] Patient-centeredness is a constellation of skills that are considered crucial elements in the provision of quality interpersonal care.[69-71] Patient-centered skills have been described as those responsive to the patient's values, needs, and preferences.[72,73] These skills include the following:

- Information-gathering skills (e.g., use of open-ended questions, particularly in the psychological domain).

TABLE 13-3

CULTURAL DOMAINS IN THE PURNELL MODEL FOR CULTURAL COMPETENCE

CULTURAL DOMAIN	RELATED CONCEPTS	CULTURAL DOMAIN	RELATED CONCEPTS
Background and Heritage	Country of origin Current residence Effects of the topography of country of origin on health Effects of current residence on health Economics Politics Migration Education status Occupations	High-risk behaviors	Drug use Alcohol use Tobacco use Use of safety equipment (e.g., seat belts, helmets) High risk behaviors Lifestyles
Communication	Dominant language Dialects Cultural communication patterns Personal space Volume and tone Eye contact Body language Facial expressions Temporal relationships Touch Time Names Greetings	Nutrition	Common foods Rituals and taboos associated with food Meaning of food to the culture How food is used in sickness and in health Limitations Deficiencies
		Pregnancy and childbearing practices	Fertility practices Birthing practices Views towards pregnancy Postpartum
Family roles and organization	Head of household Gender roles Goals and priorities Developmental tasks Roles of the aged Roles of extended family members Individual and social status in the community Alternative lifestyles	Death rituals	Views towards death Euthanasia Preparation for death Burial practices Bereavement practices
		Spirituality	Meaning of life Religious practices Use of prayer Individual strength Spirituality and health
Workforce issues	Autonomy Acculturation Gender roles Language barriers	Health care practices	Focus on health care Magicoreligious beliefs Traditional practices Individual responsibility for health Self medicating practices Views towards issues such as • Organ donation • Transplantation • Mental illness • Rehabilitation Expression of pain Sick role Barriers to health care
Biocultural ecology	Biological variation Skin color Body type Heredity Genetics Ecology Drug metabolism	Health care practitioners	Type of practitioners • Biomedical • Traditional or folk Perceptions of practitioner Gender and health care

(Adapted from Purnell D, Paulanka J, editors: *Guide to culturally competent healthcare*, Philadelphia, 2005, F.A. Davis.)

TABLE 13-4

DIMENSIONS OF HEALTH AND CULTURE

DIMENSION	QUESTIONS TO CONSIDER
Health and illness beliefs	What paradigm is used to explain illness or healing?
Decision-making style	Does decision-making rest with the individual patient, the group, family or community peers?
Healing traditions	What are the alternative or complementary approaches used for healing? What is the role of traditional healers (e.g., shamans)?
Locus of control	Is the individual responsible for his or her own destiny or is destiny predetermined?
Status and hierarchy	Is the status of head of household conferred by age, gender, or kinship? What status is attributed to physicians and healers?
Privacy	Is privacy at the level of the individual or the family?
Communication	Is there a preferred mode of communication (e.g., English, Spanish)? Is an interpreter needed? Is a cultural broker needed? Do written materials need to be provided?
Socioeconomic status	Is social status in the community conferred on the basis of family, vocation, wealth, or education?
Immigrant status	Is the patient or their family immigrants? How long have they been living in the United States? Are acculturation and generational issues at play? Is immigrant status a potential legal concern?

(From Mutha S, Allen C, Welch M: *Toward culturally competent care: a toolbox for teaching communication strategies*, San Francisco, 2002, Center for Health Professions, University of California, San Francisco.)

- Relationship skills (e.g., use of empathy, reassurance, support, and emotional responsiveness).
- Partnering skills (e.g., paraphrasing, asking for patient's opinions, negotiation, and joint problem-solving).
- Counseling (e.g., applying motivational interviewing and stages of change approaches).

Positive patient communication requires that the patient and the provider bring their unique perspectives to the clinical encounter. Effective communication underpins prevention efforts at the clinical level, when providers have the opportunity to engage in one-on-one counseling that is culturally and linguistically appropriate. Diagnoses and care plans require dental professionals to negotiate a common understanding with patients about expectations and courses of care. The quality of provider-patient communication can affect numerous indicators, including patient adherence to health recommendations and health status.[74] Appropriate information and effective communication with a provider cannot only relieve patients' anxieties but also can help patients understand their choices, allow them to participate in informed decision making, and better manage their own oral health concerns.

The RESPECT Model is an acronym for Rapport, Empathy, Support, Partnership, Explanations, Cultural Competence, and Trust. The RESPECT Model highlighted in Table 13-7 focuses on the patient centered approach to communication. Integrating simple strategies that follow the RESPECT guidelines can improve communication for patient centered oral health care, while adding little or no time to the clinical encounter. Table 13-8 outlines examples of Cross-Cultural Communication Models that can be adapted by oral health care providers in clinical practice in the public, private, and nonprofit sectors to provide culturally effective oral health care. Essential requirements for effective cross-cultural communication include self-awareness of personal communication style, and willingness to modify that style to respond appropriately to the patient.[75]

OPPORTUNITIES FOR FUTURE PRACTICE: THE CARING FRAMEWORK FOR ORAL HEALTH

Oral health teams should integrate processes that foster productive interactions with patients and families into their clinical practice. In addition,

TABLE 13-5

CULTURAL INFLUENCES AND DISEASE ETIOLOGY

CONDITION	SYMPTOMS AND DESCRIPTIONS	WHERE RECOGNIZED
Ataque de nervios (Nervous attack)	Neurotic or psychotic episode caused by a traumatic event, family conflict, or anger, intense but brief.	Among Latinos.
Amok or mal de pelea	A dissociative disorder characterized by outbursts of violent, aggressive, or homicidal behaviors directed at people or objects, usually as a consequence of real or imagined insults.	Among patients from Malaysia, Laos, Philippines, Papua New Guinea, and Puerto Rico.
Bilis (Bile, age)	Overt and obvious outburst of anger.	Among Latino communities.
Dhat	Severe anxiety and panic associated with a sense of weakness, exhaustion, and the discharge of semen. Patient believes condition may be life threatening.	Among the Indian, Chinese, and Sri Lankan patients
Falling out	Seizure-like symptoms resulting from traumatic events or stress, such as death in the family. Accompanied by dizziness and temporary inability to move while still remaining conscious.	Among African-American communities.
Ghost sickness	Weakness and dizziness resulting from the deeds of witches, evil forces, or evil spirits.	Among Native Americans.
Hwa-byung	Pain in the upper abdomen, usually in females. Fear of death, and tiredness resulting from the imbalance between reality and anger. May be caused by unsettled anger.	Among Asian communities
Pikalogktog	A dissociative disorder or episode characterized by excitement, coma, and convulsive seizures. Associated with amnesia, withdrawal, irritability, and irrational behavior such as breaking furniture and verbalization of obscenities.	Among patients from the Arctic and subarctic regions.
Taijin fyofusho	Guilt and embarrassment of offending others by awkward behaviors. Timid behavior resulting from the feeling that one's appearance, odor, or facial expressions are offensive to others.	Among the Asian communities.
Mal Puesto, Mal de Ojo, hex, root work, and voodoo death (Evil eye)	Unnatural diseases occurring from the power of people who use evil spirits. Also a hex, usually on children, that is caused by an admiring gaze, usually unconscious.	Among African Americans and Latino communities.
Susto, espanto, espasmo, and miedo (Fright-induced "soul loss")	Tiredness and weakness resulting from frightening experiences. Can be as a result of shock, depression, or anxiety.	Among Latino communities.

(Adapted from Juckett G: Cross-cultural medicine, *Am Fam Physician*, 72:2267-2274, 2005; and Salana D: *Cultural competency: a practical guide for mental health service providers*, Austin, TX, 2001, Hogg Foundation for Mental Health, University of Texas at Austin.)

TABLE 13-6

INTEGRATING CULTURAL AND SOCIAL DIMENSIONS INTO THE ORAL HEALTH CARE PROCESS

COMPONENTS OF THE ORAL HEALTH PROCESS	EXAMPLES OF SOCIAL AND CULTURAL DIMENSIONS
Communication	Effective verbal and nonverbal communication are critical aspects of all phases of the oral health care process. Patient and provider language disparity may be a significant barrier to oral health care, and the use of an interpreter may be necessary. Ideally, the interpreter and should be trained, and not a family member, for the following reasons: • The family members may be too emotionally involved to be objective. • The patient may have privacy concerns. • The patient may withhold sensitive or personal information to avoid upsetting the family member.
Assessment (personal history, health history, dental history, vital signs)	Culturally competent oral health providers explore and assess the patient's cultural values, beliefs, and health practices. During the assessment stage, the provider has the opportunity to develop rapport with the patient. The goal of the personal history is to find out as much as possible about the patient and his or her "story." To be culturally competent, the oral health provider should expand questions to include socially and culturally specific information. The use of respectful, nonjudgmental questions will assist the patients' comfort level to reveal values, needs, and concerns regarding the entire process of care. Despite the oral health provider's own perspective, he or she should not criticize or reject the patient's beliefs, concerns, and values, because this will interfere with further interaction and could compromise outcomes. The oral health care provider should make every effort to understand health from the patient's point of view, failure to do so may lead to unsuccessful outcomes. The patient's views on oral health may be culturally conditioned. Instead of relying on Western medicine, some patients from diverse cultural backgrounds may choose to use more traditional methods of care. When assessing vital signs, the oral health provider should take into consideration predisposing factors in a patient's systemic conditions to avoid contraindications.
Extraoral and intraoral examinations	Oral health providers should note the presence of any oral manifestations associated with systemic diseases in relation to sociocultural factors. The oral health provider should be cognizant that some populations may exhibit a higher rate of specific oral disease because of factors such as access to care issues, diet, and genetic variations.
Diagnosis (Care plan and informed consent)	On completion of collecting information, the oral health provider is able to make a dental diagnosis on the basis of the findings. When planning care, the oral health provider should avoid the imposition of his or her own beliefs and values on the patient. The care plan must be realistic and individualized to meet the patient's needs The patient's values, beliefs, behaviors, and knowledge should be considered in developing a care plan that reflects specific cultural and social factors.

Continued

TABLE 13-6

INTEGRATING CULTURAL AND SOCIAL DIMENSIONS INTO THE ORAL HEALTH CARE PROCESS—cont'd

COMPONENTS OF THE ORAL HEALTH PROCESS	EXAMPLES OF SOCIAL AND CULTURAL DIMENSIONS
Provision of oral health care	The oral health provider should explain the procedures that will be performed throughout the encounter. The involvement and opportunity to ask questions by the patient is especially valuable when providing culturally competent care. The more culturally competent the oral health provider has been throughout the care process, building rapport, and individualizing care, the more desirable will be the achieved outcome.

(From Carins D: The role of the dental hygienist in a multicultural society: review of the literature 1988-1993, *Probe* 27:177-181, 1993; Tamparo CT, Lindh WQ: *Therapeutic communication for health professionals*, ed 2, Clifton Park, NJ, 2000, Delmar Learning; Spector RE: *Cultural diversity in health and illness*, ed 5, Upper Saddle River, NJ, 2000, Prentice Hall; Fitch P: Cultural competency and dental hygiene care delivery: integrating cultural care into dental hygiene care process, *J Dent Hyg* 11-2,2004.)

oral health practice has evolved, requiring that cultural competency be expanded from the interpersonal level and integrated into new approaches at the community and health system levels. Models that describe systematic approaches have been developed for the provision of care for chronic conditions and children's health.[76-78] Also, novel frameworks integrate health initiatives for improvements among individuals as well as their families and communities.[79]

TABLE 13-7

RESPECT MODEL

ELEMENT	DESCRIPTION
Rapport	Connect on a social level. See the patient's point of view. Consciously suspend judgment. Recognize and avoid making assumptions.
Empathy	Remember that the patient has come to you for help. Seek out and understand the patient's rational for their behaviors and illness. Verbally acknowledge and legitimize the patient's feelings.
Support	Ask about and understand the barriers to care and compliance. Help the patient overcome barriers. Involve family members if appropriate. Reassure the patient you are and will be available to help.
Partnership	Be flexible with regard to control issues. Negotiate roles when necessary. Stress that you are working together to address health problems.
Explanations	Check often for understanding. Use verbal clarification techniques.
Cultural competence	Respect the patient's cultural beliefs. Understand that the patient's views of you may be defined by ethnic and cultural stereotypes. Be aware of your own cultural biases and preconceptions. Know your limitations in addressing medical issues across cultures. Understand your personal style and recognize when it may not be working with a given patient.
Trust	Recognize that self-disclosure may be difficult for some patients. Consciously work to establish trust.

(From Mutha S, Allen C, Welch M: *Toward culturally competent care: a toolbox for teaching communication strategies*, San Francisco, 2002, Center for Health Professions, University of California, San Francisco.)

TABLE 13-8

CROSS-CULTURAL COMMUNICATION MODELS

MODELS	SOURCES
BATHE Background (What is going on in your life?) Affect (How do you feel about what is going on?) Trouble (What troubles you most?) Handling (How are you handling that?) Empathy (This must be very difficult for you.)	Stuart MR, Liebermann JR: *The fifteen-minute hour: applied psychotherapy for the primary care physician*, New York, 1993, Praeger.
BELIEF Beliefs about health (What caused your illness/problem?) Explanation (Why did it happen at this time?) Learn (Help me to understand your belief/opinion.) Empathy (This must be very difficult for you.) Feelings (How are you feeling about it?)	Dobbie AE, Medrand M, Tysinger J et al.: The BELIEF instrument: a preclinical teaching tool to elicit patients' health beliefs, *Fam Med* 35:316-319, 2003.
Eliciting patient information and negotiating Identify core cross-cultural issues Explore the meaning of the illness Determine the social context Engage in negotiation	Carrillo JE, Green AR, Betancourt JF: Cross-cultural primary care: a patient-based approach, *Ann Intern Med* 130: 829-834,1999.
ESFT model for communication and compliance. Explanatory model Social risk for noncompliance Fears and concerns about the medication Therapeutic contracting and playback	Betancourt JR, Carrillo JE, Green AR: Hypertension in multicultural and minority populations: linking communication to compliance, *Curr Hypertens Rep* 1:482-488, 1999.
ETHNIC Explanation (How do you explain your illness?) Treatment (What treatment have you tried?) Healers (Have you sought any advice from folk healers?) Negotiate (mutually acceptable options) Intervention (agreed on) Collaboration (with patient, family, and healers)	Levin SJ, Like RC, Gottlieb JE: ETHNIC: a framework for culturally competent ethical practice, *Patient Care* 34:188-189, 2000.
Kleinman's questions What do you think has caused your problem? Why do you think it started when it did? What do you think your sickness does to you? How severe is your sickness? Will it have a short or long course? What kind of treatment do you think you should receive? What are the most important results you hope to receive from this treatment? What are the chief complaints your sickness has caused for you? What do you fear most about your sickness?	Kleinmann A, Eisenberg L, Good B: Culture, illness and care: clinical lessons from anthropologic and cross-cultural research, *Ann Intern Med* 88:251-258, 1978.
LEARN Listen with sympathy and understanding to the patient's perception of the problem Explain your perceptions of the problem Acknowledge and discuss the differences and similarities Recommend treatment Negotiate treatment	Berlin EA, Fowkes WC: A teaching framework for cross-cultural health care, *West J Med* 139:14-23, 1983.

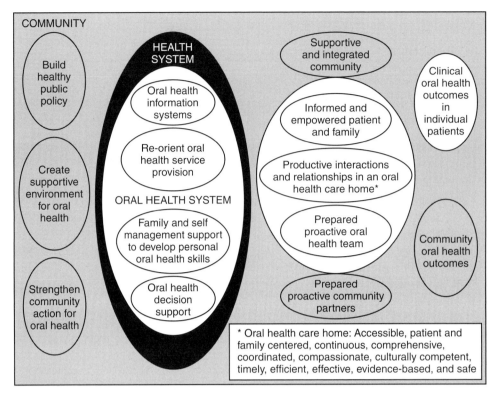

Figure 13-17 Caring framework for oral health.

The Caring Framework for Oral Health provides a visual image of the multiple factors necessary to improve oral health at the community, organization, practice, and patient levels. The outcomes described in the Caring Framework include functional and clinical indicators for individual patients and population oral health measures. The Caring Framework for Oral Health highlights key elements for positive interactions and relationships between the oral health team with the patient and family. It links the family and patient with a supportive community. Also, the oral health team is connected with community partners who are stakeholders in the health of the community and can mobilize resources to achieve oral health improvements.

In addition, the Caring Framework for Oral Health (Figure 13-17) integrates the community into the model by building healthy public policies, creating supportive environments, and strengthening community actions according to the Ottawa Charter for Health Promotion. Community resources and policies are mobilized to meet patient needs. The Caring Framework links community resources and policies promoting wellness with the health system as well as the oral health system. The Oral Health System is part of the Health System in this framework. It supports mechanisms that promote safe, high quality oral health care. The Oral Health System includes the following elements:

- Family and self-management support to develop personal oral health skills (for example, empowering and supporting parents to manage the oral health and oral health care of their children to prevent early childhood caries).
- Reorient oral health service provision (for example, reorienting the dental visit to ensure effective and efficient clinical oral health care and follow-up services that support patient self-management).
- Oral health decision support (for example, providing clinical oral health care that is evidence-based and addresses patient's preferences and needs).
- Oral health information systems (for example, systematizing oral health data and record keeping that are beneficial for patients, the community, and the system).

SUMMARY

In today's evolving society, an awareness of individuals from diverse cultures living in communities throughout the United States is vital to improving overall health status. A growing recognition exists that a multicultural society requires a system of health care whereby dental professionals provide culturally and linguistically effective oral health care.

Multicultural education is an important aspect of personal and professional development for oral health care providers. It is important to note that cultural competency is a process. It is often developed in stages by building on acquired knowledge and experiences. Reaching cultural competency is a continuous process; therefore, education in the core topics and developing skills must be ongoing. Cultural competency should be integrated into both didactic courses and clinical oral health services throughout the education process, and provide service-learning opportunities in culturally diverse communities. The acquisition of the knowledge, awareness, and skills related to culturally effective oral health care begins in institutions of higher education and continues as a part of life-long learning.

Along with the oral health care provider being culturally competent, the oral health care system should encourage and support the provision of culturally competent oral heath care to every patient regardless of race, ethnicity, gender, language preference, disability, or age. A culturally competent oral health care organization can contribute to a system that improves oral health outcomes and reduces oral health disparities. Strategies include organizational support for continuing education opportunities about cultural competency and cross-cultural issues. In addition, policies should be in place within dental offices and clinics that reduce cultural and linguistic barriers to oral health care.

Eliminating oral health disparities must become a priority of oral health organizations, government agencies, and institutions involved with the oral health professions. Oral health leaders and dental professionals in all sectors, including public health, health care organizations, foundations, and advocacy groups need to be knowledgeable, skilled, and committed, and culturally and linguistically competent. They need to understand the determinants of oral health to address cultural, social, linguistic, economic, and environmental factors that contribute to oral health disparities. Multifaceted strategies by all stakeholders in oral health, including educators, practitioners, and advocates are required to address oral health disparities and improve the oral health of the diverse populations in the United States.

References

1. Wells SA, Black RM: *Cultural competency for health professionals*, Albany, NY, 2000, American Occupational Therapy Association.

2. Cross TL, Bazron B, Dennis K et al.: *Towards a culturally competent system of care: a monograph on effective services for minority children*, Washington, DC, 1989, National Center for Cultural Competence, Georgetown University.

3. U.S. Department of Health and Human Services: *Healthy people 2010: understanding and improving health*, ed 2, Washington, DC, 2000, U.S. Government Printing Office, 2000.

4. U.S. Department of Health and Human Services: *Health care Rx: access for all chartbook*, Washington, DC, 1998, U.S. Department of Health and Human Services.

5. Beaman C, Devisetty V, Forcina Hill JM et al.: *A guide to incorporating cultural competency into medical education and training*, Los Angeles, CA, 2005, National Health Law Program.

6. American Dental Hygienists' Association: *Bylaws and code of ethics*, Chicago, 2006, American Dental Hygienists' Association.

7. Berger JT: Culture and ethnicity in clinical care, *Arch Intern* 158:2085-2090, 1998.

8. Stewart M, Brown JB, Boon H et al.: Evidence on patient-doctor communication, *Cancer Prev Control* 3:25-30, 1999.

9. Williams DR, Rucker TD: Understanding and addressing racial disparities in health care, *Health Care Financ Rev* 21:75-90, 2000.

10. Institute of Medicine: *Crossing the quality chasm: a new health system for the twenty-first century*, Washington, DC, 2001, National Academies Press.

11. Smedley BD, Stith AY, Nelson AR, editors, *Unequal treatment: confronting racial and ethnic disparities in health care*, Washington, DC, 2003, National Academies Press.

12. Stewart M, Brown JB, Weston WW et al.: *Transforming the clinical method: patient-centered medicine*, Abingdon, UK, 2003, Radcliffe Medical Press.

13. National Cancer Institute: *Theory at a glance: a guide for health promotion practice*, Bethesda, MD, 1995, National Cancer Institute, National Institutes for Health.

14. U.S. Department of Health and Human Services: *Oral health in America: a report of the Surgeon General*, Rockville, MD, 2000, National Institute of Dental and Craniofacial Research, National Institute of Health.

15. Cohen LK, Gift HC, editors: *Disease prevention and oral health promotion: socio-dental sciences in action*, Copenhagen, Denmark, 1995, Munksgaard.

16. Science Data Analysis Network, University of Michigan: Census 2000 charts and trends, Science Data Analysis Network (website): http://www.CensusScope.org. Accessed October 5, 2006.

17. American Academy of Pediatrics, Committee on Pediatric Work Force: Policy statement: ensuring culturally effective pediatric care, implications for education and health policy, *Pediatrics* 114:1677-1685, 2004.

18. Gist YJ, Hetzel LI: *We the people: aging in the United States, census 2000 special reports*, Washington, DC, 2004, U.S. Department of Commerce, Economics and Statistics Administration, U.S. Census Bureau.

19. US Census Bureau, Public Information Office: *Facts for features: 12th anniversary of Americans with Disabilities Act*, Washington, DC, 2002, U.S. Department of Commerce, Economics and Statistics Administration, U.S. Census Bureau.

20. Zola I: Toward the necessary universalizing of a disability policy, *Milbank Q* 67:401-428, 1989.

21. Centers for Disease Control and Prevention: Public health and aging: trends in aging—United States and worldwide, *MMWR Morb Mortal Wkly Rep* 52:101-106, 2003.

22. Betancourt JR, Green AR, Carrillo JE: *Cultural competence in health care: emerging frameworks and practical approaches*, New York, 2002, The Commonwealth Fund.

23. Jones NA, Smith AS: *Census 2000 brief: the two or more races population: 2000*, Washington, DC, 2001, U.S. Department of Commerce, Economics and Statistics Administration, U.S. Census Bureau.

24. Schachter J: *Geographic Mobility 2002 to 2003*, Washington, DC, 2004, U.S. Department of Commerce, Economics and Statistics Administration, U.S. Census Bureau.

25. Simmons T, O'Neill G: *Census 2000 brief: households and families: 2000*, Washington, DC, U.S. Department of Commerce, Economics and Statistics Administration, U.S. Census Bureau, 2001, September 2001.

26. Fronczek P, Johnson P: *Census 2000 brief: occupations 2000*, Washington, DC, U.S. Department of Commerce, Economics and Statistics Administration, U.S. Census Bureau, 2001, August 2003.

27. DeNavas-Walt C, Proctor BD, Lee CH: *Income, poverty, and health insurance coverage in the United States: 2005*, Washington, DC,

2006, U.S. Department of Commerce, Economics and Statistics Administration, U.S. Census Bureau.

28. U.S. Census Bureau: Poverty thresholds 2004, Washington, DC, 2005, U.S. Department of Commerce, Economics and Statistics Administration, U.S. Census Bureau.

29. National Center for Children in Poverty: *Basic facts about low-income children: birth to age 18*, New York, 2006, National Center for Children in Poverty.

30. Berstein J, Brocht, C, Spade-Aguilar M: *How much is enough? Basic family budgets for working families*, Washington, DC, 2000, Economic Policy Institute.

31. American Institute for Research: *Teaching cultural competence in health care: a review of current concepts, policies, and practices, report prepared for the Office of Minority Health, U.S. Department of Health and Human Resources*, Washington, DC, 2002, American Institute for Research.

32. Shin HB, Bruno R: *Census 2000 brief: language use and English-speaking ability: 2000*, Washington, DC, 2003, U.S. Department of Commerce, Economics and Statistics Administration, U.S. Census Bureau.

33. U.S. Census Bureau: *Data profile highlights: 2005 American community survey*, Washington, DC, 2005, U.S. Department of Commerce, Economics and Statistics Administration.

34. Kutner M, Greenberg E, Baer J: *A first look at the literacy of America's adults in the 21st century*, Washington, DC, 2005, National Center of Education Statistics.

35. Schwartzberg JG, VanGeest JB, Wang CC: *Understanding health literacy: implications for medicine and public health*, Chicago, 2005, AMA Press.

36. Institute of Medicine: *Health literacy: a prescription to end confusion*, Washington, DC, 2004, National Academies Press.

37. Kutner M, Greenberg E, Jin Y, Paulsen C: *The health literacy of America's adults: results from the 2003 national assessment of adult literacy*, Washington, DC, 2006, National Center of Education Statistics.

38. National Institute of Dental and Craniofacial Research, National Institutes of Health, U.S. Public Health Service, Department of Health and Human Services: The invisible barrier: literacy and its relationship with oral health, a report of a workgroup sponsored by the National Institute of Dental and Craniofacial Research, *J Public Health Dent* 65:174-182, 2005.

39. Prevention Institute: *The California campaign to eliminate racial and ethnic health disparities: health for all*, Oakland, CA, 2003, Prevention Institute.

40. U.S. Department of Health and Human Services: *National call to action to promote oral health*, Rockville, MD, 2003, U.S. Department of Health and Human Services, Public Health Service, National Institutes of Health, National Institute of Dental and Craniofacial Research.

41. U.S. Department of Health and Human Services: *Healthy People 2010: progress review, focus area 21, oral health*, Washington DC, 2004, U.S. Department of Health and Human Services.

42. U.S. Department of Health and Human Services: *Healthy people 2010: progress review, focus area 21, oral health—data presentation and briefing book materials*, Washington, DC, 2004, U.S. Department of Health and Human Services.

43. U.S. Government Accounting Office: *Oral health—dental disease is a chronic problem among low-income populations*, Washington, DC, 2000, U.S. Government Accounting Office.

44. U.S. Government Accounting Office: *Oral health: factors contributing to low use of dental services by low-income populations*, Washington, DC, 2000, U.S. Government Accounting Office.

45. Beltrán-Aguilar ED, Barker LK, Canto MT et al.: Surveillance for dental caries, dental sealants, tooth retention, edentulism, and enamel fluorosis, *MMWR Morb Mortal Wkly Rep Surveillance Summaries* 54:1-44, 2005.

46. Task Force on Community Preventive Services: Promoting oral health: interventions for preventing dental caries, oral and pharyngeal cancers, and sports-related craniofacial injuries: a report on the recommendations of the task force on community preventive services. *MMWR Morb Mortal Wkly Rep* 50(RR-21):1-13, 2001.

47. Fluoride Recommendations Work Group: Recommendations for using fluoride to prevent and control dental caries in the United States, *MMWR Morb Mortal Wkly Rep* 50(RR-14):1-42, 2001.

48. Institute of Medicine: *Primary care: America's health in a new era*, Washington, DC, 1996, National Academies of Sciences.

49. Steffensen JEM: Measuring progress in oral health. In Geurink KV, editor: *Community oral health practice for the dental hygienist*, ed 2, St Louis, 2005, Elsevier.

50. Centers for Disease Control and Prevention: *Data 2010, healthy people 2010 January 2006 edition*, Atlanta, GA, 2006, Centers for Disease Control and Prevention.

51. U.S. Department of Health and Human Services, Office of Minority Health: *National standards for culturally and linguistically appropriate services in health care*, Rockville, MD, 2001, U.S. Department of Health and Human Services.

52. Rowland ML, Bean CY, Casamassimo PS: A snapshot of cultural competency education in US dental schools, *J Dent Educ* 70:982-990, 2006.

53. Saleh L, Kuthy RA, Chalkley Y et al.: An assessment of cross-cultural education in U.S. dental schools. *J Dent Educ* 70:610-623, 2006.

54. Formicola A, Stavisky J, Lewy R: Cultural competency: dentistry and medicine learning from one another, *J Dent Educ* 67:869-875, 2003.

55. Beach M et al.: Cultural competence: a systematic review of health care provider educational interventions, *Med Care* 43:356-373, 2005.

56. Fortier JP, Bishop D: *Setting the agenda for research on cultural competence in health, final report*, Rockville, MD, 2003, U.S. Department of Health and Human Services, Office of Minority Health and Agency for Healthcare Research and Quality.

57. Mutha S, Allen C, Welch M: *Toward culturally competent care. A toolbox for teaching communication strategies*, San Francisco, CA, 2002, Center for the Health Professions, University of California, San Francisco.

58. The Henry J. Kaiser Family Foundation: *Compendium of cultural competence initiatives in health care*, Menlo Park, CA, 2003, The Henry J. Kaiser Family Foundation.

59. American Medical Student Association Foundation: *Achieving diversity in dentistry and medicine, cultural competency curricular guidelines for medical and dental schools*, Washington, DC, 2005, American Medical Student Association Foundation.

60. Purnell L, Paulanka B, editors: *Transcultural health care: a culturally competent approach*, ed 2, Philadelphia, 1998, F.A. Davis.

61. National Center for Cultural Competency (NCCC): *The cultural competence health practitioners assessment (CCHPA)*. Washington, DC, 2006, Georgetown University Center for Child and Human Development.

62. Kaiser Permanente: *Multicultural caring: a guide to cultural competence for Kaiser Permanente health professionals*, Los Angeles, CA, 2002, Kaiser Permanente.

63. Purnell L: A description of the Purnell model for cultural competence, *J Transcult Nurs* 11:40-46, 2000.

64. Purnell L: The Purnell model for cultural competence, *J Transcult Nurs* 13:193-196, 2002.

65. Welch S, Comer J, Steinman M: Some social and attitudinal correlates of health care among Mexican Americans, *J Health Soc Behav* 14:205-213, 1973.

66. Spector RE: *Cultural diversity in health and illness*, ed 5, Upper Saddle River, NJ, 2000, Prentice Hall.

67. de la Torre MA: Cultural competency. In Geurink KV, editor: *Community oral health practice for the dental hygienist*, ed 2, St Louis, 2005, Elsevier.

68. U.S. Department of Health and Human Services: *Communicating health: priorities and strategies for progress*, Washington, DC, 2003, Office of Disease Prevention and Health Promotion, U.S. Department of Health and Human Services.

69. Lipkin M, Putnam S, Lazare A, editors: *The medical interviews: clinical care, education, and research*, New York, 1995, Springer-Verlag.

70. Mead N, Bower P: Measuring patient-centeredness: a comparison of three observation-based instruments, *Patient Educ Couns* 39:71-80, 2000.

71. Tressolini CP, Pew-Fetzer Task Force: *Health professions education and relationship-centered care*, San Francisco, CA, 1994, Pew Health Professions Commission.

72. Lazare A, Putnam SM, Lipkin M: Three functions of the medical interview. In Putman SM, Lipkin M, Lazare A: *The medical interviews: clinical care, education, and research*, New York, 1995, Springer-Verlag.

73. Roter DL: The enduring and evolving nature of the patient-physician relationship, *Patient Educ Couns* 39:5-15, 2000.

74. Ong LM, de Haes JC, Hoos AM et al.: Doctor-patient communication: a review of the literature, *Soc Sci Med* 40:903-918, 1999.

75. Association of Reproductive Health Professionals: Communicating with patients: a quick reference for clinicians, Washington, DC, no date. http://www.arhp.org/healthcareproviders/onlinepublications/QRGPACC.cfm. Association of Reproductive Health Professionals. Accessed October 5, 2006.

76. Wagner EH: Chronic disease management: what will it take to improve care for chronic illness? *Effective Clin Pract* 1:2-4, 1998.

77. Glasgow R, Orleans C, Wagner E et al.: Does the chronic care model also serve as a template for improving prevention? *Milbank Q* 79:579-612, 2001.

78. Betancourt JR: Cultural competence and health care disparities: key perspectives and trends. *Health Aff* 24:499-505, 2005.

79. Barr V, Robinson S, Marin B et al.: *British Columbia's expanded chronic care model*, Victoria, British Columbia, 2005, Ministry of Health, Chronic Disease Management.

Part *IV*

Prevention and Practice

Chapter 14

Disease Prevention and Health Promotion

DIANE RIGASSIO RADLER AND RIVA TOUGER-DECKER

ORAL HEALTH PROMOTION AND DISEASE PREVENTION REPORTS

> The World Oral Health Report
> Surgeon General's Report on Oral Health

EVIDENCE-BASED DIETARY STRATEGIES FOR ORAL HEALTH PROMOTION

> Dietary Guidelines
> The Food Guidance System

OVERWEIGHT AND OBESITY

> Practice Recommendations

DIABETES AND CARDIOVASCULAR DISEASES

OSTEOPOROSIS

> Practice Recommendations

SUMMARY

LEARNING OBJECTIVES

Upon completion of this chapter, the learner will be able to:
- Examine an integrated common risk factor approach to oral and systemic health promotion.
- Relate dietary practices to the risk for oral diseases.
- Define Dietary Guidelines and The Food Guidance System for the interpretation, education, and promotion of nutritional principles associated with oral health promotion.
- Review common elements of dietary recommendations for risk reduction of chronic systemic and oral diseases.
- Explore obesity risk screening strategies appropriate for dental settings.
- List and describe steps to address the risk for osteoporosis.

KEY TERMS

Dietary cholesterol
Dietary fiber
Energy balance
Fat free
Food groups
Insoluble fiber
Moderate alcohol intake
Monounsaturated fat
Nutrient
Nutrient-dense foods
Polyunsaturated fat
Potassium-rich foods
Saturated fat
Simple sugars
Sodium in food
Soluble fiber
Trans fat
Whole grain

The bidirectional relationship between oral health and general health is fundamental to oral care and suggests that the association between oral diseases and some chronic diseases is based on common risk factors.[1] According to Sheiham and Watt, "health promotion is directed at the underlying determinants as well as the immediate causes of ill health."[2] These authors note two "immediate causes" or risk factors for oral infectious diseases, common to chronic diseases: diet and smoking. Healthy lifestyles, including dietary behaviors and tobacco cessation, are cornerstones of the effort to reduce the risk of cardiovascular disease, diabetes, and cancer. These same behaviors are correlated with oral health risks such as dental caries, periodontal disease associated with premature tooth loss, oral mucosal lesions, and oropharyngeal and pharyngeal cancer.[1,2]

A common risk factor approach model (illustrated in Figure 14-1) allows the dental professional to focus on systemic and oral health conditions.[2] This model suggests that a goal to target the fewest risk factors with the greatest impact on many diseases, with the greatest efficiency and effectiveness, would have the most beneficial health outcome.[2] A risk may be defined as the probability, associated with a unique condition, of developing or experiencing a change in health status. Because many risk factors are relevant to more than one chronic disease, targeting a risk factor may impact the incidence of several diseases. For example, the risk factors of excessive alcohol consumption, poor diet, and tobacco use are often seen in the same cohorts within the U.S. population. Modification of one of these risk factors can have an effect on the others. Similarly, improvement in one risk factor has an effect on multiple disease states. National and international government reports support the collaboration across health care disciplines necessary to communicate a resounding message of health promotion and disease prevention. The Prevention and Practice section of this book addresses key health promotion and disease prevention

strategies generic to chronic diseases and conditions, with a focus on their applicability to oral disease prevention and health promotion. This chapter specifically examines dietary behaviors related to oral disease risk. Other chapters address tobacco cessation, hygiene, and stress/anxiety issues.

ORAL HEALTH PROMOTION AND DISEASE PREVENTION REPORTS
The World Oral Health Report

In 2003 the World Health Organization (WHO) published the World Oral Health Report[1] to outline the current status of oral health worldwide and to highlight strategies for improving oral health in the twenty-first century. The WHO Oral Health Report recognized that oral health is a key component of general health, contributes to quality of life, and can be integral in reducing premature mortality. The Report underscored the role of diet and nutrition in oral health, and the importance of recognizing **nutrient** deficiencies and excesses associated with the divergent needs of populations worldwide. Malnutrition increases susceptibility to oral diseases, and micronutrient deficiencies may be manifested first in the

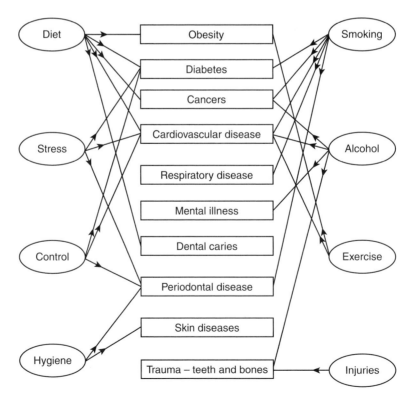

Figure 14-1 The common risk factor approach. (Redrawn from Sheiham A, Watt RG: The common risk factor approach: a rational basis for promoting oral health, *Community Dent Oral Epidemiol* 28:399-406, 1000.)

oral cavity. Alternatively, dietary excesses can lead to obesity, diabetes, cardiovascular disease, and cancer that may impact the integrity of the oral cavity.

The Report highlighted challenges to the achievement of healthy nutrition and oral health states. These challenges include advocating nutritional counseling for general health aspects and direct aspects of oral health, promoting breastfeeding practices to reduce rampant childhood caries, among other benefits to the mother and baby, decreasing the consumption of sugary drinks that contribute to dental caries and erosion, promoting a healthy diet especially in deprived or remote areas by advocating natural foods versus refined and processed foods, and advocating a diet rich in fruits and vegetables and low in alcohol to help prevent oral cancer.

The report further describes the impact of oral diseases on health and the associations between general health risk factors and those that specifically affect oral health, such as tobacco, alcohol, and poor diet. The relationships between lifestyle behaviors and risk factors for disease, and the increased risk of dental caries, periodontal disease, oral infections, oral cancers, and craniofacial defects indicate the need for an integrated approach to health promotion for oral and systemic health. The report emphasizes reducing risk factors, the burden of oral diseases, and the inequity of oral health care, while improving oral health systems and community programs to promote world health. A common risk factor approach is suggested as a way to target general health conditions and oral health risk factors through shared approaches.

Surgeon General's Report on Oral Health

Optimal health cannot be achieved independent of oral health. Although significant progress has been made during the last 60 years to improve oral health in the United States, not all Americans have benefited equally from these advancements.[3] *Healthy People 2010*, a report by the U.S. Department of Health and Human Services, emphasizes improving quality of life and eliminating health disparities.[4] The Surgeon General's Report (SGR) on Oral Health[3] reinforces the goals for prevention of disease and promotion of health. Both the SGR and the WHO Report support oral health as a vital component of overall health that must be included in all aspects of health care and health promotion.[1,3]

The mouth is identified as a mirror to the rest of the body, thus reinforcing the importance of examining the oral cavity as a component of health assessment. Furthermore, relationships between abnormal conditions of the oral tissues and acute or chronic systemic diseases can follow. The SGR delineates the staggering burden of oral diseases and disorders on children, adults, and the elderly in the U.S. population. Although dental caries and periodontal disease are the two most widespread oral

health problems, oral health promotion and disease prevention must also include reducing the risk of birth defects, craniofacial injuries, tobacco-related lesions and cancers, viral infections, disorders of the temporomandibular joint, and orofacial pain. The SGR notes the disparities in oral health care in the U.S. population, and the subsequent impact poor oral health has on individual pain and suffering, quality of life, financial loss (by lost wages and lack of reimbursement from third-party payers), and the burden to the American society.[3]

The SGR identifies multiple opportunities for improving oral health and suggests collaboration among health professionals, communities, and individuals. Safe and effective measures exist for oral health promotion and disease prevention. Related messages for oral health must be communicated to health care workers, community leaders, and the public at large to improve the overall health of the U.S. population. Advocacy for integrating oral health promotion into public policy, health care practice, and personal behaviors are a basic theme of the report.[3]

EVIDENCE-BASED DIETARY STRATEGIES FOR ORAL HEALTH PROMOTION
Dietary Guidelines

The 2005 edition of the Dietary Guidelines for Americans represents the sixth revision of the recommendations for people older than 2 years.[5] These guidelines are an authoritative resource describing optimal dietary practices and physical activity to promote health and reduce risk of chronic diseases. The first edition was published in 1980 and has been revised every 5 years by the U.S. Department of Agriculture (USDA) and the Department of Health and Human Services (DHHS). Each revision has included an analysis of current scientific information describing the effect of diet and sedentary activity on morbidity and mortality in the United States.

There are nine key recommendations for the general U.S. population listed in Box 14-1. The first three focus on attaining and maintaining a healthy body weight by consuming **nutrient-dense foods** within a balanced energy pattern, preventing weight gain, achieving weight loss when indicated, and including physical activity as a means to weight stabilization, cardiovascular conditioning, and muscle strength. The next four recommendations are associated with **food groups** and nutrients. A variety of fruits and vegetables, **whole grains**, and low-fat or fat-free dairy products are encouraged. **Trans fats** have been added to the category of those fat compounds (including **saturated fats** and cholesterol) that should be avoided in a daily diet. Fiber-rich carbohydrates are encouraged, and a specific reference to reducing the incidence of dental

BOX 14-1

DIETARY GUIDELINES FOR AMERICANS

- Consume a variety of foods within and among the basic food groups while staying within energy needs.

- Control calorie intake to manage body weight.

- Be physically active every day.

- Increase daily intake of fruits and vegetables, whole grains, and nonfat or low-fat milk and milk products.

- Choose fats wisely for good health.

- Choose carbohydrates wisely for good health.

- Choose and prepare foods with little salt.

- If you drink alcohol, do so in moderation.

- Keep food safe to eat.

(From U.S. Department of Health and Human Services and U.S. Department of Agriculture: *Dietary guidelines for Americans, 2005*, ed 6, Washington, DC, 2005, U.S Government Printing Office.)

caries is included by encouraging good oral hygiene and decreased frequent consumption of sugary and starchy foods and beverages. Sodium and potassium are highlighted, with an emphasis on choosing **potassium-rich foods** and those with less sodium. The final two recommendations of the guidelines focus on the sensible use of alcoholic beverages, and on proper food handling techniques for food safety and avoidance of food borne illness.

The Dietary Guidelines are used as a cornerstone for federal nutrition policies and education. The principles embodied in the guidelines influence national nutrition assistance programs such as the USDA's School Meals, Food Stamp Program, and the Supplemental Food Program for Women, Infants, and Children.[5,6]

The Food Guidance System

The Dietary Guidelines for Americans and the Food Guidance System replaced the Food Guide Pyramid, which was first introduced in 1992.[5,7] Key recommendations of the Dietary Guidelines are presented in an easy to use format that can be customized for the consumer. Depending on individual energy needs, specific quantities of foods from each food group are used to define potential optimal health. Furthermore, the current Food Guidance System includes physical activity assessment and recommendations for activity for the first time in the history of the Pyramid graphics.

The Center for Nutrition Policy and Promotion (CNPP), a branch of the USDA, is ultimately responsible for the promotion of the Dietary Guidelines for Americans. The "MyPyramid" (Figure 14-2), a tool designed to translate the Food Guidance System to a graphic and interactive representation, allows each person to monitor his or her food and physical activity to achieve optimum health. "MyPyramid" illustrates six recommendations including personalization, gradual improvement, physical activity, variety, moderation, and proportionality. The interactive technology afforded by the government website allows each consumer to enter his or her own age, gender, and physical activity for personal recommendations and to compare individual food intakes to the Dietary Guidelines for Americans.[5]

OVERWEIGHT AND OBESITY

In 1949 Ancel Keys stated "Under the right economic & social circumstances, obesity from overeating would be a dominant nutritional problem. While caloric intake goes up energy output goes down. The wonderful advances of technology not only free us from backbreaking toil; they make it almost impossible to get a decent amount of calorie-using exercise."[8] Overweight and obesity remain one of the primary public health problems of the twenty-first century in adults and children.[9,10] According to the WHO, a blatantly visible public health problem is mirrored in the paradoxical coexistence of undernutrition and an escalating global epidemic of overweight and obesity. The term "globesity" has become synonymous with an array of serious health disorders.[9] Changes from 1995 to 2000 in the numbers of obese adults around the globe resulted in an increase of 50%, from 200 million to 300 million, in both developed and underdeveloped countries. Approximately one in two adults was overweight and one in three adults was obese in the U.S. in 2004.[10] From 1999 to 2004 the prevalence of overweight and obesity in the United States has increased in children and men, but has remained constant among women.[11] A 37 % increase in average medical expenditures can be attributed to obesity, which translates to approximately $92.6 billion in 2002 dollars.[12]

Risk of chronic disease and select cancers has been shown to be greater in individuals who are overweight or obese.[9,10] Excess weight is considered a significant risk factor for four of the top six leading causes of death (heart disease, cancer, stroke, and diabetes).[12,13] In addition, the growing prevalence of obesity has been identified as a contributing factor in a decline in life expectancy.[14,15] The global nature of this risk has been demonstrated in the 52 Country Heart Study (INTERHEART) in which overweight and obesity, as measured by body mass index (BMI) and waist-to-hip ratio, were predictors of risk of myocardial infarction.[16]

Although international, federal, and private sectors are increasingly involved in setting policy and creating public health programs, health professionals have been encouraged to become involved on the individual consumer level to arrest this epidemic.[9,10,17-20] The U.S. Preventive Services Task Force (USPSTF) Screening for Obesity in Adults guidelines recommends that all health clinicians

Anatomy of MyPyramid

One size doesn't fit all
USDA's new MyPyramid symbolizes a personalized approach to healthy eating and physical activity. The symbol has been designed to be simple. It has been developed to remind consumers to make healthy food choices and to be active every day. The different parts of the symbol are described below.

Activity
Activity is represented by the steps and the person climbing them, as a reminder of the importance of daily physical activity.

Moderation
Moderation is represented by the narrowing of each food group from bottom to top. The wider base stands for foods with little or no solid fats or added sugars. These should be selected more often. The narrower top area stands for foods containing more added sugars and solid fats. The more active you are, the more of these foods can fit into your diet.

Personalization
Personalization is shown by the person on the steps, the slogan, and the URL. Find the kinds and amounts of food to eat each day at MyPyramid.gov.

Proportionality
Proportionality is shown by the different widths of the food group bands. The widths suggest how much food a person should choose from each group. The widths are just a general guide, not exact proportions. Check the Web site for how much is right for you.

Variety
Variety is symbolized by the 6 color bands representing the 5 food groups of the Pyramid and oils. This illustrates that foods from all groups are needed each day for good health.

Gradual Improvement
Gradual improvement is encouraged by the slogan. It suggests that individuals can benefit from taking small steps to improve their diet and lifestyle each day.

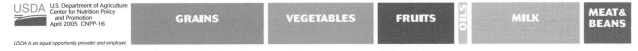

Figure 14-2   MyPyramid. (Redrawn from U.S. Department of Agriculture, Center for Nutrition Policy and Promotion: Anatomy of MyPyramid, Washington, DC, 2005, U.S. Government Printing Office; CNPP-16.)

screen adult patients for obesity.[18] Similarly, the American Academy of Pediatrics recommends that all children and adolescents be screened for risk of overweight and obesity.[21] Therefore, screenings for evidence of obesity-linked disease and disorders are the charge of all health care professionals.

The WHO advocates public health screening campaigns to alert the public and health professionals to the risks of obesity, and promotes public health measures to make "healthy choices easier."[9] The 2001 Surgeon General's "Call to Action to Prevent Overweight and Obesity" includes recommendations focused on communication, action, and research.[20] Health professionals are guided to change the perception of the disease, to educate the public (parents, expectant parents), and to provide culturally competent education programs for targeted audiences. Patient care plans focused on increasing physical activity and healthy food choices supported by the school, workplace, home and community, and advocacy for reimbursement for services for health professional's intervention are stressed. This "Call to Action" supports the need for further research into the causes and prevalence of obesity and strategies aimed at intervention, prevention, and management of this spreading problem. Because the benefits of screening and subsequent intervention by health professionals outweigh any risks, the USPTSF recommends that all health professionals in clinical care settings screen adults for obesity.[18] Outcomes as a result of weight loss include improved glucose tolerance, lipid levels, and blood pressure; all of which can impact chronic disease incidence and severity, including the risk for oral soft tissue infectious diseases.[22]

Community-based programs offer opportunities for patient referrals for those motivated to explore support to achieve a healthy body weight. The Centers for Disease Control and Prevention (CDC) Division of Nutrition and Physical Activity promotes healthful eating and physical activity to reduce overweight and obesity through funded programs in states across the United States.[23] These programs are aimed at promoting healthful lifestyles in the school setting, workplace, and community. The CDC has also developed growth charts for infants, children, and adolescents, which include calculation of BMI for age.[24]

Screening is defined as examining groups or individuals to determine those with a high probability of having or developing a specific condition or disease.[25] Simple, noninvasive, and quick techniques are usually the rule in most screening protocols. Screening for overweight and obesity includes identifying whether an individual is underweight, normal weight, overweight, or obese, and providing some level of intervention, which may be as basic as referring the individual to a registered dietitian or physician for further assessment and intervention. Anthropometric parameters used may include height and weight, body mass index (BMI), and waist and hip circumferences (see Chapter 8).

The WHO and the U.S. National Heart, Lung, and Blood Institute (NHLBI) have recommended the use of BMI to determine overweight and obesity. BMI is measured as weight in proportion to height {weight in pounds/(height in inches × height in inches)} × 703 (see Chapter 8).[9,26] Because of controversial issues in the interpretation of the BMI in different ethnic groups, however, waist-to-hip ratio appears to be a preferred measure of risk. The BMI of individuals who are very muscular may overestimate their degree of fatness because this index does not differentiate between adipose and lean body tissue. When examined across ethnic groups, BMI has been a poor predictor of disease risk, particularly for myocardial infarction. The 2005 review of the INTERHEART study demonstrated that the waist-to-hip ratio was the strongest predictor in risk of myocardial infraction across ethnicities from 52 countries.[16] In this investigation, the use of an elevated waist-to-hip ratio as a measure of obesity increased the population risk for myocardial infarction three times higher than when BMI was used. Although this is one study, its generalizability across ethnicities provides strong evidence in favor of waist-to-hip ratio, rather than BMI, as a measurement of risk for myocardial infarction.

Waist circumference provides a measure of abdominal fat and is an independent risk factor for certain chronic diseases, including dyslipidemia, type 2 diabetes, CVD, and hypertension.[26] Similarly, waist-to-hip ratio provides an estimation of abdominal fat. More precise measurements of body composition can be done with bioelectrical impedance analysis (BIA). An estimate of total body water is used to estimate an individual's **fat-free** mass and body fat with BIA instrumentation. The precision and quality of the BIA equipment combined with the expertise of the clinician and the client's state (typically fasting, at rest) impacts BIA measurements and thus may be appropriate for dental care settings.

Practice Recommendations

None of the guidelines cited herein specify the role of the dental professional in screening individuals (adults and children) for overweight or obesity.[9,18,19,26] Although limited research supports the direct relationship between overweight and obesity and oral health, the connection with other diseases associated with oral health and overall mortality is more evident. Preliminary investigations examining the relationship between oral health status and BMI have been reported in older people and in children.[27] Further research is needed to explore relationships between oral health and disease and degree of adiposity. Clinical evidence of the relationships between oral disease, degree of adiposity, and systemic health associated with chronic diseases can impact oral health.[12,13,28-30] The caloric adequacy of a varied diet is generally accepted as one index of adequate nutritional status, and provides one perspective of dietary quality. Risks associated with specific nutrient inadequacies need to be explored with additional screening and diagnostic approaches if indicated. Diagnosis of a true deficiency, however, requires a complete nutritional assessment (see Chapter 8).

Dental professionals are comprehensive care providers and as such should play a role in all health risk reduction strategies in accordance with a common risk factor approach. Just as the dental professional may encourage tobacco cessation, they can advise patients regarding diet and healthy body weight with equal assurance of the importance of these behaviors in decreasing the risk of oral and systemic diseases.

With the recent dramatic increase in type 2 diabetes mellitus in children and adolescents as a result of overweight and obesity, it is advisable for pediatric dental professionals to educate children and parents during these developmental years on weight management related to oral and systemic health and to discuss the importance of obesity prevention with parents.[29] The pediatric dental professional is in the ideal position to educate parents on the lifetime risks associated with obesity and encourage families to seek intervention from a registered dietitian. Measuring height and weight of children, calculating BMI, and educating parents are simple, noninvasive screening methods that can be used in the dental setting.

As comprehensive health care providers, dental professionals caring for adults can measure a patient's height and weight or waist circumference, calculate BMI, address the patient's degree of overweight or obesity, and make appropriate referrals to a qualified health professional specializing in weight management. Although it is outside of the scope of practice for dental professionals to provide medical nutrition therapy or weight loss counseling, they should provide general health promotion and risk reduction strategies to patients in the context of appropriate patient education.

DIABETES AND CARDIOVASCULAR DISEASES

Interactions among obesity, diabetes, cardiovascular disease, and periodontal disease have been examined in several observational studies.[30] Mechanisms among the suspected associations have not been clearly understood. Accumulating evidence suggests that chronic infections and inflammatory and immune response related to these diseases may be the linking predictor between oral and systemic health status, particularly in aging cohorts.[30] Diet and nutrition are known modulators of risks for these diseases, and modulators of optimum disease-management regimens. Numerous government and health agencies have outlined evidence-based dietary recommendations that are central to the particular management of persons with chronic diseases such as diabetes, dyslipidemia, and hypertension.[31] These are similar to the Dietary Guidelines for Americans and mirror principles of dental nutrition for the decreased risk of oral infectious diseases. Table 14-1 shows an interpretation of dietary variables across the spectrum of chronic diseases that have been investigated for links with periodontal disease and dental caries. This framework can provide a template for addressing health promotion in a dental practice.

OSTEOPOROSIS

The relationship between systemic osteoporosis and oral bone loss has not been definitively identified. Numerous studies suggest that findings on dental panoramic radiographs can be used to detect individuals with low bone mineral density (BMD).[32] Osteoporosis is defined as a systemic skeletal disease characterized by low bone mass and microarchitectural deterioration of bone tissue, with a consequent increase in bone fragility and susceptibility to fracture.[33] According to the WHO, osteopenia (low bone mass) and osteoporosis are defined on the basis of the standard deviation of the BMD score of the individual below the mean for a young adult or their T-score.[9] When bone mass declines, the risk of fracture rises, particularly of the hip, spine, and wrist. In the United States, four out of every 10 (40%) white women 50 years or older will suffer a fracture of the hip, spine, or wrist in their lifetime as compared with 13% of white men, who will sustain a fracture as a result of osteoporosis.[34] It is projected that by the year 2010, 40 million adults older than age 50 years will have osteopenia (low bone mass) with another 12 million having osteoporosis. In 2020, projections are for more than 47 million individuals with osteopenia and 14 million with osteoporosis.[35]

This increasingly prevalent disease will lead to increased health care costs, which will include oral health care.

Osteoporosis is no longer an older person's disease, but is increasing in younger generations. Risk indicators for osteoporosis are listed in Box 14-3. Physical inactivity and inadequate calcium and vitamin D intake have increased risk of this disease in the young and the elderly in both men and women. Studies have demonstrated significant relationships among tooth loss, periodontal disease, low calcium intake, and osteoporosis in older men and women who are notably at increased risk of both osteoporosis and periodontal disease.[35-40] The research, although limited, has demonstrated that total calcium intake (in part from calcium supplements) is significantly associated with the odds of tooth loss in elderly men and women, and that higher serum vitamin D {25(OH)D3} levels are associated with less loss of periodontal attachment in adults older than 50 years.[37,38] Vitamin D is necessary for calcium absorption. In osteoporosis, calcium is more easily mobilized from trabecular bone found in the distal radius, head of the femur and vertebrae, and the alveolar bone. Mandibular bone mass is highly correlated with bone mass in other parts of the body including the spine. Yoshihara found a significant relationship between periodontal disease and bone mineral density in healthy elders in Japan.[39] Others have demonstrated a significant relationship between alveolar bone loss and bone mineral density finding that those with osteoporosis lose significantly more alveolar bone than those without.[40] Despite these relationships, the scientific evidence is limited and therefore cannot be considered conclusive.[41] All health professionals, including dental professionals, have a role in promoting bone health, identifying patients at risk for osteoporosis, and providing patient education that includes strategies to reduce the risk of bone loss and fractures.

Practice Recommendations

The 2004 U.S. Surgeon General's Report on Osteoporosis supports the role of all health professionals, including dental professionals, in osteoporosis risk screening to identify individuals at risk, provide baseline risk reduction strategies, promote bone health, and refer patients to physicians for BMD density testing.[34,35]

In addition to oral hygiene, dental prophylaxis, and smoking cessation, every oral health professional can operationalize the following three key steps: (1) integrate risk factor screening into new patient and routine history and examinations; (2) stress the importance of good bone health, including weight-bearing exercise and diets rich in calcium and vitamin D; and (3) refer patients with known high-risk factors such as associated chronic diseases or long-term steroid use to physicians for assessment of osteopenia or osteoporosis.

A simple strategy for dietary screening of calcium adequacy from the National Osteoporosis Foundation is

TABLE 14-1

INTERPRETATION OF DIETARY GUIDELINES FOR PROMOTION OF GENERAL AND ORAL HEALTH

DIETARY VARIABLE	COMMON FOOD SOURCES	OBESITY	DIABETES	DYSLIPIDEMIA	HYPERTENSION	DENTAL HEALTH PROMOTION MESSAGE
Total calories		Recommend calories to promote weight and portion control and regular eating patterns.				Frequent eating increases risk of caries and weight gain.
Total fat	Fatty meats, high-fat dairy foods, and processed foods. Added fats such as spreads, oils, dressings, and sauces.	Suggest 25%-35% of total daily calorie intake. (1 g of fat = 9 calories) Example: 2000 × .30 = 600 calories ÷ 9 = 67 g			High-fat, processed foods are usually high in sodium and salt content.[1]	Choose low-fat foods and vegetable oils such as olive and canola oils that interfere with adherence of food to the tooth surface and that provide dietary sources of healthy fats.
Saturated fat	Fats from animal sources and palm and coconut oils, hydrogenated fats.			Suggest <7% of total daily calorie intake Example: 2000 × .07 = 140 calories ÷ 9 = 16 g		
Polyunsaturated fat	Vegetable oils and fats.			Suggest <10% of total daily calorie intake Example: 2000 × .10 = 200 calories ÷ 9 = 22 g		
Trans fat	Hydrogenated fats and oils.			Minimize intake to zero.		
Omega fatty acids	Fish, nut, and seed oils.			Suggest one to two servings of fish per week.		
Total carbohydrate	Fresh fruit and vegetables, breads and cereals, added sugars, and processed foods such as cake, cookies, and crackers.	Recommend choices to promote weight management and portion control. Encourage selection of a variety of 5-9 daily servings of fruits and vegetables. Promote whole-grain foods. (1 gram of carbohydrate = 4 calories) Suggest 45%-65% of total daily calorie intake. Example: 2000 × .60 = 1200 ÷ 4 = 300 g				Fruits, vegetables, and whole grains promote mastication and salivary flow and activity of antibacterial salivary components.
Dietary fiber	Fruit and vegetables, legumes, beans, and whole grain breads and cereals.	14 g per 1000 calories	20-35 g per day	10-25 g/day of soluble fiber from foods such as oats and beans.	5-9 servings fruits and vegetables. 5 servings of grains.	

Simple sugars	Brown and white sugar, corn syrup, soft drinks, candy, cakes, cookies, and sweetened dairy foods.	Restrict to <10% of total daily calories. Example: $2000 \times .10 = 20 \div 4 = 5$ g	Achieve good glycemic control. Minimize simple sugar intake.	Excessive and frequent sugar intake is associated with increased risk of caries and dental plaque.
Total protein	Meats, chicken, fish, eggs, beans, legumes, dairy foods, breads, and cereals.	Recommend 10%–35% of total daily calories on the basis of individual needs. Promote low-fat and lean choices. (1 g of protein = 4 calories) Example: $2000 \times .25 = 500 \div 4 = 125$ g	2–3 servings daily of low-fat dairy products.	Dietary protein can buffer and neutralize an acidic oral environment and promotes healthy oral tissues.
Eating patterns	Dietary eating patterns to support decreased risk of chronic diseases and to promote general and oral health encourage typical meal (breakfast, lunch, and dinner) and snacking (1 to 2 per day) patterns to include a variety of foods that are nutrient dense and spaced to allow for digestion, physical activity, and a return of oral plaque pH to neutral levels.			

(Adapted from: *Diet, nutrition, and the prevention of chronic disease. Report of a Joint WHO/FAO Expert Consultation*, Geneva, Switzerland, 2003. WHO Technical Report Series 916; Institute Of Medicine Of The National Academies: *Dietary reference intakes for energy, carbohydrate, fiber, fat, fatty acids, cholesterol, protein, and amino acids (macronutrients)*,Washington, DC, 2005, The National Academies Press; *Third report of the expert panel on detection, evaluation, and treatment of high blood cholesterol in adults (adult treatment panel III), NHLBI, NIH 2002*, NIH Publication No. 02–5215; American Diabetes Association: Clinical practice recommendations, *Diabetes Care* 29(Suppl 1):S10, 2006.)

BOX 14-3

Risk Indicators for Osteoporosis

- Women aged 65 years or older
- Family history of osteoporosis
- Immediate female family member with history of adult fracture
- Personal history of bone fracture after age 50 years
- Cigarette smoker
- Amenorrhea
- Early menopause (before age 45 years)
- Low body weight
- Physical inactivity
- Prolonged history of low dietary calcium intake
- Use of medications associated with bone loss (i.e., steroids, excessive thyroxine replacement, antiepileptic medications, immunosuppressive agents)
- Diseases associated with osteoporosis risk (i.e., hyperthyroidism, chronic pulmonary disease, endometriosis, hyperparathyroidism, cancer, chronic liver or renal disease, Cushing's disease, multiple sclerosis, rheumatoid arthritis, sarcoidosis, inflammatory bowel disease, hemachromatosis, vitamin D deficiency)

(From National Osteoporosis Foundation: *Physician's guide to prevention and treatment of osteoporosis*, Washington, DC, 2003; and Public Health Service, United States Department of Health and Human Services: *bone health and osteoporosis: a report of the Surgeon General*, Rockville, MD, 2004, Office of the Surgeon General.)

BOX 14-4

Estimating Daily Dietary Calcium Intake

STEP 1: ESTIMATE CALCIUM INTAKE FROM CALCIUM-RICH FOODS.*

PRODUCT	NO. OF SERVINGS/DAY	CONTENT PER SERVING, mg calcium, mg	
Milk (8 oz) _____	× 300	= _____
Yogurt (8 oz) _____	× 400	= _____
Cheese (1 oz) _____	× 200	= _____
Fortified foods or juices _____	× 80-1000†	= _____

STEP 2: TOTAL FROM ABOVE + 250 mg FOR NONDAIRY SOURCES = TOTAL DIETARY CALCIUM.

*Approximately 75% to 80% of the calcium consumed in American diets is from dairy products.
†Calcium content of fortified foods varies.
(From National Osteoporosis Foundation: *Physician's guide to prevention and treatment of osteoporosis*, Washington, DC, 2003.)

development and can make timely referral of patients for bone mineral density testing. Patients with osteoporosis or at risk for the disease can be referred to physicians, registered dietitians, and other health professionals for appropriate intervention.

shown in Box 14-4.[35] Dietary recommendations for calcium for adults in the United States are based on age, gender, and other disease and medication factors. In general, for healthy adults, 18 to 50 years of age, 1000 mg of calcium and 200 IU of vitamin D are the daily recommendations, with recommended increased intakes of calcium and vitamin D for those older than 51 years of age.[34] Table 14-2 shows calcium and vitamin D recommendations by age and gender, and Box 14-5 lists dietary sources of these nutrients. Dental practitioners should also question patients regarding calcium supplement use. Foods, particularly dairy products because of their high elemental calcium content and absorption rate, should be encouraged as the primary source of calcium intake. Supplements are an alternative for those unable to meet their needs through diet.[42] Calcium carbonate and calcium citrate are the calcium supplements with the highest rates of absorption.[34] Guidelines for calcium and vitamin D supplementation are listed in Box 14-6.

All health professionals, including dental professionals, can play a role in identifying osteoporosis risk early in its

TABLE 14-2

DAILY REFERENCE INTAKE OF CALCIUM AND VITAMIN D BY AGE AND GENDER

GROUPS BY AGE*	CALCIUM mg/day	VITAMIN D† mcg/day
0-6 months	210	5
7-12 months	270	5
1-3 years	500	5
4-8 years	800	5
9-18 years	1300	5
19-50 years	1000	5
51-≥70 years	1200	10
>70 years	1200	15
PREGNANCY AND LACTATION		
≤18 years	1300	5
19-50 years	1000	5

*All groups except pregnancy and lactation are male and female.
†One mcg cholecalciferol = 40 IU vitamin D.
(From Institute of Medicine, Food and Nutrition Board: *Dietary reference intakes for calcium, magnesium, vitamin D and fluoride*, Washington, DC, 1997, National Academy Press.)

BOX 14-5

DIETARY SOURCES OF CALCIUM AND VITAMIN D

CALCIUM	VITAMIN D
• Milk, nonfat, reduced-fat, and whole • Cheese • Yogurt • Sardines • Salmon • Calcium-enriched juices and beverages	• Salmon • Tuna fish • Sardines • Milk, nonfat, reduced-fat, and whole, vitamin D-fortified • Ready-to-eat cereals fortified with 10% of the daily value for vitamin D • Cod liver Oil

SUMMARY

The Surgeon General's Report on Oral Health suggests three key components as a strategic framework for action to improve oral and systemic health.[3] The signs and symptoms of oral disease or sequalae of chronic disease are often regarded as minor or less important than other

BOX 14-6

GUIDELINES FOR CALCIUM AND VITAMIN D SUPPLEMENTATION

1. Take calcium supplements that have vitamin D added.
2. Take no more than 500 mg of calcium in any single dose.
3. Do not take a calcium supplement within 4 hours of taking iron supplements or thyroid medications, because it may reduce absorption of these substances.
4. Buy products that list the amount of elemental calcium in the product in order to meet your recommended intake. Calcium carbonate is 40% elemental calcium, and calcium citrate is 20% elemental calcium. For example, if a requirement is 1000 mg a day, it will be necessary to take 5 tablets of 500 mg of calcium carbonate (500 × .40 = 200 mg Ca) throughout the day to meet needs. Calcium carbonate should be taken with meals; calcium citrate may be taken independent of meals and may be better absorbed in older adults.
5. Select supplements that meet the U.S. Pharmacopoeia standards for lead levels.

systemic symptoms. The first strategy is to change perceptions and improve the public's understanding of the relationships between the mouth and the rest of the body. Messages should target all populations, crossing language and culture barriers. The second strategy is to change policymakers' perceptions of the importance of oral health and the burdens of oral disease on the American society. The third and final strategy is to change the health providers' perceptions. The nondental provider must be educated on the importance of oral health and disease, highlighting the relationships between oral health and systemic health. Similarly, the dental professional should acknowledge the link between systemic and oral disease. Specific examples are to include an oral examination as part of the physical examination, address dietary patterns and choices, advocate for the cessation of tobacco use, and collaborate with health professionals in the interest of the patient's overall health.[3]

Health promotion and disease prevention strategies are fundamental to health care practice, yet some of the most effective and widely accepted approaches are not routinely advocated in some health care settings.[43] Barriers to preventive care result from clinicians' practice patterns, patients, and health care settings. Clinicians may have competing demands for their time or lack training in prevention, knowledge of existing services, or both. Patients may not know what to ask or not understand the relationships between risk factors and disease. Health care settings may be insufficiently reimbursed for services or may not integrate prevention to primary health care.[43] Dental practitioners have the knowledge and training to recognize the associations between oral health and general health. This enables them to collaborate with other health care team members, policy makers, patients, and the community to identify risk factors common to several diseases. Subsequently, procedures to communicate the health promotion messages may be implemented at all levels in an effort to achieve optimal health and improve the quality of life among all patients, regardless of inequities.

Oral health promotion and disease prevention strategies should be established within routine dental care environments. Screening patients for medical and drug histories, including anthropometric, dietary, and physical activity assessments, requires minimal time, yet may yield important data. The patient who perceives the dental professional as a member of the comprehensive health care team will become a member of that provider's dental family. Patient education that includes global messages about dietary choices and patterns and that is coupled with appropriate referrals for more extensive dietary counseling and intervention enhances the perceived expertise of the dental professional. Simple approaches to exploring dietary intake patterns and to providing key nutrition education messages or appropriate referrals contribute to a comprehensive and successful care plan uniquely tailored to each dental patient.

REFERENCES

1. Peterson PE: The World Oral Health Report (website): http://www.who.int/oral_health/publications/report03/en/index.html. Accessed 11-13-05.
2. Sheiham A, Watt RG: The common risk factor approach: a rational basis for promoting oral health, *Commun Dent Oral Epidemiol* 28:399-406, 2000.
3. U.S. Department of Health and Human Services: *Oral health in America: A Report of the Surgeon General*, U.S. Department of Health and Human Services, National Institute of Dental and Craniofacial Research, National Institutes of Health (website): http://www.surgeongeneral.gov/library/oralhealth. Accessed November 15, 2005.
4. U.S. Department of Health and Human Services, Office of Disease Prevention and Health Promotion: *Healthy people 2010* (website): http://www.healthypeople.gov/. Accessed December 2, 2005.
5. U.S. Department of Health and Human Services and U.S. Department of Agriculture: *Dietary guidelines for Americans, 2005*, ed 6, Washington, DC, 2005, U.S Government Printing Office.
6. U.S. Department of Agriculture: *Women, infants and children* (website): http://www.fns.usda.gov/wic/. Accessed December 2, 2005.
7. The Food Guidance System: http://mypyramid.gov, accessed November 13, 2005.
8. Keys A: The management of obesity, *Minn Med* 48:1329-1331, 1965.
9. World Health Organization: Controlling the global obesity epidemic, September 2003, (website): http://www.who.int/nut/obs.htm. Accessed September 16, 2005.
10. Centers for Disease Control and Prevention: Overweight and obesity home (website): http://www.cdc.gov/nccdphp/dnpa/obesity. Accessed September 16, 2005.
11. Ogden CL, Carroll MD, Curtin LR et al.: Prevalence of overweight and obesity in the United States, 1999-2004, *JAMA* 295:1549-1555, 2006.
12. Finkelstein EA, Fiebelkorn IC, Wang G: National medical spending attributable to overweight and obesity: how much, and who's paying? *Health Affairs Web Exclusive.* 2003;W3:219-226. Available at: http://content.healthaffairs.org/cgi/content/full/hlthaff.w3.219v1/DC1.
13. Jemal A, Ward E, Hao Y et al.: Treads in the leading causes of death in the United States, 1970–2002, *J Am Med Assoc* 294:1255-1259, 2005.
14. Flegal KM, Graubard BI, Williamson DF et al.: Excess deaths associated with underweight, overweight, and obesity, *JAMA* 293:1861-1867, 2005.
15. Olshansky SJ, Passaro DJ, Hershow RC et al.: A potential decline in life expectancy in the United States in the 21st century, *N Engl J Med* 352:1138-1145, 2005.
16. Yusef S, Hawkens S, Ounpuu S et al.: Obesity and the risk of myocardial infarction in 2700 participants from 52 countries: a case control study, *Lancet* 366:1640-1649, 2005.
17. Clinical guidelines on the identification, evaluation, and treatment of overweight and obesity in adults, National Institutes of Health, National Heart, Lung, and Blood Institute: The Evidence Report. National Institutes of Health (publication number 98-4083) (website): http://www.nhlbi.nih.gov/guidelines/obesity/ob_gdlns.htm. June 1998.
18. U.S. Preventive Services Task Force: Screening for obesity in adults (website): http://www.ahrq.gov/clinic/uspstf/uspsobes.htm. Accessed September 16, 2005.
19. U.S. Department of Health and Human Services: Weight Control Information Network (website): http://win.niddk.nih.gov/statistics/index.htm. Accessed September 16, 2005.
20. U.S. Department of Health and Human Services: The Surgeon General's call to action to prevent and decrease overweight and obesity, Rockville, MD, 2001, U.S. Department of Health and Human Services, Public Health Service, Office of the Surgeon General Available from Washington DC, Government Printing Office.
21. American Academy of Pediatrics: AAP recommendations from the prevention of pediatric overweight and obesity, *Pediatrics* 112: 424-430, 2003.
22. Beck JD, Offenbacher S: Systemic effects of periodontitis: epidemiology of periodontal disease and cardiovascular disease, *J Periodontol* 76:2089-2100, 2005.
23. Centers for Disease Control and Prevention, Division of Nutrition and Physical Activity. Physical Activity Topics (website): http://www.cdc.gov/nccdphp/dnpa/physical/index.htm. Accessed September 16, 2005.
24. Centers for Disease Control and Prevention: Growth charts, 2000 (website): http://www.cdc.gov/growthcharts/. Accessed September 16, 2005.
25. *The American Heritage Stedman's Medical Dictionary*, Boston, 2002, Houghton Mifflin Company.
26. National Heart, Lung, and Blood Institute and the North American Association for the Study of Obesity: The practical guide: identification, evaluation, and treatment of overweight and obesity in adults, Bethesda, MD, 2000, National Institutes of Health publication 00-4084 (website): http://www.nhlbi.nih.gov/guidelines/obesity/practgde.htm. Accessed September 16, 2005.
27. Kantovitz KR, Pascon FM, Rontani RMP et al.: Obesity and dental caries—a systematic review, *Oral Health Prev Dent* 4: 137-144, 2006.
28. Houpt M: Childhood obesity—a growing epidemic, *Pediatr Dent* 25:422, 2003.
29. Cara JF, Chaiken RL: Type 2 diabetes and the metabolic syndrome in children and adolescents, *Curr Diab Rep* 6:2412-2450, 2006.
30. Beck JD, Offenbacher S: Systemic effects of periodontitis: epidemiology of periodontal disease and cardiovascular disease, *J Periodontol* 76:2089-2100, 2005.
31. Mobley CC: Lifestyle interventions for "Diabesity": the state of the science, *Compendium* 25:207-218, 2004.
32. Dervis E: Oral implications of osteoporosis, *Oral Surg Oral Med Oral Pathol Oral Radiol Endod* 100:349-356, 2005.
33. Merck (website): http://www.merckmedicus.com/pp/us/hcp/diseasemodules/osteoporosis/default.jsp. Accessed September 15, 2005.
34. Public Health Service, United States Department of Health and Human Services: *Bone health and osteoporosis: a report of the Surgeon General*, Rockville, MD, 2004, Office of the Surgeon General.
35. National Osteoporosis Foundation: *Physician's guide to prevention and treatment of osteoporosis* (website): http://www.nof.org/_vti?bin/shtml.dll/physguide/index.htm. Accessed October 22, 2004.
36. Nishida M, Grossi SG, Dunford RG et al.: Calcium and the risk for periodontal disease, *J Periodontol* 71:1057-1066, 2000.
37. Krall E et al.: Calcium and vitamin D supplements reduce tooth loss in the elderly, *Am J Med* 111:452-456, 2001.
38. Dietrich T: Association between serum concentrations of 25-hydroxyvitamin D3 and periodontal disease in the US population, *Am J Clin Nutr* 80:108-113, 2004.
39. Yoshihara A, Seida Y, Hanada N et al.: A longitudinal study of the relationship between periodontal disease and bone mineral density

in community-dwelling older adults, *J Clin Periodontol* 21:680-684, 2004.

40. Payne JB, Reinhardt RA, Nummikoski PV et al.: Longitudinal alveolar bone loss in postmenopausal osteoporotic/osteopenic women, *Osteoporos Int* 10:34-40, 1999.

41. Payne JB, Reinhardt RA, Nummikoski PV et al.: Longitudinal alveolar bone loss in postmenopausal osteoporotic/osteopenic women, *Osteoporos Int* 10:34-40, 1999.

42. The role of calcium in peri- and postmenopausal women: consensus opinion of the North American Menopause Society, *Menopause* 8:84-99, 2001.

43. AHRQ: *A step-by-step guide to delivering clinical preventive services: a systems approach* (website): http://www.ahrq.gov/ppip/manual. Accessed November 13, 2005.

Chapter 15

Prevention Strategies for Dental Caries

JOHN P. BROWN AND MICHAEL W. J. DODDS

CLINICAL APPROACHES FOR CARIES PREVENTION

PROFESSIONALLY APPLIED PREVENTIVE AGENTS AND PROCEDURES

> Fluorides
> Pit and Fissure Sealants

PREVENTIVE AGENTS FOR SELF-APPLICATION: CHEMOPREVENTION

> Fluoride Gels by Prescription
> Fluoride Rinses without Prescription
> Dentifrices
> Fluoride Supplements by Prescription
> Antimicrobials by Prescription
> Xylitol and Sorbitol
> Diet and Plaque Control

RISK-BASED PREVENTION

> **Low Caries Risk**
> **Moderate Caries Risk**
> **High Caries Risk**

SUMMARY

LEARNING OBJECTIVES

Upon completion of this chapter, the learner will be able to:
- Describe differences between primary, secondary, and tertiary prevention.
- Outline the objectives of the Clinical Prevention and Population Health Framework and its relevance to caries prevention.
- Outline clinical preventive services for the treatment of dental caries.
- Detail the different types of fluoride and other products available for the prevention of dental caries and their use in prevention by professionals and individuals.
- Explain the application of risk-based preventive strategies.

KEY TERMS

Caries activity
Caries risk
Primary prevention
Remineralization
Secondary prevention
Tertiary prevention

The prevention of dental caries includes measures to prevent the occurrence of disease, such as risk factor reduction, but also to arrest the progress of disease and reduce consequences of disease once it is established.[1] **Primary prevention** is directed toward preventing the initial occurrence of disease and maintaining physiological equilibrium[2] (Figure 15-1). Primary prevention also focuses on altering the susceptibility or reducing the exposure for susceptible individuals. **Secondary prevention** addresses early detection and intervention to prevent disease progression, including nonoperative treatment. Finally, **tertiary prevention** addresses alleviation of disability and loss of function resulting from caries and attempts to restore effective functioning. In oral health practice, tertiary prevention focuses on restorative and prosthodontic methods.

Strategies for individual prevention based on risk assessment are integrated into the health professions curriculum for prevention and population health. The Clinical Prevention and Population Health Framework

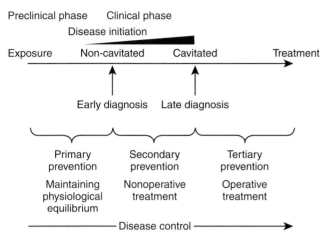

Figure 15-1 Prevention as it applies to the progression of dental caries and disease control. (Modified from Fejerskov O, Nyvad B: Is dental caries an infectious disease? Diagnostic and treatment consequences for the practitioner. In Schou L (ed): *Nordic Dentistry 2003 Yearbook*. Copenhagen, Quintessence Publishing, 2003, pp. 141-151.)

(CPPHF) has four components: (1) the evidence base of practice, (2) clinical preventive services including health promotion, (3) health systems and health policy, and (4) community aspects of practice.[3] Specifically, the clinical preventive services and health promotion component of the curriculum has the following four domains: (1) screening, including risk estimation; (2) counseling for health behavior change, to include plaque control and dietary change as needed; (3) professionally applied preventive procedures; and (4) personally applied preventive formulations, referred to here as chemoprevention. Chapter 4 provides an in-depth discussion of the first phase of the preventive process, which is detection of disease for risk estimation. The second phase of prevention, counseling, is reviewed in Chapters 10 and 11. This chapter will address both professionally applied prevention and self-applied chemoprevention of dental caries, domains (3) and (4) above.

Protocols to address prevention and treatment of the initial carious lesion were developed at the University of Texas Health Science Center at San Antonio. Although these algorithms are not definitive, they provide guidelines based on the current science. Four algorithms were developed at the caries lesion level for adults and on the basis of the tooth surface involved: fissured surfaces (Figure 15-2), approximal surfaces (Figure 15-3), smooth surfaces (Figure 15-4), and root surfaces (Figure 15-5).

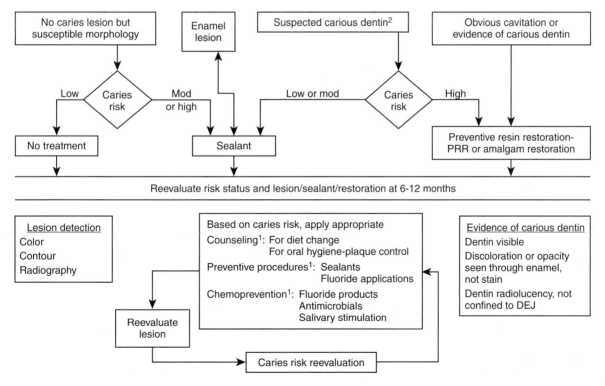

[1]Follows the schema of the curriculum framework in prevention for oral health professions. *Am J Prev Med* 27. 471-476, 2004.
[2]'Suspected' carious dentin implies no clear decision reached, despite having applied visual, radiographic and other applicable tests.

Figure 15-2 Algorithm for the assessment and management of the initial carious lesion in fissured surfaces. (Modified from Brown JP, Dodge WW, Dove SB, Summit JB, University of Texas Health Science Center at San Antonio.)

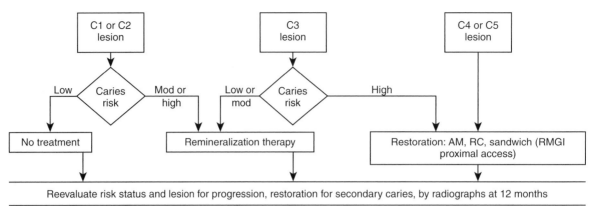

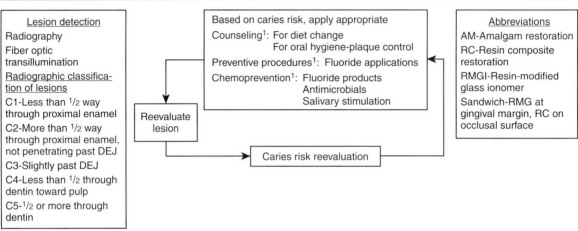

[1]Follows the schema of the curriculum framework in prevention for oral health professions. *Am J Prev Med* 27. 471-476, 2004.

Figure 15-3   Algorithm for the assessment and management of the initial carious lesion in coronal proximal surfaces. (Modified from Brown JP, Dodge WW, Dove SB, Summit JB, University of Texas Health Science Center at San Antonio.)

These algorithms have similarities in structure. The initial process involves both caries detection and risk estimation. Prevention is based on an assessment of those findings and primary, secondary, or tertiary prevention of the lesion is recommended. Primary prevention for the patient based on risk status is paramount and, although it appears separately on the algorithm, it is meant to be incorporated into the treatment plan.

CLINICAL APPROACHES FOR CARIES PREVENTION

Risk-based preventive strategies for dental caries depend on two assumptions. The first is that the patient who is at increased risk will be identified. The second assumption is that once identified, the patient will receive appropriate preventive care based on etiological factors for that person, to reduce the likelihood that the disease will either occur or progress.[4] Risk identification is discussed in Chapter 4. With Chapters 10 and 11, this chapter describes and applies the preventive strategies that are available (Table 15-1).

PROFESSIONALLY APPLIED PREVENTIVE AGENTS AND PROCEDURES

The benefits of fluoride in caries prevention extend throughout the life span. A description of these age-specific guidelines appears in Table 15-2. The Centers for Disease Control and Prevention (CDC) recommend that all persons use optimally fluoridated water when possible and brush twice daily with fluoride toothpaste.[27]

Fluorides.   Fluoride remains one hallmark of dental caries prevention. In 1942 Bibby first showed caries reductions in children when they were administered topical fluoride applications.[5] Since this early work, professional fluoride applications have been effective in reducing dental caries. Studies demonstrated that a caries reduction rate of 20% to 40% can be achieved by using these products.[6] The American Dental Association (ADA) recognizes the efficacy of topical fluoride agents in preventing dental decay. Three specific professionally applied fluoride products are most often used

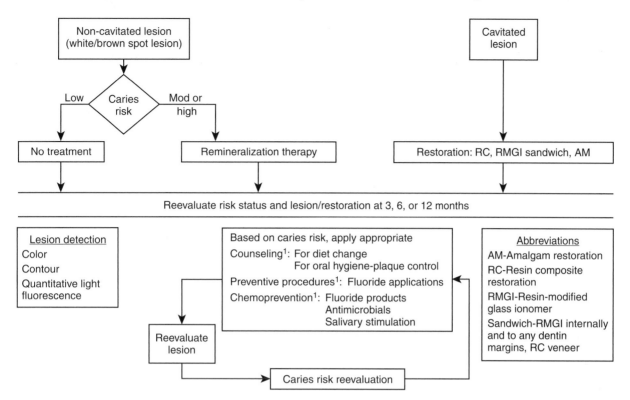

Figure 15-4 Algorithm for the assessment and management of the initial carious lesion in coronal-free smooth surfaces. (Modified from Brown JP, Dodge WW, Dove SB, Summit JB, University of Texas Health Science Center at San Antonio.)

clinically today. These are 1.23% acidulated phosphate fluoride (APF), 2% neutral sodium fluoride, and 5% fluoride varnish. The best efficacy is for 1.23% APF. The ADA Council on Scientific Affairs concluded that these agents are beneficial in reducing rates of decay.[7] Preventive products are listed in Table 15-1.

Acidulated phosphate fluoride (APF 1.23%, 12,300 ppm F, pH 3.2) is available as solution, gel or thixotropic gel, and as a foam. The thixotropic gel is preferred because of pH stability and reduced likelihood of swallowing. Brudevold (1963) developed APF by acidifying sodium fluoride (NaF) with phosphoric acid.[8] He found that the use of a phosphate-containing acid alters the equilibrium in favor of hydroxyapatite/fluorapatite formation, thereby strengthening the enamel structure. At a low pH (pH = 3.2), more than 50% of fluoride ion is present as uncharged hydrogen fluoride (HF) and this will diffuse into enamel: $H+ + F- \sim HF$. This reaction with enamel is the key benefit of APF over neutral NaF. Sodium fluoride (NaF) 2.0% (8000 ppm fluoride ion) is available as a gel or foam. It is less effective than APF because the acidulation facilitates uptake; however, the acidity in APF may etch some restorative materials. Because NaF is neutral, it is used for patients with porcelain and glass ionomer restorations; however, the efficacy is less well established than APF.

Both the APF and NaF materials are applied similarly. A minimum amount of the gel should be applied to fully coat the liner of disposable foam trays. The gel should fully coat the teeth, but not extrude from the tray. Before seating the tray, the material should be distributed using the wooden end of a cotton-tipped applicator to distribute material evenly. The trays should be inserted into the mouth and care taken to make certain that very little of the gel is swallowed. Because fluoride acidity and the tray itself stimulate salivation, suction should be used to remove saliva and excess material. The trays should be applied for 4 minutes for maximum efficacy. A 1-minute application shows equivalent fluoride uptake, but the efficacy data on actual caries reduction is lacking. Therefore, the 1-minute application is not recommended. After 4 minutes, the trays can be removed and discarded. The teeth should be completely wiped to remove retained gel, and suctioned to extract additional material. The individual should be asked to spit out any of the remaining gel. After the professional fluoride treatment, patients should be instructed to refrain from eating or drinking for at least 30 minutes.

Fluoride varnishes (5% NaF, 23,000 ppm F) can be applied to the entire mouth as a preventive measure and

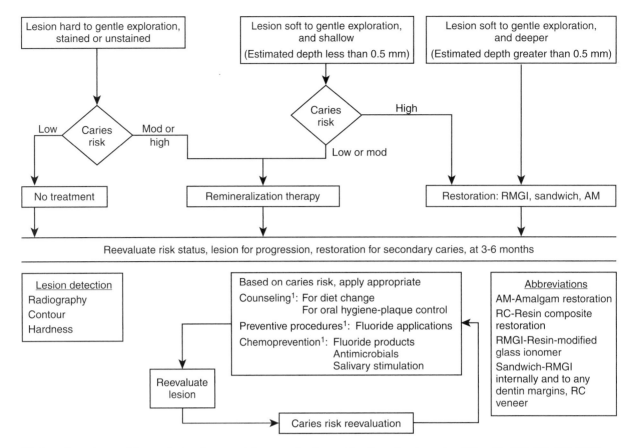

Figure 15-5 Algorithm for the assessment and management of the initial carious lesion in root surfaces. (Modified from Brown JP, Dodge WW, Dove SB, Summit JB, University of Texas Health Science Center at San Antonio.)

have caries-reducing benefits comparable to conventional APF. Varnishes come in a tube [Duraflor, Duraphat], or in unit doses (CavityShield, 0.25 ml and 0.4 ml). The advantage of using a fluoride varnish is small volume, and therefore low dose, that can be applied while administering a high concentration and, because of the adhesion to the tooth, a long application time. Because of these features, it is advocated especially for preventing/arresting early childhood caries. Children younger than 6 years are at greater risk for swallowing the gels or rinses and in these cases, fluoride varnish has a distinct advantage over the tray products. Fluoride varnish for caries prevention is used routinely, but this use continues to remain "off-label" or without FDA approval for that particular use. Canadian and European studies support the efficacy of fluoride varnish.[9,10]

Fluoride varnish application is also recommended for secondary prevention (**remineralization**) of early carious lesions on smooth surfaces. The high concentration of fluoride in the varnish may block the relatively intact enamel surface by precipitated CaF, preventing deeper remineralization in the body of the carious lesion. Remineralization of the early lesion should be considered when the lesion is noncavitated (enamel caries) and the patient is at a moderate or high risk for caries development or there is a high likelihood that the lesion is active (currently undergoing demineralization). **Caries activity** *in vivo* can only be determined by longitudinal observation.

Lesion appearance is an important criterion when considering remineralization. For remineralization of approximal surfaces, clinical caries detection methods should indicate whether the lesion is limited to enamel (see Figure 15-3). Lesions should also be considered for remineralization if slight spread is observed at the dentoenamel junction (DEJ) and the individual is at low or moderate **caries risk**. Smooth surface lesions can be remineralized if the clinical examination indicates enamel caries. Clinically, the lesions should have a chalky or matte appearance with no evidence of cavitation. Lesions that are accompanied by visible plaque deposits and/or adjacent gingival inflammation should be considered as active. When inactive, the enamel surface is less chalky and has a more polished appearance. Root surfaces can be considered for remineralization if the demineralized lesion is less than 0.5 mm in depth.

TABLE 15-1

PREVENTIVE PRODUCTS GUIDE

I. PROFESSIONALLY APPLIED PRODUCTS OR AVAILABLE BY PRESCRIPTION

PRODUCT	USE	METHOD	FORM
Sodium Fluoride supplements	Written Professional Rx Personal use	Children and teens, daily. Preferably chew, swish, and swallow. Check dose for age and water F level. (See dosage chart below)	Tabs, 0.25, 0.5, 1.0 mg. (1) as F⁻, Rx ≤120mg F mg in total For Drops conc. F varies by manufacturer. (1)
1.23% Acidulated Phosphate Fluoride	Professional APF Gel	Child & adult in foam-lined trays for 4 min without swallowing. Use minimum amount to coat liner and teeth. Remove, fully wipe teeth with gauze, H.V. suction, spit out. Moderate risk every 6 months. High risk every 3 months. 1 minute app~ not recommended, as is based on F uptake not caries reduction	Flavored (1) Do not swallow 12,300 ppm F⁻
	Professional APF Solution	For persons who do not tolerate trays, use cotton roll isolation, apply with cotton tip for 4 min.	Flavored (1) Do not swallow 12,300 ppm F⁻
2.0% Neutral Sodium Fluoride	Professional Gel	Adults. Root sensitivity. Root caries. Use cotton roll isolation, or tray. Also use neutral NaF gel to avoid etch of porcelain and GIC	Flavored "Flurocare" 2.0% NaF = 8,000 ppm F⁻
Fluoride Varnish 5% NaF	Professional Topical Varnish	Children and adults. Remineralization therapy. Certain selected high risk patients, early childhood caries. See protocol for patient selection and method (6)	"Dura-flor," "Durphat" "Cavity Shield" – unit dose of 0.25 and 0.4 ml (5-9mg F) 23 mg F⁻/mL 23,000 ppm F⁻
0.717% F⁻(NaF, SnF2, HF Solutionᴺ)	Professional application for root sensitivity	Apply to saliva moistened teeth at sites affected. Unit dose 0.6 mL	"Dentin Bloc" 7,170 ppm F⁻
Potassium Oxalate Solution	Professional application for root sensitivity	Apply to affected sites. Unit dose 0.6 mL	"Protect"
Sealants	Professional	Stained, retentive, or fissures with enamel (incipient) caries of children and young adults, preferably soon after eruption. Dry field essential	"UltraShield"—F⁻ Releasing white, light activated "Concise" —white, chemically activated (1)

Continued

TABLE 15-1

PREVENTIVE PRODUCTS GUIDE—cont'd

PRODUCT	USE	METHOD	FORM
1.23% APF prophylaxis paste or non-fluoride paste	Professional	Rubber cup—do not use this or other fluoride or oil containing products prior to placing sealants, use plain pumice	Fine or med abrasive Do not swallow

II. SPECIAL SELF APPLICATIONS BY RX

PRODUCT	USE	METHOD	FORM
0.2% Sodium Fluoride Rinse	Group use-Rx item School prevention program. in non-F area with population at risk	Elementary, junior, and high school. Weekly rinse, not for pre-school Do not swallow	"Medical Products" (1) 900 ppm F⁻
0.4% Stannous Fluoride	Personal use gel Written Rx or give gel to patient with written instructions (Rx required, but same strength SnF₂ as original 'Crest' toothpaste [no longer sold])	Adults with mod or high risk of coronal or root caries or root sensitivity. Used 1 × day on toothbrush Do not swallow Less documented efficacy than 0.05% NaF rinse	"Gel-Kam," "Omni-Gel" 0.4% SnF₂ = 1,000 ppm F Limited to 4.3 oz size Issued or prescribed for home use Flavored (1)
1.1% NaF Gel	Personal use Written RX	Adults—Daily self-appl by toothbrush for high risk Do not swallow	"Prevident" 5,000 ppm F⁻ Flavored
0.12% Chlorhexidine	Personal rinse. Rx item (i) If S. mutans ≥5.5 × 10⁵ CFU/mL and caries is still active at re-evaluation, or (ii) For persistent gingivitis	Rinse 1/2 oz.× 30 sec × 2/day × 30 days (i) Monitor S. mutans and sugar intake (ii) Special patients. Not a substitute for mechanical plaque control	"Peridex" (1) Do not swallow

III. AVAILABLE FOR PURCHASE AT STORES AND PHARMACIES – NO RX REQUIRED

PRODUCT	USE	METHOD	FORM
a) NaF 0.15% w/v F⁻; 1.3% pyrophosphate anticalculus b) Na₂PO₃F 0.15% w/v F⁻ c) NaF 0.15% w/v F⁻ 0.3% triclosan; 2.0% copolymer of methoxyethylene and maleic acid. —anticalculus, reduces gingivitis	Toothpastes for personal use Labeled as "0.15% w/v F ion" All dentifrices are approx. 1100 ppm F⁻ w/v (weight/vol)	After meals on a toothbrush For young children use small "pea-sized" amount on the brush, and supervise to limit swallowing. Preschool children at risk of caries (erupted teeth) should use 2/day.	a) e.g., "Crest" , "Colgate" "Tartar Control Gel" (1) b) "Colgate MFP" "Aquafresh" (1) c) "Colgate Total" (1)

Product	Availability / Use	Directions	Brands
a) 5% Potassium nitrate and NaF (0.15% w/v F^-) b) $Na_2PO_3F + KNO_3$ c) SrCl d) Potassium Nitrate-5% and SnF_2 (0.15% w/vF^-)	Self applied for root sensitivity. Over the counter sale (see also 0.4% SnF_2 and 1.1% NaF gels for root sensitivity)	On toothbrush for root sensitivity in adults	a) "Sensitivity Protection Crest" 1,000 ppm F^- (1) b) "Sensodyne MFP" c) Sensodyne Strontium Chloride d) "Colgate Sensitive"
0.05% Sodium Fluoride Mouthrinse	Personal use. Over the counter sale. Not for preschoolers	Children and adults at mod high risk. 1 x daily rinse x 10ml. Do not swallow	"Fluorigard" (1) "Act" "Oral B" "CVS" "Wal-Mart" 0.05% F, 225 ppm F
Waxed or unwaxed dental floss standard, extra fine, tape	Personal Use, with floss threader or holder if needed	1-2 times per day to prevent gingivitis	Various brands
Toothbrushes	Personal Use	Soft multitufted, round end nylon bristles. Child & adult size. Use after meals with fluoride toothpaste.	
Xylitol Chewing gum % xylitol not stated, first listed ingredient is highest	Child and adult	Salivary stimulant for hyposalivation. Substitute for sucrose for gum user. Reduced bacterial colonization (?)	"Carefree Koolerx" Nabisco "Dental Care" Arm & Hammer "Aquafresh" Beecham "Fresh Breath" Walgreens

Knowing F content of water is necessary for prevention planning and also before Rx F supplements (tablets, drops). Public water systems are analyzed by State and Local Dept. of Health Services. This is available from CDC at http://apps.nccd.cdc.gov/MWF/ The household water bill defines the water supplier. For water analysis of private wells only, analysis of the water for fluoride content is advised.

(Adapted table courtesy J P Brown UTHSCA) Note: References 1, 3, and 6 are cited in the table. References 2, 4, and 5 are provided as additional resources.
For more detailed information
1. Accepted by ADA Council on Scientific Affairs – "ADA Seal of Acceptance."
2. Caries Diagnosis & Risk Assessment—a review of preventive strategies & management. JADA 126;15–245 1995 Suppl.
3. ADA Guide to Dental Therapeutics. Chicago ADA Publishing 1998.
4. Dodds MWJ, Suddick RP. Caries Risk Assessment for Determination of Focus and Intensity of Prevention in a Dental School Clinic. J. Dent. Educ. 59:945–956, 1995.
5. Recommendations for Using Fluoride to Prevent and Control Dental Caries in the United States. MMWR Aug 17, 2001. 50. 1–42. CDC – USPHS. Am J. Prev. Med. 2002;23(15)16–80.
6. Protocols for Remineralization Therapy of Individual Lesions and Full Mouth Application of Fluoride Varnish in Selected High Risk Patients. UTHSCSA Department of Community Dentistry. Nov. 2001.

TABLE 15-2

AGE-SPECIFIC GUIDELINES FOR FLUORIDE THROUGHOUT THE LIFE CYCLE

AGE	FLUORIDE	COMMENTS
Pregnant women: visit dental professional during pregnancy	Fluoride supplementation is not indicated. Use fluoridated toothpaste and drink fluoridated water.	
Infants: birth-6 months	Oral supplementation is not recommended. Drink fluoridated water.	Fluoride supplement schedule (Table 15-3).
Infant: 6-12 months	Oral supplementation if prescribed by health professional. Brush with small amount of fluoridated toothpaste. Drink fluoridated water.	
Toddler: 1-24 months	Use oral supplements if prescribed. Brush with small amount of fluoridated toothpaste. Drink fluoridated water.	Use pea-sized amount of toothpaste or smear on the brush. Caregiver should conduct brushing.
Children: 2-3 years of age	Use oral supplements as directed. Professional fluoride application as needed. Brush with small amount of fluoridated toothpaste Drink fluoridated water.	Use a pea-sized amount of toothpaste or smear on the brush. Caregiver should conduct brushing. Advise against ingesting toothpaste and rinses.
Children: 3-12 years of age	Drink fluoridated water. Use fluoride toothpaste. Use oral supplements as directed. Professional fluoride application if moderate or high caries risk. Home fluoride rinse for high–caries-risk children if older than 5 years of age.	Minimal risk of fluorosis (until 8 years of age).
Adolescents, adults, elders	Drink fluoridated water. Use fluoride toothpaste. Professional fluoride application as needed. Home fluoride rinses or gels for high–caries-risk persons.	No risk of fluorosis.

(Adapted from Position of the American Dietetic Association: the impact of fluoride on health, *J Am Dietetic Assoc* 105:1620-1628, 2005.)

Fluoride varnish is applied to caries affected surfaces by using a bristle brush or cotton pellet and painted onto the tooth surfaces. Although fluoride varnish is water tolerant and will adhere to the tooth in the presence of saliva, it is best to dry the tooth surfaces and remove excess saliva from the area. For remineralization, a broad area over and around the lesion should be covered. The total volume of fluoride varnish applied should be limited to 1 mL (23 mg of fluoride ion) per appointment. In young children, the application should be limited to 0.25 mL (6 mg fluoride ion). Postoperative instructions should be provided that include the following guidelines: (1) refrain from brushing or flossing the area until the

following morning, and (2) refrain from eating high-fiber or abrasive foods for the rest of the day. Instructions for remineralization should be accompanied by an explanation of the objectives and the role that the patient should play in maintaining their own oral health, including dietary and preventive practices.

Fluoride varnish application for remineralization should be repeated in 1-2 weeks. After 90 to 120 days from the first series of applications, two additional applications of fluoride varnish, 1 week apart, should be administered and the caries reevaluated.[11] Adherence to the entire preventive plan should be reinforced at each patient visit.

Conventional practice includes continued dental prophylaxis or tooth cleaning with a professional fluoride application. A report by Ripa showed that a dental prophylaxis does not enhance F uptake or caries prevention.[12] A prophylaxis with pumice and rotating bristle brush removes oral plaque and stains, but will also remove the fluoride-rich outer layer of enamel (at the rate of approximately 0.1 to 1.0 μm per 10 seconds). The rationale for using fluoride-containing pastes is to reduce the loss of, or help to replenish the fluoride. In general, this method is preferred to simple abrasive-only systems, but no strong evidence exists that they provide more than marginal protection against caries.

Professional fluoride application is recommended every 6 months for persons at moderate risk of caries and is recommended every 3 months for individuals at high risk.[13] For patients at low caries risk with no caries activity, topical fluoride applications are not necessary. Brushing daily with fluoride toothpaste and exposure to community water fluoridation are sufficient for the low caries risk individual and recommended for all persons.

Pit and fissure sealants. Dental sealants, developed by Buonocore in the 1960s, are plastic coatings that occlude the pits and fissures of tooth surfaces.[14] Sealants are complementary to water fluoridation and other fluorides. Although the primary effects of fluoride products are on smooth surfaces, sealants prevent caries of pits and fissures. Studies demonstrate that intact sealants reduce caries by as much as 99%.[15] The 1983 National Institutes of Health (NIH) Sealant Consensus Development Conference endorsed the use of dental sealants and strong endorsements have come from the Centers for Disease Control and Prevention (CDC), NIH, and the United States Surgeon General.[16] Studies have demonstrated that bacteria in early caries beneath sealants decline in number when deprived of nutrients, but do not disappear entirely. Provided the sealant remains intact, caries does not progress, even if the disease is at a very advanced stage.[17] Pit and fissure sealants can be effectively used as a primary preventive agent and as a secondary preventive measure in early occlusal caries.

First permanent molars should be sealed soon after eruption at 6 to 7 years of age and second permanent molars at 12 to 13 years for those children who are at moderate to high risk for caries development. Premolars should be considered for sealants if the patient is at high caries risk and has a strong history of occlusal caries. Primary molar teeth may be sealed at approximately age three years in preschool children who are at high risk for developing caries. Greater use of pit and fissure sealants as a strategy in preventive practice and programs is encouraged.

The increment of new caries, including pit and fissure caries, is substantial and highest in younger and middle-aged adults.[18] This finding from the National Health and Nutrition Examination Surveys III emphasizes the importance of caries prevention in adults and not just children. Because dental caries is a disease of the life span, risk assessment should be continuous and when warranted, dental sealants should be used as a preventive strategy for all ages on the basis of caries risk status. Therefore, sealants can be strongly indicated in adults who are at high risk and who have a current history of pit and fissure caries.

Two types of dental sealant material are available commercially: light-cured sealant material and chemical-cured sealant material. Light-cured material can be manipulated until the operator cures the material with the light. The chemical-cured material sets within a short working time, thus manipulation of the material is limited. No evidence exists on the basis of efficacy (caries reduction) to show that light-cured sealants are preferable to chemically cured.

Placement of pit and fissure sealants is technique-sensitive. Success in retention of the sealant is directly related to the maintenance of a dry field. Although retention rates are operator-dependent, initial success rates of well over 90% have been demonstrated with sound application techniques. The average rate of loss (approximately 5% per year) is greatest soon after placement. This statistic compares very favorably with the success rate of restorations. Sealants that are compromised by moisture contamination are usually lost early after placement. Therefore, recall within the first year to evaluate sealant retention is important. Even if the sealant is lost, however, some caries protection is achieved.

Pit and fissure sealant application is described in detail in Waggoner and Siegal.[19] First, plaque and debris should be removed from the tooth surface. Cleaning should be accomplished with a prophy cup or bristle brush, with or without pumice, or with an explorer or a toothbrush and forceful rinsing with water. Prophy pastes should not be used to clean the surface, because the residual oils can impede adherence of the sealant to the tooth and fluoride can hamper the acid etch. In addition, no evidence exists to suggest that widening or opening the fissure will enhance caries prevention. In fact, opening the fissure will breach the integrity of the mature surface enamel and should be avoided unless a lack of bonding of the sealant is observed at placement.

Sealant success is shown to be linked to complete isolation of the tooth from saliva. Isolation with either a rubber dam or cotton rolls is effective in moisture control. Tooth selection is important to this process. Partially erupted teeth that are difficult to isolate should probably not be sealed until the gingival tissue is free from the occlusal surface. For the sealant material to adhere to the tooth, the enamel must be etched with orthophosphoric acid. Clinical studies indicate that a 15-second etch is adequate for sealant retention. Liquid or gel materials are equally effective and no differences are observed in retention.

The purpose of rinsing and drying the tooth after etching is to remove the etchant and water from the tooth surface. Once clean and dry, the sealant material can be placed on the tooth. The fissures should be covered with a thin layer of sealant material. Polymerization with the light should occur immediately after placement of the material. Chemical-cured material will harden after approximately 45 seconds. After polymerization, the sealant should be inspected to check for occlusal interferences, for adherence, for the integrity of the sealant and to ensure complete coverage of the pit and fissured surface. Slight occlusal interferences will quickly wear, as sealants are not highly-filled resins.

PREVENTIVE AGENTS FOR SELF-APPLICATION: CHEMOPREVENTION

Several products are available for personal use as prescription items or over the counter. The prescription items generally have a higher concentration of fluoride and therefore have a greater potential for toxicity. Fluoride is a pharmaceutical and the potential for overexposure in higher strength products requires that care be taken to inform patients about the risks and for dental professionals to prescribe and use them appropriately. Dental professionals should understand fluoride metabolism and toxicology and be able to calculate the dose administered either by design or inadvertently. Also, the provider should be able to diagnose and appropriately treat overdosage.[20]

Fluoride gels by prescription.   These items are recommended for patients who are at high or moderate caries risk and would experience beneficial effects from additional exposure to fluoride. Prevident is a 1.1% neutral NaF (5000 ppm F) gel. This product is prescribed for high-risk patients and should be applied daily with a toothbrush. The patient should be instructed not to swallow the gel and to expectorate the excess gel after brushing, and to avoid rinsing with water immediately after use. Application before bedtime is recommended for maximum effectiveness.

GelKam and OmniGel (0.4% SnF$_2$, 960 ppm F) are available by prescription. The strength of these products is equal to that in toothpastes. These products are self-applied either in custom trays or by toothbrush. Evidence for efficacy for the use of 0.4% SnF$_2$ in patients undergoing head and neck irradiation and in those wearing orthodontic bands has been documented; however, their general efficacy is not well established. The recommendation is to apply the product immediately before bedtime for maximum contact. After application, the patient should expectorate any residual gel, and should avoid rinsing with water. These products have also been shown to reduce dentinal hypersensitivity. The mechanism of action is the deposition of stannous fluorophosphate into the dentinal tubules.

Two products are routinely recommended for root sensitivity. Products that contain 0.4% SnF$_2$ are often advised for high caries–risk adults with root caries; however, questions remain about the scientific evidence to support this application. In addition to these gels, 0.717% F (DentinBloc) is an effective desensitizing agent for exposed root surfaces. Protect is a potassium oxalate solution that is available for root sensitivity. These agents are professionally applied and come in a 0.6-mL unit dose. These agents should be applied to saliva-moistened teeth at the sensitive sites, where gingival recession and exposed root surfaces are evident.

Fluoride rinses without prescription.   Of all self-applied agents other than toothpaste, NaF (0.05%) daily rinses have the best evidence of efficacy. These over-the-counter rinses have been shown to be effective in reducing caries in moderate-risk or high-risk patients. These products come in several brand and generic forms and are found in the dental products section of pharmacies (see Table 15-1). Although the concentration of the over-the-counter products is less than prescription items, the lower cost, ease of availability, palatable taste, and low strength contribute to efficacy and adherence. A 10-ml rinse for 30 seconds daily is recommended for these products. Again, as with all fluoride products, the rinse should be expectorated. Caries reduction has been shown to range from 30 to 50%.[21] The use of a 0.05% daily rinse should routinely be advised for moderate or high caries risk patients over the age of 5 years.

Dentifrices.   Early clinical trials of fluoridated toothpastes conducted in the late 1940s were ineffective, because calcium-based abrasives interfered with availability of fluoride ion when it was added to toothpaste that contained sodium fluoride.[22] In 1960, Crest was given provisional acceptance, and in 1964 was given full acceptance by the ADA Council on Dental Therapeutics as the first toothpaste containing fluoride as a preventive agent. Crest used a concentration of 0.4% SnF$_2$ and heat-treated calcium pyrophosphate as the abrasive. Today, the standard fluoride concentration is 0.15% weight/volume (approximately 1000 ppm) of fluoride ion.

At present, more than 95% of all toothpastes in the U.S. market are fluoridated.[23] Fluoridated toothpaste is recommended for all dentate persons, along with community water fluoridation, for the primary prevention of dental caries. All caries risk groups should brush with a fluoridated toothpaste twice daily. For young children, care should be taken to minimize the amount of toothpaste placed on the toothbrush. Young children have a tendency to swallow, rather than spit toothpaste, and are at greater risk for experiencing very mild or mild fluorosis. Currently, the recommendation is to use a "pea-sized" or smear of toothpaste for preschool children. An adult should supervise tooth brushing for preschool children, and should encourage the child to spit, not swallow, the toothpaste.

Over the years, the most common active agent transitioned from stannous fluoride (SnF_2) to sodium monofluorophosphate (MFP) (Na_2PO_3F) to sodium fluoride (NaF) as the preferred agent. Toothpastes contain one of the fluoride formulations as the active ingredient and an abrasive to assist with plaque removal and fluoride uptake. Three ADA-accepted fluoride agents are used in toothpastes.

Sodium fluoride is in toothpaste at a concentration of 0.24% NaF (1100 ppm of fluoride ion). Abrasives can include calcium pyrophosphate ($Ca_2P_2O_7$), insoluble sodium metaphosphate ($NaPO_3$), and silica (SiO_2). Toothpastes using this formulation include Crest, Colgate Tartar Control Gel, Mentadent, and Colgate Total. NaF pastes show marginally better caries reductions than other fluoride formulations.

Sodium monofluorphosphate (Na_2PO_3F), or MPF, is compatible with conventional calcium containing abrasives and contains 0.15% or 1100 ppm F-. Abrasives include aluminum oxide (Al_2O_3), dicalcium phosphate ($CaHPO_4$), and calcium carbonate ($CaCO_3$). Both Colgate MFP and Aquafresh contain this formulation.

Stannous fluoride (SnF_2) at a concentration of 0.4% (960 ppm fluoride ion) was previously used as the active ingredient in some toothpaste brands. Stannous fluoride has several properties that make it less attractive commercially. These properties include staining, alteration of taste, and incompatibility with some abrasives, especially dicalcium phosphate ($CaHPO_4$). Abrasives used with stannous fluoride toothpastes include calcium pyrophosphate ($Ca_2P_2O_7$) and insoluble sodium metaphosphate ($NaPO_3$) with silica (SiO_2). The use of SnF_2 in toothpaste has been largely discontinued.

Fluoridated toothpastes account for caries reductions in the range of 17% to 35%.[24] The preventive effectiveness of toothpaste is lower in fluoridated areas. Caries reductions are greatest for approximal surfaces of posterior teeth and for newly erupted teeth, which are undergoing posteruptive maturation of enamel. The greatest caries-preventive effect of fluoride is on smooth surfaces. Research established that the preventive effect of toothpastes is shown to be a dose-response relationship. Persons should be advised to look for the ADA Seal of Acceptance when selecting a brand of toothpaste, which indicates the active agent, efficacy or fluoride uptake, and method for use.

The preventive action of toothpastes is to increase the bioavailability of fluoride when the enamel is under acid challenge. Toothpastes also increase the fluoride content of the surface enamel.[25,26] Fluoridated toothpastes have preferential uptake in demineralized areas. By forming a less soluble, more resistant apatite crystal in enamel, fluoridated toothpastes limit demineralization and promote remineralization. Although fluorides have been shown to have an antibacterial property, the lower concentration of fluoride present in toothpaste is not likely to have antibacterial action. Some brands, such as Colgate Total, have formulations that provide some antibacterial action. This product, which contains Triclosan, for antibacterial action is used to prevent gingivitis (Chapter 16).

Fluoride supplements by prescription. Fluoride supplements or dietary fluoride supplements are recommended for children and adolescents who live in areas that do not have access to the benefits of community water fluoridation.[27] These products are prescribed in tablet or drop form. Supplements are effective if continuity of administration is achieved, with reduction in dental caries ranging from 11% to 80%, depending on the age of the patient when the regimen is initiated.[28] The prescription guidelines (Table 15-3) are based on the amount of fluoride in the drinking water and the age of the child. Because the level of exposure to fluoride in drinking water is a consideration when prescribing fluoride supplements, the dental provider must know the fluoride concentration in the water consumed. Fluoride levels for water systems are available from utilities and at *http://apps.nccd.cdc.gov/MWF/Index.asp*. This resource, My Water's Fluoride, is available on the CDC's website, as reported by state health departments. Families that obtain water from a private well will need to have the levels of fluoride measured before prescribing supplements. A State or Local Health Department or Dental School

---

TABLE 15-3

FLUORIDE SUPPLEMENT DOSAGE SCHEDULE

	Amount of Fluoride (F ion) by Water F Level		
AGE	<0.3 PPM	0.3-0.6 PPM	>0.6 PPM
Birth-6 mos	0	0	0
6 mos-3 yr	0.25 mg F	0	0
3-6 yr	0.5 mg F	0.25 mg F	0
6-at least 16 yr	1.0 mg F	0.5 mg F	0

(2.2 mg NaF =1.0 mg F ion.)
(Adapted from the *ADA Guide to Dental Therapeutics*, Chicago, IL, 1998.)

can assist with measuring fluoride levels for private well water supplies.

Fluoride drops are recommended for children younger than 2 years. The drops are supplied as 0.5, 2.0, 2.5, and 5.0 mg/mL of fluoride. Product names include Fluoritab, Pediaflor, and Luride. Dental professionals should not dispense more than 60 to 115 mg depending on the concentration, because a concentration of fluoride greater than 50 mg is the acute toxic dose of fluoride for a 1-year-old weighing approximately 10 kg.

Fluoride tablets are often prescribed for older children and adolescents by using the guidelines in Table 15-3. The following brands of tablets are available: Fluoritab, Flura-loz, Flura-tablets (1 mg fluoride), and Luride (0.25, 0.5, or 1.0 mg fluoride). Dental professionals should be careful not to prescribe more than 120 tablets at one time, each containing 1.0 mg of fluoride to reduce the risk of toxicity.

Antimicrobials by prescription. Because dental caries is a diet-dependent, vertically transmissible, infectious, bacterial disease, an antimicrobial approach to control the cariogenic bacteria is logical. One of the key determinants of caries development in children is the acquisition of the cariogenic flora from the mother. A "window of infectivity" occurs before 3 years of age.[29] Evidence suggests that when the mother's level of mutans streptococci is low, the incorporation of mutans streptococci into the infant's normal oral flora is delayed and reduced in intensity and the caries experience in these children is minimized. These findings can be implemented to reduce the burden of early childhood caries. Long-term effectiveness of antimicrobials on caries control in older children and adults is less clear, because by then, all have acquired mutans streptococci. Differences in the virulence of cariogenic bacteria are important. For adults, the application of antimicrobial therapy can be best used as a second line of prevention. If a reduction in a high count of cariogenic indicator organisms can not be achieved by behavioral and other preventive approaches, the use of antimicrobials may then be warranted.

Chlorhexidine gluconate (Peridex, 0.12%) is the antibacterial agent of choice to control oral pathogens. Other essential oil-based products are available, but are far less effective. Although chlorhexidine gluconate is effective in reducing the burden of oral bacteria, it has significant negative side effects, including staining of the teeth and alteration of taste. Adherence to the protocol can be problematic.

Chlorhexidine gluconate is only available by prescription. Patients should be advised to rinse twice per day with 0.5 oz (one capful) for 30 seconds per rinse. This product should be used only for a 30-day period, every 3 months, because substantivity provides ongoing action. Substantivity refers to the persistence of the active ingredient after application of the agent has ceased. This regimen will suppress the load of mutans streptococci when oral hygiene and dietary intervention are insufficiently applied.

Xylitol and sorbitol. Xylitol ($C_5H_{12}O_5$) is a 5-carbon (pentose) sugar alcohol. Sorbitol is a polyol found in many fruits and berries. Termed a natural sugar, xylitol is found in low levels in certain fruits, and may also be referred to as birch sugar from which it was derived. In 2001, an NIH consensus statement promoted the use of products containing noncariogenic sweeteners as one method to prevent caries initiation.[30] These sweeteners include xylitol, sorbitol, other nonnutritive sugars, sucralose (chlorinated sucrose), and aspartame (aspartic acid and phenylalanine). These sweeteners are included in a growing number of foods, including candies, gums, and drinks. The actual content of noncariogenic sweeteners may not be explicitly stated on the label, but ingredients are listed on product packaging in order of content percent.

The mechanism of action of xylitol in the oral cavity differs from other sugar alcohols. Xylitol cannot be metabolized by the typical acid-forming bacteria found in dental plaque, and bacteria cannot use xylitol as a nutrient. Xylitol is converted into xylitol 5-phosphate (X5P) after its uptake into bacterial cells and X5P may inhibit bacterial metabolism, including acid production. Thus, xylitol retards growth of *S. mutans* and *S. sobrinus* and inhibits acid production by these organisms in the presence of other sugars.[31] Observations of reduced plaque mass in subjects consuming xylitol suggest an effect of xylitol on the process of polysaccharide production that causes decreased bulk and stickiness of the plaque biofilm. Xylitol in the growth medium both reduced polysaccharides produced by *S. mutans* to a greater extent than sorbitol and decreased cell-cell (aggregation) and adhesivity of the bacteria.[32]

Xylitol and sorbitol chewing gums promote saliva stimulation and an increase in the plaque pH or a more rapid return to neutrality after a sugar challenge, or both.[33,34,35] Park et al. tested 5 commercially available gums and found no statistically significant differences in plaque pH between any of the sugar-free gums.[36] Scheie et al. were unable to detect any differences in plaque quantity or acidogenic potential after chewing either xylitol or sorbitol gums.[37] These studies suggest no increased benefit from xylitol over sorbitol in salivary stimulation or in plaque quantity and acidogenicity.

The role of xylitol in remineralization of demineralized enamel was raised by observations that xylitol can form complexes with calcium ions and may penetrate dental enamel during demineralization *in vitro*.[38] It also inhibited demineralization (lesion depth) directly and was shown to reduce free Ca2+ ion activity when added to saturated hydroxyapatite solutions. Amaechi et al. tested the *in vitro* demineralization and remineralization effects of xylitol solutions, and found no specific effect of the xylitol on either process.[39] The current science is equivocal about the specific effectiveness of xylitol in caries control versus sorbitol. The sucrose substitution effect and salivary stimulation effect by cleansing are not in question. Although some of the clinical trials support the remineralization properties of xylitol, the data provide limited evidence of efficacy.[40,41] Remineralization studies do not confirm any superiority of xylitol. The demonstrated effectiveness of salivary stimulation in caries prevention does not appear any greater for xylitol than for sorbitol. Thus, despite strong biological plausibility, the specific anticaries effect of xylitol has not been clearly established.

Diet and plaque control.   In Chapters 4 and 8, dietary factors are discussed relative to caries risk and prevention. Table 8-4 provides a list of questions that are tied to the algorithm in Figure 8-2 that is designed to guide decision-making about more in-depth nutritional assessment. Ultimately, the data gathered through the nutritional assessment methods should lead to the development of a dietary education, counseling, and follow-up plan. Table 8-12 provides a rationale that explains dietary behaviors in the context of oral health.

Throughout this book reference is made to the role of fermentable carbohydrates as a primary substrate for the initiation of dental caries. Terms used to characterize foods by specific response to cariogenic bacteria are listed in Table 15-4. The primary purpose of a preventive plan designed to address dietary variables associated with caries risk is to examine the frequency of sugar consumption, total sugar consumption, combinations of snacking and meals that exceed six times per day, the total quality of the diet as defined by variety and balance, and the introduction of anticariogenic and cariostatic foods in the daily dietary pattern.[42]

Oral health beliefs and practices are important in caries prevention. Health behaviors, including diet, oral hygiene, and use of smokeless tobacco, are integral to the caries process. Behavior modification, education, and counseling are important to dental caries prevention. These topics are addressed in chapters 10 and 11.

RISK-BASED PREVENTION

The hallmark of risk-based prevention strategies is to identify risk factors integral to the disease process for individual patients and to modulate those factors by using appropriate preventive strategies (Table 15-1).

Low Caries Risk

Patients who are at low risk for caries are successful in self-management of their oral health. Prevention strategies for both children and adults should focus on reinforcement of oral hygiene and dietary practices and the use of fluoridated toothpastes two times per day. Individuals in this risk category should be encouraged to drink fluoridated water and brush with fluoridated toothpastes. These patients should be recalled annually for risk reevaluation.

TABLE 15-4

DESCRIPTIVE RESPONSE ASSOCIATED WITH TERMS USED TO DESCRIBE FOODS AND BEVERAGES AND THEIR ROLE IN THE PROGRESSION OF CARIES

TERM	DESCRIPTION	EXAMPLES
Acidogenic	Foods/beverages that readily cause a drop in plaque pH to <5.5 within 30 minutes.	Sweet pastries, sweetened cereals.
Cariogenic	Foods/beverages that contain fermentable carbohydrates that can be metabolized by oral bacteria to cause a decrease in bacteria to cause a decrease in plaque pH to <5.5 and demineralization of tooth enamel.	Sugar-sweetened beverages sipped during an extended period. Sticky, sugary foods. Highly processed starchy foods.
Anticariogenic	Foods/beverages that can prevent cariogenic activity when eaten with/before an acidogenic product.	Xylitol gums and candies. Beverages sweetened with sugar substitutes/alcohols. Hard cheese. Nuts and seeds.
Cariostatic	Foods/beverages that cannot be easily metabolized by dental plaque. Bacteria, and therefore do not cause a significant drop in salivary pH.	High-quality proteins. Dairy foods.

CARIES PREVENTION BY RISK STATUS AND AGE GROUP "CLINICAL PREVENTIVE SERVICES INCLUDING HEALTH PROMOTION"*

Screen, Test, Examine, and Estimate Caries Risk		CHILD/ADOLESCENT	ADULT
LOW	Counseling	Preventive practices.	Preventive practices.
	Chemoprevention	Brush with fluoride toothpaste.	Brush with fluoride toothpaste.
	Clinical procedures	1-year recall.	1-year recall.
MODERATE	Counseling	Preventive practices, diet.	Preventive practices, diet, salivary stimulation.[†]
	Chemoprevention	Brush with fluoride toothpaste, fluoride mouth rinse/fluoride varnish.[‡] Fluoride supplements,[§]	Brush with fluoride toothpaste, fluoride mouth rinse/alternative fluoride gel.[¶]
	Clinical Procedures	Professional topical fluoride, sealants, remineralization therapy;[‖] 6-month recall, reassess risk and disease.	Professional topical fluoride, sealants, remineralization therapy;[‖] 6-month recall, reassess risk and disease.
HIGH	Counseling	Preventive practices, diet.	Preventive practices, diet, salivary stimulation.[†]
	Chemoprevention	Brush with fluoride toothpaste, fluoride mouth rinse/fluoride varnish.[‡] Fluoride supplements,[§]	Brush with fluoride toothpaste, fluoride mouth rinse/alternative fluoride gel.[¶]
	Clinical Procedures	professional topical fluoride, sealants remineralization therapy; 3-month recall, reassess risk and disease.	Professional topical fluoride, sealants, remineralization therapy, antimicrobial agent;[#] 3-month recall, reassess risk and disease.

*Component 2 of the Clinical Prevention and Population Health Common Framework for all health professions. The Domain "Immunization" has been renamed "Clinical Procedures" for dental application. Allan J, Barwick TA et al.: Clinical prevention and population health: curriculum framework for health professions, *Am J Prev Med* 27:471-476, 2004. This component parallels the structure of the U.S. Preventive Services Task Force: *http://www.ahrq.gov/clinic/uspstf/uspstopics.htm.*
[†]If indicated (e.g., xylitol/sorbitol gum or lozenges).
[‡]Mouth rinse not recommended for children younger than 6 years. Use fluoride varnish procedure.
[§]All persons, without regard to risk, should use fluoridated water if possible. Supplements are recommended when the water is not fluoridated to optimum levels.
[‖]If indicated by early caries lesions.
[¶]Fluoride gel on toothbrush for cervical sensitivity, root caries.
[#]If indicator bacterial levels remain elevated.

Moderate Caries Risk

Moderate risk patients should be recalled every 6 months for reevaluation and educational reinforcement of good oral hygiene and dietary practices, including use of fluoride toothpaste. Dietary assessment, counseling, and reinforcement can benefit these patients. Moderate risk patients should receive a topical fluoride application twice per year and instructions on plaque control by brushing and flossing if necessary. If the patient is at moderate risk because of smooth surface, approximal, or root caries, daily fluoride rinse (0.05% NaF) is indicated. If the patient is at moderate risk because of pit and fissure caries, the dental provider should consider the appropriate use of dental sealants.

The dental professional should carefully assess those risk factors specific to the individual patient. If salivary gland hypofunction is noted, appropriate counseling for salivary stimulation should be provided and dietary issues and methods of salivary stimulation should be reviewed. Salivary gland hypofunction can be determined from the five screening questions[43] (Chapter 4) and confirmed by testing the salivary flow rate (Chapter 9). At each recall visit, a caries risk reevaluation should be accomplished and the effectiveness of preventive interventions assessed and modified based upon adherence, risk status, and caries preventive outcomes.

High Caries Risk

Intensive preventive strategies should be considered for the high caries risk child or adult. Patients who are at high caries risk are unable to sustain their own oral health and require additional and more intensive intervention. Dietary counseling, oral hygiene instruction and reinforcement should be provided. Daily additional brushing with fluoride toothpaste should be strongly encouraged. A professional fluoride application of 1.23% APF, 2% neutral NaF or 5% fluoride varnish should be provided at 3 month intervals. Fluoride varnish is especially applicable for use in younger children at high caries risk and for special populations.

Sealants should be placed for the high caries risk patient with a history of pit and fissure caries or when enamel lesions are present. High caries–risk patients without multiple smooth surface lesions should be advised to use an over-the-counter sodium fluoride rinse (0.05% NaF).

High caries–risk individuals with multiple enamel or dentinal carious lesions require intensive fluoride therapy, and can be advised to use a high concentration of 1.1% neutral sodium fluoride gel (Prevident) daily on a toothbrush. Fluoride varnish (5% NaF) can be applied to remineralize early approximal and smooth surface lesions according to the protocols outlined in Figures 15-2 through 15-5. Antimicrobial agents should be considered if the moderate-to-high levels of mutans streptococci do not decrease after dietary and oral hygiene counseling. Re-evaluation of the effectiveness of the preventive plan and professional preventive therapy should be accomplished every 3 months for high caries risk patients. Re-evaluation is accomplished on an interim basis by evaluating preventive behaviors and practices. Long-term re-evaluation will examine preventive outcomes. The preventive plan will then be modified and reinforced. Because risk status is dynamic, all patients should be re-evaluated at regular intervals. When indicated by reduced risk, the frequency and intensity of prevention can be lowered.

SUMMARY

Dental caries is a chronic, biobehavioral disease that extends throughout the life span. Prevention of this disease in the individual can focus on increasing the ability of the host to respond to the insult, decreasing the cariogenicity of the bacterial agents, and altering the diet to be less caries promoting. To be effective, however, the dental professional should assess the caries risk of the individual and address the active etiological factors that are influenced by behavior, using a combination of clinical preventive procedures, behavioral interventions by the patient, and self-applied chemoprevention.

REFERENCES

1. World Health Organization: *Health promotion glossary*, Geneva, 1998, World Health Organization.
2. Fejerskov O: Changing paradigms in concepts on dental caries: consequences for oral health care, *Caries Res* 38:182-191, 2004.
3. Allen J, Bartwick TA, Cashman S et al.: Clinical prevention and population health. Curriculum framework for health professions, *Am J Prev Med* 27:417-422, 2004.
4. Bader JD, Shugars DA, Kennedy JE et al.: A pilot study of risk-based prevention in private practice, *JADA* 134:1195-1202, 2003.
5. Bibby BG, Zander HA, McKellegaret M et al.: Preliminary reports on the effect of dental caries of the use of sodium fluoride in a prophylactic cleaning mixture and in a mouthwash, *J Dent Res* 25:207-211, 1946.
6. Ripa LW: A critique of topical fluoride methods (dentifrice, mouthrinses, operator and self-applied gels) in an era of decreased caries and increased fluoride prevalence, *J Public Health Dent* 51:23-41, 1991.
7. The ADA Council on Scientific Affairs: Professionally applied topical fluoride. Executive summary of evidence-based clinical recommendations, *JADA* insert, May 2006.
8. Brudevold F, Savory A, Gardner DE, et al.: A study of acidulated phosphate fluoride solutions. I. In vitro effects on enamel, *Arch Oral Biol* 8:179-182, 1963.
9. Clark DC, Stamm JW, Tessier C et al.: The final results of the Sherbrooke-Lac Megantic fluoride varnish study, *J Can Dent Assoc* 53:919-922, 1987.
10. Helfenstein U, Steiner M: Fluoride varnishes (Duraphat): a meta-analysis, *Commun Dent Oral Epidemiol* 22:1-5, 1994.
11. Seppa L, Tolonen T: Caries preventive effect of fluoride varnish applications performed two or four times a year, *Scand J Dent Res* 29:327-330, 1990.
12. Ripa LW: Clinical studies of high-potency fluoride dentifrices: a review, *JADA* 118:85-91, 1989.
13. Newbrun E: Preventing dental caries: current and prospective strategies, *JADA* 123:68-73, 1992.
14. Buonocore MG: A simple method of increasing the adhesion of acrylic filling material to enamel surfaces, *J Dent Res* 34:849-853, 1955.
15. Buonocore MG Caries prevention in pits and fissures sealed with an adhesive resin polymerized by ultraviolet light: a two year study of a single adhesive application, *JADA* 82:1090-1093, 1971.
16. Dental sealants in the prevention of tooth decay. *Natl Inst Health Cons Dev Conf Summ* 4:9, 1984.
17. Mertz-Fairhurst EJ, Schuster GS, Fairhurst CW: Arresting caries by sealants: results of a clinical study, *JADA* 112:194-197, 1986.
18. Winn DM, Brunelle JA, Selwitz RH et al.: Coronal and root caries in the dentition of adults in the US 1988-91. NHANES III, *J Dent Res* 75(Special Issue)62-51, 1996.
19. Waggoner WF, Siegal M: Pit and fissure sealant application: updating the technique, *JADA* 127:351-361, 1996.
20. Bayless JM, Tinnanoff N: Diagnosis and treatment of acute fluoride toxicity, *JADA* 110:209-211, 1985.
21. Rugg-Gunn AJ, Holloway PJ, Davies TGH: Caries prevention by daily fluoride mouthrinsing, *Br Dent J* 135:353-360, 1973.

22. Muhler JC, Radike AW, Nebergall WH et al.: Comparison between the anticariogenic effects of dentifrices containing stannous fluoride and sodium fluoride, *JADA* 51:556-559, 1955.

23. Zero DT: Dentifrices, mouthwashes and remineralization/caries arrestment strategies, *BMC Oral Health* 6(suppl 1):S9, 2006.

24. Muhler JC: Effect of a stannous fluoride dentifrice on caries reduction in children during a three-year study period, *JADA* 64:216-224, 1962.

25. Von der Fehr FR, Moller IJ: Caries-preventive fluoride dentifrices, *Caries Res* 12(suppl):31-37, 1978.

26. Dijkman TG, Arends J: The role of 'CaF2-like' material in topical fluoridation of enamel in situ, *Acta Odontol Scand* 46:391-397, 1988.

27. Centers for Disease Control and Prevention: Recommendations for using fluoride to prevent and control dental caries in the United States, *MMWR Recomm Rep* 50:1-42, 2001.

28. Margolis FJ, Reames HR, Freshman E et al.: Fluoride: a ten year prospective study of deciduous and permanent dentition, *Am J Dis Child* 130:794-800, 1975.

29. Caufield PW, Griffen AL: Dental caries: an infectious and transmissible disease, *Pediatr Clin North Am* 47:1001-1019, 2000.

30. Diagnosis and management of dental caries throughout life, *NIH Consens Statement* 18:1-24, 2001.

31. Kakuta H, Iwami Y, Maganagi H et al.: Inhibition of acid production and growth of mutans Streptococci in the presence of various dietary sugars under strictly anaerobic conditions, *Caries Res* 37:404-409, 2003.

32. Soderling E, Makinen KK, Chen CY et al.: Effect of sorbitol, xylitol, and xylitol/sorbitol chewing gums on dental plaque, *Caries Res* 23:378-384, 1989.

33. Frostell G: Dental plaque pH in relation to intake of carbohydrate products, *Acta Odontol Scand* 1:3-29, 1969.

34. Muhlemann HR, Schmid R, Noguchi T et al.: Some dental effects of xylitol under laboratory and in vivo conditions, *Caries Res* 11:263-276, 1977.

35. Imfeld TN: Identification of low caries risk dietary components, *Monogr Oral Sci* 11:1-198, 1983.

36. Park KK, Hernandez D, Schemehorn BR et al.: Effect of chewing gums on plaque pH after a sucrose challenge, *ASDC J Dent Child* 62:180-186, 1995.

37. Scheie AA, Fejerskov O, Danielson B: The effects of xylitol-containing chewing gums on dental plaque and acidogenic potential, *J Dent Res* 77:1547-1452, 1998.

38. Arends J, Christofferson J, Schuthof J et al.: Influence of xylitol on demineralization of enamel, *Caries Res* 18:296-301, 1984.

39. Amaechi BT, Higham BT, Edgar WM: Caries inhibiting and remineralizing effect of xylitol in vitro, *J Oral Sci* 41:71-76, 1999.

40. van Loveren C: Sugar alcohols: what is the evidence for caries-preventive and caries-therapeutic effects, *Caries Res* 38:286-293, 2004.

41. Maguire A, Rugg-Gunn AJ: Xylitol and caries prevention— is it a magic bullet? *Br Dent J* 194:492-436, 2003.

42. Mobley CC: Nutrition and dental caries, *Dent Clin North Am* 47:319-336, 2003.

43. Fox PC, Busch KA, Baum BJ: Subjective reports of xerostomia and objective measures of salivary gland performance, *JADA* 115:581-584, 1987.

44. Caries diagnosis and risk assessment. A review of preventive strategies and management, *JADA* 126:1S-24S, 1995.

Chapter 16

Prevention Strategies for Periodontal Diseases

BECKY DeSPAIN EDEN

LEARNING OBJECTIVES

Upon completion of this chapter, the learner will be able to:
- Describe dental plaque and its development.
- Discuss the role of mechanical removal of supragingival plaque and the devices used for personal plaque control, including manual toothbrushes, powered toothbrushes, dental floss, and other devices used to maintain personal oral hygiene.
- Identify approved active ingredients in over-the-counter antiplaque/antigingivitis products.
- Explain the professional services that reduce the risk for periodontal diseases.
- Explain the objectives of education and behavior change in periodontal disease prevention.

KEY TERMS

Acquired pellicle
Antiplaque agent
Antigingivitis agent
Antimicrobial, biocide
Antiseptic

Chemotherapeutic
Dental calculus
Dental plaque: oral biofilm
Dentin hypersensitivity
Embrasure
Gingival abrasion
Gingival crevicular fluid
Gingival recession
Host modulation therapy
Mechanical nonsurgical periodontal therapy
Oral care products
Oral malodor
Oral self-care
Oral prophylaxis
Periodontal maintenance
Substantivity
Therapeutic claim
Periodontopathogens

BACKGROUND/HISTORY/STATE OF THE CURRENT SCIENCE

Periodontal diseases result from the interaction between microbial agents and a susceptible host. Host response is mediated by environmental, systemic, and socioeconomic factors. The host response and influences of the oral environment are determinants of disease severity that can be specifically addressed by dental professionals. Strategies to reduce the risk for periodontal diseases are based on these tenets. This chapter addresses the prevention of periodontal diseases using risk-based strategies.

PREVENTIVE STRATEGIES DIRECTED TOWARD MICROBIAL AGENTS

Dental plaque is the principal etiological agent of most periodontal diseases. Effective preventive strategies are **antimicrobial**, with the preponderance of scientific evidence supporting the physical removal of dental plaque through personal oral hygiene measures and periodic professional care. Combining professional and self-care with **chemotherapeutic** agents that reduce periodontal microbiota provide additional benefits for those patients at greater risk for periodontal diseases.

Dental plaque is a complex biofilm attached to teeth. The first stage in development of this **oral biofilm** is the **acquired pellicle**, which forms immediately on exposure of a clean tooth surface to saliva. The acquired pellicle allows adhesion of naturally occurring oral bacteria that produce exopolysaccharides to enhance further accumulation of bacteria. Dental plaque becomes more complex when bacteria multiply and other bacterial species replace initial colonizers. Over time, as the plaque thickens and matures,

bacterial colonies aggregate to construct a community-like structure, an interactive microenvironment. These bacterial communities increase metabolic efficiency, promote growth of organisms, and protect microorganisms in the biofilm against host defenses and antimicrobial activity.[1-4] A detailed description of this process is presented in Chapter 2.

In undisturbed areas of the dentition, plaque is detectable in 12 to 24 hours. Within 5 days, plaque is easily visible and clinical signs of gingival inflammation can be observed in localized areas. In 2 to 3 weeks, generalized gingivitis becomes apparent.[5,6] Prevention of gingivitis relies on supragingival plaque removal at appropriate, regular intervals to return the gingiva to a healthy state.

Dental plaque on the tooth surface adjacent to the gingival margin, an area sheltered from chewing forces and salivary flow by its anatomical form, expands into the subgingival tooth surface. With changes in the local environment and alterations that occur within the biofilm, the bacterial composition of subgingival plaque grows increasingly complex, to include gram-negative anaerobic bacteria. These **periodontopathogens** in subgingival plaque are responsible for the initiation of periodontitis.[2,7] Removal of subgingival plaque is necessary to manage periodontitis, but methods that remove supragingival plaque are a prerequisite. The control of supragingival plaque suppresses periodontopathogens in subgingival plaque and changes the microbial composition of the biofilm to one that is more compatible with periodontal health.[8-10]

Control of the oral biofilm is a primary objective of periodontal disease prevention. The routine removal of supragingival plaque through personal oral hygiene is the most effective, efficient, and economical means to achieve this goal.

MECHANICAL REMOVAL OF SUPRAGINGIVAL PLAQUE
Manual Toothbrushing

Toothbrushes were produced in Europe as early as the eighteenth century, and the first U.S. patent for a toothbrush was awarded in 1857. Today, the toothbrush remains the primary device for routine oral hygiene and mechanical plaque removal. Virtually everyone in the United States owns a toothbrush, and 95% report tooth brushing at least once daily.[11] In a 2003 survey, 34% of adolescents and 42% of adults in the United States ranked the toothbrush as the one invention they could not live without, ahead of the automobile, personal computer, and cell phone.[12] The marketing of toothbrushes and other oral hygiene products is a multibillion dollar industry.

Toothbrushing is one of the most studied topic areas in the field of dentistry, with hundreds of publications available on efficacy, side effects, methods of brushing, and types of brushes, documenting the health benefits of mechanical plaque removal. Toothbrushing removes plaque and food debris, reduces gingival inflammation, decreases the number of microorganisms within the biofilm, and reduces pathogens in the subgingival microbiota.[5,13-15]

Toothbrush Designs

Despite the universality of toothbrushing, individual outcomes of toothbrushing are inconsistent and depend on each person's skill, dexterity, knowledge, attitudes, and commitment. The design of manual toothbrushes has been modified and refined during the years in pursuit of more effective plaque removal and improved oral health. Numerous toothbrush types with a variety of shapes and sizes of handles, heads, and bristles are available commercially, as noted in Figure 16-1. Bristles patterns reconfigured from the traditional flat brushing plane pictured in the figure purportedly enhance interdental access, although little supporting evidence exists. Figure 16-2 depicts ergonomic handle designs that improve control of the brush and enhance manual dexterity.

Marketing claims may confuse consumers, who often seek guidance regarding **oral care products** from a dental professional. Making a specific toothbrush recommendation to a patient on the basis of sound science is not easy. Most published studies have limited value because they are short-term, use small sample sizes, or do not report health outcomes. Scientific evidence fails to confirm the advantage of any particular manual toothbrush design.[16-19] Therefore, the choice of a toothbrush is a matter of personal preference. A particular design feature may be chosen to address a specific patient need.

The U.S. Food and Drug Administration (FDA) regulates toothbrushes as medical devices. A manufacturing company is required to register each device sold and to demonstrate its safety and effectiveness. In addition, the American Dental Association (ADA) evaluates toothbrushes and other oral care products under a voluntary program.[20] ADA approval allows the manufacturer to use the ADA Seal of Acceptance, pictured in Figure 16-3, on packaging and in marketing. Approval indicates compliance with ADA guidelines using specific evaluation protocols. These include minimum requirements for the duration of the evaluative study, sample size, assessment criteria, and statistical analysis of data. Data from clinical and laboratory studies must support the safety and efficacy of the product, as well as advertising claims. Promotional claims and materials are reviewed for compliance with

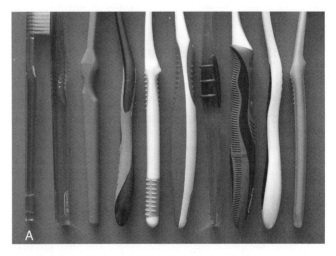

Figure 16-2 The brush labeled **A** has a traditional straight 6-in handle. The other brushes have ergonomic handles that help improve control and manual dexterity.

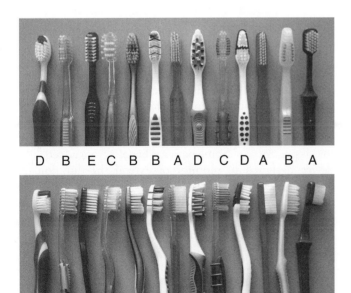

Figure 16-1 A sampling of designs of toothbrush heads and bristle trim patterns. The brushes labeled **A** have a traditional flat brushing plane. Other bristle trims include rippled (**B**), bilevel (**C**), multilevel (**D**), and domed (**E**).

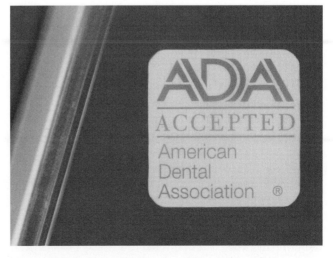

Figure 16-3 The ADA Seal of Acceptance as it appears on packaging of consumer oral health care products.

advertising standards.[21] The ADA program uses highly structured outcome criteria to qualify an approved appliance. Studies require only a 15% reduction in plaque and gingivitis from baseline in a single study using a minimum of 30 participants.[20]

Powered Toothbrushes

Powered or automatic toothbrushes were developed to improve oral hygiene and make **oral self-care** easier. The first electric toothbrush was introduced in the United States in 1959. Since then, powered toothbrushes have gone through several cycles of design, acceptance, and popularity. The third generation of powered toothbrushes is currently on the market. New technology and unique features make powered toothbrushes more effective, as well as more attractive to both consumers and dental professionals. In addition, current models are more reliable, easier to maintain, more portable, and some are more affordable than earlier models.

The safety and effectiveness of powered toothbrushes are based on evidence demonstrating that these brushes are more effective than manual toothbrushes for decreasing plaque and reducing gingival inflammation and bleeding.[22,23] Because the heads of these brushes are compact with denser bristle arrangements, interdental cleaning appears to be improved.[22,24] Although most powered brushes remove plaque more efficiently than hand brushing, the duration of brushing should not be reduced.

Powered toothbrushes either simulate manual toothbrushing with the brush head that moves from side-to-side or vibrates at a rapid speed. Other models imitate a professional polishing device through use of a circular brush head. Examples of these two types are shown in Figure 16-4. The bristles of circular brushes may rotate 360 degrees in one direction or may rotate clockwise and counter-clockwise, an action called rotation-oscillation. Another design has individual bristle tufts that rotate and counter rotate independently. The speed of the brush movement ranges from 3800 oscillations to 40,000 strokes per minute, suggesting that powered brushes remove more plaque than manual toothbrushes when time is constant.[25] Short-term evaluations show that the rotation-oscillation design removes plaque and reduces gingivitis better than manual toothbrushing.[26,27] No long-term clinical trials corroborate these findings or clarify their clinical significance.

Powered toothbrushes appear to help individuals who have difficulty maintaining an acceptable level of oral hygiene with a manual toothbrush. These include orthodontic patients, children with physical or mental impairments, adults with disabilities or limited dexterity, and institutionalized residents that have a caregiver provide their oral hygiene.[18,28] A powered brush may be beneficial for these individuals and patients who are less diligent in their oral self-care.

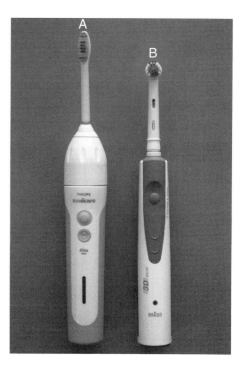

Figure 16-4   Two types of powered toothbrushes. **A** simulates manual toothbrushing but vibrates at a very rapid speed. **B** uses rotation-oscillation, that is, the brush head rotates clockwise, then counterclockwise.

Toothbrushing Methods

The early dental literature contains descriptions of several toothbrushing methods, distinguished by the direction and motion of the brush and the positioning of the bristles on the dentition. These methods have not been compared in recent clinical studies and the benefit of any one brushing method over another has not been subjected to evidence-based evaluations.

The prevalence of gingivitis indicates that toothbrushing is not as effective in practice as it is in supervised studies. The most common shortcoming of toothbrushing technique is lack of adequate time devoted to the task. Most people overestimate their actual brushing time, which is usually less than 1 minute per session. This brushing time removes only 40% to 50% of the plaque that is present.[29-32] Some patients benefit from a feedback device designed to monitor or extend the duration of brushing. Examples include using a timer or counting numbers that estimate adequate brushing time for each area of the mouth. The built-in timer on some powered toothbrushes functions in this manner.

Adverse Effects of Toothbrushing

Gingival abrasion and **gingival recession** are associated with improper toothbrushing. Gingival abrasion, or toothbrush trauma, is a localized acute injury caused by vigorous brushing, excessive brushing pressure, or hard toothbrush bristles. Depending on the depth of abrasion, this lesion may cause discomfort, but usually heals uneventfully in a few days. Gingival recession, which may be localized or generalized, is not reversible. Studies have linked gingival recession to age, malpositioned teeth, frequent toothbrushing, and use of a hard bristled toothbrush.[33-36] Although the prevalence of gingival recession is higher among those with high levels of oral hygiene, little evidence exists to indicate toothbrushing as the primary cause.[37] The major health complications of gingival recession are root caries and **dentin hypersensitivity**.

Cervical abrasion of teeth is characterized by a wedge-shaped defect in the root surface near the cementoenamel junction. Once thought to be a side effect of improper toothbrushing, cervical abrasion results from the abrasive agent in toothpaste in combination with dental erosion and occlusal factors. Toothbrush bristles alone have no deleterious effect on hard tissues.[38]

Interdental Plaque Removal

Toothbrushing does not completely remove plaque from proximal surfaces of teeth even when performed by the most adept person. Because periodontal diseases more frequently affect interproximal areas, interdental mechanical plaque removal is necessary for most patients. Dental floss is the most common means of interdental cleaning, although a much smaller proportion of the population use floss compared with brushing.[39] Other devices for interdental cleaning are available, including interdental brushes and wooden wedges. For some patients, these alternatives may be more effective at interdental cleaning than flossing.

Dental floss is available in different widths, materials, and either waxed or unwaxed, as illustrated in Figure 16-5. Plaque removal and gingival health are not dependent on the type of dental floss.[16,40] Automatic flossing devices were recently introduced as an aid to flossing. Two models are shown in Figure 16-6. The specialized forms of floss pictured in Figure 16-5 are designed to clean around abutment teeth or open interdental spaces. A floss threader, also pictured, is a device used to insert dental floss into the **embrasure** under the contact. This device is used for flossing under a fixed prosthesis, around orthodontic appliances, and between splinted teeth.

Using dental floss is a complicated skill that many people find difficult to master. Unlike toothbrushing, few people have learned how to properly use dental floss. Patients benefit from step-by-step instructions, as detailed in Box 16-1 and Figure 16-7. Because many people think that floss is used to remove food particles, patients must be advised that the objective is to remove plaque that adheres to the tooth surface. To accomplish this objective, the dental floss must be adapted to the shape of the tooth surface and carried under the margin of the gingival papilla. Floss holders, pictured in Figure 16-8, help those who cannot floss because of physical or manual dexterity challenges, limited opening of the mouth, or a strong gag reflex. These devices are as

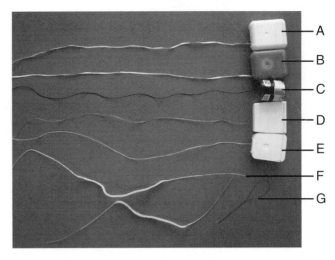

Figure 16-5 Examples of dental floss. **A** is dental tape. **B** is made of polytetrafluoroethylene (PTFE), a slippery substance that makes the floss slide easily between tight contacts and also shred-resistant. **C** is unwaxed nylon; the black color contrasts with the tooth so the user can see it. **D** is waxed dental floss flavored with mint. **E** is traditional waxed dental floss. **F** shows examples of "super floss," which is used in more open interdental spaces or under fixed bridges. Note the threader end for inserting the floss. **G** is a floss threader used to insert floss between splinted teeth, under prostheses, or around orthodontic appliances.

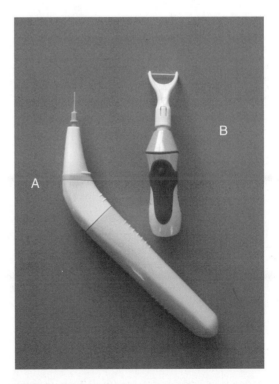

Figure 16-6 Examples of automatic flossers. **A** has a filament that is inserted between the teeth. The floss on **B** vibrates.

BOX 16-1

INSTRUCTIONS FOR THE Use OF Dental Floss

1. Use a 15- to 18-in length of floss.
2. Wrap the floss around the middle finger of each hand, leaving a 4- to-6-in section of floss between the two hands, as shown in Figure 16-7, **A**. Figure 16-7, **B** shows an alternate way to hold floss, by using a loop or circle of floss.
3. Hold the middle half inch of the floss taut between the forefingers or thumbs.
4. Rest one hand against the face and place the finger of the other on the tongue side of the teeth.
5. Place the floss on the chewing surface between the teeth, and guide the floss through the contact with a short, sawing motion.
6. Use gentle, controlled pressure on the floss to prevent snapping through onto the soft tissue.
7. Curve the floss in a "U" shape around the tooth surface and press firmly against the side of the tooth, as shown in Figure 16-7, **C**.
8. Slide gently under the gingival margin and move the floss up and down lengthwise on the tooth.
9. Clean the opposite proximal surface in the same way, as shown in Figure 16-7, **D**.
10. Remove the floss from between the teeth.
11. Move to a clean area of floss to begin the next area.

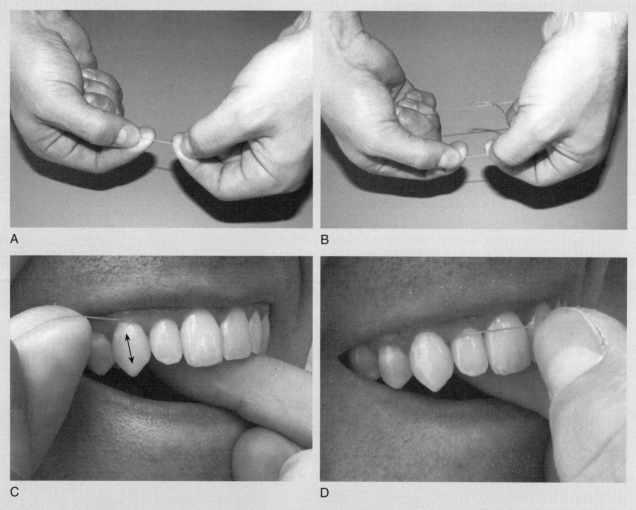

A   B

C   D

Figure 16-7 **A,** The "Spool Method" of flossing. Dental floss is spooled around the middle finger of each hand. **B,** The "Loop Method" of flossing. This method uses a circle of dental floss created by folding the floss and tying a knot 4 to 6 inches from the fold to create a circle. **C,** Floss is adapted to the curve of the tooth surface and moved along the length of the tooth. **D,** Note that the floss is moved under the gingival margin so that dental plaque removal will be complete.

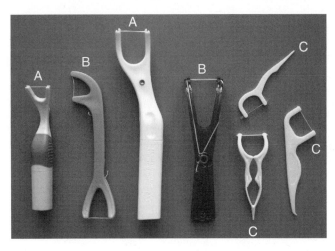

Figure 16-8 Floss holders available in several designs. The models labeled **A** have dental floss stored inside the handle. Floss is added to the holders labeled **B**. The three styles labeled **C** are one-time use, disposable flossers.

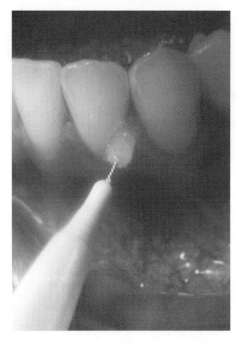

Figure 16-10 Use of an interdental brush. Note that the marginal gingiva is slightly displaced, allowing removal of subgingival plaque.

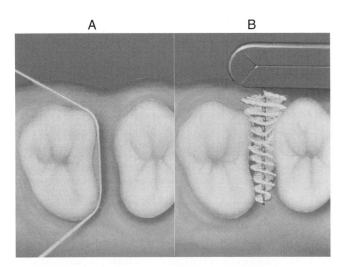

Figure 16-9 The drawing labeled **A** illustrates the limitations of dental floss on proximal root surfaces. Floss does not reach the area where a concavity exists. The bristles of an interdental brush are more likely to remove plaque in the depression, as depicted in the drawing labeled **B**.

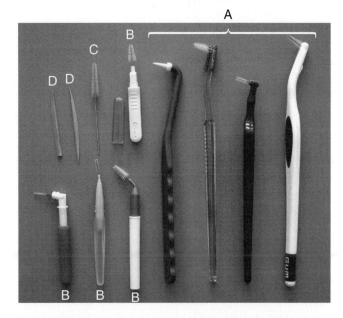

Figure 16-11 Alternatives to dental floss. **A,** Interdental brushes with replaceable brushes. **B,** Portable interdental brushes. **C,** A simple interdental brush that can be angled as needed. **D,** Interdental wooden wedges.

effective as conventional flossing methods and often preferred by the patient.[41,42]

The interdental papilla typically does not fill the embrasure between teeth affected by gingival recession. Furthermore, concavities and longitudinal depressions characterize exposed proximal root surfaces.[43] An interdental brush is more effective than dental floss for plaque removal in areas of recession or partially open or wide embrasures as shown in Figure 16-9.[44-46] Figure 16-10 illustrates the use of an interdental brush. The wide selection of interdental brush sizes and handle styles, displayed in Figure 16-11, allows this device to be individualized to

patient needs. An interdental wooden wedge, a triangular soft toothpick shown in Figure 16-9, is another alternative for interdental cleaning. Access from the lingual aspect and plaque removal near the lingual surface is limited by using this product.

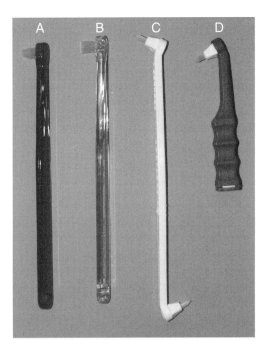

Figure 16-12 Examples of single tuft toothbrushes. **A** has a domed bristle pattern, and **B** has a flat brushing plane. **C** has a smaller brush head that fits better into interdental spaces. Differently angled brush heads adapt to facial or lingual surfaces. **D** is a portable model.

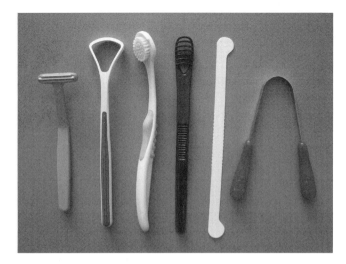

Figure 16-13 Examples of tongue-cleaning devices available commercially.

Single-Tuft Brushes

For the individual unable or unwilling to floss, the single-tuft or unituft toothbrush is a less effective option. Figure 16-12 shows several types available. The smaller brush head allows the user to direct the bristles into the interdental space. A single-tuft brush will not reach plaque under the contact.

The single-tuft brush is helpful for mechanical plaque removal from displaced or inclined teeth, exposed furcations, crowded and overlapped teeth, implants, fixed dental prostheses, and areas with limited access, including distal and lingual surfaces of posterior teeth.[17]

Tongue Cleaning

The tongue is covered with fissure and crypts. Taste receptor papillae are located on the dorsum of the tongue. This rough surface harbors large numbers of bacteria, including known periodontopathogens. The healthy tongue has a thin, pale white coating composed of microorganisms, food debris, desquamated epithelial cells, saliva, and components of blood products. This coating can be noticeably thicker, discolored, or both, ranging from yellow to nearly black. Because thicker tongue coatings have been observed in patients with periodontal diseases, the tongue is viewed as a potential reservoir for periodontal pathogens.[47] The presence and extent of this coating is associated with **oral malodor**, also known as halitosis.[48,49] For this reason, cleaning of the

tongue is an important component of oral self-care. Implements for cleaning the tongue include the toothbrush, a spoon, or a variety of commercial tongue scrapers shown in Figure 16-13.

Frequency of Plaque Control

The ideal frequency for oral self-care is not well defined. Based on observations of biofilm development, periodontal health can be maintained with complete removal of plaque every 4 days.[5,6] Few people have ideal oral health or the ability to perform perfect plaque removal, however. The effectiveness of oral hygiene depends on oral health needs, personal factors, and the presence or absence of systemic, environmental, local, and socioeconomic factors that are associated with an increased risk for developing periodontal disease. Therefore, the frequency of oral hygiene practice must be customized for each patient.

CHEMOTHERAPEUTIC AGENTS FOR PLAQUE CONTROL

The use of chemical agents to prevent periodontal diseases is based on the hypothesis that this disease follows an infectious disease model and that onset and severity are related to a consortium of pathogens. A number of dentifrices and oral rinses that contain antimicrobial agents are available to consumers. Although regulated by the FDA, most oral care products are viewed as cosmetic, creating a marketplace that is both convincing and bewildering. Advertising claims for cosmetic benefits include fresh breath, better brushing, stain removal, and tooth whitening. Even claims that oral care products "kill germs," something detergents and soaps accomplish at least temporarily, are disseminated. Any **therapeutic claim** subjects the product to more stringent regulation as a drug. The ADA Seal of Acceptance program reviews therapeutic claims, including caries prevention, antiplaque, anticalculus, or antigingivitis properties, and reduction in dentinal hypersensitivity. ADA evaluation of chemotherapeutics requires evidence of statistically and a clinically demonstrable reduction in both plaque and gingivitis, in addition to data that support the product safety.[50]

Current evidence supports the use of approved toothpastes and oral rinses only as adjuncts to mechanical plaque control. Dentifrices serve as a carrier for fluoride, which has been shown to reduce caries. For the control of periodontal disease, these products primarily benefit those who cannot achieve a level of personal oral hygiene or facilitate a sufficient level of oral hygiene to maintain periodontal health.

Two **antiseptic** oral rinses have been approved for personal plaque control, chlorhexidine gluconate (Peridex, Zila Pharmaceuticals, Phoenix, AZ.) and an essential oils combination product (Listerine, McNEIL-PPC, Inc., Morris Plains, NJ). Generic equivalents with supporting data are also approved.[51,52]

Chlorhexidine Gluconate Oral Rinse

Chlorhexidine gluconate is the most effective **antiplaque** agent currently approved. Chlorhexidine is a broad-spectrum antiseptic that is bactericidal and effective against some yeasts and viruses.[53] The effectiveness of chlorhexidine is documented in many controlled clinical trials showing a 50% to 60% decrease in plaque, a 30% to 45% reduction in gingivitis, and a reduction in the number of oral bacteria.[54,55] The efficacy of chlorhexidine stems from its ability to bind to oral tissues and slow release into the oral cavity. This characteristic, known as **substantivity**, provides a continued inhibitory effect on plaque formation for 12 to 14 hours.

In the United States, chlorhexidine is available only by prescription in 0.12% concentration for use twice a day. Some components of toothpastes, including sodium lauryl sulfate and calcium, interact with chlorhexidine to reduce its effectiveness; therefore, its use should be delayed for 30 minutes after toothbrushing.[56,57] Bitter taste of chlorhexidine and alteration in taste that may last as long as 4 hours are side effects resulting from chlorhexidine use. Other side effects include increased calculus formation, irritation of the mucosa, and staining of teeth, tongue, and restorations. Consequently, patients using chlorhexidine should be reevaluated every 6 months. The use of chlorhexidine for as long as 2 years is not associated with increased microbial resistance or disruption of the ecological balance in the oral cavity.[53,58]

Patient compliance with prescription medications is usually low and is a potential problem when the use of chlorhexidine is promoted. Other barriers to adherence of a chlorhexidine regimen include the inconvenience of obtaining the product by prescription and the associated expense.

Essential Oils Oral Rinse

A mouthwash with a combination of four phenol-related essential oils, thymol, menthol, eucalyptol, and methyl salicylate (oil of wintergreen), has been available commercially for more than 100 years. In 1988, it was the first over-the-counter oral rinse to receive the ADA Seal of Acceptance. Since then, generic equivalents have been approved. Studies demonstrate a moderate effectiveness in plaque control when this mouth rinse is used twice a day after toothbrushing. Plaque reduction ranged from 20% to 34% and gingivitis decreased by 28% to 34%.[59]

The original formulation contains 26.9% alcohol as an inactive ingredient, which is a concern because of a possible association with oral cancer, the potential for absorption through mucous membranes, and child safety. The National Cancer Institute and the FDA found no causal relationship between the incidence of oral cancer and alcohol in oral rinses.[59] In response to this concern, manufacturers introduced new formulations of essential oil rinses with reduced alcohol content.

Essential oil rinses may cause a burning sensation in the mouth but users accommodate in a short time. No other side effects have been reported. Recovering alcoholics may want to avoid mouth rinses with high alcohol content. Furthermore, a potential exists for gastrointestinal disturbance in patients who take metronidazole or disulfiram.[60]

Dentifrices

The delivery of an antimicrobial by way of a dentifrice seems ideal, given the general acceptance and wide use of these compounds. Toothpaste formulations are complex and the potential for interactions between the **biocide** and other ingredients has limited this application.

Triclosan

One dentifrice with the active ingredient triclosan (Colgate Total, Colgate Oral Pharmaceuticals, Piscataway, NJ) has been approved by the ADA as an **antigingivitis**, antiplaque agent. Triclosan, a common antiseptic used in soap and other personal care products, is a synthetic phenol derivative in a nonionic form, making it compatible with other components of toothpaste.[61] The formulation used in toothpaste contains 0.3% triclosan with 2% copolymer added to improve substantivity of the antimicrobial. Clinical trials suggest a moderate antiplaque activity and demonstrate a presence of the active ingredient in the oral environment for at least 12 hours.[62]

Stannous Fluoride

The bactericidal action of stannous fluoride was recognized when the original toothpaste was approved for caries prevention in 1955.[63] The efficacy of stannous fluoride for reducing gingivitis was confirmed years later when the product formulation was improved to stabilize the tin ion, which is responsible for the antibacterial action.[59,64,65] However, stannous fluoride dentifrices carry the ADA Seal of Acceptance only for anticaries activity. Extrinsic staining of teeth is a possible side effect of stannous fluoride toothpastes and they must be labeled accordingly.

Anticalculus Agents

Dental calculus, known commonly as tartar, is mineralized dental plaque. Calculus occurs in most people, but the extent varies widely among individuals and populations. Oral self-care, frequency of dental care, age, systemic health, diet, and ethnicity affect the formation of calculus. Calculus is a contributing factor to periodontal diseases due to the retention of dental plaque on its rough surface.

Soluble pyrophosphates in dentifrice inhibit calculus formation. Formulations with the greatest efficacy contain a combination of pyrophosphates and a copolymer. Studies show a reduction in supragingival calculus deposits ranging from 25% to 45%.[62,66] Promoted for their "tartar control" properties, these products provide greater benefits for moderate and heavy calculus formers and the anticalculus effect increases with duration of use.[67]

PROFESSIONAL CARE

The methods of oral self-care discussed have limited utility in removal of subgingival plaque, which is essential for the prevention of periodontal diseases. Professional dental care is necessary to control the subgingival biofilm. Furthermore, early identification of clinical signs of disease is crucial to arrest inflammatory periodontal diseases in susceptible individuals.

Oral Prophylaxis

The annual or semi-annual dental visit is an example of secondary prevention with a goal of early diagnosis and treatment, but these recall schedules are not based upon sound science. Typically, this "check-up" incorporates examination of the teeth and surrounding tissues for indications of periodontal diseases and conditions, periodontal probing of the gingival crevice for signs of inflammation, and traditional **oral prophylaxis** or "dental cleaning" to remove accumulated plaque and calculus from the teeth. Outcomes are enhanced when professional plaque removal includes oral hygiene instructions[68] and recall is based on estimation of future disease risk.

People who receive regular professional care have better oral health status and retain more teeth over time.[69-71] On the other hand, insufficient evidence exists to demonstrate specific periodontal health benefits of oral prophylaxis in those who are at low risk for chronic adult periodontitis.[72]

Mechanical Nonsurgical Periodontal Therapy

Mechanical nonsurgical periodontal therapy, also known as scaling and root planing or subgingival debridement, is indicated for individuals with early periodontitis and as the initial phase of treatment of moderate or advanced periodontal diseases. Scaling and root planing removes subgingival calculus and plaque, disrupts the dental biofilm, and frees the root surface of contamination from microbial byproducts. One of the most common periodontal procedures, effective nonsurgical therapy requires meticulous instrumentation of periodontal pockets. Similar results are achieved with the use of hand instruments or ultrasonic scalers.[73,74]

The primary effect of mechanical nonsurgical therapy is reducing the microbial challenge. Multiple clinical studies show that nonsurgical therapy significantly decreases the number of microorganisms in subgingival plaque and alters the subgingival microbiota to decrease the likelihood of disease progression.[75-79] Evidence supports the efficacy of scaling and root planing in reducing pocket depth through resolution of inflammation and stabilizing periodontal attachment levels.[73,74,80,81] An important outcome of reduced probing depths is an environment that permits personal oral hygiene practices to be more effective.

Antimicrobial Adjuncts to Mechanical Nonsurgical Therapy

Subgingival instrumentation is technically demanding. Pocket depths, anatomy of root surfaces, and other tooth related factors, such as furcations, affect the outcome of therapy. The procedure does not remove bacteria that invade the periodontal soft tissues or organisms found in dentinal tubules of the tooth root. The host response and systemic health factors influence the results of mechanical nonsurgical periodontal therapy. Antimicrobial agents are used to enhance the effectiveness of scaling and root planing. Antimicrobials may be delivered locally or systemic antibiotic drugs may be administered.

Locally delivered chemotherapeutics are placed in the gingival crevice to make direct contact with the site of infection. These products are called controlled- or sustained-release antimicrobials because their effectiveness is ensured only when clearance or washing away of the active ingredient by the **gingival crevicular fluid** can be countered. In a periodontal pocket, the gingival crevicular fluid turns over every 90 seconds and will quickly dilute the concentration of any medication.[82]

Four products have been approved by the FDA as an adjunct to periodontal debridement in patients with chronic adult periodontitis. Each product has an antimicrobial as the active ingredient and a delivery vehicle that improves substantivity or keeps the agent in place in the pocket. These include 10% doxycycline hyclate in a bioabsorbable polymer base (Atridox, CollaGenex Pharmaceuticals, Inc., Newton, PA), tetracycline fibers (Actisite, ALZA Corporation, Mountain View, CA.), minocycline in a powder form combined with a bioadhesive, bioresorbable polymer (Arestin, OraPharma, Inc., Warmister, PA), and chlorhexidine digluconate in a biodegradable gel wafer (PerioChip, Dexcel Pharma, Or-Akiva, Israel).

Results from clinical studies showed reductions in probing depth, decreases in selected pathogens, especially spirochetes, and slight gains in clinical attachment level.[83] When compared with scaling and root planing procedures alone, however, probing depths were reduced by less than 1 mm and significant increases in attachment levels were uncommon. Therefore, the clinical significance of the study outcomes is unclear.

One advantage of the using systemic antibiotic therapy is that the drug will treat the portions of the mouth not otherwise affected by subgingival debridement, including the tongue, throat, and oral mucosa. Tetracyclines, metronidazole, ornidazole, penicillins, and macrolides are among the systemic antimicrobials tested as adjuncts for periodontal debridement.[84,85] Possible adverse consequences of antibiotic use include colonization of the subgingival niche with drug resistant microbial strains and allergic reactions to the medication.[86] Antibiotics are not routinely used as adjuncts to periodontal debridement but are used when the patient has a poor response to therapy or for individuals with aggressive forms of disease.[75,87]

Periodontal Maintenance

Periodontal maintenance, also called supportive periodontal therapy or periodontal recall, refers to professional care for those who have previously received treatment of periodontal disease. The objective of periodontal maintenance is to prevent the recurrence of disease, to stop disease progression and, ultimately, to reduce the loss of teeth.[88] Evidence demonstrates the effectiveness of periodontal maintenance in achieving these goals.

Periodontal maintenance procedures include review of the patient's health status, complete clinical examination of the dentition and periodontium, assessment of risk for future disease, and evaluation of the patient's skills, attitudes, and self-care knowledge.[89] Mechanical nonsurgical periodontal therapy performed in sites with clinical indications of inflammation disrupts the biofilm, reduces periodontal pathogens in the local environment, and arrests disease.

Monitoring of the patient's oral hygiene performance is an important function of periodontal maintenance. Periodic review of plaque removal skills and clarification of periodontal health issues ensures adherence with recommendations and improves periodontal health.[90]

Individual needs and risk factors determine the frequency of periodontal maintenance. Conventional practice is to recall patients with chronic adult periodontitis every 3 months for periodontal maintenance, although research has shown that intervals ranging from 2 to 12 months can also be effective.[89,91,92] Timing of periodontal maintenance is reevaluated at each recall visit. For patients who maintain a high standard of oral hygiene and exhibit little inflammation, the interval may be extended gradually from 4 to 6 months.[93,94] Periodontal maintenance will be scheduled more frequently for those with clinical signs of disease progression or inadequate self-care.

Correction of Tooth-Related Local Factors

Local factors for a site-specific disease are associated with periodontal disease progression. Dental conditions that cause plaque retention or inhibit the removal of plaque contribute to a more severe clinical disease presentation. These conditions include restorations with overhanging margins, open contacts, ill-fitting dental prostheses, overcontoured crowns, food impaction sites, and malocclusion. Furcation involvement, root surface concavities and longitudinal grooves are normal anatomical characteristics and examples of local factors; however, these factors are not amenable to change. Tooth-related local factors should be corrected, when possible, through professional care as a part of comprehensive periodontal disease prevention.[95,96]

PREVENTIVE STRATEGIES AIMED AT ENVIRONMENTAL FACTORS

Environmental and systemic risk factors influence the progression of periodontal diseases by affecting the agent and host interaction. These risk factors include the use of tobacco, genetic predisposition, nutrition, and comorbidities, such as diabetes. Tobacco cessation is an integral component of a comprehensive strategy for prevention of periodontal diseases.[97]

Tobacco Cessation

The detrimental effects of smoking on periodontal health are well documented, and cigarette smoking is recognized as a major risk factor for periodontal diseases.[98-101] Smokers are three times more likely to have severe periodontitis than nonsmokers and half of adult periodontitis cases are attributable to current and former smoking.[102]

Smokers exhibit a more severe clinical presentation of disease, including greater loss of attachment, deeper pockets, more teeth affected, increased loss of alveolar bone, and more missing teeth.[103-106] Gingival bleeding is reduced in smokers, however, apparently because of impairment of the gingival vasculature by smoking.[107,108] A dose-response relationship exists between the severity of periodontitis and the duration of smoking (number of years) and intensity of smoking (the number of cigarettes).[109] Light smokers are twice as likely to have attachment loss as nonsmokers, whereas heavy smokers have approximately five times the risk of developing periodontal disease.[110] A similar pattern is observed with bone loss. Light to heavy smokers experience three to seven times greater risk of bone loss respectively when compared with nonsmokers.[111] Furthermore, smoking negatively affects the outcome of periodontal therapy, including mechanical nonsurgical therapy.[112-115]

Clearly, tobacco cessation is an important risk reduction strategy for periodontal health. Indeed, smokers who quit lose fewer teeth and have better periodontal status than current smokers.[106,116-118] Few patients understand that smoking affects periodontal health, although most patients expect dental services to include tobacco counseling.[119] Dental professionals have a responsibility to ask about patients' tobacco habits and offer tobacco cessation advice, assistance, and support with pharmacotherapy.[120] Research shows that interventions in dental offices are successful in helping patients quit tobacco.[121-123] Tobacco cessation strategies for dental practice are presented in Chapter 17.

MODULATION OF THE HOST RESPONSE

A third approach to preventing periodontal diseases is to alter the host response to the challenge of the infectious agent. This strategy is relatively new and the body of evidence somewhat limited.

An inflammatory response is triggered when pathogenic microorganisms that inhabit the dental biofilm contact the gingival tissue. Although the host response is biologically protective by design, the cytotoxic products that are produced to eliminate the insult by the bacteria result in the breakdown of the periodontium. Neutrophils and macrophages migrate into the connective tissue of the gingiva where they release cytokines, proteases, prostaglandins, and collagenase that destroy connective tissue and, ultimately, alveolar bone.[124] The rationale for host modulation is to change or block the pathway that leads to periodontal tissue destruction.

Three approaches are proposed for **host modulation therapy**: collagenase inhibitors, nonsteroidal antiinflammatory drugs, and bone-sparing agents similar to those used to treat osteoporosis. The FDA has approved the use of doxycycline hyclate (Periostat, CollaGenex Pharmaceuticals, Inc.) to suppress collagenase activity.[125] This form of tetracycline administered at a sub-antimicrobial dose is used as an adjunct to nonsurgical mechanical therapy for patients with adult periodontitis. Doxycycline produced slightly reduced probing depths and increased clinical attachment over scaling and root planing alone. These limited benefits may not justify the use of doxycycline for host modulation therapy in routine preventive services.[126]

RISK ASSESSMENT AND SELECTION OF PREVENTION STRATEGIES

Risk assessment provides the basis for developing a strategy for periodontal disease prevention for each patient (see Chapter 5). Risk assessment is a complex assessment that uses multiple sources of information, including the patient history, findings from clinical examinations, and diagnostic tests to identify disease risk factors. The risk assessment is used to establish a risk profile and classify the level of risk. This information is used to tailor preventive strategies to the patient's risk and to prioritize preventive interventions. Risk-based prevention improves the effectiveness of disease management strategies, enhances health outcomes, and increases cost-effectiveness.

Complete and ongoing patient assessment is essential for developing and adapting a preventive strategy. Dental professionals often have a bias toward the clinical examination and its use for the diagnosis and treatment planning; however, other components of patient assessment are central to the development of the preventive care plan. For example, the dental history identifies common symptoms of periodontal problems, such as loose teeth, sensitivity, or gingival bleeding, which demonstrate the effects of disease. The patient's view of their oral health, their perception of their role in their own health, satisfaction with previous care, and any past difficulties or problems associated with previous dental treatment provide insight that will allow focused communication.

Recording of plaque and calculus is especially important in risk-based prevention of periodontal disease. Such a chart displays the pattern of plaque formation and helps determine the contribution of oral hygiene to the risk for periodontal disease. For the patient, the plaque index recording is a visual aid to explain reasons for any increased probing depths recorded during the periodontal examination.

The oral self-care evaluation measures the patient's oral hygiene knowledge, attitudes, and practices. The first step is identification of the patient's oral care routine, including the identification of products and devices. Specific questions can be used to determine the duration and frequency of these oral hygiene behaviors and to evaluate the patient's understanding of the role of these practices in disease prevention. The patient's willingness to change current oral self-care behaviors should be established. Adherence to self-care practices is discussed in Chapter 11. Finally, the dental professional should observe the patient using a toothbrush and dental floss to determine the level of skill and dexterity and the effectiveness of plaque removal. Otherwise, skill deficits or other limitations may go unrecognized.[127]

When assessment is complete, the next step is to identify all risk factors and rank them in order of importance. By exploring all the possible strategies, educational and clinical approaches can be used to mitigate the effect of each risk factor.

Adherence to a preventive plan is more likely when the patient and the clinician participate as partners in its development. Such a partnership between the clinician and patient is known as a therapeutic alliance. To be active in this alliance, the patient needs the same information base as the clinician. Using the framework of a therapeutic alliance means that the patient is an active participant in the decision-making process.

The dental professional has a duty to inform the patient about his or her present oral health status, the diagnosis, findings of the clinical examination, etiology of periodontal disease, and his or her own specific risk factors. Moreover, the patient must be aware of a problem to appreciate the need for professional care, adopting new behaviors, or changing current ones. Oral health education and behavior modification are the foundation of periodontal disease prevention because the ultimate success of self-care and professional care depend on changes in the patient's behavior. Therefore, the time and effort dedicated to educational services should be equal to that committed to clinical services.

Once the initial periodontal status is clear, the patient is ready to identify oral health goals and set short-term objectives toward achieving improved periodontal health. The impact of professional services and changes in self-care should be discussed and choices agreed on.

The main undertaking in oral hygiene instruction is to ensure that the individual effectively removes plaque through self-care measures. Patient adherence is hampered because plaque is imperceptible and gingival disease is largely asymptomatic. A disclosing agent that temporarily stains the biofilm helps the patient identify areas that need attention and the time necessary to remove plaque. Many patients do not equate toothbrushing with plaque removal or understand the connection to gingival health. The majority of people say that they brush to prevent decay, and others report that they like the clean feeling, want fresher breath, or would like to improve their appearance.[11]

Improving a patient's plaque control skills takes more time and reinforcement than allowed for by most dental professionals. One role of the dental professional is to engage the patient as a partner in their own oral health, however, which can be done at intervals at each appointment. Useful strategies are described in Chapter 10. Brief interventions are positive for the patient and clinician. It is effective to focus on plaque that remains in disease sites to move the patient to improve his or her oral hygiene technique. The patient is more willing to make small changes than to completely alter an established habit. One who does not floss at all may agree to floss an unhealthy area, for example.

As a part of the therapeutic alliance, the patient should choose his or her plaque control devices and oral care products from among those available. Without pressure to comply, the patient is likely to ask for the dental professional's recommendation. Another area for collaboration is the frequency of oral self-care. The patient who does not use dental floss every day may agree to do so every other day or 3 times a week. The practitioner can facilitate the negotiation with a question beginning, "Would you be willing to?"

Follow-up sessions are essential to monitor the patient's progress in achieving short-term goals and the response to professional care. A question that begins with "What keeps you from?" helps to identify barriers to success. For example, when dental floss "is too hard to get between my teeth" the clinician may suggest a Teflon floss that slides easily or can introduce an interdental brush.

The PREVENT Model, shown in Box 16-2, offers a way to remember the basics to develop a preventive plan.[128] The purpose of the model is to establish a sequence of educational and clinical services decided on in collaboration with the patient that will be effective for reducing the risk for disease and promoting oral health.

BOX 16-2

THE *PREVENT* MODEL

The goal of the model is to establish a sequence of educational and clinical services decided on in collaboration with the patient that will reduce the risk for disease and promote oral health.

Provide complete information.
Inform the patient of the findings of the clinical examination, present oral health status, causes of periodontal disease, and personal risk factors.

Realistic goals identified.
Work with the patient to set realistic short- and long-term goals for improving oral health and changing oral health behaviors.

Explain professional care options.
Discuss the professional services available to solve current problems, maintain oral health, and reduce risk for disease.

Variety of choices offered.
Offer the patient a choice of plaque control devices, oral care products, and self-care methods.

Encourage the patient.
Increase the patient's self-confidence in changing oral self-care behaviors through encouragement, reinforcement, skill building, and other methods.

Negotiate frequency of self-care.
Support the patient in assuming responsibility for personal health and negotiate a schedule for the self-care regimen.

Time reevaluation appropriately.
Sequence appointments to reinforce new skills and evaluate progress toward achieving short-term goals.

SUMMARY

The multifactorial nature of periodontal diseases provides challenges to maintaining optimal health. Understanding those factors that place each patient at risk for future disease allows the practitioner to tailor a plan of prevention. This preventive care plan should include an assessment of risk, strategy to minimize risk and implement a professional care and self-care strategy that leads to improved periodontal health. Initiating a therapeutic alliance with the patient as a partner in their care can improve their overall periodontal health and adherence to home care regimens. Dental professionals should receive training to better understand patient behavior change and effectively provide oral health education.

Improvements in periodontal risk assessment can be achieved through a greater understanding of the causal pathway for the diseases. Continuing research to identify other organisms involved in periodontal infections, to establish the threshold levels of microorganisms necessary to initiate disease, and to elucidate the complex relationship between the infection and the host response would increase the effectiveness of preventive approaches. Host modulation therapy presents an opportunity to prevent destruction of periodontal tissues that could reduce tooth loss among susceptible adults and save precious resources devoted to restoring a functional dentition following treatment of periodontal diseases.

Evaluation of periodontal home care devices, including toothbrushes, brushing methods, and other plaque removal devices, are necessary to better inform the patient. Recommendations should be made on the basis of evidence-based science, which is unavailable for many of these products. Greater knowledge about both the etiology of periodontal diseases and preventive approaches will improve the periodontal health of our patients.

REFERENCES

1. Marsh PD: Dental plaque: biological significance of a biofilm and community life-style, *J Clin Periodontol* 32:7-15, 2005.
2. Nishihara T, Koseki T: Microbial etiology of periodontitis, *Periodontol 2000* 36:14-26, 2004.
3. Socransky SS, Haffajee AD: Dental biofilms: difficult therapeutic targets, *Periodontol 2000* 28:12-55, 2000.
4. Listgarten MA: The structure of dental plaque, *Periodontol 2000* 5:52-65, 1994.
5. Löe H, Theilade E, Jensen SB: Experimental gingivitis in man, *J Periodontol* 36:177-187, 1965.
6. Theilade E, Wright WH, Jensen SB et al.: Experimental gingivitis in man. II. A longitudinal clinical and bacteriological investigation, *J Periodontal Res* 1:1-13, 1966.
7. Mombelli A: The role of dental plaque in the initiation and progression of periodontal diseases. In Lang NP, Attstrom R, and Löe H, editors: *Proceedings of the 1(st) European workshop on mechanical plaque control*, Berlin, 1998, Quintessenz Verlag.
8. Hellstrom MK, Ramberg P, Krok L et al.: The effect of supragingival plaque control on the subgingival microflora in human periodontitis, *J Clin Periodontol* 23:934-940, 1996.
9. Katsanoulas T, Renee I, Attstrom R: The effect of supragingival plaque control on the composition of the subgingival flora in periodontal pockets, *J Clin Periodontol* 19:760-765, 1992.
10. Dahlen G, Lindhe J, Sato K et al.: The effect of supragingival plaque control on the subgingival microbiota in subjects with periodontal disease, *J Clin Periodontol* 19:802-809, 1992.
11. Gift HC: Current utilization patterns of oral hygiene practices. State-of-the-science review. In Löe H and Kleinman DV, editors: *Dental plaque control measures and oral hygiene practices*, Washington, DC, 1986, IRL Press.
12. MIT News Office: Toothbrush beats out car and computer as the invention Americans can't live without, according to Lemelson-MIT Survey, Massachusetts Institute of Technology News Office, 2003.
13. Petersilka GJ, Ehmke B, Flemmig TF: Antimicrobial effects of mechanical debridement. *Periodontol 2000* 28:56-71, 2002.
14. Haffajee AD, Thompson M, Torresyap G et al.: Efficacy of manual and powered toothbrushes (I). Effect on clinical parameters, *J Clin Periodontol* 28:937-946, 2001.
15. Cancro LP, Fischman SL: The expected effect on oral health of dental plaque control through mechanical removalm, *Periodontol 2000* 8:60-74, 2000.
16. Frandsen A: Mechanical oral hygiene practices. A state-of-the-science review. In Löe H and Kleinman DV, editors: *Dental plaque control measures and oral hygiene practices*, Washington, DC, 1986, IRL Press.
17. Brothwell DJ, Jutai DK, Hawkins RJ: An update of mechanical oral hygiene practices: evidence-based recommendations for disease prevention. *J Can Dent Assoc* 64:295-306, 1998.
18. Sicilia A, Arregui I, Gallego M, et al.: Home oral hygiene revisited. Options and evidence. *Oral Health Prev Dent* 1:407-22, 2003.
19. Claydon N, Addy M, Scratcher C et al.: Comparative professional plaque removal study using 8 branded toothbrushes, *J Clin Periodontol* 29:310-316, 2002.
20. ADA Council on Scientific Affairs: *Acceptance Program Guidelines. Toothbrushes*, Chicago, IL, 1998, American Dental Association.
21. ADA Council on Scientific Affairs: *Acceptance Program Guidelines. Determination of Efficacy in Product Evaluation*, Chicago, IL 1999, American Dental Association.
22. Heasman PA, McCracken GI: Powered toothbrushes: A review of clinical trials. *J Clin Periodontol* 26:407-420, 1999.
23. Barnes CM: Powered toothbrushes: A focus on the evidence. *Compend Contin Educ Oral Hygiene* 7:3-9, 2000.
24. Stoltze K, Bay L: Comparison of a manual and a new electric toothbrush for controlling plaque and gingivitis. *J Clin Periodontol* 21:86-90, 1994.
25. van der Weijden FA, Timmerman MF, Snoek IM et al.: Toothbrushing duration and plaque removing efficacy of electric toothbrushes, *Am J Dent* 9:S31-S36, 1996.
26. Robinson PG, Deacon SA, Deery C et al.: Manual versus powered toothbrushing for oral health, *Cochrane Database Syst Rev*, 2005.
27. Sicilia A, Arregui I, Gallego M, et al.: A systematic review of powered vs manual toothbrushes in periodontal cause-related therapy, *J Clin Periodontol* 29:39-54, 2002.
28. van der Weijden FA, Timmerman MF, Danser MM, et al.: The role of electric toothbrushes: advantages and limitations, In Lang NP, Attstrom R, and Löe H, editors: *Proceedings of the 1(st) European workshop on mechanical plaque control*, Berlin, 1998, Quintessenz Verlag.
29. van der Weijden GA, Timmerman MF, Nijboer A et al.: A comparative study of electric toothbrushes for the effectiveness of

plaque removal in relation to toothbrushing duration. Timerstudy, *J Clin Periodontol* 20:476-481, 1993.

30. Saxer UP, Barbakow J, Yankell SL: New studies on estimated and actual toothbrushing times and dentifrice use, *J Clin Dent* 9: 49-51, 1998.

31. van der Weijden GA, Timmerman MF, van der Velden U: Relationship between the plaque removal efficacy of a manual toothbrush and brushing force, *J Clin Periodontol* 25:413-416, 1998.

32. De la Rosa M, Guerra JZ, Johnson DA et al.: Plaque growth and removal with daily toothbrushing, *J Periodontol* 50:661-664, 1979.

33. Serino G, Wennstrom JL, Lindhe J et al.: The prevalence and distribution of gingival recession in subjects with a high standard of oral hygiene, *J Clin Periodontol* 21:57-63, 1994.

34. Khocht A, Simon G, Person P et al.: Gingival recession in relation to history of hard toothbrush use, *J Periodontol* 64:900-905, 1993.

35. Vehkalahti M: Occurrence of gingival recession in adults, *J Periodontol* 60:599-603, 1989.

36. Niemi ML, Sandholm L, Ainamo J: Frequency of gingival lesions after standardized brushing as related to stiffness of toothbrush and abrasiveness of dentifrice, *J Clin Periodontol* 11:254-261, 1984.

37. Litonjua LA, Andreana S, Bush PJ et al.: Toothbrushing and gingival recession, *Int Dent J* 53:67-72, 2003.

38. Addy M, Hunter ML: Can tooth brushing damage your health? Effects on oral and dental tissues, *Int Dent J* 53:177-186, 2003.

39. Bakdash B: Current patterns of oral hygiene product use and practices, *Periodontol 2000* 8:11-14, 1995.

40. Kinane DF: The role of interdental cleaning in effective plaque control: need for interdental cleaning in primary and secondary prevention. In Lang NP, Attstrom R, and Löe H, editors: *Proceedings of the 1(st) European workshop on mechanical plaque control*, Berlin, 1998, Quintessenz Verlag.

41. Carter-Hanson C, Gadbury-Amyot C, Killoy W: Comparison of the plaque removal efficacy of a new flossing aid (Quik Floss) to finger flossing, *J Clin Periodontol* 23:873-878, 1996.

42. Spolsky VW, Perry DA, Meng Z et al.: Evaluating the efficacy of a new flossing aid, *J Clin Periodontol* 20:490-497, 1993.

43. Fox SC, Bosworth BL: A morphological survey of proximal root concavities: a consideration in periodontal therapy, *J Am Dent Assoc* 114:811-814, 1987.

44. Christou V, Timmerman MF, van der Velden et al.: Comparison of different approaches of interdental oral hygiene: interdental brushes versus dental floss, *J Periodontol* 69:759-764, 1998.

45. Kiger RD, Nylund K, Feller RP: A comparison of proximal plaque removal using floss and interdental brushes, *J Clin Periodontol* 18:681-684, 1991.

46. Smukler H, Nager MC, Tolmie PC: Interproximal tooth morphology and its effect on plaque removal, *Quintessence Int* 20:249-255, 1989.

47. Yaegaki K, Sanada K: Volatile sulfur compounds in mouth air from clinically healthy subjects and patients with periodontal disease, *J Periodontal Res* 27:233-238, 1992.

48. De Boever EH, Loesche WJ: Assessing the contribution of anaerobic microflora of the tongue to oral malodor, *J Am Dent Assoc* 126:1384-1393, 1995.

49. Bosy A, Kulkarni GV, Rosenberg M et al.: Relationship of oral malodor to periodontitis: evidence of independence in discrete subpopulations, *J Periodontol* 65:37-46, 1994.

50. ADA Council on Scientific Affairs: *Acceptance program guidelines. Chemotherapeutic products for control of gingivitis*, Chicago, 1997, American Dental Association.

51. Council on Dental Therapeutics accepts Listerine, *J Am Dent Assoc* 117:515-516, 1988.

52. Council on Dental Therapeutics accepts Peridex, *J Am Dent Assoc* 117:516-517, 1988.

53. Marsh PD: Microbiological aspects of the chemical control of plaque and gingivitis, *J Dent Res* 71:1431-1438, 1992.

54. Barnett ML: The role of therapeutic antimicrobial mouthrinses in clinical practice: control of supragingival plaque and gingivitis, *J Am Dent Assoc* 134:699-704, 2003.

55. Walker CB: Microbiological effects of mouthrinses containing antimicrobials, *J Clin Periodontol* 15:499-505, 1988.

56. Barkvoll P, Rolla G, Svendsen K: Interaction between chlorhexidine digluconate and sodium lauryl sulfate in vivo, *J Clin Periodontol* 16:593-595, 1989.

57. Barkvoll P, Rolla G, Bellagamba S: Interaction between chlorhexidine digluconate and sodium monofluorophosphate in vitro, *Scand J Dent Res* 96:30-33, 1988.

58. Sreenivasan P, Gaffar A: Antiplaque biocides and bacterial resistance: a review, *J Clin Periodontol* 29:965-974, 2002.

59. Wu CD, Savitt ED: Evaluation of the safety and efficacy of over-the-counter oral hygiene products for the reduction and control of plaque and gingivitis, *Periodontol 2000* 28:91-105, 2002.

60. Claffey N: Essential oil mouthwashes: a key component in oral health management, *J Clin Periodontol* 5:22-24, 2003.

61. Rolla G, Kjærheim V, Waaler SM: The role of antiseptics in primary prevention. In Lang NP, Karring T, and Lindhe J, editors: *Proceedings of the 2(nd) European workshop on periodontology*, Berlin, 1997, Quintessenz Verlag.

62. Brading MG, Marsh PD: The oral environment: the challenge for antimicrobials in oral care products, *Int Dent J* 53:353-362, 2003.

63. Fischman SL: The history of oral hygiene products: how far have we come in 6000 years? *Periodontol 2000* 15:7-14, 1997.

64. Mankodi S, Bartizek RD, Winston JL et al.: Anti-gingivitis efficacy of a stabilized 0.454% stannous fluoride/sodium hexametaphosphate dentifrice, *J Clin Periodontol* 32:75-80, 2005.

65. McClanahan SF, Beiswanger BB, Bartizek RD et al.: A comparison of stabilized stannous fluoride dentifrice and triclosan/copolymer dentifrice for efficacy in the reduction of gingivitis and gingival bleeding: six-month clinical results, *J Clin Dent* 8:39-45, 1997.

66. Sanz M: Anti-calculus efficacy. In Lang NP, Karring T, and Lindhe J, editors: *Proceedings of the 2(nd) European workshop on periodontology*, Berlin, 1997, Quintessenz Verlag.

67. Netuveli GS, Sheiham A: A systematic review of the effectiveness of anticalculus dentifrices, *Oral Health Prev Dent* 2:49-58, 2004.

68. Needleman I, Suvan J, Moles DR et al.: A systematic review of professional mechanical plaque removal for prevention of periodontal diseases, *J Clin Periodontol* 32:229-282, 2005.

69. Kressin NR, Boehmer U, Nunn ME et al.: Increased preventive practices lead to greater tooth retention, *J Dent Res* 82:223-227, 2003.

70. Lang WP, Farghaly MM, Ronis DL: The relation of preventive dental behaviors to periodontal health status, *J Clin Periodontol* 21:194-198, 1994.

71. Boehmer U, Kressin NR, Spiro A III: Preventive dental behaviors and their association with oral health status in older white men, *J Dent Res* 78:869-877, 1999.

72. Beirne P, Forgie A, Worthington HV et al.: Routine scale and polish for periodontal health in adults, *Cochrane Database Syst Rev*, 2005.

73. Hallmon WW, Rees TD: Local anti-infective therapy: mechanical and physical approaches. A systematic review, *Ann Periodontol* 8:99-114, 2003.

74. van der Weijden GA, Timmerman MF: A systematic review on the clinical efficacy of subgingival debridement in the treatment of chronic periodontitis, *J Clin Periodontol* 29:55-71, 2002.

75. Umeda M, Takeuchi Y, Noguchi K et al.: Effects of nonsurgical periodontal therapy on the microbiota, *Periodontol* 36:98-120, 2000.

76. Cugini MA, Haffajee AD, Smith C et al.: The effect of scaling and root planing on the clinical and microbiological parameters of periodontal diseases: 12-month results, *J Clin Periodontol* 27:30-36, 2000.

77. Haffajee AD, Cugini MA, Dibart S et al.: The effect of SRP on the clinical and microbiological parameters of periodontal diseases, *J Clin Periodontol* 24:324-334, 1997.

78. Sbordone L, Ramaglia L, Gulletta E et al.: Recolonization of the subgingival microflora after scaling and root planing in human periodontitis, *J Periodontol* 61:579-584, 1990.

79. Mousques T, Listgarten MA, Phillips RW: Effect of scaling and root planing on the composition of the human subgingival microbial flora, *J Periodontal Res* 15:144-151, 1980.

80. Suvan JE: Effectiveness of mechanical nonsurgical pocket therapy, *Periodontol 2000* 37:48-71, 2005.

81. Hung HC, Douglass CW: Meta-analysis of the effect of scaling and root planing, surgical treatment and antibiotic therapies on periodontal probing depth and attachment loss, *J Clin Periodontol* 29:975-986, 2002.

82. Research, Science and Therapy Committee of the American Academy of Periodontology: The role of controlled drug delivery for periodontitis, *J Periodontol* 71:125-140, 2000.

83. Bonito AJ, Lohr KN, Lux L et al.: *Effectiveness of antimicrobial adjuncts to scaling and root planing therapy for periodontitis, vol 2, evidence tables,* AHRQ Publication No. 04-E014-3. Rockville, MD, 2004, Agency for Healthcare Research and Quality.

84. Herrera D, Sanz M, Jepsen S et al.: A systematic review on the effect of systemic antimicrobials as an adjunct to scaling and root planing in periodontitis patients, *J Clin Periodontol* 29:136-159, 2002.

85. Bonito AJ, Lux L, Lohr KN: Impact of local adjuncts to scaling and root planing in periodontal disease therapy: a systematic review, *J Periodontol* 76:1227-1236, 2005.

86. Jorgensen MG, Slots J: Responsible use of antimicrobials in periodontics, *J Calif Dent Assoc* 28:185-193, 2000.

87. Mombelli A, Samaranayake LP: Topical and systemic antibiotics in the management of periodontal diseases, *Int Dent J* 54:3-14, 2004.

88. Cohen RE: Position paper: periodontal maintenance, *J Periodontol* 74:1395-1401, 2003.

89. American Academy of Periodontology: Parameter on periodontal maintenance, *J Periodontol* 71:849-850, 2000.

90. Echeverria JJ, Manau GC, Guerrero A: Supportive care after active periodontal treatment: a review, *J Clin Periodontol* 23:898-905, 1996.

91. Renvert S, Persson GR: Supportive periodontal therapy, *Periodontol 2000* 36:179-195, 2004.

92. Hancock EB, Newell DH: Preventive strategies and supportive treatment, *Periodontol 2000* 25:59-76, 2001.

93. Rosen B, Olavi G, Badersten A et al.: Effect of different frequencies of preventive maintenance treatment on periodontal conditions. 5-Year observations in general dentistry patients, *J Clin Periodontol* 26:225-233, 1999.

94. Axelsson P, Lindhe J, Nystrom B: On the prevention of caries and periodontal disease. Results of a 15-year longitudinal study in adults, *J Clin Periodontol* 18:182-189, 1991.

95. Matthews DC, Tabesh M: Detection of localized tooth-related factors that predispose to periodontal infections, *Periodontol 2000* 34:136-150, 2004.

96. American Academy of Periodontology. Parameter on chronic periodontitis with slight to moderate loss of periodontal support, *J Periodontol* 71:853-855, 2000.

97. Parameters of Care. American Academy of Periodontology, *J Periodontol* 71(5 suppl):847-883, 2000.

98. Johnson GK, Hill M: Cigarette smoking and the periodontal patient, *J Periodontol* 75:196-209, 2004.

99. Rivera-Hidalgo F: Smoking and periodontal disease, *Periodontol 2000* 32:50-58, 2003.

100. Kinane DF, Chestnutt IG: Smoking and periodontal disease, *Crit Rev Oral Biol Med* 11:356-365, 2000.

101. Krall EA, Garvey AJ, Garcia RI: Alveolar bone loss and tooth loss in male cigar and pipe smokers, *J Am Dent Assoc* 130:57-64, 1999.

102. Tomar SL, Asma S: Smoking-attributable periodontitis in the United States: findings from NHANES III. National Health and Nutrition Examination Survey, *J Periodontol* 71:743-751, 2000.

103. Razali M, Palmer RM, Coward P et al.: A retrospective study of periodontal disease severity in smokers and non-smokers, *Br Dent J* 198:495-498, 2005.

104. Bergstrom J: Influence of tobacco smoking on periodontal bone height. Long-term observations and a hypothesis, *J Clin Periodontol* 31:260-266, 2004.

105. Haffajee AD, Socransky SS: Relationship of cigarette smoking to attachment level profiles, *J Clin Periodontol* 28:283-295, 2001.

106. Research, Science, and Therapy Committee of the American Academy of Periodontology: Position paper: tobacco use and the periodontal patient, *J Periodontol* 70:1419-1427, 1999.

107. Palmer RM, Wilson RF, Hasan AS et al.: Mechanisms of action of environmental factors–tobacco smoking, *J Clin Periodontol* 32:180-195, 2005.

108. Dietrich T, Bernimoulin JP, Glynn RJ: The effect of cigarette smoking on gingival bleeding, *J Periodontol* 75:16-22, 2004.

109. Calsina G, Ramon JM, Echeverria JJ: Effects of smoking on periodontal tissues, *J Clin Periodontol* 29:771-776, 2002.

110. Grossi SG, Zambon JJ, Ho AW et al.: Assessment of risk for periodontal disease. I. Risk indicators for attachment loss, *J Periodontol* 65:260-267, 1994.

111. Grossi SG, Genco RJ, Machtei EE et al.: Assessment of risk for periodontal disease. II. Risk indicators for alveolar bone loss, *J Periodontol* 66:23-29, 1995.

112. Labriola A, Needleman I, Moles DR: Systematic review of the effect of smoking on nonsurgical periodontal therapy, *Periodontol 2000* 37:124-137, 2005.

113. Grossi SG, Zambon J, Machtei EE et al.: Effects of smoking and smoking cessation on healing after mechanical periodontal therapy, *J Am Dent Assoc* 128:599-607, 1997.

114. Kaldahl WB, Johnson GK, Patil KD et al.: Levels of cigarette consumption and response to periodontal therapy, *J Periodontol* 67:675-681, 1996.

115. Ah MK, Johnson GK, Kaldahl WB et al.: The effect of smoking on the response to periodontal therapy, *J Clin Periodontol* 21:91-97, 1994.

116. Jansson L, Lavstedt S: Influence of smoking on marginal bone loss and tooth loss–a prospective study over 20 years, *J Clin Periodontol* 29:750-756, 2002.

117. Bergstrom J, Eliasson S, Dock J: A 10-year prospective study of tobacco smoking and periodontal health, *J Periodontol* 71:1338-1347, 2000.
118. Krall EA, Dawson-Hughes B, Garvey AJ et al.: Smoking, smoking cessation, and tooth loss, *J Dent Res* 76:1653-1659, 1997.
119. Campbell HS, Sletten M, Petty T: Patient perceptions of tobacco cessation services in dental offices, *J Am Dent Assoc* 130:219-226, 1999.
120. Fiore MC, Bailey WC, Cohen SJ et al.: *Treating tobacco use and dependence: clinical practice guidelines*, Rockville, MD, 2000, U.S. Department of Health and Human Services, Public Health Service.
121. Warnakulasuriya S: Effectiveness of tobacco counseling in the dental office, *J Dent Educ* 66:1079-1087, 2002.
122. Tomar SL: Dentistry's role in tobacco control, *J Am Dent Assoc* 132:30S-35S, 2001.
123. Cohen SJ, Stookey GK, Katz BP et al.: Helping smokers quit: a randomized controlled trial with private practice dentists, *J Am Dent Assoc* 118:41-45, 1989.
124. Kornman KS, Page RC, Tonetti MS: The host response to the microbial challenge in periodontitis: assembling the players, *Periodontol 2000* 14:33-53, 1997.
125. Oringer RJ: Modulation of the host response in periodontal therapy, *J Periodontol* 73:460-470, 2002.
126. Caton JG, Ciancio SG, Blieden TM et al.: Treatment with sub-antimicrobial dose doxycycline improves the efficacy of scaling and root planing in patients with adult periodontitis, *J Periodontol* 71:521-532, 2000.
127. DeSpain B, Niessen L: Health promotion and disease prevention, *J Esthet Dent* 7:189-196, 1995.
128. Niessen LC, DeSpain B: Clinical strategies for prevention of oral diseases, *J Esthet Dent* 8:3-11, 1996.

Chapter 17

Prevention Strategies for Oral Cancer

K. VENDRELL RANKIN AND DANIEL L. JONES

LEARNING OBJECTIVES

Upon completion of this chapter, the learner will be able to:
- List the preventable risk factors associated with oral cancer.
- List strategies to address oral cancer risk factor reduction.
- Describe the Agency for Healthcare Research and Quality (AHRQ) guidelines for tobacco cessation.
- Review recommendations or prescriptions for appropriate pharmacotherapy, or both, for tobacco cessation.
- Explain alcohol consumption evaluation strategies.
- Develop a plan for oral cancer prevention and provide preventive services appropriate to the patient's needs and desires.
- Explain follow-up care and modifications for subsequent treatment, as necessary.

KEY TERMS

CAGE questionnaire
Five "A"s
Five "R"s
Nicotine dependence
Nicotine replacement therapy
Standard drink equivalents
Withdrawal symptoms

PRIMARY PREVENTION

The etiology of oral cancer is the result of a complex interaction among factors, including the patient's immune status, genetic predisposition, gender, age and oncogenic viruses, and preventable factors including: tobacco use, alcohol consumption, and nutritional status. Primary prevention involves the implementation of strategies to reduce the risk associated with the factor(s) within the patient's control that increase risk for oral cancer. Therefore, risk reduction for intraoral cancer should include a thorough patient evaluation and use of the appropriate strategies to address tobacco use, alcohol dependence, and nutritional deficiencies. Refer to Chapter 8 for a discussion of nutritional factors.

Although viruses and tobacco have been implicated in the etiology of cancer of the lip, the primary risk factor for cancer of the lip is exposure to ultraviolet radiation. Risk reduction for cancer of the lip can be accomplished through the use of sunscreen with an SPF of 30 or greater, the use of a wide-brimmed hat that fully shades the face, or both. This practice is advocated for sun exposure for all body parts. This routine is particularly important for individuals who have fair skin, work or play outdoors frequently, or who live in areas of the country with numerous sunny days.

SECONDARY PREVENTION

The 5-year relative survival rates for oral cancer vary widely by site and stage at the time of diagnosis, ranging from 100% for localized cancers of the lip, to 80% for intraoral cancers diagnosed at the localized stage, to 15% for cancers that have metastasized to distant sites.[1] This finding has been interpreted as evidence that early detection and diagnosis improves prognosis and increases survival. Because of feasibility, human subject protection, and cost issues, no randomized clinical trials exist to demonstrate that early detection of oral cancer reduces oral cancer mortality. In the absence of such data, however, early detection, diagnosis, and treatment of precancerous lesions and diagnosis of oral cancer at localized stages are considered to be the definitive approach to secondary prevention of these cancers. The principal test for oral and pharyngeal cancers is a comprehensive clinical examination that includes a visual and tactile examination of the mouth, full protrusion of the tongue with the aid of gauze, and palpation of the tongue, floor of the mouth, and lymph nodes in the neck. The U.S. Preventive Services Task Force (1996) concluded that insufficient evidence exists to recommend for or against routine screening for oral cancers, but noted that clinicians should remain vigilant for signs and symptoms of oral cancers and premalignancy in people who use tobacco, regularly use alcohol, or both.[2] The American Cancer Society recommends that primary care physicians and dentists examine the mouth and throat as part of a

routine cancer-related screening.[3] On the basis of available evidence that early detection probably improves prognosis, several *Healthy People 2010* objectives specifically address the early detection of oral cancer. Objective 21-6 is to "Increase the proportion of oral and pharyngeal cancers detected at the earliest stage" and Objective 21-7 is to "Increase the proportion of adults who, in the past 12 months, report having had an examination to detect oral and pharyngeal cancer."[2] In addition to the recommended annual professional examination, patients should be instructed to conduct oral self-examinations on a regular basis. Dental professionals should seek to educate every patient on the risk factors for, and early warning signs of, oral cancer as studies have demonstrated that this information is not generally available in the popular media or widely known by the most adults in the United States.

STATE OF THE CURRENT SCIENCE
Tobacco

Cigarettes have been described as "the Holy Grail of drug delivery devices."[6] Nicotine from a cigarette is delivered to the brain within 19 seconds of inhaling tobacco smoke. Nicotine is a highly addictive drug that has multiple pharmacological effects and activates the reward pathway in the brain, which reinforces continued tobacco use. The principal effects of nicotine are related to release of neurotransmitters in the brain, including acetylcholine, norepinephrine, dopamine, serotonin, and beta-endorphin. The release of dopamine is involved in the reinforcing effects of nicotine and suggests the mechanism for **nicotine dependence**. The central nervous system effects are biphasic in that nicotine has a stimulating effect at lower doses but a depressant effect at higher doses. Nicotine also stimulates the sympathetic nervous system, which increases the blood pressure, heart rate, and cardiac output. Alterations in endocrine function are also stimulated, as nicotine causes the release of adrenocorticotropic hormone (ACTH) and cortisol, which affect mood and contribute to osteoporosis. Nicotine increases the metabolic rate, suppresses the appetite, and relaxes skeletal muscle.[7] Nicotine dependence is classified as nicotine use disorder, according to the *Diagnostic and Statistical Manual of Mental Disorders, Fourth Edition-Text Revised (DSM-IV-TR).*[8] The criteria for this diagnosis includes the finding of any *three* of the following seven items within a 1-year time span:

• Tolerance to nicotine with decreased effect and increase in dose to obtain same effect
• Withdrawal symptoms after cessation
• Smoking more than usual
• Persistent desire to smoke despite efforts to decrease intake

- Extensive time spent smoking or purchasing tobacco
- Postponing work, social, or recreational events to smoke
- Continuing to smoke despite health hazards

When tobacco users try to cut back or quit, the absence of nicotine typically leads to **withdrawal symptoms,** both physical and psychological. Physically, the body reacts to the absence of nicotine. Psychologically, the tobacco user is confronted with finding a new way to deal with reality without a psychoactive drug that produced a sense of well being, relaxation, reduced fatigue, and enhanced attention. Socially, the tobacco user is surrounded by cues that have become behaviorally associated with tobacco use. All of these factors should be dealt with simultaneously to increase the odds of a successful quit attempt. Withdrawal symptoms[9] can include the following:

- Depression
- Feelings of frustration and anger
- Irritability
- Trouble sleeping
- Difficulty concentrating
- Restlessness
- Headache
- Tiredness
- Increased appetite

These uncomfortable symptoms may lead the tobacco user to resume his or her tobacco use, returning blood levels of nicotine to a level at which no symptoms exist. If an individual has used tobacco regularly for a few weeks or longer and abruptly stops or cuts back, withdrawal symptoms will typically occur within a few hours of the use, and will peak at 48 to 72 hours. Withdrawal symptoms can last from a few days to as long as several weeks. The form of tobacco consumed determines the amount of nicotine delivered (Table 17-1), the peak time of delivery of nicotine to the brain and the

TABLE 17-1

AVERAGE NICOTINE CONTENT PER DOSE BY TYPE OF TOBACCO

FORM OF TOBACCO	NICOTINE CONTENT (MG)
Cigarette (filter)	1.1
Pipe	5.2
Smokeless tobacco	
Chewing tobacco	4.5
Moist snuff	3.6
Cigars	
Little cigars (Swishers)	3.8
Premium (Macanudo)	13.3
4-mg nicotine gum	1.9

sustained level of plasma nicotine. These parameters should be considered when counseling patients for tobacco cessation.

Tobacco dependence is a chronic brain disease embedded in a social and psychological context. Therefore, successful treatment requires pharmacotherapy to treat withdrawal symptoms and to focus on making appropriate and sustainable behavioral and social changes.[10]

Dentistry has a long and successful history of prevention. Persons aged 22 to 40 years are more likely to have regular dental visits than physician visits and will benefit substantially from cessation efforts. Addressing cessation with this age group is especially important for females in their childbearing years. Additionally, cessation for parents reduces the deleterious effects of second hand smoke on children and other family members. These effects of tobacco use along with the desire for cosmetic treatment provide a perfect opportunity for the practice of tobacco cessation in the dental office.[11] Furthermore, cessation programs can be integrated into frequent recall systems.

Alcohol

In 2004, the U.S. Preventive Services Task Force recommended screening and behavioral counseling interventions to reduce alcohol misuse. The task force did not recommend or endorse a specific strategy for intervention. A recent meta-analysis concluded that brief alcohol interventions in a primary care setting can significantly reduce alcohol consumption when compared with no intervention, usual care, or less than 5 minutes of intervention. The intervention should last from 5 to 15 minutes, be accompanied by written material, and provide the opportunity for the patient to schedule a follow-up visit. This has the potential to significantly reduce alcohol consumption.[12]

STRATEGIES FOR APPLICATION IN PRACTICE

Treating Tobacco Use and Dependence: Clinical Practice Guidelines

Treating Tobacco Use and Dependence, Clinical Practice Guideline[10] offers the following guidelines:

- Tobacco dependence is a chronic condition that often requires repeated intervention. Effective treatments exist that can produce long-term or even permanent abstinence. Because effective tobacco dependence treatments are available, every patient who uses tobacco should be offered treatment.
- Patients *willing* to try to quit tobacco use should be provided treatments identified as effective in the guideline.

- Patients *unwilling* to try to quit tobacco use should be provided a brief intervention designed to increase their motivation to quit.

Dental professionals have a responsibility to identify, document, and counsel every tobacco user seen in the oral health care setting. Brief tobacco dependence counseling is effective, and every patient who uses tobacco should be offered at least a brief intervention. This session, lasting as little as three minutes, can improve abstinence. A strong dose-response relationship exists between the intensity of tobacco dependence counseling and its effectiveness. The brief 3-minute intervention can be expanded on the basis of available time. The following three types of counseling/ behavioral therapies are particularly effective and should be considered for use with all patients trying to quit:

- Practical counseling: problem-solving skills/training
- Provision of social support as part of treatment
- Assistance in securing or identifying social support outside of treatment
- One or more pharmacotherapies should be recommended to all patients attempting to quit, except in the presence of contraindications

The five "As". *The Clinical Practice Guideline* offers a reliable roadmap for the clinical practice of tobacco cessation based on the five "As," which offer the following directions to health care practitioners

- **A**sk about tobacco use.
- **A**dvise tobacco users to quit.
- **A**ssess readiness to make a quit attempt.
- **A**ssist with the quit attempt.
- **A**rrang**e** follow-up care.

ASK.   Ask every patient at every visit about his or her tobacco use. Consider tobacco use as a vital sign to be obtained on every patient as a routine part of his or her medical/social history with periodic updating. This information should be a part of the standard clinical record. This can provide clinician and patient with a nonthreatening opportunity to begin a discussion about tobacco use, past quit attempts, and the chronic addictive nature of tobacco in a medical context. This approach also emphasizes the clinician's progressive, prevention-focused practice. The Tobacco Use Assessment Form and Brief Tobacco Cessation Intervention can be easily integrated into dental practice.[13]

ADVISE.   Advise patients to quit in a **clear, strong,** and **personalized** manner. Tailor the message to the patient's particular circumstance. Personalized, problem-focused advice is more effective than generic statistics or "scare tactics." Although it is tempting to assume that all tobacco users know that it is "bad for them," and it is not necessary to advise them to quit, studies suggest that the average person is not necessarily in possession of complete or accurate information. It may require the benefit of the health care professional to interpret the severity of potential harm, the probability of harm, and the difficulty of avoiding the harmful consequences of continued tobacco use.[14]

A recent study reported that smokers believe that, on average, smoking "light" and "ultra light" cigarettes confers a 25% and 33% reduction in risk, respectively, compared with regular brands.[15] In another study, 27% of smokers felt that the risk of lung cancer was lower for those who smoked light cigarettes, compared with smoking regular cigarettes.[16] These findings raise significant concerns about accurate knowledge of the consumer population and the effect of "light" and "ultra light" product labeling on public health. Since the late 1960s, many cigarette manufacturers have perforated their filters with lines of ventilation holes, which dilute the smoke as it travels through the filter. The perforations lead to lower yields of tar and nicotine from these cigarettes, according to machine-derived measurements. Tobacco manufacturers label these lower-yield products "light" and "ultra light" cigarettes. Evidence suggests smokers may be unwittingly compensating for the reduced nicotine delivery by altering their smoking behavior. To compensate for the reduction in nicotine yield, people increase the number of puffs they take from a cigarette, increase the volume of each puff, or increase the number of cigarettes smoked. They may also place their fingers or lips over the ventilation holes.

Research on light or lower-yield cigarettes has shown that the disease risk of these products is not significantly different than regular or medium-yield cigarettes.[17,18]

ASSESS.   Assess the patient's readiness to quit tobacco use. First, interpret the information the patient has provided and adapt the message to what he or she is prepared to hear and accept. Not everyone will have the same level of commitment, or readiness, to take action. Faced with change, many people are not ready to act. Furthermore, change is usually not a single step or linear process, but a cycle, in which the same step may be repeated several times before a person progresses to the next step.[19,20] Some patients may never make a quit attempt. Some are aware that they need to quit, but have tried and failed and lack the confidence to try again. Others may be considering quitting but may not have gathered the courage or information necessary to make a serious quit attempt. Some may be ready to set a quit date. Do not force patients to take action, simply let them know that help is available when and if they are ready.

To facilitate this interaction, use questions as simple as "What do you like best about smoking?" or "What do you like least about smoking?" The patient's degree of motivation may vary. If the patient is ready to set a definitive quit date within the next 30 days, the clinician should provide information on effective behavioral, cognitive and support strategies for quitting and discuss the use of pharmacotherapy. If the patient is not ready to quit, the clinician can use the **five "Rs,"** listed below, which describe the key components of motivation strategies to help move patients towards readiness. Chapter 11 provides additional information about this topic.

The Five "Rs" to Enhance Motivation for Patients Not Ready to Quit.

- *Relevance:* How is quitting most relevant to the patient? Tailor advice and the discussion to the patient's situation and readiness to quit.
- *Risks:* Provide new information on the risks of continued tobacco use specific to the individual's circumstance. Attempt to elicit suggestions from the patient on risks specific to their situation.
- *Rewards:* Suggest or elicit suggestions from the patient on the benefits of quitting that are unique to the patient.
- *Roadblocks:* Assist patients in identifying the barriers to quitting tobacco use and guide them toward solutions. Assist the patient in developing discrepancy between current behavior (tobacco use) and the desired behavior (quitting).
- *Repetition:* Reinforce your motivational message at every opportunity.

ASSIST.   Assist patients who are ready to quit. Patients are more successful when they have a well developed "quit plan" and the dental professional can assist with this task. Setting a quit date is essential to the plan. The mnemonic **"TRIPS"** offers a simple way to ensure that the plan includes the major elements for a successful quit attempt:

- **T**riggers, challenges, coping skills (discuss past quit attempts)
- **R**easons for wanting to quit
- **I**mportance/confidence in ability to quit
- **P**harmacotherapy and a quit date
- **S**ocial and emotional support

Triggers and Challenges.   Ask the patient to identify situations when they routinely use tobacco. If the patient had previous unsuccessful quit attempts, or experienced situations in which tobacco use was restricted, encourage them to recall these situations and establish coping behaviors before the event. Some examples of triggers and alternative coping behaviors are:

- Talking on the phone: holding a straw or scribbling on a pad
- Driving: chewing sugarless gum/mints
- Feeling stressed: exercising, deep breathing, calling a friend
- Waking up: changing morning routine

Research shows that using both cognitive and behavioral strategies increases a patient's likelihood of quitting.

Behavioral coping skills involve controlling the patient's environment to avoid stimuli that can trigger tobacco use. Caution patients to avoid situations associated with tobacco use. They should plan activities that exclude tobacco use and counsel them to, if appropriate, avoid friends and family who use tobacco. Cessation patients should avoid alcohol, coffee, or other substances and situations that trigger tobacco use. Cognitive skills are predetermined activities designed to help the patient deal with situations or feelings that elicit tobacco use. These may include skills such as meditation, deep breathing exercises, positive self-talk, and relaxation exercises.

Meditation helps calm the mind by focusing on one thing or word. If practiced regularly, this can help control urges to return to a previous habit such as tobacco use. The instructions to the patient would be to sit quietly and repeat a word such as "one" or "calm." If other thoughts intrude, the patient lets them go and continues repeating the word.

Deep breathing is a simple calming action that can be done anywhere and anytime. The focus is on taking slow deep breaths to help relax muscles, especially in the neck and shoulder area. This action increases oxygen in the blood. The act of inhaling and exhaling mimics the act of smoking and eases the difficulties experienced during an acute craving.

Self-talk is another strategy for changing behaviors. Monitor self-talk to eliminate negative talk (e.g., thoughts such as "I can't cope without a cigarette; I've tried before; I'm a failure; I don't care if tobacco makes my breath stink, I have to have it.") Replace negative messages with positive messages such as "I am learning new ways to cope with stress; I don't need a cigarette; I've learned from my previous quit attempts; I will be successful this time; I want to remain tobacco-free to improve my oral health; My breath is fresher; I don't need to use smokeless tobacco."

Relaxation exercises help patients learn to cope with stress in a positive way. Guided imagery, progressive muscle relaxation, or focused breathing while listening to calming music, practiced on a routine basis, will assist the patient in dealing with stress and anxiety related to cessation.

Reasons for Wanting to Quit.   The dental practitioner should urge the patient to make a list of the reasons for quitting tobacco use. Self-motivation is developed by the patient's perception of the discrepancy between continued tobacco use and his or her desire to meet stated goals.

Importance/Confidence in Ability to Quit.   The patient's belief in his or her ability to quit tobacco use is a determinant in his or her motivation to succeed in the quit attempt. The practitioner should ask the patient to rate his or her confidence in the ability to quit on a scale of 1 to 10. If confidence is low, the dental practitioner can ask what he or she can do to increase the patient's confidence.

Social and Emotional Support.   A social support network is essential during the quit attempt. This network is crucial if the patient is living in a smoking household and will be surrounded by individuals who will continue to use tobacco. Patients may need to negotiate boundaries with other smokers with whom they cannot avoid contact.

ARRANGE.   The clinician should arrange for follow-up care and patient monitoring. With each patient contact, progress should be documented in the treatment record. This record provides a starting point for subsequent discussions. Follow-up visits can be arranged in several ways.

- "Checking in" with the patient on the next visit.
- Scheduling specific follow-up visits to discuss tobacco cessation.
- Referral to a tobacco cessation group of the patient's choosing.
- With prior approval, calling the patient at home to assess progress. (If a message is left, the clinician should not indicate that he or she is calling regarding a quit attempt, because this might be private information that the patient does not want others to hear.)
- Documenting key dates (e.g., quit dates and tobacco-free anniversaries) and acknowledging important milestones.

A follow-up contact should occur within the first week after the quit date. A second follow-up is recommended within the first month. Further follow-up contacts should be scheduled as needed or indicated. During these contacts, the patient should be congratulated for successes. If tobacco use has occurred, the patient and clinician should review triggers for the event and develop future coping skills to help the patient return to total abstinence. The patient should be reminded that lapses (slips) occur as part of the normal learning process and should be viewed as such. Compliance and possible side effects of pharmacotherapy use should be discussed. When appropriate, referral to more intensive treatment should be considered.

According to the Clinical Practice Guideline, multiple patient contacts are associated with higher quit rates. Even brief interventions (i.e., asking about tobacco use and advising to quit) can increase patients' readiness to quit.[10] In a meta-analysis of trials, brief advice was associated with an increased likelihood of quitting compared with no advice or usual care (OR = 1.69). More intensive advice led to a higher likelihood of quitting when compared to more minimal advice (OR = 1.44).[21] A dose-response relationship also exists for the counseling session length and the total amount of contact time (across treatment sessions). The greater the amount of time spent with the patient, the more likely the patient is to achieve abstinence.[10]

The appropriate use of pharmacotherapy in conjunction with counseling can double the probability of a successful quit attempt.[22] Some patients may not wish to use medications in their quit attempts. Explain the options available and the benefits and contraindications, and respect the patient's choice.

Pharmacotherapy for Tobacco Cessation

The Food and Drug Administration (FDA) has approved bupropion SR (Zyban) and five forms of **nicotine replacement therapy** as first-line pharmacotherapy for the treatment of tobacco dependence. Prescribe the medication(s) requested by the patient unless contraindicated. If the patient has previously experienced an unsuccessful quit attempt while using a medication, they may be unwilling to use this particular one again. Selecting pharmacotherapy on the basis of patient needs and attributes of pharmacotherapy is described in Table 17-2. Dental practitioners should consider the following when prescribing pharmacotherapies:

- Comorbidities: Alcohol or other drugs of dependence.
- History of psychiatric disease: Should this patient be under the care of a psychiatrist during cessation?
- Concern about weight gain: Use of medications can delay weight gain, but this concern should be addressed. Consult with a registered dietitian to assist with weight management.

Nicotine replacement therapy.   Nicotine replacement therapy (NRT) is a valuable adjunct to cessation treatment for most patients making a quit attempt.[24] No evidence exists of increased cardiovascular risk with NRT, except with acute cardiovascular disease. Major medical contraindications to nicotine replacement therapy include:

- Recent myocardial infarction (within 2 weeks)
- Serious cardiac arrhythmia
- Serious or worsening angina pectoris
- Accelerated hypertension

Nicotine replacement therapy is not recommended for use in the following cases:

- Women who are pregnant or breastfeeding, except under the supervision of a physician[23]
- Adolescents, except under the supervision of a pediatrician

NICOTINE GUM.   The oldest form of nicotine replacement therapy is nicotine gum. The gum is available over the counter (OTC) in 2- and 4-mg strengths. When the 2-mg strength gum is used properly, 0.8 to 0.9 mg of nicotine is absorbed from each dose.[25] Nicotine plasma levels are lower (approximately 8 mcg/L) and peak approximately 30 minutes after chewing a 2 mg piece of nicotine gum. Compare this with smoking a single cigarette, which yields a peak nicotine level of approximately 26 mcg/L within 10 minutes.[26] The 4-mg strength gum is recommended for patients who smoke more than 25 cigarettes

TABLE 17-2

CHOOSING TOBACCO CESSATION PHARMACOTHERAPY BASED ON PATIENT NEEDS

DRUG	PATIENT NEEDS
Bupropion	Postpone weight gain. Simultaneous help with depression. Low maintenance (1 tablet, twice a day). Prescription drug (possible third-party reimbursement).
Nicotine gum	Oral stimulation; tension release of chewing. Minimal exposure to nicotine. Adjunct to another drug (e.g., bupropion, nicotine patch). Alternative to patch (e.g., skin problem, frequent swimming). Control on nicotine intake; ability to adjust dosage according to need.
Nicotine inhaler	A relatively fast burst of nicotine during craving. Hand-to-mouth motion is reminiscent of smoking. Alternative to gum when chewing is problematic. Minimal exposure to nicotine. Adjunct to another drug (e.g., bupropion, nicotine patch). Prescription drug (possible third-party reimbursement). Alternative to patch (e.g., skin problem, frequent swimming). Control on nicotine intake; ability to adjust dosage according to need.
Nicotine nasal spray	A fast burst of nicotine. Alternative to gum when chewing is problematic. Minimal exposure to nicotine when used during worst of cravings. Adjunct to another drug (e.g., bupropion, nicotine patch). Prescription drug (possible third-party reimbursement). Alternative to patch (e.g., skin problem, frequent swimming). Control on nicotine intake; ability to adjust dosage according to need.
Nicotine patch	Inconspicuous treatment. Ability to forget about treatment during the day. An even dose of nicotine throughout the day. Postponed weight gain. Prescription drug (possible third-party reimbursement). Alternative to gum when chewing is problematic. Alternative to gum, lozenge, inhaler when patient sips a lot of acidic beverages that interfere with absorption. Low-maintenance treatment (apply only in morning).
Nicotine lozenge	Oral stimulation. Alternative to gum when chewing is a problem. Minimal exposure to nicotine when used during worst of cravings. Adjunct to another drug (e.g., bupropion, patch). Alternative to patch (e.g., skin problem, frequent swimming). Control on nicotine intake; ability to adjust dosage according to need.

(slightly more than 1 pack) per day. Inadequate doses, inappropriate chewing technique, or both, are common reasons for failure of this product to relieve withdrawal symptoms.

PATIENT INSTRUCTIONS. If the patient has used this product unsuccessfully in the past or is using it for the first time, chewing instructions will avoid frustration and failure to deliver nicotine. Patients should be instructed to chew the gum very slowly several times, and to stop chewing when a slight tingling is felt (approximately 15 chews). The gum should then be "parked" between cheek and gum to allow absorption of nicotine through the buccal mucosa. Slow chewing is resumed when the taste or tingling fades. When the taste or tingling returns, the gum should again be parked, in a different place in the mouth. This cycle should be repeated over a period of approximately 30 minutes. Acidic foods or beverages 15 minutes before or during drug use will impair nicotine absorption because of lowered oral pH.

DOSAGE.   Patients using nicotine gum are more likely to succeed if they chew the gum on a fixed schedule rather than as needed. During the initial 6 weeks of therapy, patients should chew one piece of gum every 1 to 2 hours while awake. In general, this amounts to at least nine pieces of gum daily. Some smokers may require a greater amount of the drug to avoid withdrawal symptoms. The clinician should adjust dosing schedules to satisfy patient craving rather than on an as-needed, or p.r.n., basis. Exceeding the maximum dose of 24 pieces of gum per day may result in adverse effects. Patients should gradually increase the interval between doses using the following schedule:

• Weeks 7-9: 1 piece every 2 to 4 hours
• Weeks 10-12: 1 piece every 4 to 8 hours

PRECAUTIONS.   Unintentional swallowing of nicotine gum can exacerbate active peptic ulcers and should be used with caution in patients with an active history of the disease. The increased viscosity of nicotine gum compared to ordinary chewing gum may not be suitable for patients with dentures, orthodontic appliances, or a history of temporomandibular joint disease.

SIDE EFFECTS.   Chewing the gum too rapidly could result in excessive release of nicotine. Patients could experience the following side effects:

• Lightheadedness
• Nausea and vomiting
• Irritation of the throat and mouth
• Hiccups
• Indigestion

NICOTINE LOZENGE.   The nicotine lozenge was introduced as an OTC form of nicotine replacement in 2002. It is available in 2-mg and 4-mg strengths. The lozenge delivers approximately 25% more nicotine than the equivalent gum dose.[26,27] Unlike the gum, dosage selection is based on the "time to first cigarette" after waking rather than quantity of tobacco use.[28] If the first cigarette is smoked more than 1 hour after waking, the 2-mg form is an appropriate dosing choice. If the first cigarette is smoked within 30 minutes of waking, the 4-mg form should be used.

PATIENT INSTRUCTIONS.   Patients should be instructed not to chew or swallow the lozenge, but to move it to different areas of the mouth until it completely dissolves (20 to 30 minutes). As with the gum, consumption of acidic food or beverages 15 minutes before or during lozenge use will decrease the absorption of nicotine.

DOSING.   To facilitate tapering, encourage patients to use the lozenge on the following schedule:

• Weeks 1-6: Use 1 lozenge every 1 to 2 hours (use at least 9 lozenges per day for the first 6 weeks)
• Weeks 7-9: Use 1 lozenge every 2 to 4 hours
• Weeks 10-12: Use 1 lozenge every 4 to 8 hours
• Do not use more than 20 lozenges per day

PRECAUTIONS.   Unintentional swallowing of nicotine can exacerbate active peptic ulcers, and nicotine lozenges should be used with caution in patients with an active history of this disease.

SIDE EFFECTS.
• Nausea
• Hiccups
• Cough
• Heartburn
• Headache
• Flatulence
• Insomnia

NICOTINE TRANSDERMAL PATCH.   The nicotine transdermal patch is available OTC and delivers a steady dose of nicotine with the lowest addiction potential of all the NRTs. Multiple transdermal nicotine patch formulations are on the market that vary widely in formulation, design, and duration of wear (i.e., 16-hour and 24-hour).[22] Plasma nicotine levels obtained through transdermal delivery are approximately 50% lower than those achieved with cigarette smoking.[29] Lower levels of nicotine alleviate the symptoms of withdrawal, but are far less likely to lead to dependence when compared with tobacco or other forms of NRT.[30] Different brands of the transdermal patch have different dosing regimens. The clinician should select the best dosage and regimen to meet the individual patient's needs.

PATIENT INSTRUCTIONS.
• Choose an area of skin on the upper body or the upper outer part of the arm.
• To ensure that the patch will adhere well, make sure the skin is nonhairy, clean (not oily), dry, and free of creams, lotions, oils, or powder.
• Hair will interfere with the application of the patch.
• Do not shave the area, because this may cause skin irritation.
• Do not apply the patch to skin that is inflamed, burned, broken out, or irritated in any way, because these conditions may alter the amount of drug absorbed.
• Apply the patch to a different area each day.
• To minimize the potential for local skin reactions, the same area should not be used again for at least 1 week.
• Wash hands after patch application as nicotine on hands could get into the eyes or nose and cause stinging or redness.

- After 24 hours, remove old patch.
- Any adhesive remaining on the skin may be removed with rubbing alcohol.
- Shortly after applying the nicotine patch, patients may experience mild itching, burning, or tingling. This is a normal reaction to the patch, and should resolve within an hour.

Prescribed dosage schedule for the 24-hour patch is as follows:

For patients who smoke 10 cigarettes or less per day:

- 14-mg patch for 6 weeks
- 7-mg patch for 2 weeks

For patients who smoke more than 10 cigarettes per day:

- 21-mg patch for 6 weeks
- 14-mg patch for 2 weeks
- 7-mg patch for 2 weeks

SIDE EFFECTS.
- Headache
- Local skin reactions (erythema, burning, and pruritus)
- Usually caused by irritation resulting from skin occlusion or a reaction to the adhesive
- As many as 50% of patients experience this reaction, but less than 5% discontinue therapy

Patients with dermatological conditions (e.g., psoriasis, eczema, and atopic dermatitis) are more likely to experience skin irritation and should not use the nicotine patch.[31] Local skin irritation can be minimized by changing patch sites daily or by changing brand types (because different manufacturers use different adhesives) or both. If skin irritation at a site persists for more than 4 days, the patch should be discontinued. Some patients experience sleep disturbances while using the patch. Removing the patch at night can help to resolve this complaint.

NICOTINE ORAL INHALER.   The nicotine oral inhaler is one of the newest prescription aids to smoking cessation. A reusable mouthpiece holds a replaceable cartridge containing 4 mg of nicotine. According to the manufacturer, 80 deep inhalations during a 20-minute period releases 4 mg of nicotine, of which approximately 2 mg is systemically absorbed through the buccal mucosa. Peak plasma nicotine levels are achieved at about 15 minutes, delivering approximately 6 ng/mL in contrast to those seen with a cigarette, which increase rapidly and reach a maximum 49 ng/mL within 5 minutes.[32,33] The patient should be advised that continued vigorous puffing inhalations for more than 20 minutes is required to gain the full benefit of the inhaler. A benefit of this form of NRT is the substitution of the hand to mouth habit associated with smoking.

PATIENT INSTRUCTIONS.
- Align the marks on the mouthpiece.
- Pull and separate the mouthpiece into two parts.

- Press the nicotine-containing cartridge firmly into bottom of mouthpiece until the seal breaks.
- Put the top on the mouthpiece and align the marks to close.
- Press down firmly to break the top seal on the cartridge.
- Twist the top piece to misalign the marks and secure the unit.
- The nicotine inhaler is now ready for use. When inhaled or puffed through the mouthpiece, nicotine turns to a vapor that is absorbed across oropharyngeal mucosa.
- Inhale deeply into back of the throat or puff in short breaths.
- Nicotine in the cartridge is depleted after approximately 20 minutes of active puffing.
- The 20-minute supply can be used all at one time or can be used a few minutes, put down, and then picked up later for a total of 20 minutes of active puffing per cartridge.
- An open cartridge remains potent for 24 hours.
- Once opened, whether fully used or not, the cartridge should be replaced after 24 hours.
- The mouthpiece is reusable and should be cleaned regularly with a mild detergent and water.

DOSING.   Encourage patients to use at least six cartridges per day, up to a maximum of 16, for 3 to 12 weeks. After a minimum of 3 weeks, the patient should begin to gradually reduce the number used daily. Advise patients to avoid acidic foods or beverages 15 minutes before or during use. The delivery of nicotine is decreased at temperatures below 40° F.

PRECAUTIONS.
- Asthma or chronic pulmonary disease may induce bronchospasm.
- May precipitate an incident in patients with a recent history of myocardial infarction, angina pectoris, serious arrhythmia, or vasospastic disease.
- Severe renal impairment affects nicotine metabolite clearance, and can potentiate the effect.
- Delays healing in peptic ulcer disease.
- Nicotine causes release of catecholamine by the adrenal medulla and should be used with caution in hyperthyroidism, pheochromocytoma, or insulin-dependent diabetes.

SIDE EFFECTS.   Side effects are generally mild and improve with time. They include the following symptoms:

- Irritation of the nose and throat
- Coughing
- Rhinitis

NICOTINE NASAL SPRAY.   Available only by prescription, the nicotine nasal spray bottle contains 10 mL of an aqueous solution of nicotine. Each metered dose delivers a 50-μl spray (0.5 mg nicotine). The nicotine is rapidly absorbed through the nasal mucosa. The nasal spray has a faster onset of action (4 to 15 minutes) in comparison with the gum, patch, or inhaler, and as a consequence it also has the highest addiction potential of all NRTs.[34] Wide variation exists among patients in plasma nicotine concentrations from the spray. Approximately 20% of patients reach peak nicotine concentrations similar to those seen after smoking one cigarette.

PATIENT INSTRUCTIONS.
• Tilt head back slightly
• Insert tip of bottle into nostril
• Spray once in each nostril
• Do not sniff or inhale while spraying
• Wait 2 to 3 minutes before blowing nose
• Avoid contact with skin, eyes, and mouth

DOSING.[35]
• One dose = 1 mg nicotine (2 sprays, one 0.5-mg spray in each nostril)
• Instruct the patient to use one dose (one spray in each nostril) one or two times per hour, at least 8 times daily for the first 6 to 8 weeks
• Use a maximum of 5 doses per hour or 40 mg nicotine (80 sprays) per day
• Each bottle contains approximately 100 doses (approximately 1 week's supply)
• Taper gradually during an additional 4 to 6 weeks after the initial 6 to 8 week trial

PRECAUTIONS.
• Reactive airway disease (e.g., asthma and bronchospasm)
• Chronic nasal disorders (e.g., rhinitis, polyps, and sinusitis)
• Patients with a history of myocardial infarction, angina pectoris or both, serious cardiac arrhythmias, or vasospastic disease
• Hepatic or renal insufficiency because of reduced drug clearance
• Use with caution in patients with endocrine disease, because nicotine causes release of catecholamines by the adrenal medulla
• Active peptic ulcer disease because of impaired healing
• Accelerated hypertension

SIDE EFFECTS.
• Moderate to severe nasal irritation (81% to 94%)
• Nasal congestion
• Transient change in sense of smell/taste

COMBINATION NICOTINE REPLACEMENT THERAPY. Combination NRT involves the use of a long-acting formulation (nicotine transdermal patch), which produces relatively constant levels of nicotine in the body, in combination with a short-acting formulation (gum, lozenge, inhaler, or nasal spray) to allow for acute dose titration as needed for withdrawal symptoms. For relapsed smokers, combination therapy improves long-term abstinence

rates (estimated abstinence 28.6% for combined therapy, vs. 17.4% for monotherapy).[21]

Bupropion SR. Bupropion SR (Zyban) is the only nonnicotine, first-line pharmacotherapy currently approved by the Food and Drug Administration (FDA) for smoking cessation treatment. Other systemic medications have been tested, but are currently not accepted as a part of dental practice. The drug bupropion SR is marketed as Zyban for smoking cessation, and as Wellbutrin SR for the treatment of depression. Bupropion has been shown to promote long-term abstinence when compared with placebo, and to decrease the cravings for cigarettes and symptoms of nicotine withdrawal.[36] By blocking neural dopamine or norepinephrine reuptake in the central nervous system, bupropion decreases the craving for nicotine and symptoms of withdrawal. Studies indicate that bupropion in conjunction with counseling can double abstinence rates when compared with the use of a placebo.[37]

Contraindications. Bupropion is contraindicated in patients with a history of seizure disorders. Although seizures were not reported in the Zyban smoking cessation clinical trials, the incidence of seizures with the sustained-release formulation (Wellbutrin) used in the treatment of depression was 0.1% (i.e., 1/1,000) in patients without a previous history of seizures. Patients who are taking any form of medication that lowers seizure threshold should not be given bupropion without close medical monitoring. Bupropion is also contraindicated in patients with a current or prior diagnosis of anorexia or bulimia nervosa because of a higher incidence of seizures noted in patients treated for bulimia with the immediate-release formulation of bupropion.

Bupropion is the active ingredient in Wellbutrin and Wellbutrin SR, which are used in the treatment of depression, and in Zyban, which is used for tobacco cessation. These medications should not be used in combination because the incidence of seizures is dose-related. The concurrent administration of bupropion and a monoamine oxidase (MAO) inhibitor is contraindicated. Studies in animals demonstrate that the acute toxicity of bupropion is enhanced by the MAO inhibitor phenelzine. At least 14 days should elapse between discontinuation of an MAO inhibitor and initiation of treatment with bupropion.

Also, bupropion is contraindicated in patients undergoing abrupt discontinuation of alcohol or sedatives, including benzodiazepines.

The FDA has classified bupropion as a pregnancy category B drug, meaning animal studies have not shown an adverse effect on the fetus, but no adequate clinical studies exist in pregnant women. The manufacturer recommends that bupropion be used during pregnancy only if clearly needed. Further, pregnant smokers should attempt cessation by using behavioral interventions before pharmacological approaches are used.

Dosage. Treatment with bupropion should be initiated while the patient is still smoking, because approximately 10 to 14 days of treatment are required to achieve steady-state blood levels. Patients should set a quit date that falls within the first 2 weeks of treatment, usually in the second week. The starting dose of bupropion is one 150-mg tablet each morning for the first 3 days. If the initial dose is well tolerated, increase the dosage on day 4 to the recommended maximum dosage of 300 mg/day, given as two 150-mg tablets taken at least 8 hours apart. The recommended length of therapy is 7 to 12 weeks; however, some patients may need continuous treatment. Whether to continue treatment with bupropion for periods longer than 12 weeks for smoking cessation must be determined for individual patients. In some patients, maintenance treatment as long as 6 months may be appropriate. If a patient has not made significant progress toward abstinence by the seventh week of therapy with bupropion, it is unlikely that he or she will quit during the current attempt, and treatment should be discontinued. Dose tapering of bupropion is not required when discontinuing treatment. Bupropion can safely be combined with any of the NRTs.[38]

Side Effects. Common side effects include insomnia (30% to 40%) and dry mouth (11%). These side effects usually lessen with continued use. Patients should be advised to avoid taking bupropion at bedtime. Side effects that are less common but associated with discontinuation of treatment include tremors (3.4%) and rash (2.4%).

Smokeless Tobacco (ST) Cessation

The nicotine from snuff is delivered through absorption through the buccal mucosa. The following calculation provides a rough estimate of relative nicotine dose in one tin of snuff compared with one package of cigarettes.

4.8 mg nicotine/gm of moist snuff, 30 gm/can = 144 mg;
144 mg nicotine/(1.8 mg nicotine/cigarette) = 80 cigarettes;
80 cigarettes/(20 cigarettes/pack) = 4 packs;
1 can snuff = 4 packs of cigarettes.

Nicotine absorption in smokeless tobacco is affected by several factors. A finer-cut tobacco releases higher nicotine levels than the coarse, "long-cut" tobacco. The addition of ammonium bicarbonate lowers the acidity of product, which yields higher free nicotine levels. The addition of acetic acid increases salivation and enhances the absorption of nicotine.[39] The pH of snuff products available in the United States varies from a low of 5.7, which delivers approximately 3.2 g/mg of free nicotine, to a high of 8.6, which delivers 11.4 g/mg of free nicotine.[40]

The following indicators can be used to assess ST dependence:[41]

- Always swallowing tobacco juice
- Use of ST in inappropriate places
- Use of ST when ill in bed
- Nicotine content of smokeless tobacco brand (e.g., Copenhagen has a higher free nicotine level than Skoal Bandits)[40]
- Use within 30 minutes of waking
- Chewing more than 16 hours/day
- Tins or pouches/week:
  Low, less than 1/week
  Moderate, 2 to 3/week
  High, more than 3/week

Cessation recommendations and guidelines for smokeless tobacco have not been formalized. Four evidence-based recommendations include[42]:

1) Behavioral interventions that include the use of an oral examination appear to be associated with the greatest treatment effect. Oral replacement products should be discussed, and selection based on the patient's choice.
2) Bupropion, 150 mg taken orally twice a day, can be continued for 3 to 6 months.
3) Tailored nicotine patch therapy, with or without gum or lozenge for nicotine self-titration, should be tailored to individual patient needs.
4) Combinations of medications can be prescribed to alleviate withdrawal symptoms.

Strategies for Alcohol Use Evaluation and Counseling

The following guidelines are adapted from *Helping Patients with Alcohol Problems*,[43] available from the National Institute on Alcohol Abuse and Alcoholism. An alcohol intake history similar to a tobacco use history should be recorded, updated, and maintained as part of the patient record.

The following questions provide a framework for assessing and recording alcohol intake:

Weekly average:
- On average, how many days a week do you drink alcohol?
- On a typical day, how many drinks do you have?
- Drinking days per week multiplied by drinks per day = weekly intake.
- If the weekly intake is greater than 14 for men or greater than seven for women, the patient is at significantly increased risk, and should be asked the **CAGE questions** given in the text that follows.

Daily maximum:
- What is the maximum number of drinks you had on any given day in the past month?
- If the maximum is greater than four for men or greater than three for women, the clinician should proceed with the CAGE questions, given in the text that follows.

CAGE Questionnaire.

C Have you ever felt that you should **C**ut down on your drinking?

A Have people **A**nnoyed you by criticizing your drinking?

G Have you ever felt bad or **G**uilty about your drinking?

E Have you ever had a drink first thing in the morning to steady your nerves or to get rid of a hangover? (**E**ye-opener).

Follow-up and interpretation:

- If the answer is "yes" to any of the above, the practitioner should then ask, "Has this occurred in the past year?"
- If the answer is "yes" to three or four questions for the past year, the patient may be alcohol dependent.
- If the answer "yes" to one or two questions for the past year, the patient may have alcohol-related problems. Even if the patient answered "no" to all questions, the patient is still at risk because of the elevated drinking level.

The **standard drink equivalents** below provide a guideline for what should be interpreted as "one drink."

- 12 oz of beer or cooler
- 8.5 oz of malt liquor
- 5 oz of table wine
- 3.5 oz of fortified wine (sherry or port)
- 2 oz of cordial or aperitif
- 1.5 oz of brandy
- 1.5 oz of spirits (e.g., 80-proof gin, vodka, and whiskey)

Assess:

- Dependence indicators
- Medical factors
- Behavioral factors
- Family history

Advise and assist:

- State your concern
- Give your advice
- Gauge the patient's readiness to change
- Negotiate an action plan for cutting down, recommend lower limits, set a drinking goal
- For abstaining: refer to an alcohol treatment center

Arrange follow-up:

Plan to monitor patient progress or refer for treatment.

One in 5 men and 1 in 10 women in the United States who visit their primary care providers meet the criteria for at-risk drinking, problem drinking, or alcohol dependence. Estimates suggest that alcohol dependence is found in 25% of persons seen in primary care settings who drink above recommended limits of alcohol use.[44] The National Institute on Alcohol Abuse and Alcoholism (NIAAA) has proposed alcohol use guidelines to limit risks for short- and long-term drinking-related consequences by establishing age- and sex-specific recommended consumption thresholds.[45] For adult women the maximum recommended consumption is 1 or less standard drinks per day and for anyone older than 65 years of age and 2 or fewer standard drinks per day for adult men. These guidelines do not apply to adolescents, pregnant women, and persons with alcohol dependence or medical conditions or medication use, or for whom alcohol intake is contraindicated, or to circumstances (i.e., driving) in which consumption is unsafe.

For patients who are at-risk or problem drinkers but not alcohol dependent, health care providers can significantly reduce alcohol use and related problems by providing brief interventions, which consist of feedback and advice from the health care provider and agreement by the patient on a course of action.

There are limitations of quantity and frequency questions that led to the development of screening questionnaire designed for use in primary care settings that focus on the consequences of patients' drinking and their perceptions of their drinking behavior such as the CAGE questionnaire discussed previously. In a brief intervention, the health care provider follows these three basic steps:

- State the medical concern.
- Advise the patient to abstain from alcohol use (if alcohol dependent), or to cut down (if not).
- Agree on a plan of action.

Health care providers who use brief interventions can also suggest techniques to help patients modify their behavior and suggest self-help material for the patients to read. Brief interventions are a valuable resource to reduce patients' problems with alcohol. The typical effective brief alcohol intervention takes no more than 15 minutes, is accompanied by written material, and offers an opportunity for the patient to schedule a follow-up. In a meta-analysis, investigators reported positive effects sustained beyond a year and lasting as long as 48 months.[46] This finding should encourage practitioners to engage in brief interventions that have the potential to effect the morbidity, mortality, and quality of life related to excessive alcohol consumption.

SUMMARY

In addition to the well-known harmful effects of smoking on respiratory and cardiovascular systems and the cause of multiple system cancers, tobacco use has significant adverse effects on oral health. Cigarette smoking is associated with an increased incidence of oral squamous cell carcinoma (OSCC), which is 4 to 7 times greater in smokers than in nonsmokers. Quitting smoking decreases the risk for oral cancer within 5 to 10 years. Tobacco exposure is also associated with an increased prevalence and severity of periodontal disease, and smoking status is an important factor in the prognosis for periodontal therapy, oral wound healing, implant therapy, and cosmetic dentistry. Smoking results in discoloration of teeth and of dental restorations, and is associated with halitosis and diminished taste. Cessation of smoking can halt disease progression and improve outcomes of periodontal therapy.

Smokeless tobacco (ST) use has been reported to cause tooth decay and discoloration of dental restorations. Chewing tobacco, in particular, is associated with an increased risk for dental caries and increased gingival recession. Effects of ST use are typically observed at anatomical locations where the tobacco contacts the mucosa, such as the labial vestibule and adjacent periodontium. Both the prevalence and severity of tobacco-related oral lesions demonstrate a dose-response relationship with the amount, frequency, and duration of ST use. Chronic ST use in the United States has been associated in a dose-response relationship with an increased risk for oral cancer.

Brief intervention for tobacco use and alcohol abuse has been proven to be effective. Furthermore, advice from a concerned health care professional increases cessation rates for tobacco use and abstinence from alcohol. Both of these behavioral changes have major and immediate as well as long-term health benefits for the individual and his or her family. Health professionals shouldn't grade themselves on how many people they can "get to quit," but rather how many times they deliver the message when the opportunity arises. Using this criterion, there is no reason not to have an intervention success approaching 100%!

Additional research in smokeless tobacco cessation should be pursued and widely disseminated in the dental community. Formal recommendations for evaluation and counseling for oral cancer risk reduction related to alcohol use in the dental office need development and dissemination.

Even as we continue to practice the existing treatments for tobacco cessation, research is rapidly advancing. New drugs that will differ radically from the existing therapies for smoking cessation are under development. Rather than slowly weaning tobacco users off nicotine, new therapies will mimic or block nicotine's chemical effects on the body. This new drug stimulates nicotine receptors in the brain, but unlike nicotine, it is not addictive. Drugs that act as a partial nicotine receptor agonist will assist in cessation by preventing nicotine withdrawal symptoms. Other drugs under development have the potential to help millions of obese people reduce their weight, but will also play a major role in tobacco cessation by inhibiting a receptor associated with regulating the body's chemical reward system, resulting in a reduction in weight in addition to decreased tobacco dependence. The dual effects on smoking cessation and reduced weight gain make this a promising agent for treating tobacco dependence. Other firms are working on vaccines for nicotine addiction. The vaccine is designed to cause the immune system to produce antibodies that bind to nicotine and prevent it from entering the brain. The nicotine antibodies act like a sponge, soaking up nicotine in the blood stream and preventing it from reaching the brain. As a result, the positive stimulus in the brain that is normally caused by nicotine is no longer present. This removes the stimulus for smoking and consequently helps people to quit or never start.

References

1. Jemal A, Murray T, Ward E et al.: Cancer statistics, 2005, *CA Cancer J Clin* 55:11-30, 2005.
2. United States Department of Health and Human Services (USDHHS): *Healthy People 2010, ed 2, with understanding and improving health and objectives for improving health, vol 2,* Washington, DC, 2000, U.S. Government Printing Office.
3. Smith RA, Cokkinides V, Harnin JE: American Cancer Society guidelines for early detection of cancer 2006, *CA Cancer J Clin* 56:11-15, 2006.
4. Canto MT, Kawaguchi Y, Horowitz AM: Coverage and quality of oral cancer information in the popular press: 1987-98, *J Public Health Dent* 58:241-247, 1998.
5. Horowitz AM, Nourjah P, Gift HC: U.S. adult knowledge of risk factors and signs of oral cancers: 1990, *J Am Dent Assoc* 126:39-45, 1995.
6. Hurt RD, Robertson CR: Prying open the door to the tobacco industry's secrets about nicotine. *JAMA* 280:172-181, 1998.
7. Benowitz NL: Pharmacology of nicotine. In Tarter RE, Ammerman RT, editors: *Handbook of substance abuse: neurobehavioral pharmacology,* New York, 1998, Plenum Press.
8. American Psychiatric Association: *Diagnostic and statistical manual of mental disorders, fourth edition-text revised (DSM-IV-TR),* Washington, DC, 1994, American Psychiatric Association.
9. Hughes JR: Tobacco withdrawal in self-quitters, *J Consult Clin Psychol* 60:689-697, 1992.
10. Fiore MC, Bailey WC, Cohen SJ, et al.: *Treating tobacco use and dependence. Clinical practice guideline,* Rockville, MD, 2000, U.S. Department of Health and Human Services, Public Health Service.
11. Carr AB, Ebbert JO: Interventions for tobacco cessation in the dental setting, *Cochrane Database Syst Rev* 2005, Issue 1.
12. Bertholet N, Daeppen JB, Wietlisbach V et al.: Reduction of alcohol consumption by brief alcohol intervention in primary care: systematic review and meta-analysis, *Arch Intern Med* 165: 986-995, 2005.
13. Stafne EE, Bakdash B: Tobacco cessation intervention: how to communicate with tobacco using patients, *J Contemp Dent Pract* 1:1-11, 2000.
14. Weinstein ND: What does it mean to understand a risk? Evaluating risk comprehension, *J Natl Cancer Inst* 25:15-21, 1999.
15. Shiffman S, Pillitteri JL, Burton SL et al.: Smokers' beliefs about "Light" and "Ultra Light" cigarettes, *Tob Control* 10(suppl 1): 17-23, 2001.
16. Etter JF, Koslowski LT, Perneger TV: What smokers believe about light and ultralight cigarettes, *Prev Med* 36:92-98, 2003.
17. Harris JE, Thun MJ, Mondul AM et al.: Cigarette tar yields in relation to mortality from lung cancer in the cancer prevention study II prospective cohort, 1982-8, *Br Med J* 328:1-8, 2004.
18. National Cancer Institute: *Risks associated with smoking cigarettes with low machine-measured yields of tar and nicotine,* Smoking and Tobacco Control Monograph 13, Bethesda, MD, 2001, National Cancer Institute.
19. Prochaska JO, DiClemente CC, Norcross JC: In search of how people change: applications to addictive behaviors, *Am Psychol* 47:1102-1111, 1992.
20. Prochaska JO, Goldstein MG: Process of smoking cessation, *Clin Chest Med* 12:727-735, 1991.
21. Silagy C, Lancaster T, Stead L et al.: Nicotine replacement therapy for smoking cessation, *Cochrane Database Syst Rev* 4:CD000146, 2002.
22. Henningfield JE, Fant RV, Buchhalter AR et al.: Pharmacotherapy for nicotine dependence, *CA Cancer J Clin* 55:281-299, 2005.

23. Dempsey DA, Benowitz NL: Risks and benefits of nicotine to aid smoking cessation in pregnancy, *Drug Safety* 24:277-322, 2001.
24. Silagy C, Lancaster T, Stead L et al.: Nicotine replacement therapy for smoking cessation, *Cochrane Database Syst Rev* 3:CD000146, 2004.
25. Benowitz NL, Jacob P, Savanapridi C: Determinants of nicotine intake while chewing nicotine polacrilex gum, *Clin Pharmacol Ther* 41:467-473, 1987.
26. Schneider NG, Lunell E, Olmstead RE et al.: Clinical pharmacokinetics of nasal nicotine delivery. A review and comparison to other nicotine systems, *Clin Pharmacokinet* 31:65-80, 1996.
27. Shiffman S, Dresler CM, Hajek P et al.: Efficacy of a nicotine lozenge for smoking cessation, *Arch Intern Med* 162:1267-1276, 2002.
28. Heatherton TF, Kozlowski LT, Frecker RC et al.: Measuring the heaviness of smoking: using self-reported time to the first cigarette of the day and number of cigarettes smoked per day, *Br J Addict* 84:791-799, 1989.
29. West R, Hajek P, Foulds J et al.: A comparison of the abuse liability and dependence potential of nicotine patch, gum, spray and inhaler, *Psychopharmacology* 149:198-202, 2000.
30. Dale LC, Hurt RD, Offord KP et al.: High-dose nicotine patch therapy; percentage of replacement and smoking cessation, *JAMA* 274:1353-1358, 1995.
31. Gore AV, Chien YW: The nicotine transdermal system, *Clin Dermatol* 16:599-615, 1998.
32. Benowitz NL, Zevin S, Jacob P: Sources of variability in nicotine and cotinine levels with use of nicotine nasal spray, transdermal nicotine and cigarette smoking, *Br J Clin Pharmacol* 43:259-267, 1997.
33. Schneider NG, Lunell E, Olmstead RE et al.: Clinical pharmacokinetics of nasal nicotine delivery. A review and comparison to other nicotine systems, *Clin Pharmacokinet* 31:65-80, 1996.
34. Schuh KJ, Schuh LM, Henningfield JE et al.: Nicotine nasal spray and vapor inhaler: abuse liability assessment, *Psychopharmacology* 130:352-361, 1997.
35. Nicotrol NS Prescribing Information (website): http://www.nicotrol.com/ns/prescribing.asp. Accessed May 2, 2006.
36. Hurt RD, Sachs DP, Glover ED et al.: A comparison of sustained-release bupropion and placebo for smoking cessation, *N Engl J Med* 337:1195-1202, 1997.
37. Hughes JR, Stead LF, Lancaster T: Antidepressants for smoking cessation, *Cochrane Database Syst Rev* 4:CD000031, 2000.
38. Jorenby DE, Leischow SJ, Nides MA et al.: A controlled trial of sustained-release bupropion, a nicotine patch, or both for smoking cessation, *N Engl J Med* 340:685-691, 1999.
39. Richter P, Spierto FW: Surveillance of smokeless tobacco nicotine, pH, moisture, and unprotonated nicotine content, *Nicotine Tob Res* 5:885-889, 2003.
40. Centers for Disease Control and Prevention (CDC): Determination of nicotine, pH, and moisture content of six US commercial moist snuff products—Florida, January-February 1999 *MMWR Morb Mortal Wkly Rep* 48:398-401, 1999.
41. Boyle RG, Jensen J, Hatsukami DK et al.: Measuring dependence in smokeless tobacco users. *Addict Behav* 20:443-450, 1995.
42. Ebbert JO, Rowland LC, Montori VM et al.: Treatments for spit tobacco use: a quantitative systematic review, *Addiction* 98:569-583, 2003.
43. US Preventive Services Task Force: Screening and behavioral counseling interventions in primary care to reduce alcohol misuse: recommendation statement, *Ann Intern Med* 140:554-556, 2004.
44. Manwell LB, Fleming MF, Johnson K et al.: Tobacco, alcohol, and drug use in a primary care sample: 90-day prevalence and associated factors, *J Addict Dis* 17:67-81, 1998.
45. National Institute on Alcohol Abuse and Alcoholism (NIAAA): *The physician's guide to helping patients with alcohol problems*, Rockville, MD, 1995, National Institutes of Health, NIH publication no. 95-3769.
46. Bertholet N, Daeppen JB, Wietlisbach V et al.: Reduction of alcohol consumption by brief alcohol intervention in primary care: systematic review and meta-analysis, *Arch Intern Med* 165:986-995, 2005.

Chapter 18

*P*revention Strategies for Oral Components of Systemic Conditions

CYNTHIA STEGEMAN AND LINDA BOYD

TAILORED STRATEGIES FOR CLINICAL PRACTICE

Xerostomia
Oropharyngeal Candidiasis
Mucositis
Oral Lichen Planus
Recurrent Aphthous Ulcers
Gingival Tissue Enlargement
Abnormal Bleeding
Wound Healing
Alveolar Bone Loss
Dysgeusia
Dysphagia
Dental Erosion
Burning Mouth Syndrome

SUMMARY

LEARNING OBJECTIVES

Upon completion of this chapter, the learner will be able to:
- Identify systemic conditions that result in oral health issues.
- Describe the oral manifestations associated with xerostomia.
- Identify appropriate recommendations to meet the specific needs of a patient experiencing xerostomia.
- Determine the treatment protocol for an individual with candidiasis.
- Assess patients for xerostomia and provide education.
- Describe clinical manifestations of and common patient complaints for mucositis.

- Provide appropriate recommendations for patients experiencing oral lichen planus.
- Explore foods to recommend to patients that may contribute to the reduction of recurrent aphthous ulcers.
- List drugs associated with gingival overgrowth.
- Identify people who are at high risk of malnutrition and the potential for poor wound healing.
- Determine a management plan for a patient experiencing alveolar bone loss.
- Describe dysgeusia and the associated implications.
- Describe dental treatment considerations for a patient with dysphagia.
- Recommend dental therapies to protect the oral health status of patients presenting with severe dental erosion.
- Describe the progression of dental erosion.
- Discuss the treatment regimes used to treat burning mouth syndrome.

KEY TERMS

Abnormal bleeding
Alveolar bone loss
Aphthous stomatitis
Burning mouth syndrome
Candidiasis
Dental erosion
Dysgeusia
Dysphagia
Gingival enlargement
Mucositis
Oral lichen planus
Osteonecrosis
Recurrent aphthous ulcers

Wound healing
Xerostomia

Oral conditions associated with systemic diseases and disorders and iatrogenic conditions resulting from medical and dental treatment and care can be managed to achieve optimum clinical outcomes and maintenance of oral health status. Some require unique approaches and considerations. This chapter provides an abbreviated discussion of a variety of oral conditions that occur in the presence of various systemic diseases and disorders. Detailed information is available in other chapters in this book. Practical strategies for preventing and/or managing the impact on oral health status are reviewed.

Evidence regarding the association between systemic and oral disease has emerged at a rapid pace due primarily to a renewed interest in the potential impact of periodontal health on systemic disease. Some systemic conditions that may be associated with periodontal disease discussed in the literature include diabetes, preterm low-birth-weight (PLBW) babies, chronic obstructive pulmonary diseases (COPD) and pneumonia, osteoporosis, rheumatoid arthritis, cardiovascular, and cerebrovascular diseases. In many situations, periodontal and other oral health issues have an impact on the severity of the systemic condition. Treatment modalities for systemic conditions such as hypertension, autoimmune diseases, cancer, and asthma are also known to impact oral health.

A comprehensive review of the research literature identified a moderate association between heart disease and periodontal disease, but a causal relationship was not confirmed.[1] Periodontitis was 91% more prevalent in persons with cardiovascular disease (CVD) and, conversely, the severity of the periodontal infection increased the risk for CVD.[2] Periodontal pathogens such as, *Porphyromonas gingivalis*, *Prevotella intermedia*, *Eikenella corrodens* and *Treponema denticola* have been found in vascular lesions associated with atherosclerosis.[3-5] A direct relationship between periodontal pathogens and atherosclerosis was thought to be the mechanism for the association.[7]

Research suggests that gingivitis is an independent risk factor for stroke, because it increases the risk for cerebral ischemia eighteenfold.[7] In comparison, clinical attachment loss (CAL) of more than 6 mm increases the risk for stroke sevenfold.[7] Acute infection, such as respiratory infection, is a known trigger for ischemic stroke but gingivitis may also be a trigger.[7,8]

Diabetes and periodontal disease have a synergistic effect because of the propensity periodontal infection has to cause changes in blood glucose levels that impair the control of periodontal disease.[9] For example, among Pima Indians with diabetes, death rates from the complications of poorly controlled diabetes were 3.2 times higher in persons with severe periodontal disease.[10] Studies have documented marked improvements in glycemic control as an improvement of approximately 0.5% in glycosylated hemoglobin (HbA1$_c$) after nonsurgical periodontal treatment.[11]

This difference would equate to a 17% reduction in diabetes-related complications and a 12% reduction in diabetes-related deaths.[12]

A systematic review of epidemiological data indicated that persons with poor oral hygiene status were 4.5 times more likely to have COPD, and those with periodontal disease were 65% more likely to have this condition.[13] A meta-analysis of oral interventions noted improved oral hygiene and reduced bacterial load was associated with a decrease on average of 40% in incidence of nosocomial pneumonia.[14] A causal relationship has not been confirmed.

A decade of studies has demonstrated that periodontal disease is associated with occurrence of PLBW. Lopez et al. found that periodontal therapy significantly reduced the rates of these births.[15]

Although the systemic bone loss seen in osteoporosis is associated with the resorption of alveolar bone and tooth loss, no definitive evidence exists that periodontal disease and osteoporosis are directly linked.[16-18] Bisphosphonates used in treatment of osteoporosis may have a positive but controversial effect on periodontal status. Bisphosphonates are synthetic analogues of pyrophosphate used in the treatment of patients with hypercalcemia as a result of malignancy, bone metastasis, and other disorders such as metabolic bone diseases, Paget's disease, and osteoporosis. Some researchers have reported improvement in pocket depths and reduction of bone loss after periodontal procedures in animals receiving bisphosphonate therapy.[19,20] Studies with small samples of human subjects receiving the same therapy have reported no changes in clinical parameters.[21] In the last decade, however, cases of osteonecrosis, a clinical condition associated with defects in vascularization of the maxilla or the mandibular bone, have been reported in patients who either underwent head and neck radiotherapy or had a dental extraction while taking bisphosphonates.[22,23] Careful evaluation of the patients' oral health is being recommended before prescribing bisphosphonate treatment.[23]

Periodontal disease and rheumatoid arthritis appear to share pathological features independent of oral plaque deposits that are related to the dysfunction of inflammatory mechanisms.[24,25] Both diseases have similar pathophysiology in that high levels of proinflammatory cytokines are present.[24] Patients with rheumatoid arthritis are twice as likely to exhibit moderate-to-severe periodontal bone loss than those without rheumatoid arthritis.[25-27] When a group of patients were examined, those with rheumatoid arthritis had 11.6 missing teeth compared with 6.7 in a control group. Although a causal relationship has not been confirmed, one study suggested that periodontal treatment with debridement reduced the erythrocyte sedimentation rate (ESR), which is a measure of rheumatoid arthritis activity.[28] Thus, management of periodontal infection may positively augment management of rheumatoid arthritis.

Animal research dating back to 1977 suggests a relationship between obesity and the severity of periodontal disease.[29] More recent epidemiological National Health and Nutrition Examination Survey (NHANES III) data showed that in populations aged 18 to 34 years, persons with abdominal and overall obesity were twice as likely to have periodontal disease.[30,31] Others have reported significant correlations between body composition and periodontal disease, with waist-to-hip ratio the most significant anthropometric indicator.[32,33]

In addition to the emerging associations between systemic disease and periodontal disease, treatment modalities exist for diseases associated with an increased risk for caries and other oral lesions. More than 500 medications used to treat conditions such as hypertension or depression had side effects that include xerostomia. Some autoimmune diseases, such as Sjögren's syndrome, also result in xerostomia. Xerostomia impairs the buffering capacity of the saliva resulting in an increase in caries risk. Other medications (such as calcium-channel blockers and cyclosporine) can cause gingival hyperplasia, which makes oral plaque removal more difficult for patients. Conditions such as bulimia nervosa, in which individuals use regurgitation as a means of purging, and gastroesophageal reflux disease (GERD), increase the risk for caries and erosion because of exposure of the teeth to acidic gastric fluids. Finally, autoimmune diseases and cancer therapies can result in candidiasis and mucositis, which make it difficult for patients to maintain adequate oral plaque removal, leading to increased risk for caries and periodontal disease.

TAILORED STRATEGIES FOR CLINICAL PRACTICE

Xerostomia

Xerostomia is the result of salivary gland hypofunction caused by either a functional or organic disturbance. In 24 hours, a healthy adult can secrete approximately 500 mL (approximately 2 cups) of saliva by the submandibular, parotid and sublingual glands, and minor salivary glands located in the oral mucosa.[34] Saliva output is highest in the morning and stimulated by mastication and gustation. The rate of salivary flow and the composition of the saliva will vary among patients, depending on the type of stimulation.[35] Sympathetic stimulation influences salivary composition, and parasympathetic stimulation influences the amount of saliva secreted (Table 18-1).

Saliva is one of the most valuable and protective body fluids. It provides numerous physiological functions, including ease in chewing, swallowing, and digestion of food, lubrication, cleansing, and antibacterial oral environmental buffering components. It augments tooth demineralization and remineralization properties and is essential for the maintenance of oral hard and soft tissue integrity. Inadequate saliva can result in an increase in

caries incidence and susceptibility to candidiasis, bacterial and fungal infections, ulcerations, stomatitis, and glossitis. Dental professionals are tasked with relieving the causes and symptoms of xerostomia to improve the quality of life for patients.

Xerostomia has numerous etiologies, including polypharmacy, systemic diseases, antineoplastic therapies, neurological and psychological disorders, dehydration, and mouth breathing. For example, salivary flow rate typically decreases when the number of medications a patient is taking each day increases.[36]

Uncontrolled diabetes, Sjögren's syndrome, rheumatoid arthritis, systemic lupus erythematosus, human immunodeficiency virus/acquired immune deficiency syndrome (HIV/AIDS), Parkinson's disease, eating disorders, anxiety or depression, renal dialysis caused by severe fluid restrictions, and dehydration are several diseases or conditions associated with xerostomia. Radiation and chemotherapy treatment, particularly of the head and neck, changes salivary flow and composition. The location, type, and length of treatment and dosage determine the severity of xerostomic conditions.[35]

A comprehensive medical and clinical assessment of the patient is necessary to determine the cause of xerostomia. When polypharmacy is an issue, consultation with the physician is indicated to discuss possible alterations in the type, dosage, frequency, or timing of over-the-counter and prescription medications. For example, the effect of the medication taken before bed will peak while the patient sleeps, thus the patient is unaware of the dryness. A suggested strategy to take smaller doses of a medication more often to allow time for salivary stimulation should be discussed. But this should not be altered without a consultation with the physician. If this is not feasible, education of the patient with suggestions to relieve the symptoms and the oral complications associated with xerostomia should be explored (see Chapter 10).

The Food and Drug Administration (FDA) has approved pilocarpine and cevimeline to treat xerostomia. Both act directly on cholinergic receptor sites. Precautions in use of these drugs are indicated for patients with asthma, coronary artery disease, hypertension, epilepsy, and pregnancy.[37]

For patients with existing or chronic xerostomia, adequate hydration is paramount. Recommendations include avoiding products containing tobacco, alcohol, and caffeine because these substances further dry oral tissue. A decrease in dry, crumbly, salty, or spicy foods, or moistening dry food in beverages to allow for ease in swallowing, should be suggested. Moist and soft textured foods, such as applesauce or cottage cheese, are also helpful. Sucking on ice chips, frequent sips of fluids, and incorporating beverages and cold foods with meals will also aid in chewing and swallowing. Over-the-counter saliva replacement products should be recommended if they are acceptable to the patient.

Text continued on page 254

TABLE 18-1

REFERENCE GUIDE FOR PREVENTION AND MANAGEMENT OF ORAL MANIFESTATIONS ASSOCIATED WITH SYSTEMIC CONDITIONS

ORAL MANIFESTATION	ASSOCIATED CONDITION/MEDICATION	CLINICAL PRESENTATION	Prevention Strategies		Management Strategies	
			ORAL HYGIENE	NUTRITION	MEDICATIONS	
Xerostomia	Diabetes Sjögren's syndrome Salivary gland disorders Systemic lupus erythematosus Rheumatoid arthritis HIV/AIDS Parkinson's disease Scleroderma Sarcoidosis Hepatitis C Neurological impairments	Dry, crusty mucosa Dry, fissured tongue Atrophy of papilla Angular cheilosis Burning mouth syndrome Difficulty with mastication, swallowing, and speech Enlarged and/or tender salivary glands Fungal and viral infections Caries, especially root caries Poorly-fitting denture Thicker, stringy saliva Gingivitis Dry eyes, nose and/or throat	Oral self-care and routine periodontal maintenance Fluoride therapy	Adequate hydration Encourage chewy, nutrient-dense foods Promote breakfast Moderate intake of alcohol and caffeinated drinks	Pilocarpine or cevimeline Antimicrobial, antifungal, and antiviral therapies	If feasible, give drug causing xerostomia prior to bedtime, and consult with physician regarding smaller doses and/or increased frequency of drug causing xerostomia SUGGEST: Use mouth rinses that are alcohol-free Smoking cessation Use of humidifier at night Use of lip balm Avoidance of excessive alcohol, caffeine and sticky foods Intake of sour, citrus, cinnamon, or mint sugarless candy or gum, in moderation Sips of sugar-free and caffeine-free fluids
Oropharyngeal candidiasis	Long term steroid use Immunosuppressant therapy Cancer therapy Diabetes HIV/AIDS	Removable white curd-like lesions on an erythematous base Angular cheilosis Atropic tongue	Oral self-care and routine periodontal maintenance	Balanced and adequate nutrition Emphasize: dietary sources of energy, protein,	High-risk immuno-compromised patients: Intravenous Amphotericin B OR	Prescribe: Clotrimazole troche (20 mg 5 ×/day) OR Nystatin (200,000-400,000U 5 ×/day)

Continued

TABLE 18-1

REFERENCE GUIDE FOR PREVENTION AND MANAGEMENT OF ORAL MANIFESTATIONS ASSOCIATED WITH SYSTEMIC CONDITIONS—cont'd

ORAL MANIFESTATION	ASSOCIATED CONDITION/MEDICATION	CLINICAL PRESENTATION	Prevention Strategies		Management Strategies	
			ORAL HYGIENE	NUTRITION	MEDICATIONS	
		Stinging or burning mucosa Metallic taste		vitamin C and zinc	Oral fluconazole (400 mg/day)	OR Fluconazole 100-200 mg/day PO NOTE: Duration of 7-14 days after clinical improvement SUGGEST: hydration with water and decaffeinated beverages and soft, high protein foods
Mucositis	Cancer therapies: Chemotherapy Radiation therapy	Tissue edema, and atrophy Ulcerations that may be covered by a necrotic pseudomembrane Burning sensation	Oral self-care and routine periodontal maintenance Minimize use of alcohol-containing mouth rinses during therapy Use cholorhexidine only as an antiplaque and antifungal agent	Adequate hydration Adequate nutrition with emphasis on high-protein, nutrient-dense foods	Benzydamine hydrochloride (HCl) NOTE: new drugs not available but in Phase III trials include Repifermin & AES-14 (L-Glutamine)	Used for palliative care despite lack of evidence: Viscous lidocaine and Kaolin-pectin or diphenhydramine SUGGEST: avoidance of hard, crunchy, sour, acidic, spicy, or salty foods
Oral lichen planus	Psychosomatic factors Infective agents Immunologic conditions Stress	Fine white lines that form a reticular pattern or "web-like" appearance on oral soft tissue May be erosive or ulcerative	Oral self-care and routine periodontal maintenance	Adequate hydration Adequate nutrition Emphasize: Folate intake (400 µg/day) high-protein, nutrient-dense foods	Use for palliative care despite lack of evidence: Cyclosporines, Retinoids, Steroids and Ultraviolet phototherapy	SUGGEST: Avoidance of alcohol, pyrophosphates and sodium lauryl sulphate Avoidance of hard, crunchy, sour, acidic, spicy, or salty foods

Recurrent aphthous ulcers	Allergies Nutrient deficiencies Ulcerative colitis Celiac disease Crohn's disease HIV *Helicobacter pylori* Behçet's disease Endocrine disorders Stress Trauma	Circular lesions with an erythematous border and central area consisting of necrotic epithelial cells Self-limiting; 10-14 days	Oral self-care and routine periodontal maintenance	Adequate nutrition Emphasize: B-vitamins, iron and zinc, nonirritating food choices, May require high-protein liquid supplements	Topical Medication: Amlexanox Tetracycline mouthrinse (no more than 5 days) Chlorhexidine mouthrinse Beclomethasone spray Systemic medications: Levamisole (administer for 5-7 days) Prednisone 40-60 mg/day for 4-7 days, then taper dosage over 2 wks Thalidomide	SUGGEST: Avoidance of alcohol, pyrophosphates, or sodium lauryl sulphate
Gingival enlargement	Systemic Neurological and metabolic conditions requiring medications such as: Dilantin Cyclosporin Calcium channel blockers	Enlargement of Gingival tissue tends to be out of proportion to local factors (e.g., plaque) Affects papilla & anterior gingival tissue more severely	Oral self-care and professional preventive care	Adequate hydration Adequate nutrition Emphasize: Foods high in vitamins D and K, calcium and folate	Discuss alternative choices for medications with primary care provider, if possible	May require surgical intervention

Continued

TABLE 18-1

REFERENCE GUIDE FOR PREVENTION AND MANAGEMENT OF ORAL MANIFESTATIONS ASSOCIATED WITH SYSTEMIC CONDITIONS—cont'd

ORAL MANIFESTATION	ASSOCIATED CONDITION/ MEDICATION	CLINICAL PRESENTATION	Prevention Strategies		Management Strategies	
			ORAL HYGIENE	NUTRITION	MEDICATIONS	
Abnormal bleeding	Systemic conditions managed with Warfarin and NSAIDS Sickle cell anemia End stage liver or kidney disease Hemophilia von Willebrand's disease	Patient self-reports excessive bleeding during initial dental appointment or following dental treatment	Stress plaque control, caries prevention, and routine periodontal maintenance	Discuss drug-nutrient interactions with patients taking anti-coagulant medication Emphasize: Adequate vitamin K intake. Review dietary supplements taken, especially vitamins C or E or herbal supplements (e.g., ginger, gingko biloba, and ginseng)	Arrange for a consult to determine INR prior to beginning invasive treatment that may cause bleeding Advise patients to discontinue NSAIDS, vitamins, or herbal supplements 1-2 weeks prior to dental procedures	Initiate use of local hemostasis methods such as retraction cord w/coagulant if needed Educate the patient about risks associated with oversupplementation with herbal supplements and vitamins
Delayed wound healing	Cancer Therapies: Chemotherapy Radiation therapy End stage renal disease Substance abuse Eating disorders Malnutrition Gastrointestinal disorders HIV/AIDS Diabetes	Wounds that do not heal in 10-14 days History of corticosteroid or immuno-suppressant therapy and gingko biloba supplementation	Recommend a soft toothbrush with chlorhexidine	Adequate hydration Adequate nutrition Emphasize: Fruits, vegetables and high-quality protein Assess nutritional status prior to treatment Consult with dietitian and MD for medically complex patients prior to developing a care plan		Recommend maintenance of adequate high protein diet Recommend dietary liquid meal replacements if necessary, and adequate fluid to enhance wound healing Amino acids, glutamine and arginine, supplementation shows promise

Condition	Etiology	Clinical Sign	Oral Self-Care	Nutrition		
Alveolar bone loss	Osteoporosis Chronic kidney dysfunction Drug-nutrient interactions	Loss of alveolar bone as evidence by clinical attachment loss (CAL)	Oral self-care and routine periodontal maintenance Use antimicrobial agents and/or antibiotics if indicated	Stress adequate nutrition Emphasize: Dietary intake of foods rich in calcium and vitamin D Assess need for appropriate vitamin supplements	Bisphosphonates may minimize bone loss but are associated with osteonecrosis and should be discussed with the primary care provider	SUGGEST: Diet rich in calcium and vitamin D Weight-bearing physical activity
Dysgeusia	Medication induced (See Chapter 7) Upper respiratory infections Radiation therapy to head and neck GERD Crohn's disease Diabetes Pregnancy Nutrient deficiencies	Unpleasant or altered taste, sensation, and/ or metallic taste	Oral self-care and routine preventive care			Manage the causative agent as well as medication-induced xerostomia SUGGEST: Avoidance of tobacco products and chlorhexidine Avoidance of salt and sugar added to food SUGGEST: Foods with added flavoring agents and spices White meats, eggs, and cheese as sources of protein Cold foods rather than hot Plastic eating utensils for those complaining of a metallic taste

Continued

TABLE 18-1

REFERENCE GUIDE FOR PREVENTION AND MANAGEMENT OF ORAL MANIFESTATIONS ASSOCIATED WITH SYSTEMIC CONDITIONS—cont'd

ORAL MANIFESTATION	ASSOCIATED CONDITION/MEDICATION	CLINICAL PRESENTATION	Prevention Strategies		Management Strategies	
			ORAL HYGIENE	NUTRITION	MEDICATIONS	
Dysphagia	Parkinson's disease Multiple sclerosis Cerebral palsy Stroke Esophageal strictures Muscular dystrophy Esophagitis Dementia Neurogenic disorders Musculoskeletal Chronic GERD Immunocompromised	Difficulty or pain on swallowing Increased risk for aspiration, pneumonia	Oral self-care and routine periodontal maintenance Appropriate use of fluorides and sealants Complete an adequate drug history to identify use of CNS depressants and corticosteroids	Adequate hydration SUGGEST: diets of thickened fluids and mechanically altered foods Soft, nutrient-dense diet Avoidance of very hot or very cold liquids Reduced exposure to cariogenic foods	Recommend discontinuation of medications associated with the condition after discussing this with the primary care provider	Discuss management of conditions such as GERD Seat patient in semi-supine position Minimize the use of water, ultrasonic instrumentation and air polishers Suggest referral to dietitian for nutrition counseling
Dental erosion	Eating Disorders GERD	Lingual surfaces of maxillary anterior teeth are smooth and glossy Teeth are sensitive to extreme temperatures Changes in occlusion Margination of amalgams Evidence of bruxism	Oral self-care and routine preventive maintenance Fluoride therapy	Avoid excessive intake of acid-based food and beverages Follow ingestion of acidic foods with neutral foods like high quality proteins (milk, meat, cheese, nuts) Chew sugar-free gum following ingestion of acidic beverages		SUGGEST: Nonacidic products to stimulate saliva flow Restore eroded areas Repair occlusion RECOMMEND: Use of mouthguard Rinses with sodium bicarbonate Brushing or rinsing with water immediately after regurgitation Avoid use of: A hard toothbrush Abrasive toothpaste Scrubbing toothbrush method

	Associated with:		Discuss	Recommend	Recommend use of:	Stimulate saliva flow, see
Burning mouth syndrome	Allergic reactions Depression and anxiety Stress Postmenopausal candidiasis Diabetes Geographic tongue Nutrient deficiencies	Prevalent on anterior ⅔ of tongue resulting in burning sensation and bitter or metallic taste, along with xerostomia Symptoms intensify throughout the day and decrease at night and when eating	Tobacco cessation and provide support	avoidance of alcohol or allergenic foods Suggest a diet rich in B vitamins, iron, and zinc	Benzodiazepines Tricyclic antidepressants Topical capsaicin Antifungal agents if candidiasis is present.	Review management strategies for prevention and management of xerostomia and stimulation of saliva flow (p. 247)

To stimulate the flow of saliva, sugarless chewing gum and sugarless hard candy, especially citrus, cinnamon, or mint flavors, are suggested. The use of lip balm or a humidifier at night will also provide relief. Because the patient with xerostomia is at increased risk for caries, patient education regarding diet and caries prevention should be provided. Dietary counseling from a registered dietitian may be required, especially when issues related to systemic diseases, polypharmacy, or other complex conditions that require more extensive patient education are present.

Oral hygiene self-care and frequent recall appointments must be part of the patient care plan. Fluoride therapy in the office, such as fluoride varnish, may be necessary to control caries. If topical office fluorides are used, a sodium fluoride will be less irritating to the xerostomic tissues than acidulated fluoride products. A sodium fluoride home fluoride gel, rinse, toothpaste, or in combination, may also be needed. In some cases, antimicrobial, antifungal, or antiviral therapy may be indicated. Products containing xylitol, such as chewing gums, may be recommended to assist in remineralization, stimulation of saliva flow, and caries prevention.[38] Dental care should be provided with caution to minimize trauma to the oral mucosa.

Oropharyngeal Candidiasis

Oropharyngeal **candidiasis** is a fungal infection caused by the genus *Candida*, especially *C. albicans*, which can be present in as many as 65% of healthy individuals who do not exhibit signs of infection.[39] In individuals with an altered immune response, however, *Candida* organisms quickly become pathogenic and cause symptomatic candidiasis of the oral mucosa.[39] Candidiasis may be a nonlife-threatening mucocutaneous infection, but it can progress to an invasive infection that involves virtually every human organ system. Clinically, oral candidiasis presents in two forms: erythematous and pseudomembranous.[40] Pseudomembranous candidiasis is the most common and appears as removable white curd-like lesions on an erythematous base.[40] Symptoms experienced during an outbreak include angular cheilitis, stinging or burning mucosa, atropic tongue, and a metallic taste, thus making eating an unpleasant experience.[40]

In some clinical conditions and as a consequence of some medications, candidiasis can be more common. For example, candidal overgrowth occurs more frequently in those with diabetes than it does in those without diabetes, and it does not necessarily appear to be associated with the level of glycemic control.[41] Patients with xerostomia are at risk of developing candidiasis due to the loss of the antimicrobial properties of the saliva. Inhalation of corticosteroids for treatment of chronic obstructive pulmonary disease (COPD), such as asthma, can also result in oropharyngeal candidiasis.

Immunucompromising conditions predispose patients to candidal infections caused by damage to mucosal barriers from radiotherapy and chemotherapy, prolonged episodes of neutropenia, and long-term use of antibiotics and steroid therapies. Candidiasis is particularly common sequelae in HIV/AIDS, cancer therapy, and organ transplantation. Oral candidiasis is often one of the first clinical symptoms of underlying HIV infection and appears in 90% of all HIV-positive patients during the course of the condition.[40] Compared with persons on highly active antiretroviral therapies (HAART), persons on other regimens were 23% to 46% more likely to report an episode of candidiasis.[42] Of patients undergoing radiotherapy to the head and neck, 25% develop oropharyngeal candidiasis and require prophylaxis to prevent infection.[43]

Prophylactic antifungal agents to prevent invasive fungal infections during periods of risk are recommended for the following categories of patient: neutropenic patients, solid-organ transplant recipients, HIV-infected patients, and patients in intensive care units (ICUs).[44] Guidelines recommend intravenous amphotericin B or intravenous or oral fluconazole (400 mg/day) for these high-risk patients because these medications have been shown to be the most effective at preventing the onset of signs and symptoms of invasive candidiasis.[44] Multiple randomized trials of oropharyngeal candidiasis demonstrated that most patients respond to topical treatments that normally include clotrimazole troche (10 mg, 5 times/day) and oral nystatin (200,000 to 400,000 units, 5 times/day).[44]

The Infectious Disease Society of America (IDSA) recommends the azole antifungal agents for oral candidiasis. For refractory or recurrent infections, orally administered fluconazole therapy (100 to 200 mg/day) is superior to other azoles.[44] Recurrent infections tend to be most common in HIV/AIDS and cancer therapy patients. In these conditions, long-term fluconazole therapy has been shown to be more effective than episodic use in response to symptomatic candidiasis.[44] In addition, the use of fluconazole for those patients at risk for candidiasis has been shown to improve the schedule of radiotherapy in head and neck cancer patients.[45]

Compromised nutritional status is increased in the presence of candidiasis. In a study of 97 older, hospitalized individuals, those with candidiasis had lower daily energy, protein, vitamin C, and zinc intakes and low serum albumin levels indicative of malnutrition.[46] Dietary intakes improved once the candidiasis was successfully treated. Adequate nutrition of high-risk patients decreases risk of candidiasis and is particularly important during outbreaks of candidiasis. If lesions are painful, soft-textured, high-calorie, high-protein foods listed in Box 18-1 are recommended. Continuous intake of water and decaffeinated fluids should be stressed for hydration.

Adequate oral hygiene and plaque removal both from natural teeth as well as from removable prosthetic appliances is essential. Studies have demonstrated that excessive oral yeast counts and increased prevalence of oral candidiasis are associated with poor oral hygiene and neglect of adequate plaque removal from prosthetic appliances.[47]

Select High-Energy, High-Protein Foods

Eggs
Dry milk powder added to milk-based beverages
  and soups
Yogurt with additional dry milk powder
Baked and grilled fish
Fish and chicken salads
Bean and legume dips and spreads
Eggnog

Mucositis

Mucositis refers to injury to the oral mucosa that results in increased vascular permeability, tissue edema, atrophy, and eventually ulcerations covered by a necrotic pseudomembrane in some instances. Bleeding may be associated with more advanced lesions. Patients usually complain of a burning sensation and they may not be able to tolerate hot or spicy foods. These lesions tend to be self-limiting and usually subside within 2 to 3 weeks after therapy is complete.[48]

Mucositis is most often associated with chemotherapy and administration of radiation therapy in the treatment of cancer. It tends to occur in the first 2 weeks of therapy. The percentage of patients with severe mucositis is highly dependent on the chemotherapy regimen, and radiation site and dosage. Seventy-five to 80% of bone marrow transplant patients who have undergone conditioning regimens with high-dose chemotherapy and radiation experience mucositis.[49]

Prevention and management of mucositis has implications beyond oral discomfort and pain. In cancer treatment it may lead to compromised nutritional intake, a delay in drug administration, life-threatening septicemia, and increased hospital stays and costs.[50]

Evidence-based guidelines for preventing and managing mucositis developed by the Multinational Association of Supportive Care in Cancer and the International Society for Oral Oncology recommend benzydamine hydrochloride (HCl) to prevent mucositis. This nonsteroidal rinse with antiinflammatory, analgesic, antimicrobial, and anesthetic properties is being tested in Phase III drug trials and is not yet available in the United States. It appears to reduce both the severity and duration of radiation-induced mucositis.[49] Several promising new drugs also undergoing Phase III trials include Repifermin (human keratinocyte growth factor 2) and AES-14 (L-glutamine).[49] An early study of Repifermin found a significant reduction in the incidence and duration of severe oral mucositis in transplant patients. AES-14 trials have demonstrated an associated lower incidence of severe oral mucositis. Although palliative care includes viscous lidocaine and kaolin-pectin or diphenhydramine, mucoadherents to coat mucous membranes, and capsaicin, none of these agents is supported by sufficient evidence to warrant guideline statements. Although chlorhexidine mouth rinse can be used as an antiplaque and antifungal agent in oral self-care, it does not prevent or treat mucositis.[49]

Once the patient is mucositis free, he or she should continue to consume adequate amounts of fluids to maintain hydration. A high-protein, nutrient-dense diet to ensure adequate nutrient intake should be maintained. Patients should avoid hard, crunchy foods, sour or acidic foods, and spicy and salty foods, because these irritate the oral mucosa. Topical analgesics can minimize the pain from mucositis associated with eating. Antioxidants such as vitamins E, C, and selenium have been the subject of clinical trials examining modulators of free radical damage associated with radiation and chemotherapy. Findings remain contradictory.[51]

Plaque removal reduces the oral bacterial load and the incidence, severity, bleeding, and cancer-therapy related pain associated with mucositis. It prevents soft tissue infections that may lead to systemic complications.[49] Oral self-care protocols including tooth brushing, a chlorhexidine rinse, and a saline rinse reduce the incidence and severity of mucositis by 38%.[52] The use of foam toothbrushes is not recommended for plaque control in patients with mucositis and use of alcohol containing mouthwashes should be minimized.[49] More frequent professional preventive care may be necessary for patients with chronic recurring mucositis.

Oral Lichen Planus

Oral lichen planus (OLP) is a chronic autoimmune disease of unknown origin that affects 0.5% to 2% of the population.[53] OLP typically affects the oral mucosa of the cheeks, gums, and tongue, and appears as fine, white lines that form a reticular pattern or "weblike" appearance. OLP can be either asymptomatic or symptomatic, which is seen as either erosive or ulcerative tissue. Lichen planus tends to increase in severity with age, and treatment is primarily palliative.[53]

Theories regarding the etiology of lichen planus include psychosomatic, genetic, infective (viral hepatitis C), and immunological (autoimmune) factors.[54] High levels of stress, anxiety, and depression can play a role in OLP, but has not been shown to be the sole etiological factor.[55] Several drugs produce lichen planus–like allergic reactions, such as nonsteroidal antiinflammatory drugs, angiotensin-converting enzyme inhibitors, beta-blockers, thiazides, diuretics, allopurinol, lithium, isoniazid, and streptomycin.[56] No one causative agent has been identified for OLP, but it is considered to be a precancerous lesion that increases the risk of squamous cell carcinoma in 0.4% to 3.3% of cases.[56]

Standard therapies for erosive and ulcerative forms of lichen planus are primarily palliative and include cyclosporines, retinoids, steroids, and ultraviolet phototherapy.[57] The most common treatment used for OLP is topical tacrolimus, although this condition is very resistant to resolution with this approach.[57,58]

Serum levels of folate (folic acid), a B vitamin, tend to be marginal in patients with lichen planus or mucositis oral lesions.[59] Adequate folate intake is important. Fortified breakfast cereals, citrus fruit, and green leafy vegetables are good dietary sources of folate. Palliative treatment with topical analgesics may be necessary to alleviate pain and assure adequate nutrient and fluid intake.

In one study of 674 patients with oral lichen planus, it was determined that poor oral hygiene exacerbated the condition.[60] Oral hygiene products that may be irritating to the lesions, such as those that contain alcohol or sodium lauryl sulphate (SLS), should be avoided.[61] Because OLP tends to be a chronic condition, more frequent professional prevention is necessary to maintain periodontal health and minimize caries risk.

Recurrent Aphthous Ulcers

Aphthous stomatitis or **recurrent aphthous ulcers** (RAU) tend to occur singly on the nonkeratinized oral mucosa. They are circular lesions with an erythematous border surrounding necrotic epithelial cells that are self-limiting and heal in 10 to 14 days.[53] Pain associated with aphthous ulcers is dependent on the size, location, and depth of the ulcers.

Epidemiological studies indicate the prevalence of RAU in the general population to be 2% to 50%.[62] The etiology of these ulcers remains unknown, but suspected precipitating factors include stress, endocrine alterations, allergies, nutritional deficiencies, Crohn's disease, ulcerative colitis, celiac disease, HIV, trauma, and food hypersensitivity.[62] Research findings suggest there is an association between *Helicobacter pylori* infection and recurrent aphthous ulcers.[63] More than 99% of patients with Behçet's disease have oral aphthous ulcers.[64]

Topical and systemic therapies have been used to relieve pain and speed the healing of aphthous ulcers.[62] If these ulcers are suspected to be associated with a systemic disease, allergy or nutritional deficiency, these must be managed to prevent and/or reduce the incidence of aphthous ulcer outbreaks. The American Academy of Oral Medicine has recommended topical medications that have been efficacious in two or more double-blind, placebo-controlled trials. These include amlexanox, tetracycline, or chlorhexidine mouth rinse, and beclomethasone spray.[65] If these topical medications are not effective, minor aphthous ulcers can be treated with Levamisole and major recurrent aphthous ulcers can require systemic corticosteroids or thalidomide.[65]

As many as 20% of patients with RAU experience nutritional deficiencies of iron, zinc, folic acid, and other B complex vitamins.[65] The primary nutritional goal during symptomatic outbreaks of recurrent aphthous ulcers is to ensure adequate hydration and nutrient dense nonirritating foods, such as puddings, scrambled eggs, and high-protein liquid supplements.

Plaque removal, reduction of bacterial load, and removal of organisms such as *H. pylori* can reduce the incidence of aphthous ulcers. Products that may cause pain on contact with the wound or ulceration, such as alcohol, pyrophosphates, and sodium lauryl sulphate, should be avoided.

Gingival Tissue Enlargement

Gingival enlargement appears first in the papilla and more severely affects the anterior gingival tissue, resulting in significant changes in the contour and size of the gingiva.[66] Gingival enlargement is primarily drug-induced. Medications associated with gingival overgrowth include phenytoin, cyclosporin, amphetamine, and the calcium channel blockers (especially nifedipine).[67,68] Gingival inflammation in areas of enlargement tends to be out of proportion to the amount of local factors, such as plaque and calculus, and can impair the ability of patients to effectively remove dental plaque. This can increase the severity of the gingival overgrowth. In patients with severe gingival overgrowth as a result of the use of cyclosporin, a reduction of gingival overgrowth has been seen with oral hygiene instructions, supragingival and subgingival debridement, and periodontal maintenance.[68]

Gingivitis may be a predisposing factor for gingival overgrowth, thus effective plaque control and regular professional preventive care are recommended to minimize this condition.[68] Although plaque is not necessary to initiate gingival overgrowth, its presence does impact the severity of the overgrowth.[66] In more severe cases, surgical intervention may be necessary. Addressing drug/nutrient interactions can improve the patient's nutritional status and augment patient management and care plans.

Abnormal Bleeding

Abnormal bleeding can occur when any phase of normal coagulation has been disrupted by a disease process, treatment, or medications. Because some procedures performed in a dental office can initiate bleeding, assessment of bleeding time before treatment may be indicated. Excessive bleeding may occur in many diseases and conditions including sickle cell anemia, end-stage liver disease, von Willebrand's disease, leukemia, vitamin K deficiency, and disturbances of bone marrow such as thrombocytopenia. During renal dialysis, heparin is used to prevent blood clotting and this may result in excessive bleeding during dental treatment of these patients. Medication-induced abnormal homeostasis may result from antiplatelet, antithrombotic agents, nonsteroidal antiinflammatory drugs (NSAIDs), high-dose vitamin C or E supplementation, and herbal supplements (e.g., bilberry, feverfew, ginger, gingko biloba, ginseng, and garlic).[69]

Some chemotherapy regimens result in low platelet counts, which can increase the risk for excessive bleeding.

Bleeding time can be assessed with measures of prothrombin time (PT), partial thromboplastin time (PTT), and the international normalized ratio (INR), a system used to report the results of blood coagulation test. The INR was introduced by the World Health Organization (WHO) to standardize the control of anticoagulant therapy internationally and is the current recognized standard for reporting bleeding time.[70]

Consultation with the patient's physician following a review of the medical history and medications used by the patient is a necessary component of each dental visit. For patients taking antithrombotic agents, such as warfarin or Coumadin, and for patients receiving dialysis or between chemotherapy regimens, it is essential to consult with the physician, oncologist, or nephrologist regarding the current INR. Patients taking self-prescribed NSAIDs and herbal supplements should be advised to stop their use for 1 to 2 weeks before dental treatment that may result in bleeding.

In relation to abnormal homeostasis, specific recommendations exist for nutrition or hydration. Patients taking anticoagulant medications are advised to maintain a consistent intake of dark-green, leafy vegetables and other sources of vitamin K to minimize alterations in homeostasis from this source. Box 18-2 lists food sources of vitamin K. Patients with end-stage liver or kidney disease need to be referred to a physician and dietitian for individualized nutrition recommendations.

Aggressive prevention and control of oral infection and plaque is recommended to minimize caries and periodontal disease. This treatment minimizes the need for more advanced dental therapies that have a greater potential bleeding risk.

Wound Healing

Wound healing can be delayed when patients are seen with diseases and conditions including end-stage renal disease, malnutrition, gastrointestinal disorders, HIV/AIDS, and uncontrolled diabetes. Therapies such as chemotherapy or radiation therapy, and medications such as corticosteroid and gingko biloba may also impair wound healing.[69]

Additional factors that may modulate wound healing include age, comorbidities, polypharmacy, and nutritional status. In the medically compromised patient it is important to attenuate any issues with malnutrition. Consultation with the physician and registered dietitian may be necessary depending on the patient's medical condition and the extent of the wound.

In healthy individuals, protein intake is usually adequate to promote wound healing. In a medically compromised patient, however, protein adequacy may be suboptimal because of increased need, and therefore supplementation may be necessary. Groups at high risk for malnutrition include the frail elderly, substance abusers,

---

BOX 18-2

Select Significant Vitamin K Dietary Sources

HIGHER LEVELS OF VITAMIN K ARE FOUND IN THE OUTER LEAVES AND PEELS OF VEGETABLES

Kale
Collards
Spinach
Turnip, beet, and mustard greens
Brussels sprouts
Broccoli
Lettuce: iceberg, butterhead, Boston, Bibb, romaine
Asparagus
Okra
Cabbage
Cauliflower
Cucumbers and pickles
Soybeans and soybean oil
Grapes
Blueberries
Raspberries
Margarine
Tuna

(Data from U.S. Department of Agriculture, Agricultural Research Service, USDA nutrient database for standard reference, Release 16, 2003 (website): http://www.nal.usda.gov/fnic/foodcomp/Data/SR18/nutrlist/sr18w430.pdf.)

---

persons with eating disorders, those with Crohn's disease, those with inflammatory bowel disease, and patients taking immunosuppressants such as glucocorticoids. A number of individual amino acids, including glutamine and arginine, have been shown to enhance wound healing. In the healthy elderly, these nutrients were found to significantly enhance collagen synthesis.[71] Other nutrients essential in wound healing are vitamin A, vitamin E, copper, zinc, B vitamins, and vitamin C to name a few of the major nutrients involved in tissue repair. A diet adequate in fruits and vegetables and protein foods will provide these additional nutrients. If a patient is unable to eat his or her usual diet after dental treatment, liquid high-protein supplements or instant breakfast-type drinks with added powdered milk can be recommended. In addition to adequate nutrition, adequate fluid intake is necessary to maintain a sufficient blood supply to the wound.

Plaque accumulations exhibit inhibitory effects on postsurgical wound healing. Maintenance of high levels of plaque removal is a determining factor in the successful outcome of periodontal therapy.[72] Studies suggest that mechanical cleaning with a very soft toothbrush, and the use of a chlorhexidine gel or mouth rinse resulted in faster clinical healing with less postsurgical discomfort and fewer complications.[73]

Alveolar Bone Loss

Cumulative **alveolar bone loss** results in a weakening of the supporting structures of the teeth and predisposes the patient to tooth mobility and loss. It is one of the hallmarks of periodontitis. Risk factors associated with this condition include medications, systemic diseases and disorders, genetics, tobacco use, and hormone therapy.

Drug-induced bone loss can occur with the long-term use of glucocorticosteroids. These drugs stimulate metabolic responses that reduce the body's ability to convert vitamin D to an active form and ultimately leads to urinary calcium loss. Patients on drug therapies including phenytoin, phenobarbitol, primidone, lithium, valproate, and carbamazepine, also have a negative impact on bone metabolism.[69,74] Some of these drugs may be commonly used to managed psychiatric disorders (see Chapter 7).

Although an association appears to exist between alveolar bone loss and osteoporosis or systemic bone mineral density, a causal relationship remains questionable and continues to be the subject of investigations.[75,76] Because of an inability of the kidney to convert vitamin D to the active form used by the body, individuals with chronic kidney dysfunction may be seen with alveolar bone loss.

Prevention and management of alveolar bone loss is dependent upon regular periodontal tissue maintenance, tobacco cessation, and adequate daily plaque removal. Bisphosphonates, such as alendronate, have been shown to significantly increase bone mineral density.[19-21] This drug has been associated with jaw bone necrosis in medically compromised patients, however, and its use should be assessed with consultation and caution.[22,23] Nutrition counseling to maximize dietary intake of calcium and vitamin D-rich foods may minimize bone loss in patients receiving glucocorticosteroids, antiseizure medication, and antipsychotic drug therapy.

Although diet alone cannot prevent alveolar bone loss, ensuring recommended amounts of calcium and vitamin D-rich foods in the diet (3 to 4 servings per day) can assist in minimizing bone loss. The primary food sources of vitamin D are fortified foods such as milk, soy milk, and some cereals. If adequate intakes cannot be obtained from dietary sources, supplementation might be necessary (see Chapter 14).

Dysgeusia

Dysgeusia refers to a persistent, unpleasant, abnormal, or altered taste sensation, sometimes described as metallic in nature. It can be short- or long-term, depending on the etiology. A common sequelae of long-standing dysgeusia is nutritional deficiencies resulting from altered dietary intake patterns.

Common conditions and diseases associated with dysgeusia include oral infection, upper respiratory tract infection, sinus infection, irradiation of the head and neck, Bell's palsy, GERD, Crohn's disease, diabetes, pregnancy, and certain primary or secondary nutritional deficiencies. Evidence of age-associated declines in taste sensitivity have been well documented.[77] When observed, older patients possessed approximately half of the ability of younger patients to recognize blended or combinations of foods.[78]

Medications associated with taste changes include antiinflammatory agents (e.g., acetylsalicylic acid), diuretics and antihypertensive agents (e.g., captopril), antimicrobials (e.g., metronidazole), protease inhibitors, antidiabetic drugs (e.g., biguanides), Parkinson's drugs (e.g., levodopa), antiseizure agents (e.g., carbamazepine), cytotoxic agents (e.g., doxorubicin and methotrexate), and allopurinol.

Management of dysgeusia includes identifying contributing factor(s). If the cause is a result of medication-induced xerostomia, artificial saliva can minimize the effects of dysgeusia. Foods commonly not well tolerated are high-protein foods. Those that are better tolerated are white meats, eggs, and cheese. Chemotherapy often elicits taste aversions that tend to increase during the course of a day. Foods not well tolerated should be eaten in the morning hours. Cold foods are usually tolerated better than hot foods because of a reduction in odors emitted during cooking and serving. If a patient complains of a metallic taste, the use of plastic utensils and food containers can be recommended.

To avoid inadequate nutritional intake, taste perceptions can be enhanced by adding flavoring agents or spices to food. Studies have reported that the elderly tend to favor foods with higher concentrations of salt, sugar, and citric acid.[78] Dietary counseling should stress the avoidance of overindulgence in salt and sugar, however, which can increase caries risk and impact blood pressure.

The ability to perceive flavors is modulated by oral health status, the presence of dentures, and the use of tobacco products.[78] Plaque bacteria and food debris can also contribute to unpleasant taste. Regular preventive oral health care and promotion of routine self-care and healthy lifestyle can diminish degrees of dysgeusia in some patients.

Dysphagia

Dysphagia is defined as a subjective feeling of difficulty swallowing. Patients may complain of feeling that food is stuck in the throat, or they may have difficulty initiating a swallow and chewing. They may cough while eating, and experience pain on swallowing. Patients with dysphagia are at increased risk for weight loss and aspiration pneumonia.[79] It is estimated that 53% to 74% of patients in long-term care facilities have dysphagia.[80]

Conditions that commonly cause dysphagia include neurogenic disorders, such as Parkinson's disease, Alzheimer's disease, amyotropic lateral sclerosis, multiple sclerosis, cerebral palsy, and cerebrovascular accident. Patients with these conditions are at increased risk of aspiration of foods and fluids. Those experiencing esophageal strictures, secondary to radiation of the head and neck, and those with musculoskeletal disorders, such as muscular dystrophy, may also be seen with dysphagia. Conditions that predispose a patient to esophagitis, such as chronic heartburn or GERD, and immunocompromised patients with esophageal candidiasis are at risk of developing dysphagia.[79] Esophagitis can be secondary to a pill-induced condition that occurs when patients are unable to completely swallow medications, such as nonsteroidal antiinflammatory drugs, iron pills, potassium tablets, and vitamins.[79] Because of the daily polypharmacy practiced among many of the elderly, and a higher incidence of dysphagia in this cohort, they are at risk for pill-induced esophagitis.[81] Dysphagia in these situations usually resolves after the medications are discontinued.

Some causes of dysphagia cannot be prevented, but many of the causes of esophagitis can be managed to prevent dysphagia. Patients with GERD need to be alerted to the importance of effectively managing reflux to prevent dental erosion and esophagitis. Eating a soft, nutrient-dense diet, and drinking fluids with meals can relieve dysphagia caused by xerostomia.

Patients who have dysphagia because of neurogenic disorders should be managed to avoid in particular the increased risk of aspiration of foods and fluids.

Patients should be instructed to eat smaller portions of food slowly, and to avoid very hot or cold liquids. Risk for dehydration because of avoidance of liquids as a result of concerns about the difficulty in swallowing should be discussed. A special diet of thickened fluids may be required for those patients at risk for aspiration. In a 1999 to 2000 survey, approximately 35.3% of nursing home residents were on mechanically altered diets because of dysphagia.[80] Every effort should be made to minimize the alteration of the texture and consistency of foods to keep foods appetizing and to limit unintentional weight loss and malnutrition.[80, 81] As a last resort, other routes to achieving enteral nutrition, such as insertion of a nasogastric or gastrostomy tube may be necessary to bypass the need to swallow.

People with dysphagia can consistently eat a soft diet and thus increase their caries risk status. When this condition occurs with long-term intake of xerostomia-inducing medications, caries risk increases even more. Aggressive periodontal maintenance and attention to caries prevention, with appropriate use of fluorides and sealants, is essential to minimize the need for advanced periodontal or restorative needs. If a person is unable to perform adequate plaque removal, the caregiver should be trained to perform oral hygiene procedures. Dietary choices to minimize the intake of cariogenic foods within the constraints of the special dietary needs should be discussed.

To avoid aspiration of fluids that can lead to pneumonia, the patient should be placed in a semisupine position with the head turned to one side during treatment to assist in managing fluids. Minimal water should be used during treatment and suction should be used frequently. Any dental equipment that uses large quantities of water, such as ultrasonic scalers and air polishers, should be avoided.

Dental Erosion

Dental erosion is associated with a demineralization of enamel and dentin resulting from chemical or mechanical action. A chemical effect includes destruction caused by vomitus, excessive consumption of acidic foods or beverages, and GERD, which lead to a sustained decreased oral pH below 5.5.[82] Initially, a chalky appearance can be observed, progressing to a smooth, glassy surface on the lingual surfaces of the maxillary anterior teeth. The other lingual surfaces are protected at this point by the placement and movement of the tongue. As the severity of the erosion continues, teeth will change in color, shape, and length, and become more brittle and translucent. Eventually, the erosion will begin to involve the incisal edges of anterior teeth, the cusp edges of posterior teeth, and create flat occlusal surfaces. In addition, margination of amalgam restorations, and exposed pulp can develop.[83] Erosion of the enamel of deciduous teeth progresses one to five times faster than the enamel of permanent teeth.[84] The severity of erosion is determined by the length of time a medical complication leads to increased regurgitation, the frequency of regurgitation, a diagnosis of an eating behavior, and routine oral hygiene practices.

GERD is a disease in which the HCl from the stomach enters the esophagus through a relaxed lower esophageal sphincter, causing damage to the delicate lining of the esophagus. Because the esophagus is located behind the heart, a patient will experience a burning sensation in this area, commonly referred to as heartburn. Patients can have GERD for 1 to 3 years before seeking medical treatment.[85]

An eating disorder is a serious, complex, and challenging condition that affects an individual's physical and psychological health and requires a multidisciplinary treatment approach.[86, 87] The dental professional may be the first health care provider to identify the eating disorder and will need to refer the patient to the appropriate provider. When vomiting is the chosen means of purging, a decrease in the oral pH occurs, creating an environment conducive to enamel demineralization and, eventually, erosion. Treating dental patients with eating disorders will require attention to patient education and counseling approaches.

Early recognition of the destruction and cause of the erosion will prevent further damage. A thorough medical and dental assessment is indicated. Once identified, a custom mouth guard may be an appropriate appliance for a patient with erosion caused by regurgitation. A mouth guard serves several purposes. It can be used as a fluoride tray, provide protection for teeth during regurgitation, and be used as protection from bruxism, if present.[88] Sealants and restorative options will depend on the degree of tooth loss. Orthodontic treatment can be indicated when advanced erosion has led to excessive dentin exposure causing malocclusion.[89] An erosive state can be further compounded by xerostomia, because the protective neutralizing property of saliva is diminished (see the previous discussion on xerostomia in this chapter).

Habitual consumption of acidic foods and beverages increases the acidic environment in the oral cavity.[90] The dental professional should complete a dietary assessment to identify sources of acidic foods. To minimize damage to enamel, patient education and counseling should be provided to emphasize avoidance of possible foods such as sodas (diet and regular), sports drinks, carbonated flavored waters, flavored teas, and citrus and tomato-based foods and beverages. Prolonged sipping and sucking behaviors should be identified with risk for dental erosion.

Education regarding oral self-care and routine preventive dental appointments are essential. Furthermore, the goal is to stimulate and sustain an oral environment conducive to the promotion of enamel remineralization. In addition to dietary guidelines, a strict regimen of topical fluoride should be initiated. The patient is to avoid brushing after regurgitation, which will further intensify the erosion, along with discontinuing the use of a hard toothbrush, abrasive toothpaste, and a "scrubbing" tooth brushing method. Rinsing with water will reduce the buffer capacity of the saliva; however, rinsing with sodium bicarbonate will neutralize the gastric acids.

Burning Mouth Syndrome

Burning mouth syndrome (BMS) is an idiopathic and multifactorial syndrome characterized by burning and painful sensations in the hard and soft tissues in the oral cavity, in the absence of physical abnormalities. The most prevalent site for BMS is the anterior two thirds of the tongue.[91] Diagnosis is often made on the basis of patient complaints of burning, dysgeusia (often bitter, metallic, or both), xerostomia, intensification of symptoms as the day progresses, nonexistence of symptoms at night, and decrease in symptoms while eating. Allergic reactions to dental materials have resulted in symptoms of BMS. The onset of pain is typically spontaneous and may persist for years.

The etiologies of BMS are complex and not fully understood. The prevalence is significant in postmenopausal women.[91] Xerostomia (and diseases and conditions that cause xerostomia), diabetes, candidiasis, geographic tongue, dental treatment, allergic reactions, depression and anxiety, and malnutrition are also associated with BMS. This condition is sometimes a symptom of physical or psychological stress, and requires referral to the physician.

Treatment depends on the symptoms presented. For example, a patient experiencing xerostomia will be provided with methods to stimulate saliva flow to minimize oral changes. Low doses of benzodiazepines and tricyclic antidepressants are considered to reduce the symptoms of BMS.[92] Additionally, topical capsaicin has been used as a desensitizing agent. Hormone replacement therapy has been recommended for postmenopausal women experiencing BMS and an antifungal agent has been prescribed for candidiasis. Lifestyle changes such as smoking cessation and avoidance of alcohol can be helpful.

Nutrient deficiencies have been identified as a factor for BMS. Insufficient dietary intake of iron, zinc, and B complex vitamins is a possible culprit. A dietitian's consultation can identify nutritional deficiencies and provide counseling focused on appropriate food and beverage choices. Appropriate dietary supplementation to alleviate the symptoms of BMS can be explored.

SUMMARY

Oral manifestations associated with systemic diseases can occur singularly or in clusters. The medically compromised, the aging, and the medicated patient are at increased risk for the conditions discussed in this chapter. The dental professional can initiate screening and preventive care plans that will address issues and concerns that may compress opportunities for these conditions to occur. He or she can also initiate appropriate and immediate treatment.

Future new and improved drug therapies, evidence-based practice, and additional research into associations and possible cause and effect relationships will further expand our understanding of data on periodontal disease and pregnancy outcomes, the association between obesity and periodontal disease, the role of nutrition in preventing oral conditions, the role of palliative care for symptomatic oral lichen planus, and the association between alveolar bone loss and osteoporosis.[15,57,93]

These patients are at greater risk for oral diseases and should be seen at more frequent intervals by a dental professional.

References

1. Genco R, Offenbacher S, Beck J: Periodontal disease and cardiovascular disease: epidemiology and possible mechanisms, *JADA* 133:14S-22S, 2002.
2. Geerts SO, Legrand V, Charpentier J et al.: Further evidence of the association between periodontal disease and coronary artery disease, *J Periodontol* 75:1274-1280, 2004.
3. Haraszthy VI, Zambon JJ, Trevisan: Identification of periodontal pathogens in atheromatous plaques, *J Periodontol* 71:1554-1560, 2000.
4. Okuda K, Ishihara K, Nakagawa T et al.: Detection of *treponema denticola* in atherosclerotic lesions, *J Clin Microbiol* 39:1114-1117, 2001.
5. Okuda K, Kato T, Ishihara K: Involvement of periodontopathic biofilm in vascular diseases, *Oral Dis* 10:5-12, 2004.

6. Desvarieux M, Demmer RT, Rundek T et al.: Periodontal microbiota and carotid intima-media thickness: the oral infections and vascular disease epidemiology study (INVEST), *Circulation* 111:576-582, 2005.

7. Dorfer CE, Becher H, Zigler CM et al.: The association of gingivitis and periodontitis with ischemic stroke, *J Clin Periodontol* 31:396-401, 2004.

8. Grau AJ, Buggle F, Becher H et al.: Recent bacterial and viral infection is a risk factor for cerebrovascular ischemia: clinical and biochemical studies, *Neurology* 50:196-203, 1998.

9. Tsai C, Hayes C, Taylor GW: Glycemic control of Type 2 diabetes and severe periodontal disease in the US adult population, *Commun Dent Oral Epidemiol* 20:182-192, 2002.

10. Saremie A, Nelson RG, Tulloch-Reid M et al.: Periodontal disease and mortality in Type 2 Diabetes, *Diabetes Care* 28:27-32, 2005.

11. Kiran M, Arpak N, Unsal E et al.: The effect of improved periodontal health on metabolic control in type 2 diabetes, *J Clin Periodontol* 32:266-272, 2005.

12. Intensive blood-glucose control with sulphonylureas or insulin compared with conventional treatment and risk of complications in patients with type 2 diabetes (UKPDS 34). UK Prospective Diabetes Study (UKPDS) Group, *Lancet* 352:837-853, 1998.

13. Garcia RI, Nunn ME, Vokonas PS: Epidemiologic associations between periodontal disease and obstructive pulmonary disease, *Ann Periodontol* 6:71-77, 2001.

14. Scannapieco FA, Bush RD, Paju S: Periodontal disease as a risk factor for adverse pregnancy outcomes. A systematic review, *Ann Periodontol* 8:70-78, 2003.

15. Lopez NJ, Smith PC, Gutierrez J: Periodontal therapy may reduce the risk of preterm low birth weight in women with periodontal disease: a randomized controlled trial, *J Periodontol* 73:911-924, 2002.

16. Krall EA, Dawson-Hughes B, Papas A et al.: Tooth loss and skeletal bone density in healthy postmenopausal women, *Osteoporosis Int* 4:104-109, 1994.

17. Krall E: Osteoporosis and the risk of tooth loss, *Clin Calcium* 16:63-66, 2006.

18. Krall EA: The periodontal-systemic connection: implications for treatment of patients with osteoporosis and periodontal disease, *Ann Periodontol* 6:209-213, 2001.

19. Rocha ML Malacara JM, Sanchez-Marin EF et al.: Effect of alendronate on periodontal disease in postmenopausal women: a randomized controlled trial, *J Periodontol* 75:1579-1585, 2004.

20. Binderman I, Adut M, Yaffe A: Effectiveness of local delivery of alendronate in reducing alveolar bone loss following periodontal surgery in rats, *J Periodontol* 71:1236-1240, 2000.

21. El-Shinnawi UM, El-Tantawy SI: Effect of alendronate sodium on alveolar bone loss in periodontitis, *J Int Acad Periodontol* 5:5-10, 2003.

22. Merigo E, Manfredi M, Meleti M et al.: Jaw bone necrosis without previous dental extractions associated with the use of bisphosphonates (pamidronate and zoledronate): a four-case report, *J Oral Pathol Med* 34:613-617, 2005.

23. Evio S, Tarkkila L, Sorsa T et al.: Effects of alendronate and hormone replacement therapy, alone and in combination, on saliva, periodontal conditions and gingival crevicular fluid matrix metalloproteinase-8 levels in women with osteoporosis, *Oral Dis* 12:187-193, 2006.

24. Heasman PA, Seymour PA: An association between long term nonsteroidal anti-inflammatory drug therapy and the severity of periodontal disease, *J Clin Periodontol* 17:654-658, 1990.

25. Bartold PM, Marshall RI, Haynes DR: Periodontitis and rheumatoid arthritis: a review, *J Periodontol* 76(11 suppl):2066-2074, 2005.

26. Mercado F, Marshall R, Klestov A et al.: Is there a relationship between rheumatoid arthritis and periodontal disease? *J Clin Periodontol* 27:267-272, 2000.

27. Mercado FB, Marshall RI, Klestov AC: Relationship between rheumatoid arthritis and periodontitis, *J Periodontol* 72:779-787, 2001.

28. Ribeiro J, Leão A, Novaes AB: Periodontal infection as a possible severity factor for rheumatoid arthritis, *J Clin Periodontol* 32:412-416, 2005.

29. Perlstein MI, Bissada MF: Influence of obesity and hypertension on the severity of periodontitis in rats, *Oral Surg Oral Med Oral Pathol* 43:707-719, 1977.

30. Al-Zahrani MS, Bissada NF, Borawskit EA: Obesity and periodontal disease in young, middle-aged, and older adults, *J Periodontol* 74:610-615, 2003.

31. Al-Zahrani MS, Borawski EA, Bissada NF: Periodontitis and three health-enhancing behaviors: maintaining normal weight, engaging in recommended level of exercise, and consuming a high-quality diet, *J Periodontol* 76:1362-1366, 2005.

32. Wood N, Johnson RB, Streckfus CF: Comparison of body composition and periodontal disease using nutritional assessment techniques: Third National Health and Nutrition Examination Survey (NHANES III), *J Clin Periodontol* 30:321-327, 2003.

33. Saito T, Shimazaki Y, Kiyohara Y et al.: Relationship between obesity, glucose tolerance, and periodontal disease in Japanese women: the Hisayama study, *J Periodontol Res* 40:346-353, 2005.

34. Porter, S, Scully C, Hagarty A: An update of the etiology and management of xerostomia, *Oral Surg Oral Med Oral Pathol Oral Radiol Endod* 97:28-46, 2004.

35. Jensen S, Pedersen A, Reibel J et al.: Xerostomia and hypofunction of the salivary glands in cancer therapy, *Support Care Cancer* 11:207-225, 2003.

36. Närhi T, Meurman J, Ainamo A: Xerostomia and hyposalivation: causes, consequences and treatment in the elderly, *Drugs Aging* 15:103-116, 1999.

37. Gage T, Pickette F: *Dental drug reference*, ed 7, St Louis, 2006, Mosby.

38. Hayes C: The effects of non-cariogenic sweeteners on the prevention of dental caries: a review of the evidence, *J Dent Educ* 65:1106-1109, 2001.

39. Hauman CH, Thompson IO, Theunissen F et al.: Oral carriage of *Candida* in healthy and HIV-seropositive persons, *Oral Surg Oral Med Oral Pathol* 76:570-572, 1993.

40. Leigh JE, Shetty K, Fidel PL: Oral opportunistic infections in HIV-positive individuals: Review and role of mucosal immunity, *AIDS Patient Care STDs* 18:443-456, 2004.

41. Belazi M, Velegraki A, Fleva A et al.: Candidal overgrowth in diabetic patients: potential predisposing factors, *Mycoses* 48:192-196, 2005.

42. Marcus M, Maida CA, Freed JR et al.: Oral white patches in a national sample of medical HIV patients in the era of HAART, *Commun Dent Oral Epidemiol* 33:99-106, 2005.

43. Redding SW, Dahiya MC, Kirkpatrick WR et al.: Candida glabrata is an emerging cause of oropharyngeal candidasis in patients receiving radiation for head and neck cancer, *Oral Surg Oral Med Oral Pathol Oral Radiol Endod* 97:47-52, 2004.

44. Pappas PG, Rex JH, Sobel JD et al.: Infectious Disease Society of America (ISHA): guidelines for treatment of candidiasis, *Clin Infect Dis* 38:162-189, 2004.

45. Koc M, Akta E: Prophylactic treatment of mycotic mucositis in radiotherapy of patients with head and neck cancers, *J Clin Oncol* 33:57-60, 2003.

46. Paillaud E, Merlier I, Dupeyron C et al.: Oral candidiasis and nutritional deficiencies in elderly hospitalized patients, *Br J Nutr* 92:86, 2004.

47. Budtz-Jlrgensen E, Mojon P, Banon-Clement JM et al.: Oral candidiasis in long-term hospital care: comparison of edentulous and dentate subjects, *Oral Dis* 2:285-290, 1996.

48. Sonis ST, Costa JW: Oral complications. In Kufe DW, Pollock RE, Weichselbaum RR et al., editors: *Cancer medicine*, ed 6, Hamilton, Ontario, 2003, BC Decker, Inc.

49. Rubenstein EB, Peterson DE, Schubert M et al.: Clinical practice guidelines for the prevention and treatment of cancer therapy-induced oral and gastrointestinal mucositis, *Cancer* 100:2026-2046, 2004.

50. Worthington HV, Clarkson JE, Eden OB: Interventions for preventing oral mucositis for patients with cancer receiving treatment, *Cochrane Database Syst Rev* 2: CD000978, 2006; DOI:10.1002/14651858.CD000978.pub2.

51. Borek C: Dietary antioxidants and human cancer, *Integr Cancer Ther* 3:333-341, 2004.

52. Cheng KK, Molassiotis A, Chang AM, et al.: Evaluation of an oral care protocol intervention in the prevention of chemotherapy-induced oral mucositis in paediatric cancer patients, *Eur J Cancer* 2001;37:2056-2063.

53. Jackler RK, Kaplan MJ: Ear, nose and throat. In Tierney, McPhee SJ, Papadakis MA, editors: *Current medical diagnosis and treatment*, ed 44, San Francisco, CA, 2005, McGraw-Hill.

54. Carrozzo M, Brancatello F, Dametto et al.: Hepatitis C virus-associated oral lichen planus: is the geographical heterogeneity related to HLA-DR6? *J Oral Pathol Med* 34:204-208, 2005.

55. Chaudhary S: Psychosocial stressors in oral lichen planus, *Aust Dent J* 49:192-195, 2004.

56. Scully C, Beyli M, Ferreiro MC et al.: Update on oral lichen planus: etiopathogenesis and management, *Crit Rev Oral Biol Med* 9:86-122, 1998.

57. Chan ES-Y, Thornhill M, Zakrzewska J: Interventions for treating oral lichen planus. *Cochrane Database Syst Rev* 2:CD001168, 1999; DOI:10.1002/14651858.CD001168.

58. Dissemond J: Oral lichen planus: an overview, *J Dermatol Treat* 15:136-140, 2004.

59. Thongprasom K, Youngnak P, Aneksuk V: Folate and vitamin B12 levels in patients with oral lichen planus, stomatitis and glossitis, *Southeast Asian J Trop Med Public Health* 32:643-647, 2001.

60. Xue JL, Fan MW, Wang SZ et al.: A clinical study of 674 patients with oral lichen planus in China, *J Oral Pathol Med* 34:467-472, 2005.

61. Rantanen I, Jutila K, Nicander I et al.: The effects of two sodium lauryl sulphate-containing toothpaste with and without betaine on human mucosa in vivo, *Swed Dent J* 27:31-34, 2003.

62. Prolo P, Domingo DL, Fedorowicz Z et al.: Interventions for recurrent aphthous stomatitis (mouth ulcers) (Protocol), *Cochrane Database Syst Rev* 3:CD005411, 2005; DOI: 10.1002/14651858.CD005411.

63. Albanidou-Farmaki E, Giannoulis L, Markopoulos A et al.: Outcome following treatment for *Helicobacter pylori* in patients with recurrent aphthous stomatitis, *Oral Dis* 11:22-26, 2005.

64. Pipitone N, Boiardi L, Olivieri I et al.: Clinical manifestations of Behcet's disease in 137 Italian patients: results of a multicenter study, *Clin Exp Rheumatol* 22(6 suppl 36): S46-51, 2004.

65. Barrons RW: Treatment strategies for recurrent oral aphthous ulcers, *Am J Health System Pharmacy*, 58:41-50, 2001.

66. Mariotti A: Dental plaque-induced gingival diseases, *Ann Periodontol* 4:7-17, 1999.

67. Hasan AA, Ciancio S: Relationship between amphetamine ingestion and gingival enlargement, *Pediatr Dent* 26:396-400, 2004.

68. Aimetti M, Romano F, Debernardi C: Effectiveness of periodontal therapy on the severity of cyclosporin A-induced gingival overgrowth, *J Clin Periodontol* 32:846-850, 2005.

69. Ciancio SG: Medications' impact on oral health, *J Am Dent Assoc* 135:1440-1448, 2004. 70. Beers KH, Berkow R: *Merck manual*, ed 17, Whitehouse Station, NJ, 1999, Merck Research Laboratories.

71. Williams JZ, Abumrad N, Barbul A: Effect of a specialized amino acid mixture on human collagen deposition, *Ann Surg* 236: 369-374, 2002.

72. Lindhe J, Exheverria: Consensus report of Session II. In Lang NP, Karring T, editors: *European workshop on periodontology: 1(st) Proceedings of the 1(st) European Workshop in Periodontology*, London, 1994, Quintessence Publishing.

73. Heltz F, Heltz-Mayfield JA, Lang NP: Effects of post-surgical cleansing protocols on early plaque control in periodontal and/or periimplant wound healing, *J Clin Periodontol* 31:1012-1018, 2004.

74. Misra M, Papakostas GI, Klibanski A: Effects of psychiatric disorders and psychotropic medications on bone metabolism, *J Clin Psychiatr* 65:1607-1618, 2004.

75. Yoshihara A, Seida Y, Hanada N et al.: A longitudinal study of the relationship between periodontal disease and bone mineral density in community-dwelling older adults, *J Clin Periodontol* 31: 680-684, 2004.

76. Persson RE, Hollender LG, Powell LV et al.: Assessment of periodontal conditions and systemic disease in older subjects: I. Focus on osteoporosis, *J Clin Peroidontol* 29:796-802, 2002.

77. Roberts SB, Rosenberg I: Nutrition and aging: changes in the regulation of energy metabolism with aging, *Physiol Rev* 86:651-667, 2006.

78. Mathey MF, Siebelink E, de Graaf C et al.: Flavor enhancement of food improves dietary intake and nutritional status of elderly nursing home residents, *J Gerontol Biol Sci Med Sci* 56: M200-M205, 2001.

79. Hussain N, Karnath B: GI Consult: Dysphagia, *Emerg Med* 35:14-19, 2003.

80. Dorner B, Niedert KC, Welch PK: Position of the American Dietetic Association: liberalized diets for older adults in long-term care, *J Am Diet Assoc* 102:1316-1323, 2002.

81. Kamer AR, Sirois DA, Huhmann M: *Bidirectional impact of oral health and general health*. In Touger-Decker R, Sirois DA, Mobley CC, editors: *Nutrition and Oral Medicine*, Totowa, NJ, 2005, Humana Press.

82. Meurman JH, Ten Cate JM: Pathogenesis and modifying factors of dental erosion, *Eur J Oral Sci* 104:199-210, 1996.

83. Pontefract HA: Erosive tooth wear in the elderly population, *Gerodontology* 19:5-16, 2002.

84. Amaechi B, Higham S, Edgar W: Factors influencing the development of dental erosion *in vitro*: enamel type, temperature and exposure time, *J Oral Rehab* 26:624-630, 1999.

85. Malfertheiner P, Hallerback B: Clinical manifestations and complications of gastroesophageal reflux disease (GERD), *Int J Clin Pract* 59:346-355, 2005.

86. Hilsen KL: Treating dental patients with eating disorders, *Dent Today* 25:106-107, 2006.

87. Ritter AV: Eating disorders and oral health, *J Esthet Restor Dent* 18:114, 2006.

88. Chu FC, Yip HK, Newsome PR et al.: Restorative management of the worn dentition: etiology and diagnosis, *Dent Update* 29:162-168, 2002.

89. Amaechi B, Higham S: Dental erosion: possible approaches to prevention and control, *J Dent* 33:243-252, 2005.

90. Bartlett DW: The role of erosion in tooth wear: aetiology, prevention and management, *Int Dent J* 55(4 suppl 1):277-284, 2005.

91. Bergdahl M, Bergdahl J: Burning mouth syndrome: prevalence and associated factors, *J Oral Pathol Med* 28:350-354, 1999.

92. Grushka M, Epstein J, Gorsky M: Burning mouth syndrome, *Am Fam Phys* 65:615-622, 2002.

93. Scannapieco FA, Bush RB, Paju S: Associations between periodontal disease and risk for nosocomial bacterial pneumonia and chronic obstructive pulmonary disease. A systematic review, *Ann Periodontol* 8:54-69, 2003.

Chapter 19

Prevention Strategies for Special Populations

MILDRED McCLAIN AND GEORGIA DOUNIS

LEARNING OBJECTIVES

Upon completion of this chapter, the learner will be able to:
- Describe the oral health needs of childhood from pregnancy through adolescence.
- Identify preventive strategies that can be used to address the special needs of children.
- Discuss the oral health status of the elderly, including independent, assisted living, and institutionalized.
- Target preventive approaches to address the elderly.
- Describe the oral health needs of the disabled patient and preventive strategies that can be used to address these needs.

KEY TERMS

Medicare
Medicaid
Activities of daily living (ADL)
Instrumental activities of daily living (IADL)
Morbidity
Mortality
Disability

Oral health care professionals continue to seek approaches, techniques, and protocols to meet the needs of a growing and diverse population. Challenges and barriers that span the entire life course, and their impediment to accessing oral health care exist for special groups within the population. There is an enormous chronological difference between children and elderly, yet they both encounter similar challenges. Both groups may rely on others to assist them with

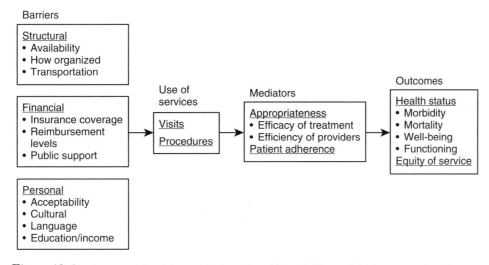

Figure 19-1   Access to health care in America. (From Millman M: *Access to health care in America: committee on monitoring access to personal health care services,* Washington, DC, 1993, National Academy Press.)

accessibility to health care needs, including proper oral health care.

The Institute of Medicine (IOM) defines access to care as the timely use of personal health services to achieve the best possible health outcomes.[1] As shown in Figure 19-1, structural, financial, or personal obstacles preclude access to oral care. The IOM provided a framework for monitoring access to care that includes behavioral elements associated with the individual choice to use and access health care services.[2,3] This model emphasizes the value patients place on their own health, their attitudes toward oral health knowledge, health literacy levels, dental habits, and their actions to seek care and adherence with recommendations. Emphasis on disease prevention and oral health promotion, including risk factor reduction (tobacco, alcohol, illicit drug use, and harmful dietary habits) is central to this model's framework. In conjunction with enabling resources, such as the ability to afford goods and services that promote healthy living, the perceived needs and personal choice to act and seek care is interrelated with the personal habits that affect outcome of care.

Dental, and craniofacial diseases and disorders are among common health problems affecting people in the United States.[3,4] Nearly 50 million Americans exhibit extreme oral health disparities.[5,6] Those at both ends of the life spectrum, children and elderly, face unique oral health needs. With changing population demographics and advances in medical and social systems, the number of people who are disabled and particularly in need of oral health services is rising dramatically.[7,8] The 2006 U.S. Census data showed approximately 51.2 million people with disabilities (18% of the total population). Additionally, 32.5 million Americans had various forms of severe disabilities (12% of the population).[7,9] This chapter addresses the oral health care needs and possible preventive strategies to reduce the oral disease burden for children and independent elders, the geriatric/nursing

home residents, independent physically disabled, mentally/emotionally disabled, and the institutionalized resident (Figure 19-2).

CHILDHOOD AND ORAL HEALTH
Prenatal

Maternal oral health has significant implications for birth outcomes and future infant oral health. Studies show that during pregnancy a range of only 23% to 43% of woman adopted oral health practices.[10] Young women, women in poverty, and women receiving Medicaid were at increased risk of not having a dental visit during their pregnancy and disproportionately failed to obtain care.[11] Maternal periodontal disease, a chronic infection of the gingiva and supporting tooth structures, has been associated with preterm birth, development of preeclampsia, and delivery of a small-for-gestational age infant.[12]

Each year, 8000 babies are born with cleft lip, cleft palate, or both, making these among the most common birth defects. Cleft lip and cleft palate interfere with normal appearance, eating, and speech.[13] Cleft lip and cleft palate have been reported at a rate of approximately one in every 1000 live births, and isolated cleft palate at a rate of approximately 0.5 to 1000 live births. These conditions are among the most common birth defects.[14,15] With advancements in science, opportunity to reduce the burden of birth defects, such as cleft lip and cleft palate in the twenty-first century may be possible.

Maternal oral flora is routinely transmitted to the infant through human contact. Increased cariogenic flora in the mother predisposes the infant to the development of caries.[16] Therefore, the opportunity to prevent early onset of dental decay can occur during prenatal counseling through discussions about diet, oral hygiene practices,

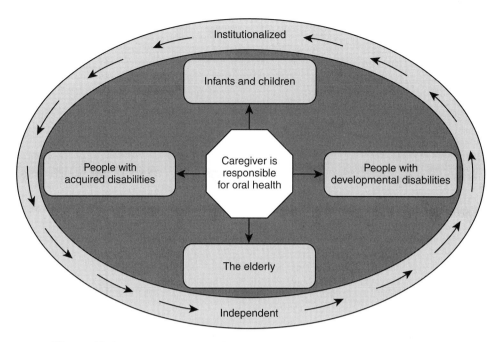

Figure 19-2   Range of special populations with unique oral health needs.

appropriate uses of fluorides, and the transmission of bacteria from parent to children. Dental visits and maintenance of daily oral hygiene are routine components of prenatal care. Pregnant women should receive prenatal care and eat a healthy diet that includes folic acid to prevent neural tube defects and possibly cleft lip/palate. Counseling to avoid tobacco and alcohol use should be included in prenatal care, and pregnant women should be advised to consult with a physician before taking any prescription medications or over-the-counter or complementary/alternative products.[13] Box 19-1 lists recommended oral hygiene practices for pregnant women and their infants and children.

Infancy

Poor oral hygiene and dietary habits have been associated with the development of caries in infants and young children.[17-19] Early childhood caries (ECC) is a diet-dependent, infectious disease of the teeth that emerges in young children between 1 and 6 years of age.[13] More than 40% of children had dental caries before they reached kindergarten.[20] ECC affects the primary teeth of infants and young children,[21] and thus it is important that these children receive early and regular oral assessments. The presence of caries in the primary dentition is a predictor of decay in permanent teeth.[22] Factors such as large family size, nutritional status of the mother and the infant, and the transfer of infectious organisms from caregiver to infant are associated with the onset of this disease.[23,24] Furthermore, mothers with low educational levels, low socioeconomic status, and those who allow their infants

to consume sugary foods frequently, are 32 times more likely to have infants with caries by the age of 3 years than infants in whom those risk factors are not present.[25]

Infant feeding practices appear to play a major role in infant oral health. Children who receive formula or other sweetened drinks or sweetened pacifiers at bedtime, especially if a child falls asleep while feeding, have experienced increased risk of ECC.[26] Prolonged exposure to sugary drinks (milk, formula, juices, and other drinks containing sugar) while a baby sleeps (when saliva flow is reduced) increases the risk of tooth decay.[13]

Adult attitudes and beliefs about the importance of the primary dentition play an important role in maintaining the child's oral health. Rather than perceiving dental caries as an infection, one common misconception is that primary teeth are not important to healthy development. This misconception stems from the fact that primary teeth are exfoliated. Before tooth eruption, an infant's gums should be wiped. As soon as the first tooth erupts, daily cleaning with a soft brush should become routine. Education and counseling of mothers during pregnancy and early in the infant's life can prevent or delay subsequent dental problems in children.[19]

Childhood

Tooth eruption times differ among children and may be delayed in those with developmental disabilities. The first primary tooth may not erupt until a child is 2 years old. Delays are often characteristic among developmentally disabled children such as those with Down syndrome.[21]

BOX 19-1

DATA FROM AMERICAN ACADEMY OF PEDIATRIC DENTISTRY AGE-SPECIFIC INSTRUCTIONS ON HOME ORAL HYGIENE

PRENATAL COUNSELING
- Counsel parents about their own oral hygiene habits and their effect as role models. Provide information to pregnant women about pregnancy gingivitis (inflammation of the gingiva caused by an exacerbated response to dental plaque related to hormonal changes during pregnancy). Review infant dental care.

INFANTS (BIRTH TO 1 YEAR OF AGE)
- Counsel parents to clean the infant's gums daily before eruption of the first primary tooth to help establish a healthy oral flora, using the following procedure:* Cradle the infant with one arm. Wrap a moistened gauze square or washcloth around the index finger of the hand of the other arm and gently massage the teeth and gingival tissues.
- Introduce a soft-bristled toothbrush during this age only if parents feel comfortable using the toothbrush. Do not use a dentifrice that contains fluoride, because fluoride ingestion is possible.

TODDLERS (1 TO 3 YEARS OF AGE)
- Introduce a toothbrush into the plaque-removal procedure (if not done earlier). Use dentifrice beginning at approximately 2 years; use only a pea-sized amount of toothpaste (apply across the narrow width of the toothbrush, rather than along its length, to decrease the chance of applying an excessive amount). Encourage the child to begin rudimentary brushing; however, parents should remain the primary caregiver in oral hygiene procedures.

PRESCHOOL-AGE CHILDREN (3 TO 6 YEARS OF AGE)
- Remind parents to continue their responsibility as primary providers or supervisors of oral hygiene procedures.
- Continue to use only a pea-sized amount of toothpaste on the child's toothbrush. Use daily flossing if any interproximal area has tooth-to-tooth contact.

*Recommended by some, but not all, dentists.
(From American Academy of Pediatric Dentistry. *Pediatr Dent* 21:18-37, 1999.)

During the past 25 years, the average number of decayed and filled teeth among 2- to 4-year-olds has remained unchanged.[5] The American Academy of Pediatric Dentistry (AAPD) and the American Dental Association (ADA) advocate that all children participate in a dental visit in the first year of life.[27] The "dental home" has been defined as a specialized primary dental care provider similar to the philosophical complex of the medical home and the primary care physician. Referring a child for an oral health examination to a dental provider who cares for infants and young children 6 months after the first tooth erupts or by 12 months of age, establishes the child's "dental home" and provides an opportunity to foster preventive oral health habits that meets each child's unique needs.[28] Starting preventive efforts early in a child's life is a critical determinant of their future health status.[29]

Risk assessment should begin at that first visit. Preventive strategies that include appropriate educational intervention should be provided to the parent. When caries appear in permanent teeth, prompt intervention should be initiated to conserve natural tooth structure. Prevention of the initial early lesion with appropriate use of fluorides and sealants is preferable to restoring the tooth after cavitation has occurred.[30]

Fluoridated toothpaste should be used sparingly until the child is 18 to 24 months of age. Parents of children younger than 6 years of age should brush the child's teeth or supervise daily tooth brushing. Because many children at this age have not learned to control the swallowing reflex, parents should teach the child to spit excess toothpaste into the sink to minimize the amount swallowed, and put only a pea-sized (0.25 g) amount or smear on the bristles of the child's toothbrush. Fluoride supplements can be prescribed for children who live in communities without optimal community water fluoridation and who are at high risk for tooth decay. For children who are younger than 6 years of age, the dental professional, physician, or other health care provider should assess risk for developing caries without introducing fluoride supplements unless necessary. Likewise, the benefit of caries prevention offered by supplements, and the potential for enamel fluorosis should be included in the decision to initiate the prescription of fluoride supplements. Consideration of the child's other sources of fluoride, especially drinking water, is essential in determining this balance (see Chapter 15 for preventive strategies for dental caries and guidelines on fluoride supplementation, sources, and use). Parents and caregivers should be educated and consulted about both the benefits and the risks of supplementation and be included in the decision to use this alternative source of fluoride. The American Dental Association supports fluoridation of community water supplies and the use of fluoride-containing products as safe and effective measures for preventing tooth decay.[32]

Children should be introduced to solid foods at approximately 6 months of age. Sharing utensils and cups should be discouraged because this promotes transmission of oral bacteria. Weaning to a cup is recommended by the American Dental Association (ADA) by the end of the first year. Exposure to sweetened beverages and *ad libidum* access to the "sippy" cup should be avoided. Both the selection of snacks and spacing of snacking/eating occasions to at least 2-hour intervals are recommended. Eating regular nutritious meals and avoiding high-sugar and starchy foods between meals will promote good oral health.[33]

Other measures to consider are dental sealants when appropriate, a helmet when bicycling, and use of protective headgear and mouth guards in other sports activities. Injuries to children, intentional and nonintentional, often involve trauma to the head, neck, and mouth. The leading causes of oral and head injuries are sports, violence, falls, and motor vehicle crashes.

Adolescence

Adolescents are defined as youths between the ages of 10 to 18 years old.[34] Caries experience is cumulative, thus higher rates of caries experience can occur among adolescents than among young children. By age 15 years, all permanent teeth other than third molars have erupted and vulnerable chewing surfaces of permanent second molars have been exposed to cariogenic factors for at least 2 or 3 years. By the age of adolescence, approximately 75% of this cohort have experienced dental decay.[30] Preventive measures including limitations of consumption of powdered drinks, colas/sodas, sport drinks, and acidic candies and foods may reduce dental erosion in this age group. Continued promotion of daily brushing and flossing, use of fluoride toothpastes and rinses, and routine dental attendance can enhance positive oral health outcomes that can be sustained throughout adulthood.[33]

Tobacco-related oral lesions occur in teenagers who use spit (smokeless) tobacco. Lesions were seen in 35% of snuff users and 20% of chewing tobacco users.[13] Tobacco cessation practices (see Chapter 17) should be initiated routinely at all dental visits and routine oral cancer screenings (see Chapter 3) should be performed. Referral to the primary care physician to assist with pharmacotherapies (see Chapter 7) and counseling should be considered when indicated.

Children With Disabilities

Access to oral health care for children with disabilities may be affected by the shortage of pediatric dental providers with training in the care of these children.[35, 36]

Consequences from the inability to access needed oral care for these children include postponed bone marrow and organ transplants, cardiac and other critical surgeries, failure to thrive, breathing difficulties, septicemia, brain abscesses, and other serious complications.[35,37]

Financial, structural, and personal barriers can limit access to health care. Financial barriers include not having health insurance, not having adequate health insurance to cover needed services, and not having the financial capacity to cover services outside of a health plan or insurance program. Structural barriers include the lack of primary care providers, medical specialists, or other health care professionals to address disabilities or the lack of health care facilities. Personal barriers, discussed in Chapter 13, include cultural or spiritual differences, language barriers, not knowing what to do or when to seek care, or concerns about confidentiality or discrimination.[38] Additional barriers may include fear of dental visits (Chapter 12), lack of providers from underserved racial or ethnic groups, and for some people with limited oral health literacy, the ability to find or understand information and services (Chapter 13).

Approximately one in four American children is born into poverty. The Federal Poverty Level (FPL) is considered as an annual income of $19,157 or less for a family of four. Children and adolescents living in poverty suffer from dental caries at twice the rate as their more affluent peers, and their disease is more likely to go untreated. Children from families without medical insurance are 2.5 times less likely than insured children to receive dental care. For every child with medical insurance, 2.6 lack dental insurance. Fewer than one in five Medicaid-covered children had a preventive dental visit during a recent yearlong study.[13]

OTHER CONSIDERATIONS

Persons of all ages are receiving professional services in the oral health care system, but more emphasis must be placed on vulnerable populations who need professional care.[39] The daily reality for children with untreated oral disease is persistent pain, inability to eat comfortably or chew well, embarrassment at discolored and damaged teeth, and distraction from play and learning. More than 51 million school hours are lost each year because of dental-related illness.[13]

HEALTHY ELDERLY (THE INDEPENDENT AND ASSISTED LIVING RESIDENT)

In the United States, a trend in the decline in the mortality rate among the elderly population has been reported.[40,41] The number of adults older than 65 years grew from 3 million to 36.5 million in 2003 and is projected to increase to 90 million by 2060 in the United States.[42]

This reflects an increase from 8% to 12%, suggesting that approximately one in five Americans will turn 65 by the year 2050.[43] Life expectancy has increased from 44 years in 1900, to 76 years in 1990, to 84 years in 2006. Medical advances have contributed to this compression of morbidity.

Older adults in the United States are living with noncommunicable chronic disorders such as hypertension (51%), arthritis (48%), heart disease (31%), cancer (21%), diabetes (16%), sinusitis (14%), and neuropsychiatric disorders (14%).[44] Treatment of these systemic conditions requires medical intervention, prescription drugs (more than 400 medications are available), and selective use of over-the-counter medications and herbal supplements. Both the chronic diseases and the medical management of these conditions have a direct or indirect effect on oral conditions. In addition, environmental and behavioral habits such as use of tobacco, alcohol, and the use of illicit drugs increases the risk of periodontal disease, xerostomia, mucosal lesions, tooth discoloration and breakdown, in addition to oral and pharyngeal cancer.[45]

More than 31.2 million noninstitutionalized elderly adults reside in community dwellings. Of this number, 1.8 million require assistance with **instrumental activities of daily living** (IADLs). **Activities of daily living** (ADLs) include those practices that healthy adults can manage for themselves. An additional 3.3 million require additional assistance with activities of daily living, including maintenance of oral hygiene, eating, and bathing.[41] The median income of adults older than 65 years in 2006 was more than $35,000, primarily from social security and other assets. Twenty-two percent reported having private dental insurance, whereas 79% reported paying out of pocket for dental care.[42] In 1991, US public health dental expenditures totaled more than $60 billion dollars, not including $451 million spent on urgent hospital admissions for dental disease. By 2002, the total dental expenditures exceeded $70 billion.[5]

Nearly 5.9 million (16%) older adults in America live at or below the poverty level with **Medicare** or **Medicaid** as the sole source of health care coverage. Medicare does not reimburse for routine oral health care and Medicaid coverage for dental procedures varies by state.[46,47] Many states do not offer Medicaid for adults, but provide support for elderly living in an institutional setting. Because of their limited financial resources, many older adults do not seek care that is sometimes critically important to maintenance of general and oral health status.[48]

Oral Health Status of the Healthy Elderly

Active and successful aging alone is not a risk for oral tissue destruction and increased dental **morbidity** and **mortality**. Oral health is an integral part of total health affected by nutrition, deglutition, digestion, speech, social mobility, employment, self-esteem, and quality of life. Dental caries and its sequelae account for more than 50%

of tooth loss. Of dentate older adults, 85% suffer from oral disease,[49] and 55% suffer from infections that lead to periodontal disease, which accounts for approximately 30% to 35% of all tooth extractions.[50,51] These conditions can have an impact on systemic health and overall quality of life.

Coronal and root caries. Dental caries is a diet-dependent multifactorial disease process that is altered throughout the life course. In the elderly, dental caries is modified by a complex medication and systemic disease history, changes in diet, and the ability to adequately maintain optimal oral hygiene. Although the same etiological factors are at play, changes in the complex interaction of biological and behavioral factors alter our risk status as we mature.[52] Amalgamation of these putative factors can trigger tooth enamel demineralization and breakdown of tooth structure. Adults older than 55 years may have a high caries risk profile because of the longitudinal exposure to multiple risk factors including higher plaque scores, multiple restored teeth, fractured teeth, and tooth loss.[53-56] Studies have indicated that tooth loss in adults 18 to 45 years old is primarily because of caries.[57]

Dental caries is a global pandemic.[58] Recent reports indicate that 96% of employed adults develop dental caries.[59] Higher mutans streptococci counts and lower buffering capacity, among other factors, contribute to the development of coronal decay.[60] The low oral acidity generated from oral bacterial sugar metabolism leads to alteration in microbial homeostasis in plaque, which leads to the selection of acid-tolerating species.[61] The occurrence of coronal decay and root caries common in older adults is summarized in Figure 19-3.

Similar to coronal caries, the development of root caries is a diet-dependent multifactorial, infectious disease.[60,62] Some studies have suggested that *Candida albicans* is a contributing factor to dentin and root caries.[63] Root caries

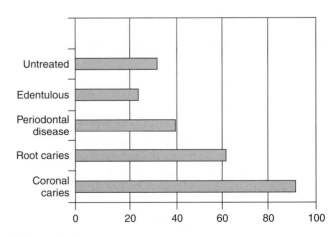

Figure 19-3 Percent of noninstitutionalized adults living in the United States older than 65 years with specific oral health conditions. (From Oral Health Resources: NHANES Findings Fact Sheets, 1999-2002.)

formation is facilitated by periodontal recession and exposure of cementum. With normal aging, an increase in gingival recession occurs in addition to cementum apposition both apically and lingually.[64] This factor, along with accumulation of plaque, may contribute to the higher incidence of facial root caries. A meta-analysis of several clinical studies that review the incidence of new caries concludes that the elderly have a higher risk of new coronal and root caries.[65] Other studies have attributed the risk of caries in this cohort to an ecological shift in tooth surface biofilm that leads to tooth mineral loss.[66]

Dental abrasion and erosion of tooth structure starts from the surface of the tooth (cementum) and extends into the dentin. This progression is enhanced by mechanical or chemical processes, thus creating an indentation in the cervical facial part of the tooth. Investigators have suggested that consumption of an acidogenic diet followed by immediate tooth brushing may be linked with this condition. The use of abrasive toothpastes and firm bristle brushes may further exacerbate the condition.[67]

Older adults are four times more likely to have untreated dental caries in comparison with school children. This is the result primarily of existing and changing financial resources that parallel the course of aging. Adults with low socioeconomic status are six times more likely to have untreated decay when compared with corresponding age groups with higher socioeconomic status.[68] Other contributing factors among poorer older adults include a prevalent history of smoking that has been associated with a higher prevalence of untreated decay (41%), untreated root caries (22%), and places them at greater risk for oral cancer when compared with a similar cohort with high socioeconomic status.[69,70] Investigators have shown an increased prevalence of tooth fractures associated with age as being caused by dentin fatigue.[71]

Periodontal disease.   Periodontal disease is identified as a disease of adulthood; however, young people can also be affected by periodontal disease.[72,73] It destroys the connective tissue and bone support, and accounts for 30% to 35% of tooth loss of those older than 45 years.[74] Advanced stages of the disease affects 10% to 15% of the population and prevalence varies with race, geographic location, and oral destructive behavioral habits. Rather than a single disease, periodontal disease is a sequelae of diseases caused by plaque accumulation on retentive tooth surfaces and bacterial infection. A susceptible host is required in addition to behavioral factors, environmental risk markers, and systemic conditions. The prevalence and severity increases with age and peaks at the age of 50 to 60 years and then subsequently declines. Men younger than 60 years with severe periodontal disease are at a higher risk (4.3 times) for a stroke, however, this appears not to be age related.[75] Periodontal disease has been linked with increased risk for hypertension, cardiovascular disease, and type 2 diabetes are associated with degrees of obesity and vitamin D deficiency.[76] These systemic

conditions, with periodontal disease, increase in prevalence with aging. Therefore, oral health professionals should consider an overall risk assessment for periodontal disease in light of other systemic conditions.

Older adults experience unique tissue changes such as thinning and decreased keratinization of the gingival epithelium. Apical migration of the junctional epithelium to the root surface results from greater attachment loss and bone loss. Physiological aging processes may not be a risk factor for the bone mass reduction, whereas systemic conditions such as osteoporosis are a contributing factor in the progression of the disease. Other risk factors for periodontal disease include cigarette smoking, use of medication, low socioeconomic status, low salivary flow and buffering capacity, and depression. These factors are discussed in Chapter 5. *Healthy People 2010* objectives challenged the dental profession to promote oral health education, prevention and application of minimal intervention to reduce permanent tooth loss due to decay and periodontal disease.[30] As with dental decay, periodontal disease is a preventable condition.

Edentulism.   The erroneous perception that increases in chronological age parallel increases in the prevalence of edentulousness is waning. The current findings show that only 25% to 30% of older adults have lost all of their natural dentition, compared with 45% in the past. This decline in the rate of edentulism is primarily the result of awareness, early disease detection, prevention, oral rehabilitation, and comprehensive dental care.[5] Most epidemiological studies indicate that the incidence of edentulism is dependent on sociodemographic variables that include race, education, geographic location, dental service use, economic status, and damaging dental health habits. Some studies suggest that many of the elderly do not believe a dental visit is necessary after they are edentulous,[77] however, these persons may be at risk for other oral conditions, including oral cancer. The cause of edentulism is the result of chronic oral infection of the teeth and the supporting structures that lead to tooth mortality.

A radiographic and visual examination of the soft and hard tissue and the present condition of the replacement prosthesis should be conducted annually. For patients who are edentulous and are at risk for oral cancer, an annual oral cancer screening is appropriate. Edentulism should not be a deterrent from recalling patients every 6 months to 1 year for an oral cancer screening when warranted. Early diagnosis and treatment is the best preventive measure, particularly for patients with chronic behavioral risks including tobacco and alcohol consumption. Lesions that do not heal shortly after denture adjustments should be considered suspect.

Complications of edentulism can be prevented. These include denture stomatitis and angular chelitis. Denture stomatitis is also known as denture-induced stomatitis, denture sore mouth, inflammatory papillary hyperplasia, and chronic atrophic candidosis. This condition is an inflammation of the edentulous mucosal tissues that is induced by *Candida* species, and it causes infection, irritation, and lesions. Many institutionalized edentulous elderly and 65% of partially and totally edentulous individuals experience this condition.[78] Transmissible opportunistic pathogens live as nonpathogenic members of the normal microflora. They grow and proliferate in response to alterations of the host's immunological and physiological responses.[79] Oral presence of these organisms starts shortly after birth; however, 28% of the colonization occurs in 60 to 69 year old adults and 72% of those older than 80 years old. Behavioral habits, including tobacco and alcohol use, promote the pathogenicity of these organisms in combination with the inability to clean the oral prosthesis. These habits enable these pathogens to proliferate on the tissue surface of the acrylic resin of the denture. These organisms are amplified in hospitalized elderly (88%) or among those who reside in long-term care facilities and who are unable to manage their oral hygiene needs.[80] Patients who are immunocompromised, suffer from malnutrition (i.e., iron, folate, or vitamin B_{12} deficiency), or have uncontrolled type 2 diabetes are most prone to this condition. Those individuals with cancer (acute leukemia, agranulocytosis) or receiving antibiotic therapy, corticosteroids, radiation therapy, or chemotherapy, are also susceptible. Continuous swallowing or possible aspiration of these pathogens from denture plaque is a risk factor for pleuropulmonary and gastrointestinal infections.[81] Denture plaque naturally adheres and accumulates on the dental prosthesis forming a dense microbial layer. The biofilm composition of this layer is similar to dental plaque with the exception of an elevated *Candida albicans* count, identified as the causal factor in denture-induced stomatitis.[82] Intraorally the fungal microbe is primarily located on the tongue and tonsillar areas or the oral cavity.[83] *Candida* biofilm and bacteria adhere in cracks and voids on the unpolished side of the denture, which may weaken the denture.[84, 85]

Continuous wearing of the denture can result in traumatic ulceration. Permeation of the oral mucosa changes the oral environment, and opportunistic pathogens line the tissue surface of the prosthesis resulting in irritation and *Candida* infection. Salivary proteins, primarily histatins, inhibit the pathogenicity of *Candida*, and can control drug-resistant antifungal infections.[86] Histatins are synthesized in the parotid and submandibular glands and provide fungicidal and bacteriocidal activity. Good oral hygiene of the edentulous mucosa and the prosthesis includes limiting the wearing of the prosthesis during resting time. This practice is advised to reduce the possibility of candidiasis.

Angular cheilitis (cracking of the lips) is often associated with *C. albicans* or *Staphylococcus aureus* and nutritional deficiencies (see Chapter 7). Excessive use of antibiotics and immunosuppressive therapies contribute to this condition. Often times the lesion will spontaneously resolve.

Recurrence is common and may require use of topical antifungals, nutritional intervention, evaluation of vertical dimension, or treatment of lesions with a soft tissue laser to prevent future recurrence.

Xerostomia. More than 400 medications prescribed to elderly adults are associated with dry mouth. Medication affects functional or organic disturbances of the salivary gland, leading to lack of normal salivary secretion. Saliva inhibits demineralization of the tooth surface and enhances remineralization. It has both buffering and lubricating capability. Furthermore, saliva is part of a natural defense system with antifungal, antiviral, and antibacterial properties. It enhances taste, bolus formation, and digestion of food.[87] When salivary flow decreases, *Candida* counts increase. Therefore, patients that suffer from xerostomia have a higher prevalence of candidal infection.[88] This can be a risk factor for elderly patients who also can experience caries and periodontal disease at increased rates or who are edentulous.

PREVENTION OF DENTAL CARIES AND PERIODONTAL DISEASE IN OLDER PATIENTS

The first step in developing a plan of prevention for older patients is to assess the patient's risk of developing oral disease. Formulation of an individualized preventive program for elderly adults requires a complete medical/social/dental history, including a medication history (see Chapters 4 to 6 for details on risk factors associated with oral disease screening). Although routine risk for disease should be considered in generating a preventive plan, it is important to consider limitations that may be associated with the older patient. These factors include xerostomia, medication history, ability to maintain oral hygiene, and gingival recession. Preventive measures should include patient counseling that stresses reduction of behaviors that are detrimental to oral health. At the conclusion of the educational session, the patient should take home self-assessment oral health criteria, including information about preventive oral care products and instruction in control of oral plaque accumulation. Professional dental prophylaxis should be provided at routine intervals, on the basis of risk, to prevent tooth mortality and exacerbate systemic conditions. For older adults that have a high prevalence of oral disease, additional diagnostic data are required to formulate an individualized preventive plan. Additional strategies can include diagnostic testing such as salivary flow rate or bacteriological count for patients both with and without a prosthesis.[60] These techniques are described in Chapter 9. Diagnostic screening for periodontal disease can be used to describe the subgingival ecology, which can indicate when broad-spectrum antibiotic therapy for periodontal disease should be applied.

Oral health status in aging adults is a dynamic condition requiring special preventive strategies important in maintaining optimum general and oral health. Choices in dietary selections, dentrifices, rinses, mouthwash, and toothbrushes can positively augment routine dental care. Those with prosthetic dentures can establish hygiene practices and dental attendance schedules, leading to optimum outcomes.

Older adults who experience permanent tooth loss have compromised masticatory function. Oral rehabilitation with an artificial prosthesis further compromises taste, diminishes chewing efficiency, and precludes consumption of nutrient rich fruits, vegetables, and some animal proteins. Many resort to consumption of diets rich in simple carbohydrates that are low in dietary fiber content. Vitamin D and calcium supplementation promotes periodontal health, reduces residual ridge resorption, reduces alveolar bone resorption and decreases tooth loss. Adequate intake of Vitamin B complex increases periodontal attachment and promotes wound healing. Chapter 8 provides a detailed description of the role of diet in oral health. Dietary counseling to address these issues can augment routine dental care. See Table 19-1 for guidelines for denture patients.

Antiseptic and Antimicrobial Mouth Rinses

Chlorhexidine gluconate, 0.12% solution, used as a 30-second rinse twice a day, is effective in reducing plaque and bleeding on probing.[89] Cetylpyridinium chloride mouth rinse has demonstrated improvement in periodontal status by significantly reducing gingival bleeding, plaque index, and gingivitis in adult patients.[90] Chlorhexidine may also be effective in hospital-associated and ventilator-associated pneumonia, especially for patients who are at high risk for oral disease.[91] For patients who have difficulty maintaining adequate home care because of compromised motor skills, antimicrobial rinses can provide additional protection from periodontal disease and dental caries.

Powered toothbrushes can be used to assist with maintenance of daily oral hygiene in patients with compromised motor control. These toothbrushes, described in Chapter 16, have significantly reduced gingivitis and plaque in older adults.

Artificial Prosthesis and Cleaning

The use of commercially available immersion denture cleaners with the mechanical removal of denture plaque is effective in inhibiting denture stomatitis.[92] Maintenance of dental prostheses are recommended routinely for all individuals with prostheses, and especially for patients residing in hospitals and long-term care facilities. The prosthesis should be soaked in sodium hypochloride overnight as an effective means to eliminate biofilm pathogens. An alternative cleaning method is microwave

irradiation, which has bacteriocidal and candidacidal properties.[93] This method is not recommended for cast-metal prostheses. Simple removal and cleaning of the denture and allowing it to air dry at night can be an adjunct to other treatment regimens.[94] Recent studies indicated that adding methacrylic to polymethymethacrylate will improve the denture surface and inhibit the adhesion of *C. albicans*.[95] Traditionally, *Candida* infections resolve with the use of amphotericin B, fluconazole, nystatin, and chlorhexidine. Some strains of *Candida* have developed resistance to these antifungals. A randomized control study comparing fluconazole and nystatin concluded that fluconazole significantly decreased oral, pharyngeal, and esophageal candidiasis. Fluconazole is the antifungal of choice for the treatment of fungal infections in immunocompromized patients.[96]

A reduction in caries was observed when geriatric patients were provided with salivary stimulants.[97] Clinical trials with acupuncture therapy concluded that this approach is a viable alternative therapy for xerostomia.[98] The use of sugarless or xylitol-containing gums or mints can be recommended for xerostomic patients to stimulate saliva production. Alteration of diet to include more chewy foods can also increase salivary flow. NovaMin is a calcium phosphate product that uses bioactive glass as a stabilizer instead of casein. This releases calcium phosphate into saliva, and the dentin acts as a core for formation of hydroxyl carbonate apatite. NovaMin is primarily used to desensitize exposed areas.

Periodic dental office visits for the prevention of dental disease are recommended for older adults on the basis of their risk status. During this visit, a complete dental examination should be performed and followed by in-office fluoride applications. Daily fluoride use is one of the most effective practices in dental disease prevention.[99-104]

GERIATRIC NURSING HOME RESIDENTS

Older adults are healthier, better educated, and have benefited from medical, preventive, pharmaceutical, and surgical advancements when compared to previous generations. It is projected that a decline in the estimates of disabled elderly will occur, and thus a decline in the associated dependency and institutionalization rates.[105] Currently, only 1.56 million (4.5%) older adults are institutionalized. The oral health status of these residents is dependent on several variables: medical status, side effects of prescription medication, nutritional intake, oral hygiene practices, the self-perceived need for oral care, the caregiver's perceptions of oral health, and a lack of interest in this population from oral health care professionals. Quality-of-life indicators are associated with oral health in institutionalized older adults. In general, they

TABLE 19-1

DIETARY GUIDELINES FOR DENTURE PATIENTS

FOOD GROUP	BEST OPTIONS	RECOMMENDED METHODS OF PREPARATION	RATIONALE
Dairy	Low-fat and fat free milk, cheese, cottage cheese, dairy desserts, and yogurt.	Add to cooked vegetables and grains. Use as a base for mixed dishes.	Major source of high-quality protein, B vitamins, and calcium.
Meat, fish, eggs, and meat substitutes	Lean, ground meats; fish; eggs; beans; and tofu.	Use moist heat to prepare meats; add to stews, salads, and mixed dishes. Adhere to principles of chewing meats on both the left and right sides of the mouth.	Aging is paralleled by dietary increased need for protein to maintain the immune system.
Vegetables and fruits	A colorful variety of fruits and vegetables can include bananas, melons, citrus, vegetable purees, and fruit/vegetable juices.	Combine fruit and dairy. Add canned/frozen/steamed/stewed vegetables and fruit in side dishes, breads, and desserts. Add juices to soups, stews, and beverages.	A major source of essential vitamins, minerals, and antioxidants, essential in maintaining oral and tissue health and tissue integrity. Provides a source of dietary fiber important in decreasing the risk for chronic disease and maintaining gastrointestinal health.
Breads, grains, and cereals	Whole grain breads and cereals.	Add milk to soften dry cereals. Choose cooked cereals and grains. Adhere to biting and chewing principles.	Major source of dietary fiber and essential vitamins and minerals.
Fats, oils, and simple sugars	Salad dressings, sugar, honey, molasses, syrup, gravies, and sauces.	Limit intake to what is essential to only improve flavor and acceptability.	Essential fats are available in foods like fish and some vegetables. Additional fats and sugars can increase caloric intake while providing minimal nutrient value. Vegetable fats, such as olive and canola oil, are better choices for added sources of fat than animal fats, such as butter and hydrogenated fats.

Adapted from Mobley CC: Nutrition and oral health, *Quintessence Int* 36:627-631, 2005.)

have higher plaque indices, more restored teeth, and higher mutans streptococci and lactobacilli counts than their noninstitutionalized counterparts.[106-108] Multiple studies reported dental decay is more prevalent in dependent institutionalized residents. In one study, it was reported that more than 78% of the elderly residents living in long-term care facilities had at least one carious lesion, 50% had coronal decay, and 68% had root caries, with an average of 3.8 carious teeth per resident.[109,110]

Oral health status in this cohort is dependent on self-perception of individual oral health status and needs, and the caregiver's and the oral health care provider's perceptions. Furthermore, the community/cultural perceptions of the importance of oral health maintenance are a determining factor. Some define perception of oral health needs of institutionalized adults as accessibility to dental insurance coverage.[46]

THE PHYSICALLY, MENTALLY, OR EMOTIONALLY HANDICAPPED DENTAL PATIENT

The Americans for Disabilities Act of 1990 defines a person with a **disability** as one who experiences a physical or mental impairment limiting one or more major life activity.[9] Individuals with disabilities present unique challenges to medical and dental professionals. Many disabled patients have complicated medical histories with accompanied undiagnosed and/or untreated dental conditions.[111] Furthermore, some of these patients may be developmentally disabled. Developmental disabilities are defined as conditions identified in early childhood that are likely to continue throughout an individual's life, and result in functional limitations requiring planned care and treatment.[112] Compared with the general population, these individuals experience a higher incidence of dental disease, missing teeth, and greater difficulty in obtaining dental care.[111]

In addition, many genetic syndromes associated with developmental disabilities have characteristic developmental dental alterations. These syndromes include the presence of extra teeth, congenital absence of multiple teeth, unusually shaped teeth, and abnormalities in tooth mineralization. Malocclusion (an overbite), an increased risk for dental decay (caries), or both, accompany these developmental disabilities.[113]

Children with disabilities and medical impairments are at greater risk for oral diseases. Examples of dysfunction include difficulty eating, chewing, and swallowing. Speech and communication are sometimes challenging. Drooling and malocclusion can contribute to poor oral health.[114] Oral health care for the child with a developmental disability is the same as it is for a typically developing child. Prevention through home dental care and regular dental attendance is the same.[113] In 2002, annual dental visits were documented for 37% of children and adults with disabilities. This finding is compared with 46% among children and adults without disabilities.[115] *Healthy People 2010* goals included elimination of health disparities among different segments of the population.[116] Children in particular are at high risk for dental disease that may affect their overall health and development. This observation is more profound in those who are developmentally disabled.[113] Many children with disabilities tend to have poor oral hygiene, excessive gingivitis, and a greater prevalence and severity of periodontal disease than children without disabilities.[117]

The Centers for Disease Control and Prevention (CDC) identified several factors (environment, behavioral practices, and access to routine preventive care) that influence health outcomes for people with disabilities.[118] Because children with disabilities frequently experience heavy plaque accumulation, controlling plaque in these individuals is an important issue in health care planning and preventive programs. Children with disabilities require increased preventive care.[117]

Access to dental services is more difficult for disabled individuals than the general population.[111] The financial burden of other medical and therapeutic expenses may preclude available resources for dental care. Chronically ill health or disabilities may limit mobility and impede travel to receive oral health care. Disabled persons may be isolated or institutionalized which impacts their ability to seek oral health care.[119] People living in institutions has decreased by 75% during the past 20 years. Many of the people who were living in institutions now live in community settings.[120] Among those with special needs, however, both the disability and the restriction associated with institutionalization continue to affect the prevalence of oral diseases.[121,122]

Other limitations may be the result of individual disabilities associated with mental or physical limitations, or both. The definition of physical frailty refers to impairment in the physiological domains that include mobility, balance, muscle strength, motor processing, cognition, nutrition, endurance, and physical activity. The definition of mental retardation refers to cognitive limitations. Currently, the average life span of persons with mental retardation is 66 years. These individuals have visual and hearing impairment, poor oral health, epilepsy, and asthma. Many times these chronic conditions even if identified are not appropriately addressed. In the aging population, untreated systemic conditions might include osteoporosis, osteoarthritis (bone fractures), pulmonary hypertension, congenital heart disease, acquired heart disease, and joint pain leading to agitation and possible violence.[123]

Individuals diagnosed with an intellectual disability have an increased prevalence of caries and genetic predisposition for periodontal disease in comparison with healthy adults. Oral care in a traditional dental setting may be challenging, because these persons may be uncooperative. Studies have shown that the use of 0.12%

chlorhexidine mouth rinse decreased plaque indices for one month but reverted to baseline after 12 months in institutionalized, cognitively impaired patients.[124] Proper oral hygiene and oral health promotion programs decrease the incidence of caries in MR patients, however, excessive oral bacterial counts and plaque remain unchanged.[125]

Although the American Dental Association (ADA) requires that private dental offices serve persons with disabilities and provide access to care, many dental professionals are not trained or are not willing to provide care to those with the complex medical, social, and behavioral problems experienced by many individuals in special needs groups.[111,126] Few dentists are engaged in institutional or public health dentistry.[127] The U.S. Surgeon General's report stresses the need for assessment and analysis of the determinants of oral health status among people with disabilities.[5,128] Possibly because of more pressing and medical issues, dental care is usually not a priority for the special needs population.[129] Oral health care for disabled individuals is challenging for family caregivers and dental providers.[118,130,131]

SUMMARY

Oral Health in America: A Report of the Surgeon General finds that oral health disparities exist in the United States that are not addressed.[5] Groups that rely on others to provide their oral health care or those who experience greater barriers to accessing oral health care are the most vulnerable. In addition, these groups tend to have unique oral health needs that impact their overall health. These groups include children, the developmentally disabled, the physically disabled, and the elderly, both independent or assisted living and institutionalized. This chapter addresses the needs of these groups and the impact of these needs on the prevention of oral diseases.

Improving access to care for these groups would help to alleviate their burden of oral disease. Some of the barriers described in the chapter include improving access to dental insurance, increasing the number of dental professionals trained to care for these patients, and providing greater support for preventive services to reduce the burden of disease. Certainly, the oral health needs of these groups demand greater attention than they have received in the past.

REFERENCES

1. Millman M: *Access to health care in America*, Washington DC, 1993, National Academy Press Institute of Medicine.
2. Lillian G, Ronald MA, Barbara D: The behavioral model for vulnerable populations: application to medical care use and outcomes for homeless people, *Health Serv Res* 34:1273-1302, 2000.
3. Ronald A: Revisiting the behavioral model and access to medical care does it matter? *J Health Soc Behav* 36:1-10, 1995.
4. Slavkin HC: The surgeon general's report and special-needs patients: a framework for action for children and their caregivers, *Spec Care Dent* 21:88-94, 2001.
5. U.S. Department of Health and Human Services: *Oral health in America: a report of the Surgeon General*, Rockville, MD, U.S. 2000, Department of Health and Human Services, National Institute of Health.
6. Pamuk E, Makuc D, Heck K et al.: *Socioeconomic status and health chartbook. Health, United States, 1998*, Hyattsville, MD, 1998, National Center for Health Statistics.
7. U.S. Department of Commerce, Economics and Statistics Administration: *U.S. Census Bureau. 2000 Brief. Disability Status 2000*, Washington, DC, Department of Commerce, 2003.
8. Ohmori I, Awaya S, Ishikawa F: Dental care for severely handicapped children, *Int Dent J* 31:177-184, 1981.
9. Americans With Disabilities Act of 1990: Public Law 101-336 (website): http://www.usdoj.gov/crt/ada. Accessed February 15, 2007.
10. Lydon-Rochelle MT, Krakoiak P, Hujoel PP et al.: Dental care use and self-reported dental problems in relation to pregnancy, *Am J Public Health* 94:765-771, 2004.
11. Mangskau KA, Arrindell B: Pregnancy and oral health: utilization of the oral health care system by pregnant women in North Dakota, *Northwest Dent* 75:23-28, 1996.
12. Boggess KA, Edelstein BL: Oral health in women during preconception and pregnancy: implications for birth outcomes and infant oral health, *Matern Child Health J* 10:169-174, 2006.
13. National Center for Chronic Disease Prevention and Health Promotion Oral Health Resources (website): http://www.cdc.gov/OralHealth/. Accessed February 15, 2007.
14. Slavkin HC: Meeting the challenges of craniofacial-oral-dental birth defects, *J Am Dent Assoc* 127:126-137, 1998.
15. Tolarova M, Cervenka J: Classification and birth prevalence of orofacial clefts, *Am J Med Genet* 75:126-137, 1998.
16. Boggess KA, Edelstein BL: Oral health in women during preconception and pregnancy: implications for birth outcomes and infant oral health, *Matern Child Health J* 10:169-174, 2006.
17. Alaluusua S, Malmivirta R: Early plaque accumulation—a sign for caries risk in young children, *Commun Dent Oral Epidemiol* 22:273-276, 1994.
18. Lewis DW, Ismail AI: Periodic health examination, 1995 update: 2. Prevention of dental caries, *CMAJ* 152:836-846, 1995.
19. Sanchez OM, Childers NK: Anticipatory guidance in infant oral health: rationale and recommendations, *Am Fam Physician* 61:115-120,123-124, 2000.
20. Pierce KM, Rozier RG, Vann WF Jr: Accuracy of pediatric primary care providers' screening and referral for early childhood caries, *Pediatrics* 109:E82-2, 2002.
21. Ismail AI, Sohn WA: A systematic review of clinical diagnostic criteria of early child hood caries, *J Public Health Dent* 59:171-191, 1999.
22. Mouradian WE, Wehr E, Crall JJ: Disparities in children's oral health and access to dental care, *JAMA* 284:2625-2631, 2000.
23. Horwitz HS: Research issues in early childhood caries, *Commun Dent Oral Epidemiol* 26:67-81, 1998.
24. Milnes AR: Description and epidemiology of nursing caries, *J Public Health Dent* 56:38-50, 1996.
25. Nowak AJ, Warren JJ: Infant oral health and oral habits, *Pediatr Clin North Am* 47:1043-1066, 2000.
26. Reisine S, Douglass JM: Psychosocial and behavioral issues in early childhood caries, *Commun Dent Oral Epidemiol* 26:32-34, 1998.
27. Houpt MI: AAP policy statement on dental home, *Pediatr Dent* 25:4, 2003.
28. Oral Health Risk assessment timing and establishment of the dental home, *Pediatr Dent* 111:1113-1116, 2003.

29. Nevada State Health Division, Bureau of Family Services: *Burden of oral disease in Nevada—2005 report.*

30. The Office of Disease Prevention and Health Promotion, U.S. Department of Health and Human Services: *Healthy People 2010* (website): http://www.health.gov/healthypeople. Accessed January 5, 2007.

32. American Dental Association: Fluoride and fluoridation (website): http://www.ada.org. Accessed January 5, 2007.

33. Mobley C: Nutrition needs and oral health in children, *Top Clin Nutr* 20:200-210, 2005.

34. National Institute of Dental and Craniofacial Research: *Practical oral care for people with developmental disabilities,* Bethesda, MD, 2004, National Oral Health Information Clearinghouse, NIH Publication No. 04-5193, 2004.

35. National Institute of Dental and Craniofacial Research: *Practical oral care for people with developmental disabilities,* Bethesda, MD, 2004, National Oral Health Information Clearinghouse, NIH Publication No. 04-5193, 2004.

36. Romer M, Dougherty N, Amores-Lafluer E: Predoctoral education in special care dentistry: paving the way to better access? *ASDC J Dent Child* 66:132-135, 1999.

37. Hollister MC, Weintraub JA: The association of oral status with systemic health, quality of life, and economic productivity, *J Dent Educ* 57:901-909, 1993.

38. U.S. Department of Health and Human Services: *Healthy people 2010: leading health indicators,* Office of Disease Prevention and Health Promotion, Office of Public Health and Science, Rockville, MD, (website): http://www.healthypeople.gov/LHI/default.htm. Accessed January 5, 2007.

39. Pezzementi ML, Fisher MA: Oral health status of people with intellectual disabilities in the southeastern United States, *JADA* 136:903-912, 2005.

40. Wilmoth JM et al.: Demographic trends that will shape U.S. policy in the twenty first century, *Res Aging* 28:269-88, 2006.

41. Knickman JR, Smell EK: The 2030 problem: caring for aging baby boomers, *Health Serv Res* 37:4, 2002.

42. U.S. Department of Health and Human Services Administration on Aging: A statistical profile of older adults aged 65+, Administration on Aging Fact Sheet, November 2006.

43. He, Wan, Sangupta W. 65+ in the United States: 2005. Current Population Reports Special Studies. US Census Bureau Current Population Report, P23-209, U.S. Government Printing Office.

44. Schoenborn CA, Vickerie JL, Centers for Disease Control and Prevention National Center for Health Statistics: Health characteristics of adults 55 years of age and over: United States 2000-2003, *Adv Data* 370:1-31, 2006.

45. Parkin DM, Bray F, Ferlay J et al.: Global cancer statistics 2002, *CA Cancer J Clin* 55:74-108, 2005.

46. Adegbembo AO, Leake JL, Main PA et al.: The influence of dental insurance on institutionalized older adults ranking their oral health status, *Spec Care Dent* 25:275-285, 2005.

47. McCluskey-Schwab A: Open wide—I meant your pocketbook: repercussions of the dental exclusion to the Medicare Act, *Spec Law Dig Health Care Law* 9:83-108, 2001.

48. Borrell LN, Burt BA, Neighbors HW: Social factors and periodontitis in an older population, *Am J Public Health* 94:748-754, 2004.

49. Beck JD, Hunt JR, Hand JS et al.: Prevalence of root and coronal caries in noninstitutionalized older population, *J Am Dent Assoc* 111:964-967, 1985.

50. Fitzgerald RJ: Dental caries in gnotobiotic animals, *Caries Res* 2:139-146, 1968.

51. Keyes PH: Research in dental caries, *J Am Dent Assoc* 76:1357-1373, 1968.

52. Marsh PD, Percival RS: The oral microflora—friend or foe? Can we decide? *Int Dent Journal* 56:(4 suppl 1), 233-239, 2006.

53. Petersson GH, Fure S, Twetman S et al.: Comparing caries risk factors and risk profiles between children and elderly, *Swed Dent J* 28:119-128, 2004.

54. Trovik TA, Klock KS, Haugejorden O: Trends in reasons for tooth extractions in Norway from 1968-1998, *Acta Odontol Scand* 58:9-96, 2000.

55. Gilbert GH, Antonsen DE, Mjor IA et al.: Coronal caries, root fragments, and restoration and cusp fractures in US adults, *Caries Res* 30:101-111, 1996.

56. Curzon MEJ: Risk groups: nursing bottle caries/caries in the elderly, *Caries Res* 38:14-33, 2004.

57. Trovik TA, Klock KS, Haugejorden O: Trends in reasons for tooth extractions in Norway from 1968-1998, *Acta Odontol Scand* 58:9-96, 2000.

58. Edelstein BL: The dental caries pandemic and disparities problem, *BMC Oral Health* 6(suppl 1):S2, 2006.

59. National Institute of Dental Research: *Oral health of United States adults: the national survey of oral health in U.S. employed adults and seniors: 1985-86,* Bethesda, MD, 1987, NIH Publication No. 87-2868.

60. Loesche WJ, Schork A, Terpenning MS et al.: Factors which influence levels of selected organisms in saliva of older adults, *J Clin Microbiol* 33:2550-2557, 1995.

61. Bradshaw DJ, McKee AS, Marsh PD: Effects of carbohydrated pulses and pH on population shifts within the oral microbial communities in vitro, *J Dent Res* 68:1298-1302, 1989.

62. Shen S, Samaranayake LP, Yip HK et al.: Bacterial and yeast flora of root surface caries in elderly, ethnic Chinese, *Oral Dis* 8:207-217, 2002.

63. Schneinin A, Pienihakkinen K, Tiekso J et al.: Multifactorial modeling for root caries prediction: 3-years follow-up results, *Commun Dent Oral Epidemiol* 22:126-129, 1994.

64. Solheim T: Dental cementum apposition as an indicator of age, *Scand J Dent Res* 98:510-519, 1990.

65. Griffin SO, Griffin PM, Swann JL, et al.: Estimating rates of new root caries in older adults, *J Dent Res* 83:634-638, 2004.

66. Fejerskov O: Changing paradigms in concepts on dental caries consequences of oral health care, *Caries Res* 38:82-191, 2004.

67. Bartlett DW, Shah P: A critical review of non-carious cervical (wear) lesions and the role of abfraction, erosion, and abrasion, *J Dent Res* 85:306-312, 2006.

68. Drury TF et al.: Identifying and estimation oral health disparities in U.S. adults (website): http://www.nidr.nih.gov/research/healthdisp/disp-estimation.pdf. Accessed January 5, 2007.

69. Beltran-Aguilar ED, Baker LK, Canto MT et al.: Surveillance for dental caries, dental sealants, tooth retention edentulism and enamel fluorosis United States, 1988-1994 and 1999-2002, *MMWR Surveill Summ* 54:1-44, 2005.

70. Featherstone JDB: The caries balance: the basis for caries management by risk assessment, *Oral Health Prev Dent* 2:259-264, 2004.

71. Bajaj D, Sundaaram N, Nazari A et al.: Age, dehydration and fatigue crack growth in dentin, *Biomaterials* 27:2507-2517, 2006

72. Cogen RB, Wright JT, Tate AL: Destructive periodontal disease in healthy children, *J Periodontol* 63:761-765, 1992.

73. Loe H, Brown LJ: Early-onset periodontitis in the United States of America, *J Periodontol* 662:608-616, 1991.

74. Trovik TA, Klock KS, Haugejorden O: Trends in reasons for tooth extractions in Norway from 1968-1998, *Acta Odontol Scand* 58:29-96, 2000.

75. Grau AJ: Periodontal disease as a risk factor for ischemic stroke, *Stroke* 35:296-401, 2004.

76. Zitterman A: Vitamin D in preventative medicine: are we ignoring the evidence? *Br J Nutr* 89:552-572, 2003.

77. Garcia JA, Juarez RZ- Utilization of dental services by Chicanos and Anglos, *J Health Soc Behav* 19:428-43, 1978.

78. Budtz-Jorgensen E: Oral mucosal lesions associated with the wearing of removable dentures, *J Oral Pathol* 10:65-80, 1981.

79. Soll DR: Candida commensalism and virulence the evolution of phenotypic plasticity, *Acta Tropica* 81:101-110, 2002.

80. MacEntee MI, Glick N, Stolar E: Age, gender, dentures and oral mucosal disorders, *Oral Dis* 4:32-36, 1998.

81. Budtz-Jorgensen E: Etiology, pathogenesis, therapy, and prophylaxis of oral yeast infections, *Acta Odontol Scand* 48:61-69, 1990.

82. Nikawa H, Hamada T, Yamamoto T: Denture plaque—past and recent concerns, *J Dent* 26:229-304, 1998.

83. Grimoud AM, Lodter JP, Marty N et al.: Improved oral hygiene and Candida species colonization level in geriatric patients, *Oral Dis* 11:163-169, 2005.

84. Webb BC, Thomas CJ, Willcox MD et al.: Candida-associated denture stomatitis. Aetiology and management: a review. Part 3. Treatment of oral candidosis, *Aust Dent J* 43:244-249, 1998.

85. Ramage G, Tomsett K, Wicks BL et al.: Denture stomatitis: a role for Candida biofilms, *Oral Surg Oral Med Oral Pathol Oral Radiol Endodont* 98:53-59, 2004.

86. Kavanagh K, Dowd S: Histatins: antimicrobial peptides with therapeutic potential, *J Pharm Pharmacol* 56:285-289, 2004.

87. VanNieuw Amerongen A, Bolsher JG, Veerman EC: Salivary proteins: protective and diagnostic value in cariology, *Caries Res* 38:247-253, 2004.

88. Torres SR, Peixoto CB, Caldas DM: Relationship between salivary flow rates and Candida count in subjects with xerostomia, *Oral Surg Oral Med Oral Pathol Oral Radiol Endod* 93:149-154, 2002.

89. Southern EN, McCombs GB, Tolle SL: Comparative effects of 0.12% chlorhexidine rinse and herbal oral rinse on dental plaque induced gingivitis, *J Dent Hygiene* 80:12, 2006.

90. Stookey GK, Beiswanger B, Mau M et al.: A 6-month clinical study assessing the safety and efficacy of two cetylpyridinium chloride mouthrinses, *Am J Dent* 18:24A-28A, 2005.

91. Kollef MH: Prevention of hospital-associated pneumonia and ventilator associated pneumonia, *Crit Care Med* 32:1396-1405, 2004.

92. Harrison Z: An in vitro study into the effect of a limited range of denture cleaners on surface roughness and removal of Candida albicans from conventional heat cured acrylic resin denture base material, *J Oral Rehabil* 31:460-467, 2004.

93. Webb BC, Thomas CJ, Willcox MD: Candida-associated denture stomatitis: aetiology and management: a review. Part 3. Treatment of oral candidosis, *Aust Dent J* 43:244-249, 1998.

94. Lombardi T, Budtz-Jorgenson E: Treatment of denture-induced stomatitis: a review, *Eur J Proshthodont Rest Dent* 2:17-22, 1993.

95. Park SE, Periamthamby AR, Loza JC: Effect of surface-charged poly(methyl methacrylate) on the adhesion of Candida albicans, *J Prosthodont* 12:249-254, 2003.

96. Lumbreras C, Cuervas Mons V, Jara P et al.: Randomized trial of fluconazole versus nystatin for the prophylaxis of candida infection following liver transplantation, *J Infect Dis* 174:583-588, 1996.

97. Mäkinen KK, Mäkinen PL, Pape HR: Conclusion and review of the Michigan Xylitol Programme (1986-1995) for the prevention of dental caries, *Int Dent J* 46:22-34, 1996.

98. Blom M, Dawidson I, Angmar-Mansson B: The effect of acupuncture on salivary flow rates in patients with xerostomia, *Oral Surg Oral Med Oral Path* 73:293-298, 1992.

99. Frame PS: Preventive dentistry: practitioner's recommendations for low-risk patients compared with scientific evidence and practice guidelines, *Am J Prev Med* 18:159-162, 2000.

100. Loesche W, Taylor GW, Dominguez LD et al.: Factors which are associated with dental decay in the older individual, *Gerodontology* 16:37-46, 1999.

101. Peterson GH, Fure S, Twetman S et al.: Comparison caries risk factors and risk profiles between children and elderly, *Swed Dent J* 28:119-128, 2004.

102. Beltran-Aguilar ED, Barker LK, Canto MT et al.: Surveillance for dental caries, dental sealant, tooth retention, edentulism, and enamel fluorosis—United States 1988-94 and 1999-2002, *MMWR Surveill Summ* 54:1-44, 2005.

103. Griffin SO, Griffin PM, Swann JL: Estimating rates of new root caries in older adults, *J Dent Res* 83:634-638, 2004.

104. Griffin SO Griffin PM, Swann JL et al.: New coronal caries in older adults: implications for prevention, *J Dent Res* 84:715-720, 2005.

105. Kubzsansky LD, Berkman LF, Glass TA et al.: Is educational attainment associated with shared determinants of health in the elderly? From the Macarthur Studies of Successful Aging, *Psychosom Med* 60:578-585, 1998.

106. MacEntee MI, Hole R, Stolar E: The significance of the mouth in old age, *Soc Sci Med* 45:1449-1458, 1997.

107. Locker D, Clarke M, Payne B: Self-perceived oral health status, psychological well-being, and life satisfaction in an older adult population, *J Dent Res* 79:970-975, 2000.

108. Loesche WJ, Taylor GW, Dominguez LD et al.: Factors which are associated with dental decay in the older individual, *Gerontology* 16:37-46, 1999.

109. Wyatt CCL: Elderly Canadians residing in long-term care hospitals: Part I. Medical and dental status, *J Can Dent Assoc* 68:353-358, 2002.

110. Wyatt CCL: Elderly Canadians residing in long-term care hospitals: Part II. Dental caries status, *J Can Dent Assoc* 68:359-363, 2002.

111. Christensen GJ: Special oral hygiene and preventative care for special needs, *JADA* 136:1141-1143, 2005.

112. White AB, Maupomé G: Making clinical decisions for dental care: concepts to consider, *Spec Care Dentist* 23:168-172, 2003.

113. Acs G, Ng MW, Helpin ML et al.: Dental care: promoting health and preventing disease. In: Batshaw ML: *Children with disabilities*, ed 5, Baltimore, MD, 2002, Paul H. Brookes Publishing.

114. Tesini DA: An annotated review of the literature of dental caries and periodontal disease in mentally retarded individuals, *Spec Care Dent* 1:75-87, 1981.

115. U.S. Department of Health and Human Services: *Disability and health in 2005: promoting the health and well-being of people with disabilities*, U.S. Department of Health and Human Services, Office of the Surgeon General, 2005.

116. Pezzementi ML, Fisher MA: Oral health status of people with intellectual disabilities in the southeastern United States, *JADA* 136:903-912, 2005.

117. Waldman HB, Perlman SP: Children with both mental retardation and mental illness live in our communities and need dental care, *J Dent Child* 68:360-365, 2001.

118. Nowak AJ: Patients with special health care needs in pediatric dental practices, *Pediatr Dent* 24:227-228, 2002.

119. Oredugba FA: Use of oral health care services and oral findings in children with special needs in Lagos, Nigeria, *Spec Care Dent* 26:29-65, 2006.

120. Boraz RA: Dental care for the chronically ill child, *Pediatrician* 16:193-199, 1989.

121. Desai M, Messer LB, Calache: A study of the dental treatment needs of children with disabilities in Melbourne, Australia, *Aust Dent J* 46:11-50, 2001.

122. Tesini DA: An annotated review of the literature of dental caries and periodontal disease in mentally retarded individuals, *Spec Care Dent* 1:75-87, 1981.

123. Fisher K, Ketti P: Aging with mental retardation. Increasing population of older adults with MR require health intervention and prevention strategies, *Geriatrics* 60:26-29, 2005.

124. McKenzie WT, Forgas L, Vernino AR et al.: Comparison of a 0.12% chlorhexidine mouthrinse and an essential oil mouthrinse on oral health in institutionalized mentally handicapped adults: one-year results, *J Periodontol* 63:187-193, 1992.

125. Mojon PA: Effects of an oral health program on selected clinical parameters and salivary bacteria in a long-term care facility, *Eur J Oral Sci* 106:827-834, 1998.

126. Guarde RDE O, Ciamponi AL: Dental caries prevalence in the primary dentition of cerebral-palsied children, *J Clin Pediatr Dent* 27:287-292, 2003.

127. Dougherty N, MacRae R: Providing dental care to patients with developmental disabilities: an introduction for the private practitioner, *N Y State Dent J* 72:29-32, 2006.

128. Reid RC, Chenette R, Macek MD: Prevalence and predictors of untreated caries and oral pain among Special Olympic athletes, *Spec Care Dent* 23:139-142, 2003.

129. Perlman S: Helping special Olympics athletes sport good smiles: an effort to reach out to people with special needs, *Adv Sports Dent* 44:221-229, 2000.

130. Baens-Ferrer C, Roseman MM, Dumas HM et al.: Parental perceptions of oral health-related quality of life for children with special needs: Impact of oral rehabilitation under general anesthesia, *Pediatr Dent* 27:137-142, 2005.

131. Waldman HB, Perlman SP: Children with both mental retardation and mental illness live in our communities and need dental care, *J Dent Child* 68:360-365, 2001.

5-year relative survival rate - Percentage of the population diagnosed with a disease that does not succumb to that disease within a defined period of time (5 years).

Abnormal bleeding - Occurs when any phase of normal coagulation has been disrupted by a disease process, treatment, or medications.

Acquired pellicle - Forms immediately on exposure of a clean tooth surface to saliva. The acquired pellicle allows adhesion of naturally occurring oral bacteria that produce exopolysaccharides to enhance further accumulation of bacteria.

Activities of daily living (ADL) - Activities routinely performed daily by the average person in a given society. Rehabilitation after illness or injury often aims to help patients achieve independence in performing these activities, which include eating, bathing, and dressing.

Age-adjusted - Rates/ratios that are standardized on the basis of a specific characteristic (age). Age adjustment controls for the effect of age on the rates/ratios and allows comparison among populations.

Allergy - A hypersensitive reaction of the body to an allergen. An antigen-antibody reaction is manifested in several forms: anaphylaxis, asthma, hay fever, urticaria, angioedema, dermatitis, and stomatitis.

Alveolar bone loss - Loss of the bone that supports the root of the teeth. Results in a weakening of the supporting structures of the teeth and predisposes the patient to tooth mobility and loss.

Andragogy - An educational approach that targets adult learning and is characterized by learner-centeredness, self-direction, and a humanist philosophy.

Annual incidence rate - Estimate of the impact of a defined exposure in a population that occurs within a 1-year period.

Anthropometrics - Measurements of physical characteristics such as height, weight, and change in weight.

Anticoagulant - A drug that delays or prevents coagulation of blood.

Antigingivitis agent - Pharmacotherapy that reduces the onset or severity of inflammation of the gingival tissues.

Antimicrobial - Substance that inhibits the growth of microorganisms, including fungi, bacteria, and viruses.

Antiplaque agent - Compound that inhibits, controls, or kills organisms associated with dental plaque formation.

Antiseptic - An antimicrobial agent for application to a body surface, usually skin or oral mucosa, in an attempt to prevent or minimize infection at the area of application.

Aphthous stomatitis - Circular lesions with an erythematous border surrounding necrotic epithelial cells that are self-limiting and heal in 10 to 14 days. Pain associated with aphthous ulcers depends on the size, location, and depth of the ulcers.

Assessment modalities - Comprehensive examination processes that generate pertinent data regarding a dental professional's knowledge, clinical judgment, and patient management skills in his or her current or intended area of practice.

Bacteria - 1. Small, unicellular microorganisms of the kingdom Monera. 2. The phylum in which these microorganisms are classified.

Behaviorism - A branch of psychology that bases its observations and conclusions on definable and measurable behavior and on experimental methods.

Bidi - Small, hand-rolled cigarettes imported from India and other Southeast Asian countries. They can be flavored (e.g., chocolate, cherry, and mango) or unflavored. Bidis have significantly higher concentrations of tar, nicotine, and carbon monoxide than conventional cigarettes sold in the United States.

Biocide - A product used to kill different forms of microorganisms.

Biofilm - A very thin layer of microscopic organisms that covers the surface of an object.

Biopsy - The removal of a tissue specimen or other material from the living body for microscopic examination to aid in establishing a diagnosis.

Brush biopsy - A procedure that uses a specially designed brush that obtains cells from all epithelial layers that are assessed by microscopic screening.

Burning mouth syndrome (BMS) - An idiopathic and multifactorial syndrome characterized by burning and painful sensations in the hard and soft tissues in the oral cavity, in the absence of physical abnormalities.

CAGE questionnaire - Have you ever felt that you should **C**ut down on your drinking? Have people **A**nnoyed you by criticizing your drinking? Have you ever felt bad or **G**uilty about your drinking? Have you ever had a drink first thing in the morning to steady your nerves or to get rid of a hangover? (**E**ye-opener).

Candidiasis - An infection by *Candida albicans*.

Candidiasis - The presence of white, irregular patches or pseudomembranes that can be easily wiped off, and fungal hyphae confirmed by routine microscopy.

Caries activity - Occurs when plaque deposits on a tooth surface and causes demineralization to the underlying tooth enamel.

Caries progression - The enlargement of an existing carious lesion, which usually extends from the enamel into the dentin that occurs through continued demineralization of the mineralized tissue. Progression is determined through longitudinal evaluation of the lesion.

Caries risk - Probability that caries activity will result in a clinical lesion within a defined period of time.

Caries risk assessment - A systematic process based on the patient's past and present caries experience and known risk factors or indicators for disease that attempt to categorize persons into risk groups with respect to the potential to develop new carious lesions over time.

Central nervous system (CNS) - The portion of the nervous system consisting of the brain and spinal cord. The portion of the nervous system beyond the brain and cord is known as the peripheral nervous system.

Chemotherapeutic - A chemical of natural or synthetic origin used for its specific action against disease, usually against infection.

Classical conditioning - A type of learning in which two stimuli, one neutral and one fear-eliciting, are paired.

Cognitive behavior therapy - Based on a set of principles and procedures that assume a synergistic interaction between cognitive mental processes and behavior without emphasizing causation.

Cognitivism - A psychological school of thought concerned with a person's internal representations of the world and with the internal or functional organization of the mind.

Comprehensive patient-centered counseling programs - Programs to enhance patient adherence have been described within numerous frameworks.

Cultural competence - A set of congruent behaviors, knowledge, attitudes, and policies that come together within a system or organization or among professionals that enables effective work in cross-cultural situations.

Culturally and linguistically appropriate services (CLAS) - Guidelines issued by the Department of Health and Human Services that are intended to guide recommended practices by targeting actions of individual practitioners and support mechanisms that are necessary within organizations to ensure access to health services that are culturally and linguistically appropriate.

Culture method - A method of bacteriological testing that relies on saliva as the vehicle for the testing. Saliva is plated on agar, incubated, and colonies counted.

Deep sedation - An induced state of depressed consciousness accompanied by partial loss of protective reflexes, including the inability to continually maintain an airway independently, respond purposefully to verbal command, or both.

Dental calculus - Mineralized dental plaque; commonly known as tartar.

Dental erosion - Demineralization of enamel and dentin that results from chemical or mechanical action.

Dental plaque - Oral biofilm—a complex biofilm attached to teeth.

Dentin hypersensitivity - Short, transient, sharp pain with a rapid onset that arises from exposed dentin. It usually occurs in response to an external stimuli, typically thermal, tactile, evaporative, osmotic, or chemical, and can not be linked to any other dental pathology.

Diabetes mellitus - A metabolic disorder caused primarily by a defect in the production of insulin by the islet cells of the pancreas, resulting in an inability to use carbohydrates. Periodontal manifestations can include recurrent and multiple periodontal abscesses, osteoporotic changes in alveolar bone, fungating masses of granulation tissue protruding from periodontal pockets, a lowered resistance to infection, and delay in healing after periodontal therapy.

Diagnostic and Statistical Manual of Mental Disorders (DSM-IV) - A manual that recognizes a broad class of anxiety disorders, including panic attack, panic disorder, agoraphobia, specific phobia, social phobia, obsessive-compulsive disorder, posttraumatic stress disorder, acute stress disorder, and generalized anxiety disorder.

Dietary assessment - Methods of dietary assessment include 24-hour food recalls, food records or diaries, diet histories, food frequency recalls, and simple brief dietary screeners.

Dietary cholesterol - The cholesterol in the food eaten that is present only in foods of animal origin, not those of plant origin. Dietary cholesterol, like dietary saturated fat, raises blood cholesterol, which increases the risk for heart disease.

Dietary fiber - Found only in foods of plant origin, dietary fiber is a group of substances exhibiting various degrees of resistance to human digestion. Cellulose, lignin, hemicellulose, pectin, and gums are the five main types of dietary fiber. Crude fiber represents the cellulose portion of dietary fiber.

Digital imaging fiber optic transillumination (DIFOTI) - Uses visible light to identify early interproximal caries in which demineralized areas of enamel or dentin will scatter light to a greater degree than sound areas. DIFOTI allows the images from all tooth surfaces to be digitally captured and stored. The images can then be used to provide a longitudinal assessment of the early carious lesion.

Disability - A physical or mental impairment that substantially limits or restricts the condition, manner, or duration under which an average person in the population can perform a major life activity, such as walking, seeing, hearing, speaking, breathing, learning, working, or taking care of oneself.

Dysgeusia - An abnormal or impaired sense of taste.

Dysphagia - A subjective feeling of having difficulty swallowing.

Embrasure - The space between the curved proximal surfaces of the teeth.

Endotoxin - A nondiffusible, lipid polysaccharide-polypeptide complex formed within bacteria (some gram-negative bacilli and others). When released from the destroyed bacterial cells, endotoxin is capable of producing a toxic manifestation within the host.

Energy balance - The relationship between potential cellular energy consumed from food sources and the cellular energy produced to maintain life and physical activities.

Epigenetics - The study of how a gene function may be altered without altering DNA or changing DNA sequences.

Erythema multiforme - A disorder characterized by the occurrence of target-type lesions of the skin and multiple areas of intraoral necrosis; also known as *Stevens-Johnson* syndrome.

Erythroleukoplakia - A white patch with a red component.

Erythroplakia - A distinct disease of the oral mucosa distinguished by red, patchy lesions.

Ethnocentrism - The inability to see beyond one's own culture and to understand why someone may act the way they do. A judgmental attitude that one's own cultural attitudes and behaviors are the only right way of seeing and doing things.

Exposure therapy - Various psychotherapeutic techniques designed to diminish conditioned fears by repeatedly exposing a patient, in the absence of an adverse experience, to a stimulus associated with stress.

Extinction - A classical conditioning theory that contends that the learned association between the neutral and fear-eliciting stimuli can be unlearned if the neutral stimulus is repeatedly presented without the fear-eliciting stimulus.

Facultative anaerobic species - Organisms that can survive in the absence, as well as presence, of oxygen.

Fat free - A food containing less than 0.5 grams of fat per serving is considered to be fat free.

Fiber optic transillumination (FOTI) - Uses visible light to illuminate the approximal surface from which a lesion can be observed through the marginal ridge.

Five "A"s - Ask about tobacco use, advise tobacco users to quit, assess readiness to make a quit attempt, assist with the quit attempt, arrange follow-up care.

Five "R"s - Relevance: How is quitting most relevant to the patient? Tailor advice and the discussion to the patient's situation and readiness to quit. Risks: Provide new information on the risks of continued tobacco use specific to the individual's circumstance. Attempt to elicit suggestions from the patient on risks specific to their situation. Rewards: Suggest or elicit suggestions

from the patient on the benefits of quitting that are unique to the patient. Roadblocks: Assist patients in identifying the barriers to quitting tobacco use and guide them towards solutions. Assist the patient in developing discrepancy between current behavior (tobacco use) and the desired behavior (quitting). Repetition: Reinforce your motivational message at every opportunity.

Flooding - Another form of exposure therapy that involves exposure to a maximum-intensity, fear-producing situation for an extended time.

Food groups - The major categories of foods defined by the USDA that provide major sources of essential nutrients important in establishing a healthy daily dietary intake.

Gene polymorphism - The occurrence together in the same population of more than one allele or genetic marker at the same locus with the least frequent allele or marker occurring more frequently than can be accounted for by mutation alone.

Genetics - The science that deals with the origin of the characteristics of an individual.

Gingival abrasion - A localized acute injury caused by vigorous brushing, excessive brushing pressure, or hard toothbrush bristles; also known as *toothbrush trauma*.

Gingival crevicular fluid (GCF) - Serous exudate or transudate that collects in the gingival sulcus and, in periodontal health, provides an active mechanism to maintain homeostasis in the gingival sulcus. The interchange of fluid between the vasculature in the gingival tissue and the gingival sulcus allows immune cells to be delivered to the site. In response to inflammation, GCF provides a vehicle for the collection of immune cells and cytokines into the sulcus in response to the microbial challenge.

Gingival enlargement - A swelling of the attached gingivae that obliterates the gingival contours; also referred to as *gingival overgrowth* and previously known as *gingival hyperplasia*.

Gingival enlargement - A swelling of the gingival tissues and papillae.

Gingival recession - The apical migration of the gingival tissue.

Gingivitis (gingival inflammation) - An inflammation of the soft tissue without apical migration of the junctional epithelium. It is reversible, nondestructive in nature, and does not result in the loss of periodontal structures.

Gram-negative bacteria - Having the pink color of the counterstain used in Gram's method of staining microorganisms. Staining property is a common method of classifying bacteria. Gram-negative bacteria are more pathogenic and have an outer membrane that consists of lipopolysaccharide.

Health disparity - Differences in rates of mortality, morbidity, incidence, prevalence, burden of disease, and other adverse health conditions among specific population groups; also refers to differential rates of access and use of services in the health care system.

Health education - Instructional activities delivered in a variety of settings and using a variety of media to influence health behaviors.

Health promotion - Measures designed to change individual lifestyles and associated behaviors to achieve a state of optimum health.

Herbal supplements - Components of natural plants used by some individuals to supplement traditional medical treatments. They are not considered to be drugs, and therefore are not regulated by the Food and Drug Agency (FDA). This absence of regulation means that the effectiveness, quality, and quantity of the ingredients have not been independently verified.

Hookah - Waterpipe smoking.

Host modulation therapy - Periodontal therapies (including chemotherapeutics) that are applied to modulate the destructive aspects of the host response.

Humanism - An affirmation of the inherent dignity and worth of every human being that asserts individual responsibility for the realization of aspirations.

Immunoglobulin - Serum protein synthesized by plasma cells that act as antibodies and are important in the body's defense mechanisms against infection. Main classes are designated as IgG, IgA, and IgM.

Inflammatory mediators - Molecules that are released by cells in response to an invasion of the host by harmful agents. These agents, produced by immune cells, facilitate the response of the host to the challenge.

Initiator - A chemical agent added to a resin to initiate polymerization.

Insoluble fiber - A crude fiber, such as cellulose and lignins, that is not soluble in water, but with passive water-attracting properties that can help to increase bulk, soften stools, and shorten transit time through the intestinal tract.

Instrumental activities of daily living (IADL) - More complex activities that are not necessarily done every day but that are important to independent living. Indicators of functional well-being that measure the ability to perform complex tasks. Activities include cooking, driving, writing, housekeeping, using transportation, and managing money.

Kretek - A tobacco alternative popular for a unique smell, taste, and appearance. They typically contain a mixture of tobacco, cloves, and other additives; also known as *clove cigarettes*.

Leukoplakia - A raised white patch on the mucosa that cannot be scraped off.

Lichenoid reactions - Ulceration and desquamation of the oral mucosa, frequently associated with lichen planus-like white striae on the buccal mucosa.

Lipopolysaccharide (LPS) - A compound or complex of lipid and carbohydrate.

Malnutrition - States of undernutrition, including intake of insufficient nutrients to meet requirements and overnutrition, intake of nutrients in excess of requirements, nutrient insufficiency, and nutrient imbalances.

Mechanical nonsurgical periodontal therapy - Also known as scaling and root planing or subgingival debridement. This treatment is indicated for individuals with early periodontitis and as the initial phase of treatment of moderate or advanced periodontal diseases. Scaling and root planing removes subgingival calculus and plaque, disrupts the dental biofilm, and frees the root surface of contamination from microbial byproducts.

Medicaid - A program sponsored by the federal government and administered by individual states that is intended to provide health care and health-related services to low-income individuals.

Medicare - A Federal health insurance program for people age 65 years and older and for individuals with disabilities.

Microorganisms - A minute living organism, such as a virus, yeast, fungus, rickettsia, or bacterium.

Moderate alcohol intake - Recommendations suggest that women have no more than one drink a day and men no more than two drinks per day. One drink is a 12-oz bottle of beer, a 5-oz glass of wine, or a 1 ½-oz shot of liquor.

Modifiable risk factor - One that the individual may be able to control. Modifiable risk factors are primarily associated with environmental and behavioral choices. These include, for example, tobacco and alcohol use.

Monounsaturated fat - A type of fat found in large amounts in foods from plants, including olive, peanut, and canola oil.

Morbidity - The incidence or prevalence of a disease or of all diseases in a population.

Mortality - Pertaining to death. The total number of deaths from a given disease in a population during a specific interval of time, usually a year.

Mortality rate - The death rate.

Motivational interviewing - A patient counseling approach that is closely aligned with change theory, but uniquely defined as being patient-centered. The specific techniques and strategies used in this approach include the expression of empathy by the counselor, the development of discrepancies among pros and cons of a behavior, rolling with resistance so as not to exert external pressure on the patient, and support for self-efficacy, as identified by the patient.

Mucositis - Injury to the oral mucosa that results in increased vascular permeability, tissue edema, atrophy, and eventually ulcerations covered by a necrotic pseudomembrane in some instances.

Nicotine dependence - A condition characterized by both tolerance and withdrawal symptoms in relation to nicotine use. Nicotine dependence can occur with cigarette smoking, smokeless tobacco use, cigar or pipe use, or prescription medications, such as the nicotine replacement transdermal patch or gum.

Nicotine replacement therapy (NRT) - A smoking cessation method intended to reduce nicotine cravings and ease the symptoms of withdrawal by substituting another source of nicotine, such as specially formulated lozenge, gum, nasal spray, inhalant, or skin patch for tobacco products.

Nonmodifiable risk factor - Indicators that influence the patient's disease that can not be reduced or controlled, such as genetic predisposition to disease.

Nutrient - An element or compound necessary for human metabolism and growth that can provide energy or other support for metabolic processes in the body (or both). Some are essential because they cannot be synthesized in the body and must be obtained from a food source.

Nutrient-dense foods - Food that provides substantial amounts of essential nutrients relative to caloric content is categorized as being nutrient-dense.

Nutritional assessment - An attempt to identify current nutritional status and related nutrient recommendations and requirements. Provides baseline data for patient monitoring and for evaluation of the quality of care provided over time.

Nutritional screening - Provides a snapshot of the dietary factors of interest, defines germane nutrition education goals, guides recommendations for dietary supplements, and identifies referral needs to either social services for resource or a registered dietitian for consultation.

Oral care products - Category of products involved primarily in oral cleansing. These products do one or more of the following: prevent cavities, prevent gum disease, freshen breath, reduce plaque/calculus, or whiten teeth. These products come in multiple forms, including paste, powder, or mouth rinse, and can be therapeutic or cosmetic.

Oral lichen planus (OLP) - A chronic autoimmune disease of unknown origin appearing as fine white lines that form a reticular pattern or "weblike" appearance; typically affects the oral mucosa of the cheeks, gums, and tongue.

Oral malodor - An offensive odor of the breath resulting from local and metabolic conditions; also known as *halitosis*.

Oral prophylaxis - Dental cleaning.

Oral self-care - Individual practices that promote oral health that include toothbrushing, interdental cleaning (flossing), and other oral hygiene interventions.

Osteonecrosis - Caused by therapy with bisphosphonates, corticosteroids, or antineoplastic agents. Clinical signs and symptoms of osteonecrosis can include pain, swelling, purulence, denuded bone, mobility, and complaints of dysesthesia.

Pack year - The number of years of smoking, multiplied by the number of packs of cigarettes smoked per day.

Patient characteristics - The patient's age, gender, academic performance, socioeconomic status, self-esteem, lifestyle, cognitive abilities, and mood.

Patient/parent relationship - The established role relationship between a patient, who is a minor or child, with their parent.

Patient/provider relationship - Relationship established between the patient and health care provider, which is based on mutual respect.

Periodontal disease (periodontitis) - An inflammatory disease of the supporting tissues of the teeth caused by specific microorganisms or groups of microorganisms, which results in a progressive destruction of the periodontal ligament and alveolar bone with pocket formation, recession, or both.

Periodontal maintenance - Professional care for those who have previously received treatment of periodontal disease; also called *supportive periodontal therapy* or *periodontal recall*. The objective of periodontal maintenance is to prevent the recurrence of disease, to stop disease progression, and, ultimately, to reduce the loss of teeth.

Periodontopathogens - Microorganisms that have been linked with an increased risk for developing periodontal disease.

Polymorphonuclear leukocytes (PMN) - White blood cells with nuclei of various forms.

Polyunsaturated fat - A type of fat that is found in large amounts in foods from plants that includes safflower, sunflower, and corn oil. This fat is essential for human health (e.g., omega 3 or omega 6).

Potassium-rich food - Natural plant foods are usually high in potassium compared with many processed foods, which are often low in potassium but high in sodium. These natural foods include fruits, vegetables, and their juices.

Predictive factors - A situation or condition that can increase the risk of an individual experiencing a certain disease or disorder.

Primary prevention - Preventing the initial occurrence of disease and maintaining physiological equilibrium. Primary prevention focuses on altering the susceptibility or reducing the exposure for susceptible individuals.

Probiotics - Live microbial-fed supplements that beneficially affect the host animal by improving its intestinal microbial balance. In humans, lactobacilli are commonly used as probiotics either as single species or in mixed culture with other bacteria.

Promoter - A substance or agent, known to cause the development or increase the incidence of cancer, that acts in later stages of the disease.

Quantitative light fluorescence (QLF) - Used for both the detection and monitoring of dental caries, QLF serves as an indirect measure of enamel porosity and lesion severity. QLF relies on the natural fluorescence of the tooth to distinguish between carious and sound enamel.

Recurrent aphthous ulcers - See *aphthous stomatitis*.

Reinforcement - A form of learning in which a neutral stimulus (the dental professional or office) is paired with a stimulus that reflexively elicits anxiety (pain or social embarrassment).

Relative risk - A measure of the degree to which the exposure to a certain factor increases the risk of experiencing a specific disease when compared with someone without the exposure.

Relaxation therapy - A form of therapy that focuses on promoting a deep muscle relaxation response because it is seen as incompatible with anxiety.

Remineralization - The reintroduction of complex mineral salts into bone, enamel, dentin, or cementum.

Risk - A factor, course, circumstance, or element that increases the possibility of suffering harm, disease, or loss.

Risk assessment - Identification of specific factors/ indicators and an evaluation or judgment of their impact on the individual. The goal of risk assessment is to develop and implement strategies in those identified as being at risk for disease that will either (1) prevent them from developing disease or (2) improve the prognosis for those with existing disease.

Risk factor - A risk factor is something that increases the probability that an individual will experience a disease.

Risk indicators - Elements that can affect the course or progression of a disease without truly being causal.

Salivary components - Includes the fluid produced from glands that contains a number of glycoproteins, peptides, and nonglycosolated proteins that contribute to important roles in maintaining the health of the oral cavity.

Salivary diagnostics - Method of oral disease detection in which saliva is the sole diagnostic biofluid.

Salivary gland hypofunction - Diagnosed if an individual's unstimulated salivary flow rate is less than 0.2 mL/min.

Saturated fat - Fatty acids that usually come from animal foods such as whole dairy foods, meats, eggs, fish, and poultry but that are also present in coconut and palm oils. They are usually solid at room temperature.

Secondary prevention - Addresses early detection and intervention to prevent disease progression, including nonoperative treatment.

Self-assessment - An evaluation of communication, values, attitudes, and environmental factors related to promoting culturally effective oral health care.

Simple sugars - Monosaccharides and disaccharides are known as simple sugars because the body quickly digests them. Examples of foods that contain simple sugars are sweet-tasting foods that include ingredients like sugar, honey, or fructose corn syrup. These sugars are also found naturally in fruit and vegetables.

Sodium in food - On average, the natural salt content of food and salt added at the table or while cooking provides a small percentage of sodium in the average diet. The recommendation is to consume less than 2300 mg (approximately 1 tsp of salt) of sodium per day.

Soluble fiber - Soluble indicates a fiber source that would readily dissolve in water, such as pectins and gums.

Stage-based models - Assumes that change is not a continuous process but something that occurs in different stages, in which barriers to change may differ.

Staging - A method to describe the growth of a tumor, the rate at which it metastasizes, and its prognosis. The four stages are evaluated according to size and whether or not the lymph nodes are involved.

Standard drink equivalents - A guideline for what should be interpreted as "one drink."

Stevens-Johnson syndrome - See *erythema multiforme*.

Subgingival plaque - Tooth-adherent plaque that forms beneath the gingival margin and may bind to either the tooth, cementum, or to the epithelial surface of the gingiva. The composition of the bacteria tends to mature from gram-positive to gram-negative species and exhibit greater pathogenicity.

Subgingival temperature - Measured as a correlate for inflammation. An increase in temperature is believed to reflect an ongoing inflammatory response, which is a response to the infection.

Substantivity - The efficacy of chlorhexidine, which stems from its ability to bind to oral tissues and slow release into the oral cavity. This provides a continued inhibitory effect on plaque formation for 12 to 14 hours.

Systematic desensitization - A form of behavior modification in which the patient is taught a series of muscle tensing and relaxing exercises intended to generate a state of deep muscle relaxation. Anxiety and deep muscle relaxation are believed to be incompatible.

Taste alterations - Changes in the sensation of taste can take several forms, from ageusia (loss of the sensation of taste), to dysgeusia (altered taste sensation), and hypogeusia (diminished sensation of taste). Most cases involve bitter or metallic taste.

Technological advance - Changes in scientific development and understanding that refer to objects of use to humanity (machines, hardware, and utensils), but the concept can also encompass broader themes, including systems and techniques.

Tertiary prevention - Addresses the alleviation of disability that results from disease and attempts to restore effective functioning. In oral health practice, tertiary prevention focuses on restorative and prosthodontic methods.

Tetracycline antibiotics - A broad-spectrum antibiotic that is effective against a wide range of bacteria. Its administration during tooth formation can lead to enamel discoloration.

Tetracycline staining - An intrinsic, permanent staining of the tooth that occurs during formation. The staining results from the administration of tetracycline during tooth development.

Therapeutic claim - A claim associated with a therapeutic goods or services or any goods and services that claim a therapeutic purpose defined as relief from or reduction of a medical condition or disease.

Toluidine blue - A chemical substance used to identify potentially malignant mucosal deviations. Use as a mouth rinse or apply over the affected area with a cotton swab.

Trans fat - A trans fatty acid (commonly shortened to trans fat) is an unsaturated fatty acid, the molecules of which contain trans double bonds between carbon atoms, resulting from hydrogenation of a liquid fat to increase its solid state.

Whole grain - Cereal grains that retain the bran, germ, and endosperm, in contrast to refined grains, which retain only the endosperm. Common whole-grain products include oatmeal, popcorn, brown rice, whole-wheat flour, sprouted grains, and whole-wheat bread.

Withdrawal symptoms - Somatic and psychosomatic symptoms recognizable after the abrupt termination of regular drug or substance use. The types of symptoms are specific to the type of withdrawn substance.

Wound healing - Restoration of the normal structure after an injury.

Xerostomia - The subjective complaint of dry mouth, which may be accompanied by significant salivary gland dysfunction.

Index

Page numbers followed by b indicate boxes, f indicate figures, and t indicate tables.

MDAS. *See* Modified Dental Anxiety Scale (MDAS)
Mean corpuscular volume blood (MCV), 119t
Measurement systems to diagnose periodontal disease, 19-22
Medical-centered models (MCM), 125, 127t
Medical Expenditure Panel Survey (MEPS), 164
Meditation, 234
MEPS. *See* Medical Expenditure Panel Survey (MEPS)
Metabolism, 95-96
Metaphors, 124
Methylxanthine, 83t
MGI. *See* Modified Gingival Index (MGI)
Microbiological testing for caries, 112-13
Micronutrient status testing, 119t
Microorganisms. *See* Bacteria
Miedo, 174t
Migraine drugs, 86t
Million Adolescent Personality Inventory, 136
Mobility, geographic, 160-61
Models, caries risk assessment, 50-54
Modified Dental Anxiety Scale (MDAS), 147-48
Modified Gingival Index (MGI), 20-21, 60
Monitoring patient adherence, 138-40
Monounsaturated fat, 187b
Morphology, tooth, 54
Motivational interviewing techniques, 52, 140-42
MRI. *See* Magnetic resonance imaging (MRI)
Mucositis, 41, 248t, 255
Multiracial persons, 160
Muscle relaxants, 83t, 86t
Mutans streptococci, 48, 54, 112-13
MyPyramid.gov, 187f

N

NaF. *See* Sodium fluoride (NaF)
Narcolepsy, 86t
Nasal sprays, nicotine, 236t, 239
National Cancer Institute, 33
    Dietary Questionnaire, 103t
National Center for Cultural Competence (NCCC), 169
National Center for Education Statistics (NCES), 161-62
National Health and Nutrition Examination Survey, 2, 5, 8
    cardiovascular disease and, 117
    Healthy People 2010 and, 12
    nutritional assessment, 94
    periodontal measures, 21
    of smokers, 58
National Institute of Dental and Craniofacial Research, 6
NCCC. *See* National Center for Cultural Competence (NCCC)
NHANES. *See* National Health and Nutrition Examination Survey
Nicotine replacement therapy, 83t. *See also* Tobacco use
    bupropion, 236t, 239-40
    combination, 239
    gum, 235-37
    inhalers, 236t, 238
    lozenges, 236t, 237
    nasal sprays, 236t, 239
    patches, 236t, 237-38
    smokeless tobacco, 240
Nitrous oxide, 152
Nonmodifiable risk factors for oral cancer, 69-70
Non-native English speakers, 161-62
Nonsteroidal anti-inflammatory drugs, 80t, 85t
Nonverbal communication, 128, 129-30
NovaMin, 272
NSI. *See* Nutrition Screening Initiative (NSI)
Nursing caries, 5
Nursing home residents, 167, 272-74
Nutrient-dense foods, 187b
Nutritional screening and assessment
    biochemical data in, 108
    body mass index in, 101-7
    components, 94-108
        dietary measures, 95-101
        historical survey measures, 94-95
    food diaries in, 99
    interpretation of findings in, 108

Nutritional screening and assessment—cont'd
    physical findings in, 107-8
    programs, 186-88
    in risk reduction, 93-94
    web sites, 103t
Nutrition and diet. *See also* Food
    caries formation and, 4, 49-50, 53, 60, 92-93
    for denture patients, 273t
    education, 108, 109t
    evidence-based strategies for oral health promotion, 185-86
    Food Guidance System, 186
    oral cancer and, 73
    osteoporosis and, 189
    plaque control and, 209
    supplementation, 60
    terminology, 187b
Nutrition Data System, 103t
Nutritionist Pro, 103t
Nutrition Screening Initiative (NSI), 94, 97-98f
Nystatin, 80

O

Obesity and overweight, 186-89, 246
Occlusal caries, 5
OGTT. *See* Oral glucose tolerance test (OGTT)
OHIS. *See* Oral Health Information Suite (OHIS)
OHI-S. *See* Simplified Oral Hygiene Index (OHI-S)
OLP. *See* Oral lichen planus (OLP)
Omega fatty acids, 190t
Ophthalmic drugs, 83t, 86t
Opioid analgesics, 86t
Oral cancer
    age and, 35f, 39f, 68, 70
    alcohol use and, 72, 232
    chronic hyperplastic candidiasis and, 73-74
    chronic irritation and, 74
    clinical presentation, 32-33
    defined, 27-28
    dental care for patients with, 41
    detection of, 41, 74
    erythroplakia and, 32-33
    gender and, 34, 38t
    immune system deficiencies and, 41, 73
    incidence of, 28-29, 33-36, 37f, 74
    malignant transformation, 30
    metastases, 29
    mortality, 29-30, 33-36, 37f, 39f
    oral epithelial dysplasia and, 31
    oral health promotion and, 41
    oral leukoplakia and, 32
    oral lichen planus and, 33, 74
    oral squamous cell carcinoma and malignant transformation, 30-31
    population-based research, 28
    prevention
        primary, 231
        secondary, 231
    race and, 35t, 36-40
    recurrence, 70
    risk factors, 29, 69-74
        modifiable, 70-74
        nonmodifiable, 69-70
    strategies for application in practice, 40-41
    sunlight exposure and, 72
    surveillance, 33-41
    testing, 116
    tobacco use and, 59, 70-72, 74-75, 132, 231-32
    trends, 36
    tumor, node, metastases clinical staging and prognosis, 31
    viruses and, 73
Oral glucose tolerance test (OGTT), 117t
Oral health
    access to care, 163-67
    caring framework for, 173-78
    disparities in health and, 163
    education, 131-32